The Advanced Practitioner in Acute, Emergency and Critical Care

The Advanced Practitioner in Acute, Emergency and Critical Care

Edited by

Sadie Diamond-Fox

MCP ACCP (FICM ACCP Member), BSc (Hons) RN, PGCAHP, NMP (V300), FHEA.

Advanced Critical Care Practitioner (ACCP) & ACCP Programme Co-Lead, Newcastle upon Tyne Hospitals; Advancing Practice Specialty Advisor for Critical Care, NHS England, North East and Yorkshire. Assistant Professor in Advanced Critical Care Practice and Subject Lead for Advanced Practice Programmes, Northumbria University, Newcastle upon Tyne, UK

Barry Hill

MSc Adv Prac, PGCAP, BSc (Hons) CCRN, DipHE/O.A. Dip, SFHEA, TEFL, NMC RN RNT/TCH V300.

Associate Professor of Nursing and Critical Care; Employability Lead for Nursing, Midwifery and Health, Northumbria University, Newcastle upon Tyne, UK

Sonya Stone

MSc ACP FICM ACCP Member FHEA.

Associate Professor of Advanced Clinical Practice; Director of Postgraduate Taught Education (School of Health Sciences); Faculty Director of Higher Degree Apprenticeships (Medicine & Health Sciences); ACP, Cardiac Intensive Care Unit, Nottingham University Hospitals NHS Trust; Faculty of Intensive Care Medicine (FICM) Clinical Lead for e-ICM

Caroline McCrea

MSc Cardiorespiratory nursing, PG Dip ACCP (FICM), BN (Hons), NMC RN and V300.

Advanced Critical Care Practitioner (ACCP) at Portsmouth University Hospital Trust

Natalie Gardner

MSc Critical Care, FICM ACCP Member, BSc (Hons) Physiotherapy, PG Cert Clinical Education, FHEA, MAcadMEd, HCPC Physiotherapist and V300.

Trust Clinical Lead for Advanced Clinical Practice and Non-Medical Prescribing; Advanced Critical Care Practitioner; Co-Chair FICM ASC Physiotherapist; Kings College Hospital NHS Foundation Trust

Angela Roberts

MSc Advanced Critical Care Practitioner (FICM ACCP Member), NMP V300, BSc (Hons) Adult Nursing.

Advanced Nurse Practitioner at Southern Health, Petersfield Hospital

Series Editor: Ian Peate

WILEY Blackwell

Registered Offices
John Wiley & Sons, Inc., 111 River Street, Hoboken, NJ 07030, USA
John Wiley & Sons Ltd, The Atrium, Southern Gate, Chichester, West Sussex, PO19 8SQ, UK

For details of our global editorial offices, customer services, and more information about Wiley products visit us at www.wiley.com.

Wiley also publishes its books in a variety of electronic formats and by print-on-demand. Some content that appears in standard print versions of this book may not be available in other formats.

Library of Congress Cataloging-in-Publication Data

Names: Diamond-Fox, Sadie, editor.
Title: The Advanced Practitioner in Acute, Emergency and Critical Care /
  [edited by] Sadie Diamond-Fox, Barry Hill, Sonya Stone, Caroline McCrea,
  Natalie Gardner, Angela Roberts.
Description: First edition. | Hoboken, NJ : Wiley-Blackwell, [2024] |
  Includes index.
Identifiers: LCCN 2023016544 (print) | LCCN 2023016545 (ebook) | ISBN
  9781119908289 (paperback) | ISBN 9781119908302 (adobe pdf) | ISBN
  9781119908296 (epub)
Subjects: MESH: Critical Care–methods | Emergency Treatment–methods |
  Acute Disease–therapy | Health Personnel | United Kingdom
Classification: LCC RC86.7 (print) | LCC RC86.7 (ebook) | NLM WX 218 |
  DDC 616.02/8–dc23/eng/20230727
LC record available at https://lccn.loc.gov/2023016544
LC ebook record available at https://lccn.loc.gov/2023016545

Cover Design: Wiley
Cover Image: © Mutlu Kurtbas/Getty Images

Set in 10.5/13pt STIXTwoText by Straive, Pondicherry, India
Printed and bound by CPI Group (UK) Ltd, Croydon, CR0 4YY

C9781119908289_311023

Contents

About the Editors

Sadie Diamond-Fox, Barry Hill, Sonya Stone, Natalie Gardner, Caroline McCrea, Angela Roberts and Ian Peate (Series Editor)

Angela Roberts
Advanced Critical Care Practitioner (FICM ACCP Member), NMP (V300), BSc Adult Nursing
Angela qualified as an adult nurse in 2007 (MMU) and has since worked at Pilgrim Hospital, Boston, Basingstoke, and North Hampshire Hospital Intensive Care Units after qualifying.

Since 2007, she has progressed as an Advanced Critical Care Practitioner (ACCP) in 2017 and is a non-medical prescriber. Due to family commitments, she left the ICU to become an Advanced Nurse Practitioner at Southern Health, Petersfield Hospital.

Angela has always been passionate about education and supporting others through postgraduate healthcare.

Barry Hill
Associate Professor of Nursing andCritical Care; Director of Employability for Nursing, Midwifery, and Health
PhD, MSc, PGCAP, BSc (Hons), DipHE, OA Dip, RN, NMC RNT/TCH, SFHEA. Associate Professor, and Director of Employability, Northumbria University, Consultant Editor for *International Journal of Advancing Practice (IJAP)*; Clinical Editor for the *British Journal of Nursing (BJN)*.

Barry is an experienced leader, academic, educator, researcher, and clinical nurse. His current role is Associate Professor and Director of Employability for Nursing, Midwifery, and Health. He has a demonstrated history of working within academia in Higher Education (HE). Barry is a senior fellow (SFHEA) and an HEA mentor, a certified Intensive Care Nurse, with an MSc in Advanced Practice (Clinical); NMC Registered Nurse (RN), NMC Registered Teacher (TCH), and NMC registered independent and supplementary prescriber (V300). He is skilled in clinical research and clinical education, and is passionate about higher education, especially nursing science, advanced clinical practice (ACP), critical care, non-medical prescribing (NMP), and pharmacology. Barry's clinical career was at Imperial College NHS Trust, London. Barry is a strongly education-focused professional who has published 9 books, 60 book chapters, and 100 peer-reviewed journal articles. He is the Consultant Editor for the *International Journal of Advancing Practice (IJAP)* and the Clinical Editor for the 'At A Glance' and 'Advanced Clinical Practice' series within the *British Journal of Nursing (BJN)*.

Caroline McCrea
MSc Cardiorespiratory nursing, PG Dip ACCP (FICM ACCP Member), BN (Hons), NMC RN and V300
Caroline qualified as a nurse in 2008 and began her career in Cardiac Nursing. The first eight years of her career were spent in specialist Cardiothoracic Nursing roles. In 2014, she completed her MSc in Cardiorespiratory Nursing and went on to become a Cardiothoracic Nurse Practitioner and non-medical prescriber. Following on from this specialist role, she progressed further to become an

Advanced Critical Care Practitioner (ACCP) and was awarded Faculty of Intensive Care Medicine (FICM) Membership. Caroline has always had a great passion for education, and continues to compliment her clinical work with teaching across a variety of disciplines. Her key interests are ECHO, Simulation, advanced level practice, and medical education.

Natalie Gardner
MSc Critical Care, FICM ACCP Member, BSc (Hons) Physiotherapy, PG Cert Clinical Education, FHEA, MAcadMEd, HCPC Physiotherapist and V300

Natalie is the Trust Lead for Advanced Clinical Practice and Non-Medical Prescribing at King's College Hospital in London, and works clinically as an Advanced Critical Care Practitioner. Natalie started her ACCP training at King's in 2017, and has sat on the Faculty of Intensive Care Medicine ACCP Sub-Committee since 2020, of which she is now the ACCP Co-Chair. Prior to this, Natalie has worked as a physiotherapist specialising in respiratory and critical care, since 2007. Natalie also serves as an Army Reserve Officer in the Royal Army Medical Corps, with significant prior service in the Royal Logistic Corps, since 2008. Natalie has served overseas in Afghanistan, Africa, and on a UN Peace Keeping Mission, and upon Commissioning at the Royal Military Academy Sandhurst in 2017, Natalie was presented the prestigious MacRobert Sword of Honour by Major General Ranald Munro.

Sadie Diamond-Fox
MCP ACCP (FICM ACCP Member), BSc (Hons) RNA, PGCAHP, Fellow (HEA) NMC RN & V300

Sadie has developed a portfolio career in advanced practice since beginning her training as an Advanced Critical Care Practitioner (ACCP) in 2012. She continues to work clinically as an ACCP at Newcastle upon Tyne Hospitals and more recently has taken a position as trainee ACCP education co-lead. Sadie is Subject Lead for Advanced Practice programmes, Assistant Professor in Advanced Critical Care Practice (FHEA) and PhD candidate ('ImpACCPt' study) at Northumbria University. She is also Advancing Practice Training Programme Director (AP TPD) for Critical Care for Health Education England's Advancing Practice Faculty in the North East and Yorkshire. Her external positions also include Honorary Assistant Professor in Advanced Clinical Practice (ACP) at Nottingham University, External Examiner for Advanced Clinical Practice Programmes at University of Southampton; Intensive Care Society (ICS) Education Committee member; Advanced Practitioners in Critical Care (APCC) Professional Advisory Group (PAG) member to the ICS; Co-Founder and Co-Lead Advanced Critical and Clinical Practice Academic Network (ACCPAN); Editor for Wiley publishing Advanced Practice series, and most recently Editorial Board member for the *International Journal of Advancing Practice (IJAP)*.

Sonya Stone
BSc, MSc, RN, ACCP, FICM ACCP Member, FHEA

Sonya is an Associate Professor of Advanced Clinical Practice at the University of Nottingham, and Advanced Clinical Practitioner in Cardiac Intensive Care at Nottingham University Hospitals. Sonya trained as a nurse in Nottingham and spent much of her nursing career in Intensive Care. She trained as an advanced critical care practitioner in Portsmouth in 2016 and took her first academic post at the University of Southampton as a clinical teaching fellow in 2018.

Sonya is an experienced leader, clinician, and academic, with an interest in critical illness and maternal critical care. She leads postgraduate taught education and CPD in the school of health sciences and is faculty academic director for higher degree apprenticeships. Sonya is an educationalist, with a passion for advancing practice and multi-professional learning.

Ian Peate

OBE FRCN EN(G) RGN DipN(Lond) RNT Bed (Hons) MA(Lond) LLM

Editor in Chief British Journal of Nursing

Consultant Editor Journal of Paramedic Practice

Consultant Editor International Journal for Advancing Practice

Visiting Professor Northumbria University

Visiting Professor St George's University of London and Kingston University London

Professorial fellow University of Roehampton

Visiting Senior Clinical Fellow University of Hertfordshire

Ian began his nursing career at Central Middlesex Hospital, becoming an enrolled nurse practising in an intensive care unit. He later undertook 3 years' student nurse training at Central Middlesex and Northwick Park Hospitals, becoming a staff nurse and then a charge nurse. He has worked in nurse education since 1989. His key areas of interest are nursing practice and theory. Ian has published widely. Ian was awarded an OBE in the Queen's 90th Birthday Honours List for his services to nursing and nurse education and was granted a fellowship from the Royal College of Nursing in 2017.

Notes on Contributors

Name	Bio
Alexandra Gatehouse	**MSC, PG Dip ACCP (FICM ACCP member) BSc (Hons) Physiotherapy, CSP member and V300, Advanced Critical Care Practitioner** Alex Gatehouse qualified as a physiotherapist in 2000, and, following Junior Rotations in the Newcastle Trust, she specialised in Respiratory Physiotherapy in Adult Critical Care, also working within New Zealand. In 2012, she trained as an Advanced Critical Care Practitioner, completing a Masters in Clinical Practice in Critical Care and a non-medical prescribing qualification. Alex continues to rotate within all of the Critical Care Units in Newcastle Upon Tyne, also enjoying teaching on Advanced Life Support courses, Regional transfer courses, and within the units. Her interests are transfer, advanced airway management, ECHO, and education.
Andrew Lee	**MSc, BSc (Hons), DipHE** Andrew is an Advanced Clinical Practitioner specialising in respiratory care. His medical journey was initiated in 2002 at Stoke Mandeville Hospital, Buckinghamshire, on a spinal and orthopaedic ward as a Health Care Assistant. He earned his nursing qualification from De Montfort University in 2007, progressing to work on a Vascular Surgery ward. His passion for respiratory care was ignited at Glenfield Hospital, where he served in a respiratory and cardiology admissions unit, subsequently advancing to the position of Critical Care Outreach Nurse. In 2018, Andrew completed his advanced practice master's degree at the University of Nottingham, and since then, he has been diligently serving as a respiratory ACP in Nottingham. With a special interest in pulmonary vascular disease, Andrew manages a pulmonary embolism follow-up clinic. Demonstrating his leadership skills, he is currently chairing the Respiratory ACP Network, working collaboratively with a remarkable team of respiratory ACPs.
Angela Roberts	**Advanced Critical Care Practitioner (FICM ACCP Member), NMP (V300), BSc Adult Nursing** Angela qualified as an adult nurse in 2007 (MMU) and has since worked at Pilgrim Hospital, Boston, Basingstoke, and North Hampshire Hospital Intensive Care Units after qualifying. Since 2007, she has progressed as an Advanced Critical Care Practitioner (ACCP) in 2017 and is a non-medical prescriber. Due to family commitments, she left the ICU to become an Advanced Nurse Practitioner at Southern Health, Petersfield Hospital. Angela has always been passionate about education and supporting others through postgraduate healthcare.

Barry Hill

Associate Professor, Critical Care; Director of Employability for Nursing, Midwifery, and Health Programmes

PhD, MSc, PGCAP, BSc (Hons), DipHE, OA Dip, RN, NMC RNT/TCH, SFHEA. Associate Professor, and Director of Employability, Northumbria University, Consultant Editor for *International Journal of Advancing Practice (IJAP)*; Clinical Editor for the *British Journal of Nursing (BJN)*.

Barry is an experienced leader, academic, educator, researcher, and clinical nurse. His current role is Associate Professor and Director of Employability for Nursing, Midwifery, and Health. He has a demonstrated history of working within academia in Higher Education (HE). Barry is a senior fellow (SFHEA) and an HEA mentor, a certified Intensive Care Nurse, with an MSc in Advanced Practice (Clinical); NMC Registered Nurse (RN), NMC Registered Teacher (TCH), and NMC registered independent and supplementary prescriber (V300). He is skilled in clinical research and clinical education, and is passionate about higher education, especially nursing science, advanced clinical practice (ACP), critical care, non-medical prescribing (NMP), and pharmacology. Barry's clinical career was at Imperial College NHS Trust, London. Barry is a strongly education-focused professional who has published 9 books, 60 book chapters, and 100 peer-reviewed journal articles. He is the Consultant Editor for the *International Journal of Advancing Practice (IJAP)* and the Clinical Editor for the 'At A Glance' and 'Advanced Clinical Practice' series within the *British Journal of Nursing (BJN)*.

Caroline McCrea

MSc Cardiorespiratory Nursing, PG Dip ACCP (FICM ACCP Member), BN (Hons), NMC RN and V300

Caroline qualified as a nurse in 2008 and began her career in Cardiac Nursing. The first eight years of her career were spent in specialist Cardiothoracic Nursing roles. In 2014, she completed her MSc in Cardiorespiratory Nursing and went on to become a Cardiothoracic Nurse Practitioner and non-medical prescriber. Following on from this specialist role, she progressed further to become an Advanced Critical Care Practitioner (ACCP) and was awarded Faculty of Intensive Care Medicine (FICM) Membership. Caroline has always had a great passion for education, and continues to compliment her clinical work with teaching across a variety of disciplines. Her key interests are ECHO, Simulation, advanced level practice, and medical education.

Clare Allabyrne

Clare Allabyrne is currently the Associate Professor and Professional Lead for the MSc Advanced Clinical Practice Mental Health (ACPMH) at London Southbank University and a Fellow of the Higher Education Academy

A dual qualified nurse (Adult and Mental Health) by profession, her areas of expertise include advanced clinical practice in mental health, child and adolescent mental health, forensic psychiatry, liaison psychiatry, substance use, physical health care in mental health, service user involvement/people participation, multi-agency/partnership working, leadership, service creation, and innovation. Clare worked for 35 years in the NHS across physical and mental health care services in clinical, therapeutic, senior operational, clinical academic, and corporate/strategic leadership roles.

David Thom   **MSc DipIMC(RCSEd) BSc(Hons) MCPara SRParaNMP(V300), Anaesthesia Associate and Advanced Practitioner – Critical Care**
David qualified as a Paramedic in 2013 working in the West Midlands and the Southeast while completing his BSc in Pre-Hospital and Emergency Care. He has worked in a range of domains, including frontline services, the Isle of Man TT, major public events, and sport. He subsequently trained as a FICM Advanced Critical Care Practitioner, completing his MSc and Non-Medical Prescribing. Subsequently, he worked on the Dorset and Somerset Air Ambulance and passed the DipIMC(RCSEd) by examination. More recently, he is undergoing training as an Anaesthesia Associate on the PGDip pathway. Interests include Pharmacology, Education, and Critical Care.

Francesca Riccio   **Paediatric Consultant Anaesthetist, FRCA, Bachelor of Medicine**
Francesca is a paediatric anaesthetist working in University Hospital Southampton. She has always had a keen interest in teaching, in particular, simulation. Throughout her training she has watched the development of advanced practitioners, particularly in the acute setting and believes they are hugely valuable to an ever expanding and demanding healthcare system.

Emma Toplis   **Advanced Clinical Practitioner**
Emma is a Registered Nurse who began her career in older people's care. In 2015, she embarked on her journey as a trainee Advanced Clinical Practitioner (tACP). This transition allowed her to explore various clinical specialities, build a comprehensive knowledge base and enhance her skills in advanced practice. Among the several specialities, Emma fosters a deep passion for respiratory medicine. She has since developed a sub-specialist interest in interstitial lung disease. Additionally, she has become an instrumental figure in the quest for quality improvement within respiratory care, cementing her role as a core member of the In-hospital Quality Improvement for Respiratory (InQuIRe) quality improvement faculty. Emma also successfully completed a quality improvement project on improving tobacco dependency management with the Respiratory team at the University Hospitals of Derby and Burton. This project was presented at the BTS 2022 summer conference and awarded the first prize. Through the respiratory Advanced Clinical Practitioner network, Emma finds an excellent opportunity to champion and share best practices in her speciality.

Emma Underdown   **MSc Advanced Clinical Practice, PGDip Advanced Clinical Practice, BSc (Hons) Intensive Care Practice, DipHE Adult Nursing, NMC RN and V300 Independent Non-Medical Prescriber**
Emma qualified in 2011 as a nurse and began her career initially as a surgical specialty nurse before moving into Critical Care. She worked for four years as an Intensive Care nurse, gaining her post-graduate degree in Intensive Care Practice. She later spent three years working as a Senior Sister in Critical Care Outreach. She commenced her Advanced Clinical Practice training in 2019 within Emergency Medicine, where she continues to work.

Emma is a keen clinician and clinical educator who delivers education and training across various disciplines and specialties. Her areas of interest include Advanced Life Support, Medical Education, service development, and PoCUS.

Hannah Conway

MSc, DipHE, AFHEA, A/Professor Advanced Clinical Practice, Advanced Critical Care Practitioner (AHP)

Hannah specialises in critical care echocardiography and ultrasound and sits on the committee for Focused Ultrasound in Intensive Care (FUSIC), taking a lead role in FUSIC Heart (FICE). Hannah is an approved supervisor and examiner for multiple accreditations and has over a decade of experience in ultrasound education.

Hannah is a keen clinical researcher and is currently conducting a study into the use of telemedicine to aid echocardiography mentoring in intensive care. Another area of research interest is the characterisation of right ventricular (RV) injury. Hannah is co-chair of PRORVnet, an international, RV-centric research network.

National roles:

Intensive Care Society (ICS) Council Member, FUSIC and Education Committee Member

Chair ICS Advanced Practitioners in Critical Care (APCC) Professional Advisory Group

Co-Chair Advanced Clinical Practitioners Academic Network (ACPAN)

Co-Chair of Protecting the Right Ventricle Network (PRORVnet)

Honorary Secretary National Association of Advanced Critical Care Practitioners (NaACCP)

Jill Bentley

MSc Adv Prac, FICM ACCP Member, MSc Pain Management, BSc, DipHE, PGCAP, FHEA, RN (Adult) IP (v300), Lecturer / ACCP

Jill qualified as a nurse in 2001 and started her career in theatres, working in Anaesthesia, Recovery, and Outreach. She then moved into a clinical specialist role, working at a large tertiary centre in acute and chronic pain management. After gaining her masters in this specialty, she took the next step to complete her ACP training in critical care, gaining a second MSc in 2012, followed by gaining the award of FICM membership as the ACCP evolved. Jill has a keen interest in education, having worked in a lecturer practitioner role for several years. Her areas of special interest are medication safety, prescribing in advanced practice, pain management, and critical care.

Jill Featherstone

National Professional Development Specialist and Medical Education Lead

Jill is a National Lead Professional Development Specialist for NHS Blood and Transplant, responsible for medical education and working alongside national clinical leads in organ donation. Her earlier critical care career was in cardiac, general, and neurology centres in Bristol, Swindon, and South Tees, including some paediatric work and as a specialist nurse in organ donation for four years. She is passionate about supporting good family experiences, teamwork, simulation, and innovation using a wide variety of forums to have as much impact and reach as possible, including leading the much-respected multidisciplinary National Deceased Donation Course for ICM trainees and conference sessions.

Joe Wood

BSc (Hons) Physiotherapy, MSc Advanced Practice, PgCert Clinical Education

Joe began his career as a Physiotherapist in Kent, with a focus on Respiratory intervention and tracheostomy management. Developing his interest in acute care, he then completed an MSc in Advanced Practice in Critical Care to become an Advanced Critical Care Practitioner. A PgCert in clinical education followed – investigating the role of simulation in healthcare education. He continues to work towards higher accreditation in medical ultrasound and acts as mentor and supervisor for point-of-care ultrasound accreditation for AHP and Medical colleagues across acute medicine, emergency, and critical care.

John Wilkinson

MBBS PGCertMedEd, Anaesthetics Registrar

John is an anaesthetics registrar at the Northern School of Anaesthesia and Intensive Care Medicine. Following studying medicine at Newcastle University and completing Foundation Training in Newcastle Trust Hospitals, he has trained in anaesthetic and critical care departments across the North of England, including as a Clinical and Education Fellow in Critical Care. He has a particular interest in Multidisciplinary Team simulation training, including creating resources for sessions involving medical, nursing, and midwifery students from Newcastle and Northumbria Universities.

Joseph Tooley

MPharm, PG Dip (Hospital Pharmacy), IP (Clinically enhanced), Lead Critical Care Pharmacist

Joseph qualified as a pharmacist in 2012 and has been a specialist pharmacist for critical care and theatres for the last seven years, working in both general ICUs and previously in neurosciences. He has contributed to the national programme for postgraduate pharmacy training with HEE and regional training on acute kidney injury with CPPE. He is currently the lead pharmacist for critical care, theatres, and surgery at Portsmouth Hospitals University NHS Trust. His interests are pharmacokinetics in critical illness, dosing drugs with renal replacement therapy, neuroscience, and critical care nutrition.

Kathryn Thomas

Advanced Clinical Practitioner and Clinical Educator

As a Registered Nurse (RN) specialising in critical care, Kathryn brings a decade's worth of experience, having trained and subsequently qualified as an Advanced Clinical Practitioner (ACP). Throughout this journey, She has had the opportunity to rotate across several specialties, with a particular emphasis on specialist medicine, and has enhanced her skills within advanced respiratory care. Her professional engagements extend across the four pillars of advanced clinical practice. Her previous roles include being a divisional lead ACP for medicine and cancer care. She also imparts her knowledge as a clinical educator for the school of medicine at Nottingham University. Actively engaged in furthering her research, she continuously seeks to enhance her advanced practice role and contribute more significantly to her discipline and level of practice.

Kirstin Geer **BSc (Hons) MSc (Advanced Clinical Practice) PGDip (Advanced Critical Care Practice) FICM ACCP Member**
Kirstin qualified as a nurse in 2005 and has worked in Emergency Admissions and Critical Care Outreach. Became a qualified ACCP in 2016. Special interests include Critical Care Transfer and Simulation.

Kirsty Laing **MSc Advanced Practice, PgDip in Respiratory Medicine, BA(Hons) Nursing Studies, HND Biomedical Science, NMC RN and V300 Independent Prescriber**
Kirsty qualified as a registered nurse with the Nursing and Midwifery Council (NMC) in 2004, working in medical admissions, coronary care, and critical care outreach. She later embarked on her MSc in Advanced Practice. Kirsty completed her MSc in 2013, gaining a wealth of experience as an Advanced Clinical Practitioner (ACP) in various fields, including acute medicine, frailty, gastroenterology, cardiology, community rehabilitation, and respiratory medicine. Kirsty currently specialises in pleural disease and has successfully established an ACP pleural service. As an enthusiastic member of the Pleural Society and the Respiratory ACP Network, she values and thrives in collaborative, multi-professional environments. Kirsty works diligently to improve the quality of services delivered to patients, using education and supervision as primary tools for development and enhancement.

Mark Cannan **MCP ACCP, BSc (Hons), Dip HE**
Mark gained a diploma as an ODP in 2013 (University of Central Lancashire), having witnessed the work of an ODP first-hand in the theatres of Camp Bastion. He completed an Honours Degree in Acute and Critical Care (University of Cumbria). Having excluded career progression in managerial or educational roles, the ACCP role seemed to best fit his aspirations. Mark qualified as an ACCP (Northumbria University) in 2019 and has since completed his Master's Degree. He has specialist interests in advanced airway management, regional anaesthesia and transfer of the critically ill patient. He is also on the national working group working towards legislation change to allow ODPs who have progressed into advanced practice the ability to undertake non-medical prescribing.

Natalie Gardner **MSc Critical Care, FICM ACCP Member, BSc (Hons) Physiotherapy, PG Cert Clinical Education, FHEA, MAcadMEd, HCPC Physiotherapist and V300**
Natalie is the Trust Lead for Advanced Clinical Practice and Non-Medical Prescribing at King's College Hospital in London, and works clinically as an Advanced Critical Care Practitioner. Natalie started her ACCP training at King's in 2017, and has sat on the Faculty of Intensive Care Medicine ACCP Sub-Committee since 2020, of which she is now the ACCP Co-Chair. Prior to this, Natalie has worked as a physiotherapist specialising in respiratory and critical care, since 2007. Natalie also serves as an Army Reserve Officer in the Royal Army Medical Corps, with significant prior service in the Royal Logistic Corps, since 2008. Natalie has served overseas in Afghanistan, Africa, and on a UN Peace Keeping Mission, and upon Commissioning at the Royal Military Academy Sandhurst in 2017, Natalie was presented the prestigious MacRobert Sword of Honour by Major General Ranald Munro.

Nick Fox

BSc(Hons), MSc, RN & V300
Following an early career in Critical Care, Nick, along with two colleagues was asked to set up the Critical Care Outreach Team at the hospital where he worked. Nick has overseen the expansion of the Critical Care Outreach Team from an initial five day a week service to a 24 hours, seven days a week service. Nick has supported the delivery of the MSc in Advanced Clinical Practice at the University of Lincoln and facilitated in-house sessions on advanced clinical examination at the hospital where he worked. Nick has written articles on safe IV therapy, SpO2 monitoring and Critical Care Outreach, and has also contributed to national guidance on standards for level 1 care.

Ollie Phipps

Course Director for Non-Medical Prescribing and MSc Advanced Clinical Practice
Ollie is a Course Director for Non-Medical Prescribing and MSc Advanced Clinical Practice (ACP) at Canterbury Christ Church University. He continues to work clinically as a Consultant Nurse in Acute Medicine and as an ACP in an Emergency Department in Kent. Ollie has led Health Education England and the Royal College of Physicians ACP Credential development for Acute Medicine and Respiratory Medicine. He is a published author on the subject of Advanced Practice within multiple texts and is an international keynote speaker on the subject. Ollie continues to be a national subject matter expert for Advanced Practice.

Padma Parthasarathy

Respiratory Advanced Clinical Practitioner
Padmavathi Parthasarathy is an Advanced Clinical Practitioner in Respiratory Medicine currently working at University Hospitals of Leicester. Padma is certified with an MSc in Advanced Clinical Practice, a PG Diploma in Critical Care, a PG Diploma in Respiratory Medicine, and a BSc in Nursing Studies. She is a Co-Chair of the Nurse Specialist Advisory Group (SAG) within the British Thoracic Society (BTS) and Vice Chair of the Respiratory ACP network. She is also a member of the Standards of Care Committee and the Education and Training Committee of BTS. Padmavathi has completed her BSc in Nursing in India and worked in various roles overseas and in the UK. She has worked as a Clinical Instructor, staff nurse, ward sister, and nurse practitioner in critical care outreach and out-of-hours service before moving into her current role as a Respiratory Advanced Clinical Practitioner.

Phil Broadhurst

RN BSc (Hons) MSc PGCE, FICM ACCP Member, MAcadMEd
Phil is an Advanced Critical Care Practitioner at Stockport NHS Foundation Trust and has significant experience in intensive care nursing. He has an MSc in Advanced Clinical Practice from the University of Salford as well as his non-medical prescribing qualification (V300). He is credentialled by the HEE Centre for Advancing Practice and is a member of the Faculty of Intensive Care Medicine. His special interest is in medical education; thus, he leads the Trust's acute illness management training programme and is an ALS instructor. He has been awarded membership in the Academy of Medical Educators and holds a PGCE in medical education.

Phil Evans

BN(Hons) MSc DipHE CertHE RN
Phil Evans is a consultant nurse in acute medicine working at Portsmouth Hospitals University NHS Trust. Phil has had a diverse and varied career, and since 2005, has been working in various independent practice roles, which have developed a broad skill set. His experience includes intensive care, emergency medicine, pre-hospital care as well as acute medicine. The majority of his time is now spent on direct clinical service provision and the development of the ACP role. His remaining time is split between education, research, and service development.

Rachel Allen-Ashcroft

MSc ACP, BSc Hons, PGCE Med.Ed, FHEA, RNT, V300, PhD Candidate XR Technology and Clinical Education
Rachel qualified as a Nurse in 2004 and has over 19 years of clinical experience within Intensive and Critical Care environments across four large NHS trusts, including a tertiary transplant centre. Rachel qualified as an ACCP in 2016 and then moved full-time into academia as a senior lecturer delivering on advanced practice MSc pathways at two HEIs. She continues to practice as an ACP within acute/emergency care. Rachel is driving forward the Advanced Practice agenda by leading collaborations with NHS partners to develop and deliver specialty advanced practice education in her role as the Associate Director of Partnerships and International at LSBU.

Rachel Wong

BMedSc, MBChB, FRCA, FFICM
Dr Rachel Wong is a Senior Clinical Fellow and ST7 specialising in cardiothoracic anaesthesia, intensive care medicine, and extracorporeal membrane oxygenation (ECMO). She is a dual anaesthetic and intensive care medicine registrar who recently completed a cardiothoracic fellowship at the prestigious Royal Papworth Hospital. Currently, in her final year of training, Dr Wong holds a keen interest in medical education, point-of-care ultrasound, and both trans-oesophageal and trans-thoracic echocardiography. Her expertise is widely recognised, as evidenced by her regular contribution to nationally focused ultrasound for intensive care (FUSIC) courses. Throughout her career, she has passionately advocated for advanced practice roles, dedicating time to supervising and developing advancing and advanced practitioners.

Rebecca Chamoto

Divisional Director of Nursing Medicine and Urgent Care, Stockport Foundation Trust; Respiratory Advanced Clinical Practitioner; Honorary Lecturer for Advanced Practice, Manchester Metropolitan University; NMC Independent and Supplementary Prescriber V300, NMC Registered Nurse, MSc Advanced Practice, BHSc Nursing Studies
Rebecca qualified as a Registered Nurse with the Nursing and Midwifery Council in 2003, working primarily in the medical and urgent care specialities before branching out to specialise in Respiratory and Critical Care. Later in her career, she undertook an MSc in Advanced Practice, gaining extensive experience and exposure in multiple specialities before settling as a Respiratory Practitioner. Rebecca continued to specialise in Pulmonary Hypertension, with Pulmonary Embolism being her area of interest. Rebecca is very passionate about leadership, development, quality improvement, and engaging and working collaboratively with multi-disciplinary teams to deliver the highest standard of care to patients.

She is involved in the teaching programme of Advanced Clinical Practitioners of the Future with one of her local Health Education Institutions. Rebecca has recently taken on the role of Divisional Nurse Director, covering Medicine and Urgent Care, leading services to deliver high-quality care to meet the needs of patients across a broad spectrum of specialities.

Rebecca Connolly **MSc(ACP), MSc(Psych), BA(Hons), DipHE NMP GMBPsS MCPara MCMI MIEDP**

Rebecca works as a Consultant ACP (Paramedic) in a large NHS Trust, where she is a senior clinical and strategic leader responsible for a large group of multidisciplinary clinicians across a number of sites, including Resuscitation, Sepsis, Critical Care Outreach, and Children and Young People Resuscitation and Sepsis. She is currently undertaking both a clinical doctorate and her separate PhD studies. She has a national profile relating to healthcare for gender-diverse patients, and has delivered keynote speeches at a number of national conferences. She previously lived and worked in Japan, and also as a police officer. Her interests include ultrasound, stigma and sickness, neuropsychology, consciousness, and how psychedelic agents can be used as adjuvant therapy in resistant depression.

Rebecca Kurylec **Advanced Clinical Practitioner**

Rebecca Kurylec is a distinguished Registered Nurse who initiated her nursing journey in Nottingham in 2011. Specialising in respiratory medicine for over a decade, she currently serves as an Advanced Clinical Practitioner (ACP) at Nottingham University Hospitals. Rebecca's extensive training includes Advanced Life Support, and she has assumed significant roles such as the resuscitation link nurse. As an ACP, her expertise encompasses patient consultation, meticulous history-taking and thorough physical examinations, underpinned by her astute decision-making capabilities. Additionally, she possesses proficiency in radiological interpretation, both independent and supplementary prescribing, and diagnosis. Rebecca is unwavering in her dedication to the field, anticipating a bright future for ACPs and consistently advocating for ongoing professional development and excellence.

Rebecca Stacey **Advanced Clinical Practitioner**

Rebecca Stacey commenced her healthcare career as a registered physiotherapist, quickly specialising in respiratory medicine. Progressing her career, she became an integral part of a team addressing complex breathlessness. Building on her expertise, she qualified as an independent prescriber, particularly in managing asthma and chronic obstructive pulmonary disease. Her academic achievements are highlighted by her co-authored paper in *European Respiratory Review*, and the British Thoracic Society has duly recognised her for her notable research. Currently serving as an Advanced Clinical Practitioner (ACP), Rebecca is central to outpatient care in general medicine and Long Covid services. Beyond her clinical duties, she passionately advocates for the broader recognition and development of the ACP role in clinical and research domains.

Sadie Diamond-Fox	**MCP ACCP (FICM ACCP member), BSc (Hons) RNA, PGCAHP, Fellow (HEA) NMC RN & V300** Sadie has developed a portfolio career in advanced practice since beginning her training as an Advanced Critical Care Practitioner (ACCP) in 2012. She continues to work clinically as an ACCP at Newcastle upon Tyne Hospitals and more recently has taken a position as trainee ACCP education co-lead. Sadie is Subject Lead for Advanced Practice programmes, Assistant Professor in Advanced Critical Care Practice (FHEA) and PhD candidate ('ImpACCPt' study) at Northumbria University. She is also Advancing Practice Training Programme Director (AP TPD) for Critical Care for Health Education England's Advancing Practice Faculty in the North East and Yorkshire. Her external positions also include Honorary Assistant Professor in Advanced Clinical Practice (ACP) at Nottingham University, External Examiner for Advanced Clinical Practice Programmes at University of Southampton; Intensive Care Society (ICS) Education Committee member; Advanced Practitioners in Critical Care (APCC) Professional Advisory Group (PAG) member to the ICS; Co-Founder and Co-Lead Advanced Critical and Clinical Practice Academic Network (ACCPAN); Editor for Wiley publishing Advanced Practice series, and most recently Editorial Board member for the *International Journal of Advancing Practice (IJAP)*.
Sarah Henry	**BSc (Hons), MSc Advanced Practice (Distinction), MCSP** **Lead Advanced Clinical Practitioner in Acute Medicine, Harrogate and District NHS Foundation Trust** Sarah's current role includes working on an Acute Medical Unit and within Same Day Emergency Care. Having trained as a Physiotherapist at St George's Hospital Medical School, she completed a variety of rotational jobs. Then she specialised as a Respiratory Physiotherapist and, subsequently, as an Acute Medicine Physiotherapist. From there, Sarah became interested in Advanced Clinical Practice and embarked on her career as an Advanced Clinical Practitioner. She completed both an MSc in Advanced Clinical Practice at the University of Leeds and Clinical Competencies within Acute Medicine. Previously, she was an Advanced Clinical Practitioner Representative on the Society for Acute Medicine Council and a member of the core group working nationally with the Royal College of Physicians developing the Acute Medicine Advanced Clinical Practice Curriculum, published in April 2022.
Sean Buchanan	**BScHons; HDipCompSci, PGDip (AdvClinPrac), MScMed (Emergency Medicine), MSc (Critical Care Medicine)** Sean became a paramedic immediately after completing school in South Africa and worked for the emergency services as well as in the emergency department. He worked in various roles, including firefighter, ambulance paramedic, trauma nurse, and mountain search and rescue officer. After 14 years in the profession, he became a critical care paramedic. Two years later, he became a flight paramedic with a helicopter emergency medical service. He went on to develop several emergency medicine training courses and delivered these across southern Africa. He later immigrated to the UK and took a post as an ACP in the emergency department of a DGH. Looking for a return to critical care medicine, he completed the ACCP training program. He continues to work as an ACCP and has a research interest in the application of AI in trauma.

Sonya Stone

BSc, MSc, RN, ACCP, FICM ACCP Member, FHEA

Sonya is an Assistant Professor of Advanced Clinical Practice at the University of Nottingham, and Advanced Clinical Practitioner in Cardiac Intensive Care at Nottingham University Hospitals. Sonya trained as a nurse in Nottingham and spent much of her nursing career in Intensive Care. She trained as an advanced critical care practitioner in Portsmouth in 2016 and took her first academic post at the University of Southampton as a clinical teaching fellow in 2018.

Sonya is an experienced leader, clinician, and academic, with an interest in critical illness and maternal critical care. She leads postgraduate taught education and CPD in the school of health sciences and is faculty academic director for higher degree apprenticeships. Sonya is an educationalist, with a passion for advancing practice and multi-professional learning.

Stephanie Shea

MSc ACP, BSc (Hons) Adult Nursing, PDTN from LSHTM, NMC RN and V300, Advanced Level Nursing Practice Credential (ALNP) with Royal College of Nursing

Stephanie has been a registered nurse since 2008. During this time, she has worked in various roles within critical care, travel health, expedition medicine, film/television, emergency medicine, and pre-hospital care. She progressed to senior sister and practice educator in urgent and emergency care before moving into advanced practice. Since 2017, she has been an ACP in emergency medicine and, as of 2022, the organisational lead. Stephanie is passionate about the vital role advanced practitioners play in the workforce, and strategies to support them are the current focus of her doctoral studies. Raising their voice and providing a national platform has been at the heart of her work and led her to be elected as the East of England Rep for RCEM ACP Forum. Her key areas of interest are emergency care, pharmacology, clinical skills, and advanced level practice.

Stevie Park

MSc ACCP (FICM ACCP Member), V300

Stevie Park is an Advanced Critical Care Practitioner (ACCP) with Faculty of Intensive Care Medicine Membership (FICM ACCP Member) at the Queen Elizabeth Hospital in Birmingham. Stevie has an MSc in ACCP and is a registered independent and supplementary prescriber (V300). She is well published in organ donation, transfer medicine, and ultrasound. Outside of work, she is fortunate to have a very understanding husband and son, without which her writing would not be possible.

Stuart Cox

MSc ACCP, BSc (Hons Nursing Science)

Stuart Cox works as a senior Advanced Critical Care Practitioner (ACCP) at University Hospitals Southampton NHS and Dorset and Somerset Air Ambulance. Prior to this he was employed as a Senior Charge Nurse ICU at Southampton and Senior Nurse CEGA Air Ambulance. He graduated with a BSc (Hons) in Nursing Science and completed his MSc in ACCP in 2018. Stuart is a Registered Nurse with the Nursing and Midwifery Council (NMC), an independent prescriber (V300), and an ACCP with membership with the faculty of intensive care medicine (FICM). Stuart has co-authored and developed national guidelines on critical care transport drawing on his experiences on pre-hospital critical care and global repatriations and retrievals.

Tracey Maxfield

MSc Advanced Practice (clinical practitioner), PGCert (Medical Imaging Reporting), DCR(R), HCPC registered diagnostic Radiographer

Tracey qualified as a diagnostic Radiographer in 1991 and has worked in Radiology departments across West Yorkshire. In 1996, she gained a PG Cert in medical imaging reporting and went on to establish the Radiographer plain film reporting service at her current NHS Trust of employment.

In 2017, she had the opportunity for a part-time secondment in the acute assessment unit of her current Trust. She developed non-Radiographic clinical skills, enabling her to apply for a training post in advanced clinical practice in acute medicine, and successfully completed an MSc in Advanced Clinical Practice in 2021. Now qualified, Tracey works full time clinically as an ACP in acute medicine and is passionate about using advanced practice to develop service to patients and to strengthen existing medical teams across urgent care, primary care, and community settings.

Tracey is an experienced presenter at conferences, study days, and university lectures both locally and nationally. Her unconventional career pathway from her background profession has been a topic she has been invited to speak and write about many times. She continues to use her Radiography skills in her new role for the benefit of patients and colleagues.

Writing for publication began earlier in her Radiography career, but latterly she has written for medical journals, submitted posters for conferences, and contributed to advanced practice textbooks.

Victoria Metaxa

MD, PhD

Dr Victoria Metaxa is a full-time Critical Care and Major Trauma Consultant, at King's College Hospital in London. She is a King's College London Honorary Clinical Senior Lecturer, and has a PhD in neurosciences and an MA in Medical Ethics and Palliative Care from Keele University. Her clinical interests include bioethics, end-of-life care, critical care outreach, and the management of patients with haematological malignancies. Dr Metaxa is a member of the European Society of Intensive Care (ESICM) Ethics section, and the representative of the section in the ESICM e-learning committee. She is the UK National Outreach Forum board Secretary and a member of the Legal and Ethical Advisory Group of the UK Intensive Care Society (ICS).

Vikki-Jo Scott

RN, MA Learning & Teaching, SFHEA

Vikki-Jo has a background in Critical Care Nursing and returned to clinical practice to work in Critical Care during the initial peaks of the COVID-19 pandemic. Since working in academia, she has focused on Continuing Professional Development for Health and Social Care professionals. She teaches on many courses, including those focussed on quality improvement and the application of learning to practice, as well as leading the Advanced Clinical Practice programmes. She is a Senior Fellow of the Higher Education Academy and, up until 2020, was the Dean of the School of Health and Social Care at the University of Essex, England. She is currently undertaking a PhD focussed on Advanced Clinical Practice and is a reviewer for the Centre for Advancing Practice accreditation processes.

Preface

Advanced practitioners are integral to the interdisciplinary team's successful care and improved outcomes for acutely ill patients in intensive care units and emergency departments. There has been an expansion of advanced practitioner roles expanding across most clinical specialties. In the context of this acute, emergency, and critical care textbook, trainee ACPs, advanced level practitioners across all disciplines, and consultant level practitioners working in emergency medicine and critical care, are the target audience. This acute emergency and critical care advanced practice book is one of several in the Wiley advanced practice series. It is written by Advanced Practitioners for Advanced Practitioners with the aim of ensuring that the services we offer people are safe and effective, and responsive to needs in your locality, from a national perspective and globally.

Advanced practice is a level of practice associated with health and care professions such as physiotherapy, nursing, pharmacy, paramedics, and occupational therapy. This is a level of practice and not necessarily a job title or role, which is designed to transform and modernise pathways of care, enabling the safe and effective sharing of skills across traditional professional boundaries. Advanced practice is delivered by experienced, registered health and care practitioners. It is a level of practice characterised by a high degree of autonomy and complex decision-making. This is underpinned by an advanced academic award or equivalent expert and autonomous experience that encompasses the four pillars of clinical practice, leadership and management, education, and research, with demonstration of core capabilities.

Activity has been undertaken at local, national, and international levels to determine how advanced practice is regulated. It is acknowledged that advanced practice brings with it considerable benefits to patients, in terms of patient satisfaction, improvement in standards of care and clinical outcomes, however, there remains discrepancy in the regulation of advanced practice within contemporary health and care systems. This enduring concern needs to be addressed by key stakeholders as advanced practice gains momentum around the world.

All health and care professionals working at the level of advanced practice have developed their skills and knowledge to an expert level. One example would be Advanced Practitioners working within a clinical context would have the freedom and authority to act, making autonomous decisions in the assessment, diagnosis, and treatment of people. Advanced practice embodies the ability to manage clinical care in partnership with individuals, families, and carers. It includes the analysis and synthesis of complex problems across a range of settings, enabling innovative solutions to enhance people's experience and improve outcomes. Advanced Practitioners are required to operate as autonomous practitioners who can make sound judgements in the absence of full information and manage varying levels of risk when there is complex, competing, or ambiguous information or uncertainty. Importantly, all Advanced Practitioners will have developed their skills and theoretical knowledge to the same standards and should be empowered to make high-level decisions of similar complexity and responsibility. Consequently, all advanced practice posts will contain elements of each of the four pillars of advanced practice. The composition of individual roles will be determined locally.

Leadership and management include identifying the need for change and innovation within clinical practice, developing the case for change, creating a strategic vision, and building a coalition of effective individuals to effect any change. Managing change and service improvement is essential in advanced practice, alongside team development, negotiation, and influencing others. Advanced Practitioners are expected to initiate, evaluate, and modify a range of interventions, which may include prescribing medicines, therapies, providing lifestyle advice, and delivering care.

Education is the cornerstone to improving practice within both the clinical and education sectors. Within advanced practice, it is necessary for practitioners to apply the principles of teaching and learning across their role with patients/service users, carers, and staff alike, promoting an inclusive and creative learning environment. Developing service user/carer education materials, as well as teaching, mentoring, and coaching staff, are essential for continuing to improve standards and the quality of care. Practitioners must be aware of the evidence underpinning subject-specific competencies, i.e., they must have the knowledge, skills, and behaviours relevant to their role and scope of practice, and how to apply these, acting as a role model for other team members. Advanced Practitioners are equipped with effective communication skills to support colleagues in making decisions, planning care, or seeking alternatives as part of the process of making positive changes.

Research and evidence-based practice are crucial for the advancement of clinical practice. This includes not only practitioners' ability to access research and use the information, but also their involvement in research, to bring about improvements and change in practice and to disseminate their findings. Advanced Practitioners can demonstrate clinical proficiency, which embodies the ability to manage clinical skills holistically, using clinical decision-making and clinical reasoning skills. They must apply analytical skills when treating people with complex problems and use evidence-based knowledge and skills; they must practise with competence and maintain ethical conduct, to enhance people's experience and improve patient outcomes.

Acknowledgements

Sadie Diamond-Fox

My dedications are extensive, but I make no apologies for this, because making a book 'come alive' does not happen overnight, nor does it happen without an extensive team by your side. To my family and friends, without whom this most definitely wouldn't have been possible, particularly my Husband. To my little boy, Oscar, I hope that if/when you read Mummy's name on the spine of a book, you will realise that it is possible to achieve your dreams with the right support and mentorship. I hope that you will never let anyone convince you otherwise. Please always remember to try and "lift as you climb", my little love. To Barry Hill and Professor Ian Peate, thank you for your continued support and for believing in my abilities as both a contributor and now an editor. You both continue to be an inspiration, thank you for being such great mentors. To my editorial team, thank you for your time, hard work, and patience throughout this process. I hope it has been an enriching experience for you all and that this will act as a springboard for you in to further publication projects for our workforce. To our contributors, without whom this book wouldn't reflect the diversity, sheer determination, and in-depth knowledge that our collective workforce boasts – thank you! I hope you consider working with us again as we continue this journey with Wiley-Blackwell. To the entire team at Wiley-Blackwell who have been fundamental to getting this book (and others in the series) onto bookshelves, you are all such fantastic people to work with, thank you! A special thank you to Tom Marriott, Charlie Hamlyn, and Ella Elliott, you have been a guiding light for me, not just for this text, but for others in this series. Thank you for being so patient.

Barry Hill

I would like to dedicate this book to the expert chapter contributors and my co-editors. You have shown tenacious commitment and enthusiasm throughout this publication journey and are fantastic individuals. Thank you to my dear friend Ian Peate and Wiley for your continued support in my development and also allowing us to shine the light on advancing practice. A special recognition to my Jose, my mum Tina and my sisters Mel and Sonia, and also my best friend Leanne. Thank you, dad, for watching over me and keeping me safe. You have all inspired me and motivated me in my academic journey.

Sonya Stone

This is for my wife, Tamsin, and my son, Rudi. You're my inspiration, my passion, and my everything, every day. And to my 'team', you know who you are, thank you.

Natalie Gardner

Dedicated to my loving partner Ben, who unwaveringly supports me in all I do. Thank you to my co-editors and chapter contributors, what a journey it has been.

Caroline McCrea

This is for my father-in-law Stuart McCrea who unexpectedly passed away at the start of this project. A fantastic father, gaga and husband who is sorely missed. Thank you for everything you did for us. I also want to thank my amazing husband and little son Joshua, you are my inspiration and I hope I make you proud. Also a big thanks to my phenomenal mother and sister. Thank you for everything you do to support me. To my expert editorial team it's been such a blast and an unforgettable experience. Thank you for taking me on this journey.

Angela Roberts

I dedicate this to the Roberts-Margett bubble – to Will for always believing in me, and to Emilia and Freddie for all the cuddles and smiles that kept me going. What a magnificent journey. Thank you to the amazing editorial team, working with you has been a blast.

How to Use Your Text Book – Pedagogical Features Contained Within Your Textbook

A standard pedagogical format has been applied to this text. The boxed pedagogical content appears throughout this text where it is relevant to the chapter content. This may vary throughout the text.

- **Learning outcomes** give a summary of the topics covered in each chapter.
- **Self-assessment questions** provide the reader with a set of questions specifically designed to help you review your own knowledge base prior to reading the chapter.
- **Multi-professional framework (MPF) for advanced clinical practice guidance for professional development** and **Accreditation considerations:** Each chapter begins with a link to each relevant accrediting organisation/Royal College accreditation document via the boxes.
- **Clinical investigations boxes** provide a link to relevant investigations that pertain to the content of the chapter.
- **Examination Scenarios** provide a link to relevant clinical examination scenarios that pertain to the content of the chapter. They also encourage the reader to reflect upon their knowledge bases concerning the scenario being presented.
- **Fields of practice – Paediatrics** provides an application of the chapter content to the field of paediatric and child health.
- **Fields of practice – Learning Disabilities** provides an application of the chapter content to the field of learning disabilities.
- **Fields of practice – Mental Health** provides an application of the chapter content to the field of mental health.
- **Learning Events** promote reflection on chapter content.
- **Pharmacological principles** directly links the main principles of pharmacology to the content of the chapter.
- **Red flags – Pathological Considerations** are specific attributes derived from a patient's medical history and the clinical exam that are usually linked with a high risk of having a serious disorder.
- **Orange flags – Psychological Considerations** alert the reader to important psychological considerations in relation to the chapter content.

- **Green flags – Social and Cultural Considerations** alert the reader to specific social and cultural issues in relation to the chapter content.
- **Case Study** presents challenging case studies that relate to the chapter content. They are data-led encouraging the reader to analyse the data, make clinical decisions, and apply the decisions to practice.
- **Take Home Points** are a succinct summary of the main points of the chapter.

UNIT 1

CONTINUOUS PROFESSIONAL DEVELOPMENT, APPRAISAL AND REVALIDATION

CHAPTER 1

Governance

Ollie Phipps

Aim
The aim of this chapter is to explore the governance required to support advanced clinical practice, the role of professional bodies, developing an advanced practitioner's scope of practice, the required indemnity, and to understand the concept of professional identity.

LEARNING OUTCOMES

After reading this chapter the reader will:

1. Understand the need of governance within advanced practice.
2. Be aware of their own scope of professional practice and how they should develop and grow it safely, within the law, supported by an appropriate governance framework.
3. Understand the need for practitioners to be clinically competent and to demonstrate this through capabilities in practice using the correct knowledge, skills, and behaviours.
4. Acknowledge the concept of interprofessional working, but understand the concept of professional identity and differences in practice.

SELF-ASSESSMENT QUESTIONS

1. How does one safely develop their scope of practice?
2. As an advanced practitioner assessing a pregnant lady – when would you need to refer to a midwife or medical practitioner?

The Advanced Practitioner in Acute, Emergency and Critical Care, First Edition. Edited by Sadie Diamond-Fox, Barry Hill, Sonya Stone, Caroline McCrea, Natalie Gardner, and Angela Roberts.
© 2024 John Wiley & Sons Ltd. Published 2024 by John Wiley & Sons Ltd.

3. How do you deem yourself competent with the correct knowledge, skills, and behaviours to assess and treat an individual?
4. What requirements should be in place to protect you from litigation?

INTRODUCTION

Advanced practice within the United Kingdom (UK) is experiencing significant development which has seen changes in traditional professional boundaries. Due to this, multi-professional advanced practitioners must be aware of the professional, legal, and ethical considerations that they may face. Advanced Practitioners are a developing part of the modern healthcare workforce (HEE 2021). These Advanced Practitioners make a vital contribution to patient care (NHS 2020) and consist of registered practitioners from a variety of healthcare professional (HCP) backgrounds who have advanced-level capabilities which embrace the four pillars of practice, as set out in the Multi-professional Framework (MPF) for Advanced Clinical Practice in England (HEE 2017).

THE MULTI-PROFESSIONAL FRAMEWORK (MPF)

The MPF expands the definition of advanced clinical practice in England (HEE 2017). The framework is designed to enable a consistent understanding of advanced clinical practice, building on work carried out previously across England, Scotland, Wales, and Northern Ireland. The core capabilities of advanced clinical practice are articulated in this framework, and these will apply across all advanced clinical practice roles, regardless of the health and care professional's setting, subject area, or job role (HEE 2017). The MPF requires that health and care professionals working at the level of advanced clinical practice have developed and can evidence the underpinning competencies (knowledge, skills, and behaviours) applicable to the specialty or subject area (HEE 2017). It must be recognised that every practitioner is responsible and accountable for their actions and omissions. This is reflected within each HCP's code of conduct (NMC 2015; HCPC 2016). The NMC Code is 2018 – Please change this from 2015.

Multi-professional Framework (MPF) for Advanced Clinical Practice Guidance for Professional Development (HEE 2017)

This chapter maps to the following statements within the MPF:

1. Clinical Practice:	1.1	1.2	
2. Leadership and Management:	2.2	2.10	2.11
3. Education:	3.1	3.2	3.8
4. Research:	4.6		

Source: Adapted from Health Education England (2017).

Accreditation Considerations

This chapter maps to the following statements within the following national accreditation documents:

Curriculum for Training for Advanced Critical Care Practitioners Syllabus V1.1 (The Faculty of Intensive Care Medicine 2018)		
3.3	4.12	

Advanced Critical Care Outreach Competencies (The Intensive Care Society, Critical Care Networks – National Nurse Leads and The National Outreach Forum 2022)			
A4	C2	C6	D1

Emergency Medicine Advanced Clinical Practitioner Curriculum 2022 – Adult (The Royal College of Emergency Medicine 2022)
Theme 2: Educational governance and leadership SLO 12: Manage, administer, and lead

Advanced Clinical Practice in Acute Medicine Curriculum Framework (Health Education England 2022)
Core CiPs: 1, 2, 5

GOVERNANCE

Many advanced titles exist in healthcare for people working at an 'advanced level', such as 'Advanced Clinical Practitioner' (ACP), 'Advanced Nurse Practitioner', 'Advanced Paramedic', and 'Advanced Practice Therapeutic Radiographer'. It is essential to note that some professionals have adopted or been given the term 'advanced' but may not have the correct credentials or simply are not working at an 'advanced' level for many reasons (HEE 2017). With the development of Advanced Practice across the UK, the four nations have taken a different approach to its implementation. It is essential that local clear governance structures must exist to support the development, implementation, and ongoing strategy for both the employer and advanced practice employee (HEE 2017). There should be policies highlighting the clear difference between base registration, enhanced practice, and advanced practice which explore the agreed scope of practice and freedom to act (HEE 2017).

Employers may need to review their workforce to ensure there is no misunderstanding for colleagues, and more importantly, the public. Appropriate governance meetings of an Advanced Practice Assurance Group, or similar, should exist with a reporting route to the trust board or similar. An executive should be identified to hold the portfolio of advanced practice and an Advanced Practice Lead should be appointed, where possible, to steer the development of advanced practice within an organisation. To embed Advanced Practice ensuring that it is fit for purpose, it is essential that governance is in place and should consider the following:

- Practice governance and service user safety requirements
- Adherence to legal and regulatory frameworks
- Support systems and infrastructure for delegated roles (e.g. requesting diagnostic tests, administering medicines)
- Professional and managerial pathways of accountability
- Continued assessment against, and progression through, the capabilities identified within this framework
- Location of advanced clinical practice within a career framework that supports recruitment and retention, and succession planning to support workforce development
- Regular constructive clinical supervision that enables reflective practice together with robust annual appraisal.

(HEE 2017)

REGULATION STATEMENTS OF STANDARDS AND CODE OF CONDUCTS

Each HCP is responsible to uphold their individual professional code of conduct and professional standards. This is even more important when working as an advanced practitioner given higher-level decision-making, undertaking procedures with potential risks, and making possible discharge decisions. Each professional code must be understood.

NURSING AND MIDWIFERY COUNCIL (NMC)

'The Code presents the professional standards that nurses, midwives, and nursing associates must uphold in order to be registered to practise in the UK. It is structured around four themes – prioritise people, practise effectively, preserve safety, and promote professionalism and trust. Each section contains a series of statements that taken together signify what good nursing and midwifery practice looks like' (NMC 2015).

HEALTH AND CARE PROFESSIONS COUNCIL (HCPC)

'The role of the standard of conduct, performance, and ethics sets out how we expect registrants to behave and outlines what the public should expect from their health and care professionals. They help us make decisions about the character of professionals who apply to our Register and we use them if someone raises a concern about a registrant's practice. Our registrants work in a range of different settings, which include direct practice, management, education, research, and roles in industry. They also work with a variety of different people, including patients, clients, carers, and other professionals' (HCPC 2016).

General Pharmaceutical Council (GPhC)

'The standards apply to all pharmacists and pharmacy technicians in Great Britain. There are nine standards that every pharmacy professional is accountable for meeting. The standards for pharmacy professionals describe how safe and effective care is delivered. They are a statement of what people expect from pharmacy professionals, and also reflect what pharmacy professionals have told us they expect of themselves and their colleagues' (GPhC 2017).

Legal Issues with Advanced Practice

Advanced Practice will often involve exploring new ways of working and touching upon roles that were traditionally performed by other professional groups, for example medical staff. Therefore, it is essential that any legal implications are fully explored to ensure that new areas of practice are appropriate for the obligations of current legislation and statutes. It must be noted that ignorance of the law is not an appropriate or sufficient defence. The law relates to rules that govern and oversee our society, with the purpose of maintaining justice, upholding social order, and preventing harm to both, individuals and property. The UK parliament can implement laws across the four countries (England, Wales, Scotland, and Northern Ireland). However, the devolved nations all have powers and judicial systems to implement laws that affect an individual country on devolved issues, and health is one of them.

Scope and Capability

Defining Scope of Practice

For HCPs, acknowledging one's scope of professional practice is important, as it defines the limit of their knowledge, skills, and experience. This scope is supported by the professional activities undertaken in their working role, and essential boundaries must be identified, acknowledged, and maintained. It is acknowledged that a professional's scope will change over time as their knowledge, skills, and experience develop.

With the evolution of advanced practice and the expansion of entrustable professional activities, traditional professional boundaries, for example, of the nurse, paramedic, and physiotherapist have significantly changed, and this is demonstrated as the multi-professional workforce comes together at an advanced level.

The provision of healthcare has evolved and is incorporated into many healthcare settings, from primary care to secondary care, from a generalist stance or within specialities. This variability and breadth have meant that advanced practice has become immersed in attempts to define and provide structure.

As this level of practice is unique to the work setting, it is acknowledged that no one profession can encompass all the expertise needed to treat and care for patients. For all, it must include the four fundamental strands of advanced practice: a clinical element, a research element, an educational element, and a management/leadership element. Technological and clinical advances across all sectors have brought about changes in practice and have contributed to the level and quantity of post-qualification education required to advance.

Often contentious is the definition of what advanced practice is. Not one definition will fit perfectly to all advanced practitioners or indeed some work environments. Advanced practice is occasionally described as a blurring of the lines of boundaries of traditional roles or registered HCPs. Yet, this 'blurring' of boundaries implies assuming aspects of a variety of roles and is needed to provide better, more holistic care to all which can be seen as a positive evolution of healthcare.

Competency versus Capability

Competency and capability are two terms that pertain to human ability. Capability is the term used to describe the quality of being capable. Does the individual have the ability to acquire the knowledge and skills required, and is it within their capacity? Capability can also be used to describe a person's implied abilities, or abilities that are not yet developed. With experience, time, and practice, a person's capabilities can develop into competence. Capabilities serve as the starting point of being able to do something and gradually becoming more adept in performing the task. Competence describes the quality of an individual's work. Competence can also be applied to the improvement or development of one's abilities and skills. Once competence has been met, it can result in an increased quality of work and/or performance. Competence can include a combination of knowledge, skills, abilities, behaviours, and attitude.

Knowledge, Skills, and Behaviours

Employers, Higher Education Institutions, Capability Frameworks and Curriculums must set out the knowledge, skills, and behaviours required to be competent.

- **Knowledge** – the information, technical detail, and 'know-how' that someone needs to have and understand to successfully carry out the required duties. Some knowledge will be more specific, whereas some may be more generic.
- **Skills** – the practical application of knowledge needed to successfully undertake the duties. They are learnt through on- and/or off-the-job training or experience.
- **Behaviours** – mindsets, attitudes, or approaches needed for competence and working as a professional. Whilst these can be innate or instinctive, they can also be learnt. Behaviours tend to be very transferable. They may be more similar across occupations than knowledge and skills. For example, team worker, adaptable, and professional.

Competence

Each advanced practitioner must possess the correct knowledge, skills, and behaviour to undertake their role and to demonstrate competence, professionally and educationally. Although embracing the four pillars of advanced practice, as experts, advanced practitioners must be professionally mature and have significant experience of practice. They must always work within their scope of professional practice and acknowledge their professional limitations and restrictions.

Multi-professional Registrations and Scope of Practice

Advanced clinical practice is multiprofessional, which differentiates it from other health and care provision by registered professionals (HEE 2021). Developing a level of advanced clinical practice will be complex as each practitioner will have different professional starting points reflecting different professional registrations, prior practice, and previous supervision and assessment experience. It must therefore be acknowledged that there is no single underpinning, pre-registration professional training for professionals developing to work at an advanced level of practice. The scope of practice for different registered professions varies; not all professional registrations extend to independent or supplementary prescribing (HEE 2021).

Credential Resources

As Advanced Practice has evolved, several professional organisations, supported by HEE and other key stakeholders, have created specialty-specific curriculum and capability frameworks to provide a standardised national structure that assists employers in the training and appointment of regulated healthcare workers in advanced clinical practice roles across England. The purpose of these curriculum frameworks is to develop ACPs who have the correct knowledge, skills, and behaviours, and to acknowledge their scope of practice and level of competence. On successful completion, learners will be able to demonstrate to their employer that they are entrusted to undertake the role of ACP within the National Health Service (NHS) and/or other health and social care settings (HEE 2021).

Core and Specific Capabilities

The capabilities in practice (CiPs) within curriculum frameworks will be mapped to the MPF but will outline specific capabilities required for specialist areas of practice. As part of the holistic development of responsible clinicians, these professional capabilities must be demonstrated at every stage of training (HEE 2021). Higher Education Institutions provide high-quality Masters level courses in advanced practice; however, these do not usually include specialty-specific competencies or nationally defined curricula. There is variation in the range of competencies acquired, and no standardisation of the level of competence of the practitioner for a specific area of practice. Specific ACP credential resources provide an opportunity for standardisation and consistency in a specific clinical area.

Royal College of Emergency Medicine – Emergency Care ACP

In 2015, the Royal College of Emergency Medicine (RCEM) opened a pilot scheme for credentialing Advanced Clinical Practitioners in Emergency Medicine. The pilot completed in summer 2017, and the process is now an accepted part of RCEM. Emergency Care ACPs (ECACPs) have developed a curriculum that enables them to care for patients with a wide range of pathologies, from life-threatening to self-limiting. On completion of the programme, ECACPs can identify the critically ill and injured, providing safe and effective immediate care. They have expertise in resuscitation and are skilled in practical procedures. As such, ECACPs can rapidly establish differential diagnoses, initiate or plan definitive care; and working with in-patient and supporting specialties, as well as primary care and pre-hospital services, correctly identify admission and discharge needs. Through completion of the RCEM credential curriculum ECACPs will acquire the requisite skills to meet both the core and area-specific requirements of ACPs and will be competent to manage complete episodes of care within their clinical specialty.

Fields of Practice – Paediatrics

Those working with and treating children must ensure that they are competent to undertake such a role. The person must possess the correct knowledge, have the right skills, and exhibit professional behaviours. Those working with children must ensure that they have the correct indemnity and insurance to cover paediatric practice. Currently, an ACP Paediatric curriculum is being developed. Health Education England, working with the Royal College of Paediatrics and Child Health (RCPCH), is creating a curricular framework that will consist of key capabilities and learning outcomes across 11 domains which map across five patient groups: non-hospital paediatrics, hospital paediatrics, neonatal, critical care, and child with complex needs.

Faculty of Intensive Care Medicine

The Faculty of Intensive Care Medicine (FICM) have created an Advanced Critical Care Practitioner (ACCP) curriculum that has identified the aims and objectives, content, experiences, outcomes, and processes of postgraduate specialist training leading to a Postgraduate Diploma/Masters qualification in Advanced Critical Care Practice or equivalent. The curriculum promotes a set structure, with expected methods of learning, teaching, feedback, and supervision. The curriculum and assessment process sets out the key requirements of knowledge, skills, and behaviours the ACCP trainee will achieve. The FICM has used the traditional medical assessment process to monitor the ACCP trainee's progress through various stages of training. The objective of the programme is to produce high-quality patient-centred practitioners with appropriate knowledge, skills, and attitudes to enable them to practice in Intensive Care Medicine. On successful completion of training and when performing in the role of an ACCP, there is a requirement to consolidate, maintain, and extend the knowledge, skills, and competence as defined by the FICM ACCP Curriculum.

Fields of Practice – Mental Health

The field of mental health is a specialist area (HEE 2020a). A minimal standard of practice has been created. HEE has developed a capability framework to support the training of Advanced Practitioners working in the specialty of Mental Health. This curriculum allows the Advanced Practitioner in Mental Health (AP-MH) to deliver high-quality, effective care for people experiencing mental health illnesses/conditions. It enables regulated HCPs to develop theoretical knowledge and clinical skills to practice in the specialist areas of mental health. The framework enables practitioners to develop their knowledge, skills, and professional behaviour to work autonomously in providing care to patients requiring complex assessment and treatment. Practitioners will also learn to develop their leadership and management skills to support the wider mental health team and contribute to organisational learning. Finally, the curriculum is designed to promote and share evidence-based knowledge to enhance mental health services and person-centred care (HEE 2020a).

Expanding Scope and Scope Creep

Those training, and those working, at an advanced level must be aware of their competence and capability. With various curriculums and capability frameworks being developed and implemented, advanced practitioners have guidance on where their knowledge, skills, and professional behaviour must sit. However, someone beginning their advanced practitioner journey must acknowledge that it will take years to acquire the knowledge, skills, and experience to work at an advanced level. For some, advanced practice touches upon the traditional knowledge and skills which were traditionally associated with medicine, however with the development of the multi-professional workforce, bringing a different set of knowledge and skills, the advanced practitioner is seen as being 'value added' rather than a role substitute.

Learning from the Airedale Inquiry

The Airedale Inquiry (2010) has steered how a scope of practice should be reviewed. The inquiry focused on a group of senior nurses who worked outside of their scope of practice and inadvertently caused harm to patients. The senior nurses recorded what they were doing in clinical records, prescription charts, and medical notes. It is unlikely that they deliberately set out to harm patients. They were utterly convinced of their own clinical prowess, which went well beyond the boundaries of acceptable nursing practice at that time and beyond the boundaries of their own clinical understanding and capability. The inquiry believes that when the scope of practice for any HCPs' roles is extended, the impact on patient care needs to be assessed. Organisations should ensure that clear lines of responsibility are in place, that training and development plans are fit for purpose, that there is appropriate evaluation of the effectiveness of the role within the organisation, and that there is effective dialogue and engagement with patients, carers, and the public (Airedale Inquiry 2010).

The Advanced Practitioner and The Pregnant Patient

The Royal College of Nursing issued guidance in 2021 regarding advanced practitioners treating pregnant ladies. It must be highlighted that the care of the pregnant woman is the domain of midwives and medical practitioners, as outlined in legislation. However, this is not in isolation from other HCPs, including advanced-level practitioners. It is imperative that all HCPs understand their own roles, limits and boundaries of practice always considering their registration and work within their scope/competence (RCN 2021). It is advisable that non-midwives and non-medical practitioners ask all pregnant women to seek advice from their named midwife at their earliest convenience, even if the condition appears to be unrelated to the pregnancy.

Fields of Practice – Learning Disabilities

Those working with and treating people with learning disabilities and autism must ensure that they are competent to undertake such a role. The person must possess the correct knowledge, have the right skills, and professional behaviours. Those working with people with learning disabilities and autism must ensure that they have the correct indemnity and insurances to cover this type of practice. In 2020, Health Education England launched the 'Advanced Clinical Practice: Capabilities framework when working with people who have a learning disability and/or autism'. This framework sets out to provide a definition of advanced clinical practice for Allied Health Professionals (AHPs) and Nursing staff in learning disabilities and autism services (HEE 2020b). In recent years, the learning disability and autism workforce has been the focus of much attention, not least because of the national Transforming Care Programme, which aims to develop health and care services so that people with a learning disability and/or autism can live as independently as possible, with the right support, and close to home. More recently, the Learning Disabilities Mortality Review (LeDeR) Programme has highlighted the persistence of preventable health inequalities and that people with a learning disability die, on average, 15–20 years sooner than people without a learning disability. The ACP framework sets out the capabilities (including knowledge, skills, and behaviours) characterised by a high degree of autonomy, complex decision-making, and management of risks. The LeDeR programme has highlighted the need for:

- healthcare coordination for people with complex or multiple health conditions
- assurance that effective reasonable adjustments are being provided for people with a learning disability and their families
- mandatory learning disability awareness training for all staff supporting people with a learning disability (HEE 2020a).

Workforce Integration and Professional Identity

Historically, advanced practice roles have been developed within professional groups without a set standard for each clinical background resulting in a large amount of discrepancy and variation (Lawler et al. 2020). It must be acknowledged that the introduction of the new ACP role may interfere with pre-existing professional identities and hierarchies. Existing and new roles have been confused by discrepancies between competencies, training, and qualifications (Lawler et al. 2020). Health Education England (2017) has attempted to standardise and clarify the advanced practitioner level of practice and associated role. However, there seems to be a dichotomy developing in terms of the implementation of the HEE framework by employers between advanced clinical practice as a level of practice of the registered professional and advanced clinical practitioner as a novel omni professional role framed in the medical model as opposed to advancement of professional practice (Lawler et al. 2020). Many advanced practitioners are rostered onto medical rotas rather than advanced practitioner rotas. A common theme exists where experienced practitioners become novice practitioners (trainees) within the medical model. Advanced practice is a level of practice, although it is used as a role. Employers should avoid advanced practitioner training to be carried out at the same time as their original job (e.g. ward sister or rotational physiotherapist).

The transition from a practitioner (nurse/physiotherapist/paramedic) to an advanced practitioner has been described as an 'overwhelming' process that is defined by straddling two identities and 'transition shock' is common. This can result in a struggle to form an identity and feeling like an imposter (Lawler et al. 2020). The transition from being experienced in a previous role to novice in a new role is a period of adjustment, and requires significant support (HEE 2021). There is a clear need for further clarity and structure for advanced practice education and role development, which HEE has started to implement. There is a need for advanced practitioners and their employers to acknowledge professional identity differences and for professional bodies (NMC, HCPC, GPhC) to issue clear guidance. Research is required to explore the specific professional differences within the ACP role. FICM, RCEM, and HEE have created processes, such as credentials, to set minimum standards of expected education and clinical capabilities in practice. These are essential for patient safety and governance. Recruitment processes should take professional identity into consideration, and need to be thorough enough to ensure candidates with the correct qualities, capabilities, and credentials are selected.

Development and Regulation

As this evolution of an alternative 'arm' to provide healthcare in the UK continues, mechanisms of governance have been difficult to hone due to the variability in roles and environments in which advanced practice can be found. In 2008, a call to have new parts added to the NMC and HCPC registers was not authorised as the Council for Healthcare Regulatory Excellence (CHRE) deemed that regulators should ensure that their codes of conduct adequately reflect the requirement for health professionals to stay up-to-date and operate safely within their areas of competence. In addition, organisations are encouraged to develop local governance frameworks, policies, and procedures to support and regulate advanced practice, taking support and guidance from the relevant advisory groups for the disciplines involved.

All these factors play a pivotal role in the continued expansion and prevalence of advanced practice roles and all professionals involved in these roles. There is a need to ensure awareness and the ability to address them all. Encompassing the four fundamental strands of advanced practice is essential nonetheless interpersonal skills and insight are equally important ensuring that advanced practice is a sustainable development in the future workforce planning and longevity of the NHS.

Responsibility and Accountability

All healthcare practitioners working either at their base registration or at an advanced level must understand that they are both responsible and accountable for the decisions they make. Expanding one's scope of practice should be done following the correct preparation, education, and experience. The concepts of accountability and responsibility are closely linked and are at the centre of the codes of conduct for those professionally regulated by the Nursing and Midwifery Council (NMC 2015) and the Health and Care Professions Council (HCPC 2016). Advanced Practitioners have an obligation to undertake their role, and associated tasks, using sound professional judgement. As their level of practice expands, they should realise that this will increase the level of responsibility. Regulated HCPs are responsible for maintaining their competence in practice. They are answerable for their decisions made within their professional practice, and the consequences of those decisions. Advanced Practitioners should be able to justify their decisions and understand the associated legislation, ethical principles, professional standards, guidelines, including evidence-based practice.

Dunning-Kruger Effect

The Dunning-Kruger effect is pertinent in advanced practice. Here, incompetence and metacognitive defects can lead to an over-estimation of an individual's abilities and performance. People in this group find it a challenge to recognise genuine levels of competence when applied to themselves or (objectively) in more competent peers. Gaining insight into one's own limitations and inadequacies is also a challenge by social comparison demonstrating an inability to 'see' their own deficits in relation to their peer's performance. The presence and prevalence of this effect in advanced practice must be recognised and challenged to counterbalance the effect of imposter syndrome, thus creating a balanced, objective practitioner.

Imposter Syndrome

Imposter syndrome is a common phenomenon amongst advanced practitioners and can be interpreted both positively and negatively. Here, the practitioner doubts their credentials, their ability to function, and is often plagued by a fear of being exposed as inadequate. This phenomenon is driven by anxiety and self-doubt, or because of attempted perfection. Often, it is associated within high-pressure environments, especially in healthcare, and associated with comparing oneself to another colleague. Within imposter syndrome, is the sense that someone else is better than you, however competent HCPs possess the same skills, knowledge, and experience.

Professional Issues

Advanced practitioners are pioneers of a new style of practice which challenges the traditions associated with professional roles. With the development of the advanced practitioner role, which is undertaken by members of the multi-professional workforce, working within professional silos has significantly changed. Within areas such as acute and emergency care, nurses, physiotherapists, and paramedics, for example, despite keeping their own professional identities, will work together, undertaking the same role, undertaking the same procedures, and working alongside one another. Each profession brings its own dimension of expertise to the patient, while embracing its own scope of practice. This is seen as being 'value added' for both the patient and the healthcare team. However, each professional group has their restrictions, often associated with legislation or their professional regulator i.e. independent prescribing.

Learning Events

- You are asked to review a patient who is acutely unwell. Although you have managed many acutely unwell patients, this patient is pushing your knowledge and clinical acumen to your limitations. Your supervisor believes you are capable and pushes you to continue your assessment and management. How would you ensure patient safety and ask for help? Are you concerned about imposter syndrome?

- An Advanced Practitioner has just completed an MSc in Advanced Clinical Practice which has been accredited by Health Education England. Some concerns have been raised about their clinical practice and there is a possibility that they are working outside of scope of practice, seeing patients independently, and starting inappropriate treatments. They do not discuss their cases with a senior clinician. How should this be handled? How should the practitioner and their supervisor manage this situation? How should the practitioners develop their scope of practice and demonstrate their capability in practice?

- A patient presents with shortness of breath. An advanced practitioner reviews the patient's chest x-ray and notes it as 'unremarkable – nothing abnormal detected'. Four hours later, the patient collapses, has a cardiac arrest, and dies. The coroner asks the advanced practitioner to demonstrate their capability in the management of the patient's initial presentation and to state how competent they are to interpret a chest x-ray. How would you respond in this situation?

CLINICAL INVESTIGATIONS

Radiology (IR(ME)R)

The Ionising Radiation (Medical Exposures) Regulations (IR(ME)R) (2017) stipulate measures for the protection of patients from unnecessary or excessive exposure to medical x-rays. They also have specific guidance for Employers, Practitioners, Operators, and Referrers in their responsibilities as Duty Holders. The Employer is responsible for putting into place a system of policies, protocols, and procedures which will govern referrals, ensure that justification of exposures takes place, and that a clinical evaluation of all radiographs is recorded. The aim is to ensure that radiation doses to patients are kept as low as is reasonably practicable. The Employer is responsible for ensuring that the diagnostic findings and clinical evaluation of each medical exposure is recorded in the patient's notes. Over recent years, advanced practitioners have been prevented from ordering investigations primarily due to a misunderstanding of their role. Therefore, in 2021, the RCEM created a protocol titled: 'Radiology Requesting Protocol for Extended and Advanced Clinical Practitioners in the Emergency Department' (RCEM 2021) to set out the clear standards which were supported by the Clinical Radiology Faculty of the Royal College of Radiologists.

Blood Tests

Clinicians requesting blood investigations must acknowledge that the responsibility for ensuring that results are acted upon rests with the person requesting the test. That responsibility can only be given to someone else if they accept by prior agreement; this includes discharging patients before results are back and forwarding to primary care colleagues (BMA 2020). Patients should be kept informed, in a sensitive and appropriate manner, of the findings of investigation results, the actions taken as a result, and in a manner that is in keeping with the principles of Duty of Candour (RCEM 2021).

Indemnity

Legal accountability involves advanced practitioners being responsible for ensuring they have professional indemnity insurance in case there is a substantiated claim of professional negligence. Regulators need to ensure that registrants have this indemnity arrangement in place, and it is now a condition of their registration. The indemnity insurance must be appropriate for their level of practice undertaken. If you are employed, your employer has vicarious liability for your actions and omissions while in their employment and is responsible for your actions. However, the practitioner must have been working within their level of competence and following their organisation's policies, procedures, and guidelines.

Indemnity Insurance

Healthcare professionals, by law, must have in place an appropriate indemnity arrangement in order to practise and provide care in the UK. It is your responsibility as a registered HCP to ensure that appropriate cover is in place for your whole scope of practice. The requirement for professional indemnity is to make sure that if someone has suffered harm through the negligent action of a practitioner, they will be able to claim any compensation to which they are entitled. Regulators know that the professionals on their registers take this obligation very seriously. Professionals do not need to hold an arrangement, but it is your responsibility as a professional to ensure that appropriate cover is in place for your whole scope of practice. If you practise without an appropriate indemnity arrangement in place, you may be removed from your professional bodies register and will be unable to practise until appropriate indemnity cover is in place. If you are an employee in the NHS or independent sector, your employer will normally have indemnity arrangements that will cover your work.

Appropriate cover is an indemnity arrangement which is appropriate to your role and scope of practice. It must take into account the nature and extent of the risks of practising in your role. The cover must have enough financial resources to meet an award of damages for a range of situations if a successful claim is made against you, including the costs of a large claim or several smaller claims. If your indemnity provider does not have enough resources to meet the cost of a claim, then you will have to secure alternative indemnity cover to meet the indemnity requirement. To help you to decide whether you have appropriate cover you should think about what your job involves and where you work; who you provide care to and the level of care you provide; the risks involved with your practice; and the possible size of any claim for damages. You could seek advice from your professional body, trade union or insurer to inform your decision. As noted above, if you are an employee in the NHS or independent sector, your employer will normally have indemnity arrangements that will cover your work but it is your responsibility to check. If you work for the NHS, you will already have an appropriate indemnity arrangement. The NHS insures its employees for work carried out on their behalf, which means you will be covered if a successful claim is made against you in that employment. Outside the NHS, many employers are likely to have professional indemnity arrangements that will provide appropriate cover for all the relevant risks related to your job and scope of practice. Arrangements may vary between employers and it is your responsibility to check with them.

Organisations

The MPF gives clear direction for organisations employing advanced practitioners. They must consider where advanced clinical practice roles can best be placed within health and care pathways to maximise their impact and should define clear purposes and objectives for advanced roles. Employers must recognise and accept the responsibilities and greater accountability in relation to governance and support for new advanced roles and the associated level of practice. Governance is essential and applies to all healthcare registrants and is cited within each respective professional code of practice. Each employer carries responsibility and vicarious liability for practitioners, and must be responsible for ensuring that all advanced clinical practice roles, whether existing or future, do not compromise safety (HEE 2017). Policies will need to be developed and processes introduced to reflect this. Without these, there is a significant risk of 'unconscious incompetence', which is likely to compromise safe person-centred care, as well as the reputation of advanced clinical practice (HEE 2017).

Case Studies

1. An ACP has recently been signed off as competent to insert a seldinger intercostal chest drain. The procedure is undertaken on a 50-year old man, who suddenly becomes breathless, with chest pain and is acutely unwell. The procedure is abandoned and taken over by a colleague.
   - What should be required to deem someone capable and competent to undertake a procedure?
   - Who should be able to assess this?
   - What governance framework should be in place?
2. An experienced Advanced Practitioner joins your team. She has been signed off on many practical procedures and has regularly attended in-hospital cardiac arrests as part of the critical care team. She is not FICM or RCEM credentialed or similar.
   - What is required within your organisation to enable this practitioner to practice safely?
   - What governance is required and how should it be implemented for practitioners to work at an advanced level and to be part of a senior decision-making rota?
   - How do you ensure members of your team are capable and competent to carry out the required role?
3. A newly appointed advanced practitioner is undertaking their MSc in ACP and working through their capability framework (FICM, RCEM, HEE ACP). They have several years of clinical experience in their area of specialty and, as such, have a depth of knowledge and skills related to the patient group. However, they have never been responsible for making diagnosis and planning patient management.
   - What would be the first steps for the trainee to achieve the required capabilities in practice for the advanced role for which they are training?
   - What are the responsibilities of their supervisor, and how might they support the trainee to achieve the capabilities in practice?
   - What is the role of university tutor in facilitating the trainee to achieve the competencies for their advanced role?

Take Home Points

- Multi-professional advanced practitioners must be aware of the professional, legal, and ethical considerations that they may face.
- Those training, and those working, at an advanced level must be aware of their competence and capability.
- To practice effectively and within your professional registration, you must possess the correct knowledge, skills, and professional behaviours to undertake your role. This includes working within your role as a newly qualified registrant, as a specialist practitioner, and as an advanced practitioner.
- Advanced practitioners must be able to demonstrate a critical understanding of their broadened level of responsibility and autonomy. They must acknowledge the limits of their own competence and professional scope of practice, including when working with complexity, risk, uncertainty, and incomplete information.
- Advanced practitioners must be aware of the risk of scope creep, and the professional legalities associated with this.
- The advanced practitioner is seen as being 'value added' rather than a role substitute, as in a developing health service under pressure, we should ensure the right person, with the right skills and knowledge, sees the right patient.

REFERENCES

Airedale Inquiry (2010). *Opiate Death Inquiry Calls for Stricter Controls* [online]. Available from: https://www.nursingtimes.net/archive/opiate-death-inquiry-calls-for-stricter-controls-15-06-2010 [accessed 20 June 2023].

British Medical Association. (2020). *Duty of Care When Test Results and Drugs Are Ordered by Secondary Care* [online]. Available from: www.bma.org.uk/advice-and-support/gp-practices/communicationwith-patients/duty-of-care-when-test-results-and-drugs-are-ordered-by-secondary-care#:~:text=The%20responsibility%20for%20ensuring%20that,between%20hospital%20team%20and%20GP [accessed 20 June 2023].

General Pharmaceutical Council. (2017). *Standards for Pharmacy Professionals* [online]. Available from: https://www.pharmacyregulation.org/sites/default/files/standards_for_pharmacy_professionals_may_2017_0.pdf [accessed 5 May 2022].

Health and Care Professions Council. (2016). *Standards of Conduct, Performance and Ethics* [online]. Available from: https://www.hcpc-uk.org/standards/standards-of-conduct-performance-and-ethics [accessed 5 May 2022].

Health Education England (HEE). (2022). *Advanced Clinical Practice in Acute Medicine Curriculum Framework – Credentials* [online]. Available from: https://advanced-practice.hee.nhs.uk/our--work/credentials [accessed 20 June 2023].

Health Education England (HEE). (2017). *Multi-professional Framework for Advanced Clinical Practice in England* [online]. Available from: https://www.hee.nhs.uk/sites/default/files/documents/multi-professionalframeworkforadvancedclinicalpracticeinengland.pdf [accessed 20 June 2023].

Health Education England. (2020a). *Advanced Practice Mental Health Curriculum and Capabilities Framework* [online]. Available from: https://www.hee.nhs.uk/sites/default/files/documents/AP-MH%20 Curriculum%20and%20Capabilities%20Framework%201.2.pdf [accessed 15 February 2022].

Health Education England. (2020b). *Advanced Clinical Practice: Capabilities Framework When Working with People Who Have a Learning Disability and/or Autism* [online]. Available from: www.skills forhealth.org.uk/wp-content/uploads/2020/11/ACP-in-LDA-Framework.pdf [accessed 5 May 2022].

Health Education England. (2021). *The Centre for Advancing Practice – Workplace Supervision for Advanced Clinical Practice: An Integrated Multi-professional Approach for Practitioner Development* [online]. Available from: https://www.hee.nhs.uk/sites/default/files/documents/Workplace%20 Supervision%20for%20ACPs.pdf [accessed 15 February 2022].

Lawler, J. Maclaine, K. and Leary, A. (2020) *Workforce Experience of the Implementation of an Advanced Clinical Practice Framework in England: A Mixed Methods Evaluation. Human resources for health* [online]. Available from: https://human-resources-health.biomedcentral.com/articles/ 10.1186/s12960-020-00539-y [accessed 20 June 2023].

NHS. (2020). *We Are the NHS: People Plan 2020/21 – Action for All of Us* [online]. Available from: https://www.england.nhs.uk/wp-content/uploads/2020/07/We_Are_The_NHS_Action_ For_All_Of_Us_FINAL_24_08_20.pdf [accessed 15 February 2022].

Nursing & Midwifery Council. (2015). *The Code* [online]. Available from: www.nmc.org.uk/ globalassets/sitedocuments/nmc-publications/nmc-code.pdf [accessed 3 March 2022].

The Faculty of Intensive Care Medicine. (2018). *Curriculum for Training for Advanced Critical Care Practitioners – Syllabus. V1.1* [online]. Available from: www.ficm.ac.uk/media/6896 [accessed 20 June 2023].

The Intensive Care Society, Critical Care Networks – *National Nurse Leads and The National Outreach Forum.* (2022). *Advanced Critical Care Outreach Competencies* [online]. Available from: https://ics.ac.uk/ asset/43B8C11B-4512-41D0-B97768FABA2C30B2 [accessed 20 June 2023].

The Ionising Radiation (Medical Exposure) Regulations. (2017). *The Ionising Radiation (Medical Exposure) Regulations 2017* [online]. Available from: www.legislation.gov.uk/uksi/2017/1322/ contents/made [accessed 20 June 2023].

The Royal College of Emergency Medicine. (2022). *Emergency Medicine Advanced Clinical Practitioner Curriculum 2022 (Adult)* [online]. Available from: https://rcem.ac.uk/wp-content/uploads/ 2022/09/ACP_Curriculum_Adult_Final_060922.pdf [accessed 20 June 2023].

The Royal College of Emergency Medicine (2021). *Radiology Requesting Protocol for Extended and Advanced Clinical Practitioners in the Emergency Department.* RCEM.

The Royal College of Nursing. (2021). *Advanced Level Nursing Practice and Care of Pregnant and Postnatal Women* [online]. Available from: www.rcn.org.uk/clinical-topics/Medicines-management/ Prescribing-inpregnancy [accessed 20 June 2023].

CHAPTER 2

Continuous Profession Development (CPD), Appraisal and Revalidation

Vikki-Jo Scott

Aim

The aim of this chapter is to provide an overview of the key aspects of continuing professional development, including appraisal and revalidation, as it relates to Advanced Practice within Emergency and Critical Care settings. It provides links to relevant policy and guidance as well as suggested tools, case studies, and further support and reading to help develop your understanding of this topic.

LEARNING OUTCOMES

After reading this chapter the reader will:

1. Recognise the importance of ongoing personal professional development for Advanced Practice and its impact on addressing evolving and novel aspects of population need and its contribution to patient safety.
2. Understand the contribution that can be made by Advanced Practitioners (APs) working in emergency and critical care settings to developing a team to work effectively.
3. Be aware of the contribution that can be made to the development of Advanced Practice beyond the local context.
4. Be able to plan the next steps in their professional development, including appraisal, revalidation, and progress towards consultant level.

SELF-ASSESSMENT QUESTIONS

1. What policy documents should you refer to when planning your development as an AP?
2. What tools can you use to plan and structure professional development?
3. Who will play a role in influencing the effectiveness of your and your team's development and achievement of goals, expectations, and requirements?
4. What networks/forums should you access to contribute and learn from the development of AP at a regional, national, or international level?

INTRODUCTION

The goals of advanced practice roles are to manage clinical care in partnership with individuals, families, and carers. It includes the analysis and synthesis of complex problems across a range of settings, enabling innovative solutions to enhance people's experience and improve outcomes. This is certainly apparent in emergency and critical care where, complexity, clinical risk, and time sensitivity often add pressure to the application of knowledge and skill for patient-centred problem solving. Transitioning into an autonomous role as an AP is therefore both daunting and a cause for celebration (Skills for Health 2020).

This chapter will explore different aspects of continuing professional development within this field to enable the Acute, Emergency or Critical Care (AECC) Advanced Practitioner (AP) to navigate their way through the requirements, expectations, and aspirations for their role.

The Multi-professional Framework (MPF) for Advanced Clinical Practice (HEE 2017) provides helpful guidance on the expectations for APs at each layer of professional development.

Multi-professional Framework (MPF) for Advanced Clinical Practice Guidance for Professional Development (HEE 2017)

This chapter maps to the following statements within the MPF:

1. Clinical Practice:	1.1	1.2	1.3	1.11	
2. Leadership and Management:	2.4	2.11			
3. Education:	3.1	3.2	3.4	3.6	3.7
4. Research:	4.8				

Accreditation Considerations

This chapter maps to the following statements within the following national accreditation documents:

Curriculum for Training for Advanced Critical Care Practitioners Syllabus V1.1
(The Faculty of Intensive Care Medicine 2018

3.21	3.23	4.12	

Advanced Critical Care Outreach Competencies
(The Intensive Care Society, Critical Care Networks – National Nurse Leads and The National Outreach Forum 2022)

C1	C4	C5	

Emergency Medicine Advanced Clinical Practitioner Curriculum 2022 – Adult
(The Royal College of Emergency Medicine 2022)

Section 9: Continuing Professional Development (CPD) and revalidation

Advanced Clinical Practice in Acute Medicine Curriculum Framework
(Health Education England 2022a)

Section 9: Continuing Professional Development (CPD) and revalidation

PROFESSIONAL DEVELOPMENT AND TRANSITION IN ADVANCED PRACTICE

When considering professional development in advanced practice, it is important to recognise that this goes beyond just the individual's development. Advanced Practitioners are rarely 'sole operators' and commonly work in emergency and critical care settings within a multi-professional team situated within an employing organisation. The individual's development will impact the broader team and organisation in which they work. At an advanced level of practice, it is also expected that individuals contribute to the broader development of the Advanced Practice community, which is diverse, multi-professional, and evolving fast. It is therefore helpful when looking at this topic to consider the 'personal', the 'team', and the 'AP community' and how the development of one will radiate out to the other layers (see Figure 2.1).

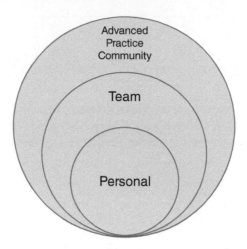

FIGURE 2.1   Layers of professional development and transition in advanced practice.

PERSONAL PROFESSIONAL DEVELOPMENT

Personal professional development is lifelong. We never stop learning, and the nature of advanced practice is that it is evolving, adapting to population needs. It is an innovative role often moving into unchartered territories which require that we use new or unfamiliar approaches or apply knowledge, skills, and behaviours in novel contexts.

In order to develop, you need to remember where you have developed from and recognise how much was learnt along the way to provide confidence and a direction for future development. While it might be useful to think about this as a journey, as depicted in Figure 2.2; where you set a goal to reach, work towards it, and then step on the podium at the end and take your medal, the race is actually never over!

For the duration of our working lives there are always new goals that we can choose to reach for. Sometimes this is because we want to push ourselves in a different direction, and sometimes it is because the world around us has changed and to keep up with this change we need to 'adjust our sails' and set new goals.

This is particularly the case in emergency and critical care, which, as we have seen over recent years in response to the COVID-19 pandemic, had to make rapid changes to the functions, structure, locations, and ways in which APs practised. This created a new challenge for APs to operate in ways that had not been encountered before, or at least not at the scale of demand that has previously been 'routine' in these settings. With the increasing demands on community services, a backlog of health interventions, and people now seeking support at a later stage in their disease due to the pandemic, we have continued to see changes and an adapted focus within the AECC services. The 'business as usual' is not the 'usual' as we would once have known it. In an online survey published by Health Education England (2020), they noted how APs were reporting being utilised in ways they had not experienced before, making more use of the full scope of their knowledge, skills, and experience.

It is important to remember that we are never starting from zero each time a new goal is set. All of your learning and experiences to date will have shaped what you are, and often lessons learnt from these can be applied or adapted to help you in achieving your next goal. The hard part, though, is often remembering what we have learnt along the way.

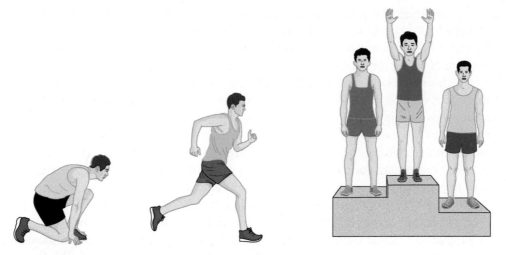

FIGURE 2.2   The professional development journey.

Think about how difficult it is to explain to someone a task that you do now unconsciously. To be successful at this you need to break it down into its constituent parts, or stages of the process. Some will seem familiar and easily transferable to a new skill, and others appear quite specialised, which took practise or different approaches, resources, or knowledge to master . . . but you did get there in the end!

As an AP you will have started in a particular profession. You will have learnt the relevant skills to master and practice within this profession, applying the knowledge and evidence base to underpin your actions, and have continued to build upon these through experience. All professions that work within the definition of 'Advanced Practice' are regulated. This means that educational standards have been set for the approval of an individual to enter that profession, and a monitoring and revalidation process is required for them to continue to practice. All regulatory requirements for healthcare professions provide scope for and a requirement to continually develop and enhance practice. Advanced practice development is therefore not outside or in addition to the requirements of professional revalidation; it is the way in which you can demonstrate how you are encompassing the requirements of your profession's specific regulatory body to continually develop.

As you develop within a specific field of practice, you will have continued to cultivate and apply the knowledge and skills gained from initial registration within a profession to the area in which you work. This will have led you to an 'enhanced' level of practice within your specialist field of emergency or critical care. Often, clinicians working in this field will describe themselves as specialists rather than generalists due to the range of presentations, conditions, complications, and body systems that they need to support for patients that come into their service. This is a specialist set of knowledge and skills in itself; to be able to consider holistically the different aspects of the patient's presentation and to balance the impact of one condition, symptom, or intervention against another.

CREDENTIALS, CAPABILITIES, OR COMPETENCIES

Within specialist areas of practice, there are organisations and professional bodies which provide resources, support, and benchmark standards that are expected for those working in these fields. For acute care, this is provided by the Health Education England Advanced Clinical Practice in Acute

Medicine Curriculum Framework (2022a); for emergency care, this is provided by the Royal College of Emergency Medicine (2022); and for critical care, this is provided by the Faculty of Intensive Care Medicine (2019). In addition, there may be profession- or location-specific networks that can be accessed (e.g. the Royal College of Nursing forum or the regional Critical Care networks). These organisations provide clear direction for those working in these fields as to the scope of practice that can be expected, and for many employers, it is expected that you provide evidence of meeting their requirements to be able to work at different levels in this field.

The standards that are used by these organisations are commonly referred to as 'credentials', 'capabilities', or 'competencies'. Work is also underway through the Centre for Advancing Practice to develop, validate, and publish credentials for particular specialisms. You should continue to look out for credentials that are relevant to your field of practice, and think about what evidence you can provide or need to gain to demonstrate you meet the expectations for the specialism in which you work.

The FICM provides a curriculum that sets out the expectations regarding recognition by them to practice as an Advanced Critical Care Practitioner (ACCP). Within their handbook, they note that the outcome from their training programme 'is such that mastery of the specialty to the level required to commence autonomous practice in a specific post is achieved by the end of training as knowledge, skills, attitudes, and behaviours metaphorically spiral upwards. Following qualification, the continuing professional development of the ACCP will follow the same model'. Their ACCP advisory group has also produced a CPD and appraisal pathway (FICM 2020) by which ACCPs can plan, institute, maintain, and evidence their ongoing clinical academic and professional learning.

They note this is in addition to regulatory body requirements regarding revalidation (with the NMC or HCPC) and includes a 'medical style' appraisal, as clinical supervision of ACCPs sits with the Consultant Medical Staff in Critical Care and clinical leads for ACCPs.

Within the 'CC3N Step Competency Framework' for critical care nurses, they also highlight the need to 'demonstrate your advanced theoretical knowledge and provide the relevant evidence base for your established practice. You are advised to keep a record of any supportive evidence and reflective practice to assist you during progress and assessment reviews'. This framework specifies the competencies and form in which evidence should be recorded to demonstrate practice at this advanced level. This includes assessment and development plans, action plans, and annual competency review alongside reflection in preparation for revalidation with the NMC (CNN 2015).

In the Royal College of Emergency Medicine (RCEM) 'Emergency Care Advanced Clinical Practitioner Curriculum (Adult and Paediatric)' (2022) (page 29), they also note the need to address the requirements for CPD as set out by the relevant regulatory body that apply to the particular profession you originally registered in (NMC or HCPC). However, in the 'common competencies' they also make reference to particular behaviours that are expected. This includes the need to 'Keep up to date with national reviews and guidelines of practice (e.g. NICE and SIGN)' under the 'common competency for Evidence and Guidelines.

In the 'Acute Medicine' credential validated by the Centre for Advancing Practice (and co-produced with the Royal College of Physicians), they set out the core, specialty, and generic capabilities that are expected for this field of practice (CiPs) (HEE 2022a). The eligibility criteria, expected duration of training, content of learning, learning outcomes, key clinical presentations and conditions/issues, and practical procedures this credential can apply to, teaching and learning methods, assessment methods, assessment criteria, and expected evidence are provided in this credential for advanced clinical practitioners (ACPs) working in acute medicine. These are furthermore linked to the Multi-professional Framework for Advanced Clinical Practice in England, to demonstrate how achievement within this credential can provide evidence within the MPF-expected capabilities (HEE 2022a).

> **Learning Event**
>
> Consider what evidence you think you need to collect, review, evaluate, and act upon to demonstrate ongoing development to meet your relevant regulatory, professional, and specialist credential standards.

This evidence should relate to your current job, specialist field, and level of practice. As a starting point you might find it helpful to look at your job description or the job description of a role you are aiming for. This is likely to give you particular expectations around your role, including relevant competencies and capabilities, tasks, and responsibilities. These can then be mapped to the expectations around Advanced Practice by looking at the capabilities in the Multi-professional Framework for Advanced Clinical Practice in England (HEE 2017) and any other credentialling, capability, or competency frameworks that are applicable to your field of practice (e.g. FICM, Acute Medicine, CC3N, or RCEM, as listed above).

So when starting out on your own personal professional development, it is helpful to identify:

- What are the expectations you should be working to?
- Who governs these expectations?
- How can/must you demonstrate that you meet these expectations?

SUPERVISION

Requirements for CPD within regulatory, professional, or credentialling bodies are often linked to expectations around supervision. Successful professional development is much more likely to be achieved where an individual is supported and guided in their practice, with opportunities for assessment, feedback, and discussion. Certain criteria may be set down by your employer or your regulatory, professional, or credentialling body regarding:

- What type, model, and volume of supervision should be expected?
- Who can act as an appropriate supervisor?
- Whether they have a role to play in assessing and confirming your progress and achievement?

For Advanced Practice, the document produced by Health Education England sets out the minimum expected standards regarding supervision (HEE 2022b). This should be referred to when planning to embark on the development as an AP and as you continue to develop in this role. It is a guide you can also use as you develop your own skills to support and supervise others, including the next generation of APs.

In addition to the HEE expectations regarding supervision, and where any credentialling, competency, or capability frameworks apply, reference should also be made to the expectations regarding supervision in these documents. These may provide additional insight or more specific requirements regarding the types of supervision, learning or assessment, and criteria for supervisors that are expected in particular fields of practice.

For example, in the CC3N Step Competency Framework for nurses working in critical care, the requirements for 'lead assessors' and 'critical care lead/Nurse manager' are set out and additional resources for mentors to guide the implementation of the framework are provided.

As you may expect, the HEE 'Acute Medicine' credential refers to the roles of co-ordinator of education and associate supervisor, which are also set out in the 'minimum expectations' document that applies more broadly to the Multi-professional Framework for Advanced Clinical Practice in England. However, the detail provided on teaching, learning, and assessment methods to be applied for this credential provides more specific direction for the particular types of supervision activity that will be expected of supervisors and those seeking recognition as an ACP in this field of practice.

In the ACCP Trainer Guidance provided by FICM, they set out the role that educational supervisors, practice mentors, and ACCP leads are expected to take in providing supervision, support, and learning opportunities to develop competence and mastery in the field of critical care advanced practice. Here, they provide specific direction regarding the types and expected timing of supervisory activity.

The Royal College of Emergency Medicine also provides information in their credentialling curriculum regarding how supervision is expected to support the development of EC-ACPs and provide links to access supervisor training. It is important to note that, as with the above, there are expectations for EC-ACPs about how, when, and who can provide final 'sign off' to say an individual has demonstrated the expected criteria to be recognised in this specialist field of practice.

It is important therefore to ensure, before embarking on seeking accreditation for emergency or critical care, that the appropriate people and correct level, types, and supervisory activities and documentation are in place in order to meet the criteria required. Fundamental to this is that both the 'trainee' and their supervisor are clear about what is to be expected by referring to the relevant accreditation documentation.

Establishing an effective supervisory relationship is key to success. It can have a significant influence on your development and your experience of the process, which may in turn affect how well you feel able to support others. You may or may not have some choice about who your supervisor will be. Getting the right balance between someone you feel you can talk to easily and someone you feel will be honest without repercussions on friendship or working relations can be difficult! Be aware of the professional relationship status that supervision holds, know what to expect and know who else you can turn to if the supervision is not working as it should.

Coaching may or may not be an approach taken within your supervision but is strongly encouraged as a reflective challenge for your practice and to develop your leadership capability. Many employers will have a people development team with some leadership coaches who would be happy to support you.

However, remember that YOU are the person that is most invested in your development. Others (including employers, supervisors, and coaches) will have their own agenda and will not necessarily appreciate the complexity of your journey to where you are today and the rich texture of how you perform at your best. A key expectation of Advanced Practice is developing autonomy. This includes taking personal responsibility for driving your progress forward in the way that works best for you, which is a necessary adjunct to effective supervision.

It is important to consider here the differences between types of supervision roles such as a line manager, coach, expert in the field, mentor, critical friend, and appraiser (see Table 2.1). Each role will have a different focus, goal, and expected outputs and may use a different approach to effectively achieve the expected goals and outputs. For example, while not exhaustive, Table 2.1 suggests an idea of who in what role may be best to approach for particular supervisory activities and purposes. The different roles may overlap at times, but being clear with supervisors about what the purpose is and picking the right person for the activity you are undertaking is key to productive supervision. For example, a workplace supervisor may be best to provide opportunities to develop confidence and competence for specific clinical tasks. A line manager may be helpful to identify potential opportunities (including potential supervisors to work with) to gain experience to achieve the expectations required and give direction on the types of evidence or performance they would expect to see. A coach (or sometimes an appraiser depending on the approach used for appraisal in your organisation) may be particularly helpful in identifying realistic goals and establishing a time-limited route map with you of how you are going to achieve these.

TABLE 2.1 The differences between types of supervision roles.

Role ✓	Line manager	Coach	Mentor	Appraiser	Expert	Critical friend
Aim/Purpose						
Permission and structure to learn	✓			✓		
Enhancing learning, making it apply to real practice, and giving learning an anchor/benchmark for practice			✓		✓	✓
Signposting and problem solving	✓		✓	✓		
Horizon scanning and development planning	✓	✓		✓		
Activity						
Reflection		✓	✓			✓
Case study review				✓	✓	
Assessment	✓			✓		
Role shadowing			✓		✓	

Learning Events

Review the bullet points below and think about who would be best to utilise to achieve these.

- What are the expectations you should be working to?
- Who governs these expectations?
- How can/must you demonstrate that you meet these expectations?

CONTINUING PROFESSIONAL DEVELOPMENT-USING APPRAISALS EFFECTIVELY

Healthcare and population needs are always changing, so professional development in advanced practice may never feel like it ends, as there are always going to be new knowledge and skills to learn. However, by setting clear objectives for your development and career aspirations, targets, and goals, you will be presented with more opportunities to make a conscious decision of what changes you want, rather than just being dragged along with the flow of change.

To do this, establish what the barriers or facilitators to change are and identify allies that will help you facilitate your development. Revisit Table 2.1 of potential people you can gain support from and consider who would be best from this list to be your ally to address barriers/facilitators. You should also take time to understand how your objectives align with intrinsic motivators (e.g. what gives you meaning, a sense of belonging, or self-esteem) and extrinsic motivators (e.g. rewards, competition, how you are seen by others) as well as organisational strategic objectives.

Every organisation will undertake an annual appraisal for all staff. This provides a golden opportunity to articulate and negotiate your achievements and aspirations, and to seek endorsement from your line manager for your plans. As you develop as an AP you should use this to synthesise your personal aspirations, your organisational objectives, and the requirements to grow in your advanced practice capabilities. The structure and prescribed format for appraisal documentation will vary from place to place but they may include, or be supplemented with the use of a number of skills and tools that you can use to identify, plan, and sustain your learning.

Undertaking a learning needs assessment will provide dedicated time and space to decide what you need to focus on for your development. From this you can be more targeted on the actions you choose to undertake to address your learning needs. Within learning needs analysis, it is helpful to get a variety of perspectives on the areas you may need to consider as a development goal. Using a self-assessment tool, alongside gathering feedback (perhaps through a 360-degree appraisal) can help to discern what is needed. We are not always the best judge of how we are perceived by others and tend to over- or underemphasise our strengths and weaknesses. Learning needs analysis does not need to be complicated; asking simple questions such as 'What are your goals?', 'What are your desired outcomes?', 'What knowledge/ skills do you already have?', and 'What do you need?', can help identify the gaps and prioritise actions.

Using a goal-setting tool such as 'SMART' can also help to clearly and concisely identify objectives and the actions, resources, and time scale needed to achieve your objectives. Think about, write out, and where possible discuss and agree with your supervisor:

- **S – Specific** – Write a clear aim and why it is significant. Try to keep it simple (you can break down complex aims into smaller chunks to help keep them specific enough for actions to be taken).
- **M – Measurable** – How are you going to meaningfully measure achievement of your aim. What will tell you that you have been successful?
- **A – Action** – What are the achievable and agreed actions you are going to undertake to address your aim?
- **R – Resources** – What resources are you going to need to achieve your goal? (This could be money, people, or access to a resource such as a course or online learning). Consider whether these are realistic (if not you may need to adjust, or stagger your goal or actions) and be clear about how these will help you achieve your goal.
- **T – Time**- Set a specific date by which you expect to achieve your goal. This may include setting dates for interim points for when actions need to be carried out, and when review is needed to check you are on track (or if you need to adjust your plan). This could be linked with a job plan, which is a helpful way of laying out time to facilitate your own development and ensure that you are meeting all four pillars of advanced practice.

Using other planning tools, such as a Gantt chart, can also be helpful to clearly set out timelines and actively plan for regular review points. Passively relying on an annual review may mean momentum is lost, or changes in circumstances derail your goals rather than adjusting to the circumstances while still keeping the ultimate goal in mind. These tools are also helpful as they encourage you to break a 'master plan' or an overarching goal into smaller, more manageable chunks. At different times you may need to break your actions down to smaller tasks to keep moving forward. For example, what can you do in the next 15 minutes towards your goal rather than in the next month? Gantt charts tend to be used as a basic structure for Personal Development Plans, where you should identify short-, medium-, and long-term goals.

Reflective tools or models are well known and used in healthcare, particularly within initial training or more formal education. You could try a few different ones to find the one that feels the best fit for you and until it feels familiar and easy to use. A key principle of reflection is that it is an 'active' rather than passive process, where you set aside time and head space to engage with your experience and consider how that may help you in the future. All reflective models will encourage you to not just keep your reflective thoughts in your head. Writing it down and discussing it with someone (e.g. a coach, supervisor, or colleague you are utilising for revalidation processes) helps expose your thoughts; it can help to provide a definitive frame of reference for your goals and plans, and from this, gives you the driving force to turn this into tangible physical action. You may also find the National Health Service (NHS) leadership model (2023) helpful as a structure for reflection. It provides prompts to explore different aspects of leadership (which is a key pillar of AP) and provides tools for self- and peer-assessment and a way in which to record your experiences, plan your development, and track your progress.

ATTITUDES TO LEARNING

Your attitude to learning can also have an impact on success. In studies that talk about a 'growth mindset', they noted that people who believed if they worked hard they could learn and achieve more, were actually more successful. Although the research has largely been based on children, this can also apply to adults, this is explored further in Carol Dweck's TED talk 'The power of believing that you can improve' (Dweck 2022). By remaining open to learning and believing that putting some effort into learning can help you to achieve your goals, you are more likely to achieve what you are aiming for. Being passive and expecting the 'learning to come to you' are much less likely to be successful.

This is one of the reasons why there has been a shift away from using lectures as the primary way of delivering education. Just being present in a lecture theatre or gathering together a portfolio of attendance certificates will not automatically guarantee that learning has been achieved – it requires some active engagement by the learner for the transfer of knowledge from one person or source to another to happen. Verification of learning and capability in Advanced Practice takes note of this. For example, in the Advanced Clinical Practice Apprenticeship Standards for End Point Assessment (Institute for Apprenticeships & Technical Education 2018), and in the HEE e-portfolio (supported) Route (2023) for evidencing that a person adequately meets the capabilities expected for working at this level of practice, a range of evidence is required. The portfolios and assessments used will expect not just a collection of certificates, but articulation of how a particular learning event or experience has contributed to your development and can be evidenced in your practice as an AP. This requires engagement with reflection on learning and within this, clear articulation of how this applies to your practice as an AP within the emergency or critical care setting. For this reason, you will need to engage in a range of work-based assessments, which include external observation and endorsement of your capabilities as well as the use of case studies to provide examples of how learning has been applied and the expected outcomes of learning achieved.

Log books, structured training reports, and mini clinical evaluation exercises are expected within the RCEM credential for EC-ACPs, and Direct Observation of Procedural Skills, Case-based Discussions, and Multi-source Feedback are required by FICM for ACCPs. Within this process, and noting the 'growth mindset' approach, this requires that you acknowledge weakness as well as strengths, drawing upon both positive and negative feedback and experiences to plan and then demonstrate your development.

There is sometimes a temptation to feel you have to do everything to a perfected level before pushing yourself forward into new roles/tasks/contexts. In reality, though we are continually developing, you can never be fully and perfectly prepared, but you can be open to learning along the way, adapting as needed. Sometimes you do need to 'just go for it'. Opportunities come by every now and again, and if you do not allow time away from the day-to-day tasks, you will miss the opportunities that occasionally pass by that could propel and boost your progress.

Finally, when considering your personal development, remember to look after yourself! Research has shown that healthcare worker wellbeing, organisational change, and patient safety are linked (Montgomery et al. 2020). There has been significant discussion of 'building resilience' and efforts to reduce burnout in healthcare workers, with the COVID-19 pandemic particularly highlighting the negative long-term impact this can have. Advanced Practitioners are not immune to this! In fact, you may be more at risk due to the emerging nature of AP roles where established support networks and a clear role identity, scope of practice, and legitimised autonomy can be a challenge. A (usually unjustified) sense of needing to prove yourself due to imposter syndrome has been noted to be a common feature of people's experience, particularly where they are working in innovative ways or in new teams or services. Investing time in your own development and wellbeing is consequently worthy of attention, not least because it contributes to patient safety. This is, of course, a priority all can agree on as important.

SUPPORTING PROFESSIONAL DEVELOPMENT WITHIN A TEAM

It is unlikely that as an AP you will be working in isolation. Commonly, Aps work within a multi-disciplinary team. Within this environment, it is important that as part of your CPD you develop your professional identity. All team members are not expected to work the same or bring the same knowledge, skills, and experience with them to the role they play within a team. Each team member should be encouraged to draw on others' strengths to complement what they contribute, thus allowing the service to adapt to address the needs of the patients, carers, and organisations they work with.

From the team perspective of professional development, it is therefore important to recognise the strengths of others. As an AP you are also likely to be leading a team, and supporting trainees. You should take a facilitatory approach to identifying where individuals may need support to develop their contribution/expertise, as well as identifying where, as a team, there may be areas that need developing.

CONTRIBUTION TO BROADER DEVELOPMENT OF AP

Within the Multi-professional Framework for Advanced Clinical Practice in England, a core capability of the 'research' pillar is that Aps are engaging and using networks to support their practice. This should be seen as your wider community of practice (beyond those you directly work with).

A Community of Practice (COP) is defined as a group of people who share a concern or a passion for something they do and learn how to do it better as they interact regularly (Wenger 2000). They usually have an agreed domain or identity shared by an area of interest and an agreed community in order to build relationships, learn from each other, and share resources on their practice. There are a number of organisations developing AP in specific areas, such as the National Association of Advanced Critical Care Practitioners, The ACP Forum, and many in between.

Identifying and engaging with a community of practice is likened to 'finding your tribe'; somewhere you feel you belong. It can be an incredibly helpful resource for shaping and supporting professional development and role transition at a personal and team level. It can help to 'calibrate' your ideas about what Advanced Practice is, what it can achieve, and what further opportunities there are to explore in this exciting field of practice.

A resounding feature of Advanced Practice is that it is diverse and often shaped by the local context. This can lead to a belief that the local way to operate is the only way; however by tapping into the diverse population of Advanced Practice, you can draw upon a wealth of experiences to open up the potential options available. By the types of work that Aps engage with and the position that this role affords, Aps are often in the position of being trailblazers and innovators, having to create new solutions or deal with new problems to solve. This creates a need for and provides an opportunity to view the situation beyond the boundaries of your particular experience to date, your profession, team, or service.

WHAT NEXT?

As you hopefully will have gathered by now, CPD is iterative. There is always further development to be undertaken. It is also the case that once you have achieved recognition or accreditation as an AP in emergency or critical care, there are expectations that you periodically revalidate your credentials to work in this field.

As noted above, each of the credentialling bodies also provides direction regarding what is expected if you want to continue to work at the advanced level in emergency or critical care.

For FICM, it is expected that the meetings and assessments that have been used within the training programme are built upon to allow regular review and overall competency progression (e.g. meetings two or three times per year with the ACCP local clinical lead). Annual appraisal can be combined with the Annual Review of Competency Progression (ARCP) while in training, and can also be utilised going forward to review progress and set development plans (including meeting any regulatory body requirements to remain registered in your profession). While there are no specific requirements set beyond the completion of the training by FICM, it is noted that the ACCP should continue to consolidate, maintain, and extend knowledge. They note that the ACCP clinical lead is expected to play a key role in supporting career progression and agreeing on any additional dimensions to service delivery that are required.

For RCEM, again they do not provide specific direction regarding requirements to retain accreditation beyond what is expected for revalidation with your relevant regulatory body. They do note that all ACPs should engage in CPD and maintain a portfolio of evidence to ensure they meet the requirements for professional revalidation.

In the CC3N Step Competency Framework, this is more specifically (and understandably) linked into the requirements for revalidation with the NMC (which is once every three years). This includes use of reflection, evidence of professional indemnity arrangements and CPD, practice hours, and feedback log books. In addition, they provide a structure for annual competency review, which should accompany local annual appraisal systems and documentation to ensure the nurse continues to demonstrate themselves as a safe and competent critical care practitioner.

The Centre for Advancing Practice have not yet agreed on a process for registering or providing continued, or renewed accreditation (as of December 2022) for validated credentials (including for Acute Medicine). In the next few years, regulatory bodies may review whether Advanced Practice will come more directly under their remit as a regulated professional title. This may have implications for people that have followed credentialling programmes and wish to maintain this status. However, all of the above organisations already draw attention to the need for registered professionals to maintain and adhere to the requirements of their regulatory body.

In many large organisations (including at Integrated Care Board [ICB] level) there are opportunities being created for leadership in Advanced Practice. It may seem tempting to see working as an Advanced Clinical Practitioner as the ultimate destination. However, taking a lead AP role can allow you to continue to develop and influence others at a broader organisational, or community of practice level.

A fundamental feature of leadership is that you are supporting others to take their journey of development and hopefully make it a positive experience for them. This requires that you share your knowledge, skills, and experiences. Actively looking for ways in which to disseminate the work you are doing as an AP should therefore always be a part of your development plan.

Sharing your experience (e.g. through publication, presentation at conference or network meetings, and reporting at a higher organisational level) can significantly increase the impact that the work you do has across many different fields of practice. Through engaging with dissemination activities at a community of practice level, you will find this is paid back in kind through the connections and networks you make, which will help to sustain your development as an AP. As an example, the Centre for Advancing Practice runs an annual conference for sharing good practice, presenting your work, and learning how others are continuing with professional development and transition.

Take Home Points
- Professional development is a continuous process and should be addressed at a personal, team, and community level.
- There is significant diversity in Advanced Practice; bespoke, individualised plans for development are needed.
- As an AP, you need to be personally active in the process of development and identify and work effectively with those who can support you.

REFERENCES

Critical Care Networks. (2015). *National Competency Framework for Registered Nurses in Adult Critical Care, Step 3 Competencies.* Cited December 2022. Available from www.cc3n.org.uk/step-competency-framework.html [accessed 20 June 2023].

Dweck, C. (2022). *The Power of Believing that You Can Improve,* TED Talk [online]. Available from: https://www.ted.com/talks/carol_dweck_the_power_of_believing_that_you_can_improve?language=en [accessed 20 June 2023].

Faculty of Intensive Care Medicine (FICM). (2020). *Advanced Critical Care Practitioners CPD & Appraisal Pathway* [online]. Available from: https://www.ficm.ac.uk/sites/ficm/files/documents/2021-10/ACCP%20CPD%20Appraisal%20Pathway%20-%20Version%202.2%20-%20March%202020.docx.pdf [accessed 26 June 2023].

Health Education England. (2017). *Multi-professional Framework for Advanced Clinical Practice in England* [online]. Available from: https://www.hee.nhs.uk/sites/default/files/documents/multi-professionalframeworkforadvancedclinicalpracticeinengland.pdf [accessed 20 June 2023].

Health Education England. (2020). *Analysis of the Online Workshop to Consider the Impact of COVID-19 and the Implications for the Future of Advanced and Consultant Practice* [online]. Available from: https://www.hee.nhs.uk/our-work/advanced-practice/reports-publications/impact-covid-19-future-advanced-consultant-practice [accessed 20 June 2023].

Health Education England. (2022a). *Advanced Clinical Practice in Acute Medicine Curriculum Framework – Credentials* [online]. Available from: https://advanced-practice.hee.nhs.uk/our-work/credentials [accessed 20 June 2023].

Health Education England (HEE). (2022b). *Advanced Practice Workplace Supervision – Minimum Standards for Supervision* [online]. Available from: https://advanced-practice.hee.nhs.uk/resources-news-and-events/reports-and-publications [accessed 20 June 2023].

Health Education England (HEE). (2023) *ePortfolio (supported) Route* [online]. Available from: `https://advanced-practice.hee.nhs.uk/our-work/eportfolio-route` [accessed 26 June 2023].

Institute for Apprenticeships & Technical Education. (2018). *End Point Assessment Plan Integrated Degree Apprenticeship for Advanced Clinical Practitioner at Level 7* [online]. Available from: `https://www.instituteforapprenticeships.org/apprenticeship-standards/advanced-clinical-practitioner-integrated-degree-v1-0` [accessed 26 June 2023].

Montgomery, A., van der Doef, M., Panagopoulou, E., and Leiter, M.P. (2020). *Connecting Healthcare Worker Well-being, Patient Safety and Organisational Change – The Triple Challenge.* Springer.

National Health Service (NHS). (2023). *Healthcare Leadership Model* [online]. Available from: `https://www.leadershipacademy.nhs.uk/healthcare-leadership-model/` [accessed 26 June 2023].

Skills for Health. (2020). *Advanced Clinical Practice: Capabilities Framework When Working with People Who Have a Learning Disability and/or Autism* [online]. Available from: `www.skillsforhealth.org.uk/images/services/cstf/ACP%20in%20LDA%20Framework.pdf` [accessed 20 June 2023].

The Faculty of Intensive Care Medicine. (2018). *Curriculum for Training for Advanced Critical Care Practitioners – Syllabus. V1.1* [online]. Available from: `www.ficm.ac.uk/media/6896` [accessed 20 June 2023].

The Intensive Care Society, Critical Care Networks – National Nurse Leads & The National Outreach Forum. (2022). *Advanced Critical Care Outreach Competencies* [online]. Available from: `https://ics.ac.uk/asset/43B8C11B-4512-41D0-B97768FABA2C30B2` [accessed 20 June 2023].

The Royal College of Emergency Medicine. (2022). *Emergency Medicine Advanced Clinical Practitioner Curriculum 2022 (Adult)* [online]. Available from: `https://rcem.ac.uk/wp-content/uploads/2022/09/ACP_Curriculum_Adult_Final_060922.pdf` [accessed 20 June 2023].

Wenger, E. (2000). *Communities of Practice.* Learning, Meaning and Identity: Cambridge University Press.

UNIT 2

COMPLEX DECISION MAKING

CHAPTER 3

Ethics and Legal Principles

Nick Fox

Aim

The aim of this chapter is to understand the ethical and legal implications of advanced practice and the impact this has on decision making and professional judgement.

LEARNING OUTCOMES

After reading this chapter the reader will:

1. Understand the four main principles of healthcare and advanced practice ethics.
2. Understand the ethical and legal implications of consent.
3. Understand the legal and ethical implications of withholding or withdrawing treatment.
4. Understand the ethical and legal implications of patient safety.

SELF-ASSESSMENT QUESTIONS

1. What are the four principles of medical ethics?
2. Which components make up the four-box approach to clinical ethics?
3. What is the criteria for a notifiable safety incident?
4. Can you define duty of candour?

INTRODUCTION

Morality is a value system which differentiates actions, decisions, and intentions as either right or wrong. Morality is founded on the principles of fairness, respect, loyalty, care, and authority.

The Advanced Practitioner in Acute, Emergency and Critical Care, First Edition. Edited by Sadie Diamond-Fox, Barry Hill, Sonya Stone, Caroline McCrea, Natalie Gardner, and Angela Roberts.
© 2024 John Wiley & Sons Ltd. Published 2024 by John Wiley & Sons Ltd.

Ethics is a system of moral behaviours, beliefs, and values that affect how people make decisions, also known as moral philosophy.

Healthcare has consistently been presented with complex challenges, and part of the evolving skill set of advanced practice is not only to recognise and adapt to the challenges but also to manage and mitigate any potential harm that may occur. Developing ethical awareness enables advanced practitioners as individuals, and as a part of the wider organisation, to act as moral agents in order to provide safe, effective, and ethical care.

Multi-professional Framework (MPF) for Advanced Clinical Practice Guidance for Professional Development (Health Education England 2017)

This chapter maps to the following statements within the MPF:

2. Leadership and Management:	2.1	2.11

Accreditation Considerations

This chapter maps to the following statements within the following national accreditation documents:

Curriculum for Training for Advanced Critical Care Practitioners Syllabus V1.1
(The Faculty of Intensive Care Medicine 2018)

3.15	3.18	4.9	4.12

Advanced Critical Care Outreach Competencies
(The Intensive Care Society, Critical Care Networks – National Nurse Leads and The National Outreach Forum 2022)

C6

Emergency Medicine Advanced Clinical Practitioner Curriculum 2022 – Adult
(The Royal College of Emergency Medicine 2022)

- SLO 7: Deal with complex and challenging situations in the workplace
- SLO 10: Participate in research and managing data appropriately

Advanced Clinical Practice in Acute Medicine Curriculum Framework
(Health Education England 2022)

- Core Learning Outcome 2
- Core CiPs 2 & 5

Prior to the 1970s, healthcare ethics was principally concerned with maximising the benefits of medicine and minimising the risks of harm and disease. However, this was a paternalistic approach to ethics with the focus being on the healthcare professional rather than the patient. In 1976, Beauchamp and Childress, proposed a framework of four principles that has become the cornerstone of present day medical ethics:

- autonomy
- non-maleficence
- beneficence
- justice

Autonomy is the right of an individual to act in what they consider to be their best interest. In medicine, a key component of autonomy is the ability of the patient to make an informed choice about their care. Informed choice requires that the patient has access to information, which may be verbal or written, pertaining to the risks and benefits of proposed interventions and therapies. The patient must have the ability to understand these risks and benefits. However, there will be situations whereby the patient is unable to make an autonomous decision, such as when mental capacity is impaired or in emergency, life-threatening situations.

Non-maleficence is the duty not to inflict intentional harm or allow harm to be caused to the patient through neglect. However, all therapies and interventions involve some harm, even if minimal; for example, an x-ray will expose the patient to radiation. Therefore, the advanced practitioner must weigh the benefits against the burdens of proposed interventions and treatments to choose the best course of action.

Beneficence is the moral duty to promote a course of treatment and intervention that is in the best interests of the patient. However, as advanced practitioners it is important to ensure that the plan of care is proportionate to the medical problem and the expectations of the patient.

Justice is the moral obligation to distribute the benefits, risks, and costs fairly. The advanced practitioner has to consider whether a course of action is compatible with the rights of the patient and that the plan of care is fair, appropriate, and equitable. In essence, that patients in similar positions are treated in a similar manner.

Veracity or truth telling can be added to the four principles advocated by Beauchamp and Childress. Truth telling as a professional obligation has only achieved prominence in the last 25 years, as a result of improved treatment options and the changing focus on the rights of the patients most notably the duty of candour.

While the pinnacles of healthcare ethics provide key points to be considered when contemplating an ethical dilemma, it can be helpful to use a more focussed approach when managing this situation. One approach developed by Jonsen and Sieger, advocates a four-box model to frame the ethical decision-making process (see Table 3.1).

There are other clinical ethics models that can be used to rationalise a dilemma and support the decision-making process. However, each situation is unique and it is important to remember that one solution for a given situation may not necessarily be appropriate for another similar situation.

TABLE 3.1   The four-box approach to clinical ethics.

Medical indication	Patient preference
• Medical problem – acute, chronic, emergent • Goals of treatment • Treatment options and alternatives • Likely success of treatment	• Informed of risks • Understands benefits • Patient has decisional capacity • Preferences • Surrogates
Quality of life	**Contextual features**
• Baseline functionality • Current lifestyle and independence • Expected time of recovery • Possible deficits resulting from treatment	• Conflicts of interest • Personal interests • Financial incentives • Professional bias • Hospital pressures • Research conflicts

Source: Adapted from Jonsen et al. (2015).

PATIENT SAFETY, ETHICS AND ADVANCED CLINICAL PRACTICE

The challenge of the principle of non-maleficence in medical ethics is that healthcare organisations and professionals should ensure that the care they provide is safe. The preservation of patient safety is viewed as a key component of a high-quality healthcare system.

While we are all familiar with various patient safety guidelines and quality care standards, we are probably less familiar with the ethical and legal dimensions underpinning these documents and declarations.

Patient safety can be studied as a practical value, in the sense that the main focus is the positive outcomes and benefits. It can also be studied as a moral value by focussing on the protection and promotion of humanity and human dignity (Kadivar et al. 2017).

The ethical challenge of ensuring patient safety supports healthcare professionals in taking all practical steps to prevent errors and injuries to patients. Healthcare professional are required to respond appropriately when things go wrong and to find new methods to prevent recurrence and new ways of working. The requirement is for honesty, transparency, and openness in dealing with our patients when things go wrong and taking responsibility for ensuring that all our colleagues are safe and competent (Leape 2005).

Advanced clinical practice is a level of practice characterised by a high degree of autonomy and complex decision-making. This level of practice embodies the ability to manage clinical care in partnership with individuals, families, carers, and other healthcare professionals. It includes the analysis and synthesis of complex problems across a wide range of settings, enabling innovative solutions to enhance people's experience and improve outcomes.

The codes of conduct that guide our practice are essentially instructions to always consciously act with ethics as a core value of our lifelong practice. As independent advanced clinical practitioners, we are not only aware of our skills, competence, and abilities but also our limitations.

The development of advanced clinical practice is not just concerned with maximising the potential of healthcare professionals, but also the key component of patient safety. Patient safety has an ethical dimension which informs our practice and behaviours. The four pillars of the framework of advanced clinical practice have at their core, the provision of safe and ethical care:

1. Clinical practice
2. Leadership
3. Education
4. Research

CONSENT

Consent is a legal and ethical principle, and where possible, all patients should be involved in making informed decisions concerning their treatment and care. Communication between the advanced practitioner and patient is fundamental to good decision-making and patient safety. A key objective of advanced practice is to prevent harm and act as an advocate to the patient. The advanced practitioner has the duty to provide the patient with information at a level they can comprehend and to ensure that their questions are answered truthfully so that they can make an informed choice about their care.

TREATY OF OVIEDO ON HUMAN RIGHTS AND BIOMEDICINE

The legal principles of consent are enshrined in the Treaty of Oviedo (1997), more often referred to as the European Convention on Human Rights and Biomedicine (ETS No164). This treaty was implemented to preserve human dignity, rights, and freedoms through a series of principles in relation to the misuse of advances in medicine. Article 5 of this treaty states that, "An intervention in the health field may only be carried out after the person concerned has given free and informed consent."

In 2020, the General Medical Council (GMC) published guidance on decision-making and consent (see Table 3.2). This publication although primarily aimed at medical staff is pertinent to advanced practice professionals who are required to obtain consent as part of their role.

TABLE 3.2   Guidance on professional standards and ethics for doctors.

One	All patients have the right to be involved in decisions about their treatment and care and to be supported in making those decisions if they are able.
Two	Decision-making is an ongoing process focussed on meaningful dialogue: the exchange of relevant information specific to the individual patient.
Three	All patients have the right to be listened to, and to be given the information they need to make a decision, and the time and support they need to understand it.
Four	Healthcare professionals must find out what matters to patients so they can share relevant information about the benefits and harms of proposed options and reasonable alternatives, including the option to take no action.
Five	Healthcare professionals must start from the presumption that all patients have the capacity to make decisions about their treatment and care. A patient can only be judged to lack the capacity to make a specific decision at a specific time, and only after an assessment in line with legal requirements.
Six	The choice of treatment or care for patients who lack capacity must be of overall benefit to them, and decisions should be made in consultation with those close to them or acting as their legal advocate.
Seven	Patients whose right to consent is affected by law should be supported to be involved in the decision-making process, and to exercise choice where possible.

Source: Adapted from GMC (2020).

Consider this: an advanced nurse practitioner following assessment of a patient in a general ward environment is discussing with the patient and his close family whether admission to critical care would be in his best interests. The patient is made aware of what he can reasonably expect to happen to him on the critical care unit. When asked whether this is something he would consider, one of the family members states he wants to go to critical care. What are the issues in this scenario?

The advanced nurse practitioner has provided the patient with information on which the patient can make an informed choice. However, the family member has intervened to state that the patient should be admitted to the critical care unit. This is an emotive situation where the wishes of the family may or may not mirror the wishes of the patient. For consent to be valid, the patient should be able to act freely and without coercion.

A key component of consent is the capacity of the individual to understand and make an informed decision concerning their care. Where capacity may be impaired, the actions of the advanced practitioner are guided by five key principles of the mental Capacity Act:

- A presumption of capacity.
- The right to be supported when making decisions.
- An unwise decision cannot be viewed as a wrong decision.
- Best interests must be at the heart of all decision-making.
- Any intervention must be with the least restriction possible.

The duty of care of the advanced practitioner includes a duty to provide the patient with advice and sufficient information upon which to reach a rational decision, whether to accept or reject treatment (Brazier and Cave 2016). Failure to provide adequate information about a proposed intervention may be viewed as negligence.

In England and Wales, the Mental Capacity Act (2005) sets out the legal position relating to determination of capacity and the principles for treating adults who lack capacity. The Act is applicable to people to people aged 16 years and over and states that capacity should be assumed unless it is established that he or she lacks capacity. In Scotland, the Adults with Incapacity Act (2000) sets out the legal framework. There is no statutory legislation governing consent for children under the age of 16 years, but there is clear case law to guide practitioners. A further key piece of legislation in relation to consent to treatment is the Mental Health Act (2007) which provides the legal framework for treating adults without their consent in carefully specified circumstances of mental illness (United Kingdom Clinical Ethics Network).

There are also psychological aspects which may require consideration for informed consent. A patient may be emotionally overwhelmed by their current illness experience and by the complexity and implications of the situation that they now face. Patients who are emotionally overwhelmed may require additional support to ensure an autonomous decision has been reached. This may be achieved by extending the time frame of the decision-making process and by involving friends, family, and loved ones, though with the latter you would need to protect the patient from coercion.

With the emergence of new technologies, a patient's ability to provide informed consent may be overwhelmed by the complexity and volume of information involved in the decision. The capacity of the patient is limited due to the information itself. In this situation an extended time frame for the decision-making process and providing the information in small sections may be useful (Bester 2016).

WRITTEN CONSENT

Consent form 1 documents the patient's agreement to proceed with a proposed investigation or treatment. It is not a legal waiver however, and if the patient has received inadequate information on which to base their decision, then the consent may be invalid, even though the form has been signed.

Consent form 2 is specific to children and young persons. Everyone aged 16 or more is presumed to be competent to give consent for themselves unless the opposite can be demonstrated. However, a child under the age of 16 can legally give consent if they have sufficient understanding and intelligence to fully understand what is proposed. If children are not able to give consent for themselves, someone with parental responsibility may do so on their behalf. People with parental responsibility for a child include: the child's birth mother; the child's father if married to the mother at the child's conception, birth, or later; a legally appointed guardian; and the local authority if the child is on a care order.

Consent form 3 is designed for procedures and/or investigations where the patient is expected to remain alert throughout and an anaesthetist is not involved in their care.

Consent form 4 is specific to those adult patients who lack capacity to give informed consent for a procedure. The healthcare professional must ensure that:

- The patient is unable to retain or comprehend information pertinent to the decision, or
- The patient is unable to use this information in the decision-making process, or
- The patient is unconscious.

In the situation where the lack of capacity may be temporary, consideration should be given as to whether the planned procedure is time-critical and whether it can be delayed until the patient has regained capacity.

The responsibility for determining whether a procedure for an incapacitated patient is in their best interests lies with the health professional performing the procedure. However, it is best practice to consult with those close to the patient (spouse/partner/parents/carer/advocate) unless you have good reason to believe that the patient would not have wished particular individuals to be consulted or the urgency of the situation prevents this.

VERBAL (EXPLICIT) AND NON-VERBAL (IMPLIED OR IMPLICIT) CONSENT

Sometimes verbal consent might be referred to as 'explicit' consent, and non-verbal may be referred to as 'implied' or 'implicit' consent.

An example of non-verbal or implied consent would be where a person, after receiving appropriate information, holds out a hand so the blood pressure can be recorded. However, the person must have understood what intervention or treatment is intended, and why, for such consent to be valid.

An example of verbal or explicit consent would be where a health professional performs an arterial puncture for blood gas analysis and informs the patient what they want to do and asks them if they agree to such an examination. If the patient agrees then this is explicit consent (verbal consent).

BEST INTERESTS PRINCIPLE IN EMERGENCY SITUATIONS

An 'emergency exception' applies when a patient is unable to provide consent (cardiac arrest, traumatic brain injury, unconsciousness, delirium, etc.) and when intervention is deemed necessary to save life, prevent deterioration or preserve health, and prevent disability. The moral imperative of beneficence is central to the best interests principle, to do good and act in the best interests of the patient. The emergency exemption is based on consent implied in law, the presumption that a reasonable person would consent to an intervention to save life and preserve health if they were able to provide consent. The limitations to this principle are that the intervention must be the least restrictive to the patient's future choices. Consideration should be given to the time-critical nature of the situation. If the patient has the potential to regain capacity to give consent without undue detriment to the well-being of the patient the best interests principle should not be applied (EUSEM 2019). Best practice dictates that any intervention undertaken using the best interests principle should be documented in the patient record.

ELECTRONIC CONSENT (E-CONSENT)

Electronic consent has been advocated for patients who have agreed to participate in research or clinical trials. Using electronic consent offers a number of potential benefits, such as:

- improving understanding
- testing and reinforcing participant comprehension
- providing feedback on how consent materials could be improved
- improving patient recruitment process and reducing dropout rates
- enabling process efficiencies.

In all cases, staff should be aware of the different types of consent and the importance of ensuring that the person understands what is going to happen to them and what is involved. Staff should also be aware of and understand what to do if people refuse care or treatment or when consent is not valid or is no longer valid.

Advanced practice requires practitioners to maintain up to date knowledge on the ethical and legal frameworks for consent. As advanced practitioners, there will be reasonable expectations to practice as experts and act as a role model for junior nursing staff and medical staff (MHRA and HRA 2018).

Case Study – A Competent Patient Refuses Treatment

Mr. A is 45-years old and is in need chemotherapy following cancer surgery. He is refusing treatment because he is scared of the side effects of the treatment. He has been counselled about the nature of the treatment; there are no other options that would be of practical benefit. He is competent to make decisions regarding his treatment. He understands that if he refuses treatment, he will die. His treating clinician feels very strongly that he should receive chemotherapy as the potential outcome is very favourable, but despite numerous attempts to persuade Mr. A, he refuses.

Mr. A is competent and has the capacity to make decisions regarding his treatment. If respect for autonomy is given the highest value, then his refusal to undergo treatment should be respected despite the resulting harm.

It is important that Mr. A is making an informed decision; a decision made without full information and at a level he can understand is not autonomous. Could more be done to support him with the treatment decision? Could he have discussions with patients who have undergone the same treatment? However, we then need to consider issues of paternalism; excessive discussions trying to change the decision Mr. A has made may be construed as coercion, which goes against his autonomy to make an informed decision.

Therefore, his refusal must be respected. If through lack of treatment his condition deteriorates and he is no longer competent to make an informed choice, his previously expressed wishes should be respected.

DUTY OF CANDOUR

The duty of candour or truth-telling arose out of the inquiry led by Robert Francis QC into the breakdown of care at Mid Staffordshire NHS Foundation Trust. Following the publication of the Francis Report in 2013, care organisations now have a legal as well as ethical obligation to be open and honest with patients and their families when something goes wrong that appears to have caused or could lead to harm in the future. Professionals and organisations are expected to acknowledge errors and offer an apology when mistakes have occurred.

It is important to remember that an apology is not an admission of guilt. To fulfil the duty of candour, the patient is offered an apology for the harm caused, regardless of fault. In some cases, it is the lack of an apology which is the impetus to take legal action.

The NMC guidance on the duty of candour states that the healthcare professional must:

- inform the patient when something has gone wrong
- apologise to the patient
- offer an appropriate support to put things right
- explain to the patient the short- and long-term effects of what has happened.

Healthcare professionals must also be open and honest with their colleagues, employers, and not stop someone from raising concerns.

There are parallels with the duty of candour and consent. When something has gone wrong, it is easier to undertake a candid discussion when the risk and consent have formed part of the clinical relationship between patient and advanced practitioner (Department of Health 2014). Part of consent is informing the patient of the risks and gaining their agreement to accept these risks.

There are two elements to the duty of candour as stated by the Department of Health (2014), low-harm incidents or professional duty of candour (see Table 3.3) and notifiable safety incidents or statutory duty of candour (see Table 3.4).

Notifiable safety incidents must meet the following criteria:

- It must have been unintended or unexpected.
- It must have been during the provision of a regulated activity.
- In the reasonable opinion of a healthcare professional, the incident has or might result in death, or severe or moderate harm to the patient receiving care.

TABLE 3.3   Disclosure process for low-harm incidents (Professional Duty of Candour).

Step 1 Incident detection and assessment	• Detect safety incident • Where possible, act immediately to put things right for the patient and prevent harm • Make an assessment of the severity of harm and report the incident through local processes
Step 2 Notification and open disclosure	• Notify the patient about the incident as soon as possible with explanation of known facts • Offer an apology • Explain the short- and long-term effects of the incident • Offer an appropriate support to put things right • Explain the steps that will be taken to prevent recurrence of the incident • Record discussion in patient's clinical notes

Source: Adapted from Department of Health (2014).

TABLE 3.4   Building a culture of candour.

Step 1 Incident detection and initial response	• Detect safety incident • Where possible, act immediately to put things right for the patient and prevent harm • Assess severity of harm and report through the local processes • Acknowledge the incident to the patient with explanation of facts and offer an apology • Explain that you will follow up with more information and further investigation
Step 2 Team discussion	The multidisciplinary team (MDT) should meet a soon as possible after the incident • Get facts straight • Assess the severity of harm • Identify the investigations required and nominate a person to communicate with the patient • Identify options for patient support • Identify options for staff support
Step 3 Notification and open discussion	• Notify the patient about the incident as soon as possible with explanation of known facts • Offer an apology • Explain the short- and long-term effects of the incident • Provide explanation of investigation • Assure patient that outcome of investigation will be shared with them • Offer an appropriate support to put things right • Explain the steps that will be taken to prevent recurrence of the incident • Record discussion in patient's clinical notes
Step 4 Follow up	• Provide written notification with apology • Arrange a follow-up discussion with the patient

Source: Adapted from Department of Health (2014).

DISCLOSURE PROCESS FOR NOTIFIABLE SAFETY INCIDENTS (STATUTORY DUTY OF CANDOUR)

Underpinning the duty of candour is a learning behaviour so that errors or mistakes are not repeated. This out of necessity requires the patient to be supported so that they continue to have confidence in the care being offered to them.

On an organisational level, processes and policies should be in place so that any concerns the patient may have are dealt with in an effective, efficient, and compassionate manner. On a more individual level, the duty of candour encompasses accountability and learning from the incident.

Case Study – Duty of Candour

Mrs. B was an in-patient awaiting a cardiac procedure; she was duly consented for this procedure, and her anticoagulation was stopped two days prior to the procedure. Unfortunately, the planned procedure had to be postponed at short notice, and a further date for the procedure was planned in two weeks. During this time period, Mrs. B deteriorated; it was initially thought that she had developed a chest infection but there was no radiological evidence to support this diagnosis. Despite this, antibiotics were prescribed which had no effect and Mrs. B continued to deteriorate. Following a referral to an Advanced Nurse Practitioner it was identified that the anticoagulation therapy had not been restarted following postponement of the initial cardiac procedure. An ECG and D-dimer blood test supported a provisional diagnosis of a pulmonary embolism; this was confirmed by CT pulmonary angiogram and therapeutic anticoagulation was commenced. Mrs. B subsequently made a full recovery and underwent her cardiac procedure at a later date.

This omission was discussed with the patient in that the failure to restart her anticoagulation had contributed to her developing a small pulmonary embolism. The patient and relatives accepted the explanation and the verbal apology and declined a written apology. Notes were made of the incident, how it was managed and the content of the discussion with the patient. It was agreed by the clinical and managerial staff that this was an adverse incident, and in line with the Trust's policy an action plan was drawn up and shared to prevent the incident happening again.

WITHHOLDING AND WITHDRAWING TREATMENT

In April 1989, Anthony Bland was caught in a crowd stampede at Hillsborough during an FA cup semi-final. He suffered crush injuries and a severe anoxic brain injury leading to a persistent comatose state from which he would not recover. In 1992, the Hospital trust applied to the Court to lawfully withdraw life-sustaining treatment including hydration, nutrition, and ventilation by artificial means. Initially, this application was granted but subsequently was then appealed to the House of Lords by the solicitor appointed to act on Tony's behalf. He argued that the withdrawal of artificial life-sustaining treatment would inevitably lead to his death and would therefore constitute murder.

The House of Lords rejected the appeal, thereby permitting Tony's doctors to lawfully withdraw treatment. While omission of care when there is an imperative to act to save a patient may be regarded as unlawful, in this instance there was no such duty when continued treatment was not in the best interests of the patient and futile. Tony was the first patient in the UK to die from the withdrawal of artificial hydration and nutrition.

This very tragic case demonstrates the ethical and legal complexities of withholding and withdrawing treatments. More recent cases have seen these most challenging ethical and legal dilemmas ultimately resolved in the Law courts.

The issue of withholding and withdrawing treatment would appear to be at odds with the ethical principle of non-maleficence and the Hippocratic Oath. One of the guiding principles of the oath is *primum non nocere*, first do no harm. However, if commencing a treatment is likely to cause more harm than perceived benefit, should that treatment be offered? Or should we continue the treatment if it is of no benefit? Consent to proposed treatment and availing the patient with the relevant information is crucial to rational decision-making. Examples of this may be the patient who decides against further chemotherapy when they are terminally ill or the patient with advanced lung disease who has limitations on what interventions are offered when they are acutely ill.

The issue of withholding or withdrawing treatment is easier when the patient has the mental capacity to be involved in the decisions regarding his care. However, when the patient lacks the capacity to be engaged with decisions regarding his care the ethical and legal issues are challenging and significant. Decisions about commencing or withdrawing treatment should be based on considerations of the patient's rights and welfare, and therefore on the benefits and burdens of the treatment.

Many professionals and family members feel more comfortable and confident with the decisions to withhold treatment. Perhaps decisions to withdraw treatment are more challenging. Because it is an acknowledgement that the planned treatment has not had the desired outcome. However, Beauchamp and Childress (2013) argue that the distinction between withholding and withdrawing treatment is morally irrelevant. Treatment can always be permissibly withdrawn if it can be permissibly withheld.

Take Home Points
- Part of the role of the Advanced Care Practitioner is to manage difficult and complex situations to ensure delivery of safe and effective patient care, sometimes under challenging circumstances. How we respond to these situations can have a positive or negative effect; therefore adopting an ethical approach to support decision-making can be of great benefit.
- The codes of practice which govern our behaviours and practice are based on ethical principles of beneficence, non-maleficence, autonomy, justice, and veracity.
- The Advanced Practitioner needs to understand the four main principles of medical ethics and how these relate to advanced clinical practice.
- The Advanced Practitioner needs to understand the different types of consent and the ethical and legal implications of consent and the professional, legal, and ethical implications of the duty of candour.

REFERENCES

Beauchamp, T.L. and Childress, J.F. (2013). *Principles of Biomedical Ethics*, 7e. Oxford: Oxford University Press.

Bester, J. (2016, 2016). Limits of informed consent for an overwhelmed patient: clinician's role in protecting patients and preventing overwhelm. *AMA Journal of Ethics* 18 (9): 869–886.

Brazier, M. and Cave, E. (2016). *Medicine Patients and the Law*, 6e. Manchester: Manchester University Press.

Department of Health (2014). *Building a Culture of Candour*. London: Department of Health.

European Society of Emergency Medicine. (2019). *Ethics Committee Recommendations on Informed Consent for European Emergency Departments for Adults and Children* [online]. Available from: `https://eusem.org/images/Patient_Informed_Consent_in_the_ED-FINAL.pdf` [accessed 20 June 2023].

GMC (2020). *Guidance on Professional Standards and Ethics for Doctors – Decision Making and Consent*. General Medical Council.

Health Education England (HEE). (2022). *Advanced Clinical Practice in Acute Medicine Curriculum Framework – Credentials* [online]. Available from: `https://advanced-practice.hee.nhs.uk/our-work/credentials` [accessed 20 June 2023].

Health Education England (HEE). (2017). *Multi-professional Framework for Advanced Clinical Practice in England* [online]. Available from: `https://www.hee.nhs.uk/sites/default/files/documents/multi-professionalframeworkforadvancedclinicalpracticeinengland.pdf` [accessed 20 June 2023].

Jonsen, A.R., Sieger, M., and Winslade, W.J. (2015). *Clinical Ethics: A Practical Approach to Ethical Decisions in Clinical Medicine*, 8e. New York: McGraw-Hills.

Kadivar, M., Manookian, A., Asghari, A. et al. (2017, 2017). Ethical and legal aspects of patient safety: a clinical case report. *Journal of Medical Ethics & History of Medicine* 10: 15.

Leape, L. (2005). Ethical issues in patient safety. *Thoracic Surgery Clinics* 15 (4): 493–501.

MHRA & HRA (2018). *MHRA & HRA Joint Statement on Seeking and Documenting Consent Using Electronic Methods (EConsent)*. London: Health Research Authority, DoH.

The Faculty of Intensive Care Medicine. (2018). *Curriculum for Training for Advanced Critical Care Practitioners – Syllabus. V1.1* [online]. Available from: `www.ficm.ac.uk/media/6896` [accessed 20 June 2023].

The Intensive Care Society, Critical Care Networks – *National Nurse Leads and The National Outreach Forum*. (2022). *Advanced Critical Care Outreach Competencies* [online]. Available from: `https://ics.ac.uk/asset/43B8C11B-4512-41D0-B97768FABA2C30B2` [accessed 20 June 2023].

The Royal College of Emergency Medicine. (2022). *Emergency Medicine Advanced Clinical Practitioner Curriculum 2022 (Adult)* [online]. Available from: `https://rcem.ac.uk/wp-content/uploads/2022/09/ACP_Curriculum_Adult_Final_060922.pdf` [accessed 20 June 2023].

SUGGESTED READING

European Society for Emergency Medicine. *Ethics committee recommendations on informed consent for European emergency department (adults and children)* [online]. Available from: `www.eusem.org` [accessed 20 June 2023].

United Kingdom Clinical Ethics Network [online]. Available from: `www.ukcen.net` [accessed 20 June 2023].

NMC (updated 2022). *Openness and honesty when things go wrong: the professional duty of candour* [online]. Available from: `https://www.nmc.org.uk/globalassets/sitedocuments/nmc-publications/openness-and-honesty-professional-duty-of-candour.pdf` [accessed 20 June 2023].

Thompson J.J. (1985). The trolley problem. *Yale Law Journal*, 94(8), pp. 1395–1415.

CHAPTER 4

Communication Skills and Breaking Bad News

Phil Broadhurst and Emma Underdown

Aim

The aim of this chapter is to introduce the reader to the key concepts of communication and provide helpful structures for breaking bad news and interprofessional communication.

LEARNING OUTCOMES

After reading this chapter the reader will:

1. Understand verbal and non-verbal communication.
2. Be able to implement the use of communication tools in practice.
3. Have considered how poor communication can lead to a breakdown of trust.
4. Consider barriers to communication.

SELF-ASSESSMENT QUESTIONS

1. What are human factors and how can they create barriers to communication?
2. What are the steps of the SPIKES tool? How can they be used in practice?
3. What is patient-centred communication? Why does it matter?
4. What are the key considerations when communicating with children?

The Advanced Practitioner in Acute, Emergency and Critical Care, First Edition. Edited by Sadie Diamond-Fox, Barry Hill, Sonya Stone, Caroline McCrea, Natalie Gardner, and Angela Roberts.
© 2024 John Wiley & Sons Ltd. Published 2024 by John Wiley & Sons Ltd.

INTRODUCTION

Communication in the healthcare environment is crucial to ensuring effective outcomes, primarily for patients, and is also a key part of teamwork and productivity. Communication is the cornerstone of developing a therapeutic relationship with patients (Chichirez and Purcărea 2018). The ability to communicate with patients effectively fosters trust and mutual respect. The clinician is able to obtain an appropriate history, formulate an accurate plan of care, and importantly address the concerns of the patient. Effective communication often requires more than merely the dynamic between clinician and patient in order to succeed, including the views of others, such as family members or wider members of the multidisciplinary team playing key roles within the continuum of patients' health journeys. This chapter will seek to introduce strategies and key considerations to help advanced clinical practitioners (ACPs) communicate well at times when the situation can be difficult.

Multi-professional Framework (MPF) for Advanced Clinical Practice Guidance for Professional Development (HEE 2017)

This chapter maps to the following statements within the MPF:

1. Clinical Practice:	1.1	1.4	1.5	1.6	1.9	1.10
2. Leadership and Management:	2.1	2.2	2.6	2.8	2.10	
3. Education:	3.3					
4. Research:	4.7	4.8				

Accreditation Considerations

This chapter maps to the following statements within the following national accreditation documents:

Curriculum for Training for Advanced Critical Care Practitioners Syllabus V1.1
(The Faculty of Intensive Care Medicine 2018)

3.6	3.11	3.12	3.13	3.14	3.15	3.21	4.12

Advanced Critical Care Outreach Competencies
(The Intensive Care Society, Critical care Networks – National Nurse Leads and The National Outreach Forum 2022)

A1	B1

Emergency Medicine Advanced Clinical Practitioner Curriculum 2022 – Adult
(The Royal College of Emergency Medicine 2022)

- Domain 2: Professional skills (Communication and interpersonal skills)
- Key Capability (KC) 6

Advanced Clinical Practice in Acute Medicine Curriculum Framework
(Health Education England 2022)

- Core CiPs: 3
- Generic Clinical CiPs: 1, 2, 4, 6
- Specialty Clinical CiPs: 1, 4, 5

VERBAL AND NON-VERBAL COMMUNICATION

The words and phrases we use are key to mutual understanding in both our professional and personal encounters. As healthcare professionals, we need to consider our choice of vocabulary and how we present this. Although medical jargon is acceptable when conversing with colleagues, it may not be understood by patients and their families and we may need to consider using alternative language to explain their illness, needs, and treatments. The choice of words we use can also convey a subconscious message and we should consider how they could be interpreted. The result of our words should be to promote understanding and gather information, not to cause unnecessary harm or distress (Bennett 2016, Lloyd et al. 2018).

Good communication requires more than merely spoken words, however. Although the language we use is important, it is estimated that 80% of how we communicate is related to the non-verbal signalling of messages. For example, the way we stand, how we gesture, the use of eye contact, and a smile or frown can convey a powerful message that makes or breaks an encounter, and it is impossible to avoid non-verbal communication (Bhat and Kingsley 2020; Blanch-Hartigan et al. 2018; Duggan and Parrott 2001).

PATIENT-CENTRED COMMUNICATION

Research has shown that communication works best when patients believe that there is a sense of partnership and understanding of their individual needs (Deledda et al. 2012). As healthcare providers, the way we express partnership and empathy can speak louder than the plans we make (reflect on the way the paragraphs up to this point have been written – we are not telling you how to communicate or being impersonal; we are walking the journey together as partners). Within healthcare encounters, this is known as 'patient-centred communication'.

Patient-centred communication happens when the relationship between healthcare practitioners and patients is structured in such a way that empowers patients to feel that their needs, values, and preferences are at the heart of all decision-making (Lloyd et al. 2019). When done effectively, patient-centred communication enables 'shared decision-making', allowing the practitioner and patient to agree on a plan that is realistic and achievable for both. Shared decision-making requires another skill as well as the ability to impart information – it also requires active listening. There is a significant difference between hearing and listening to what the patient is saying; listening involves a conscious attention and the willingness to understand the meaning and emotions involved in the information being offered (Rifkin and Lazris 2014).

The conversations that happen within Acute, Emergency and Critical Care can understandably carry a high-emotional burden, both for patients and clinicians. Ensuring communication is patient-centred at these times, for example, when discussing end-of-life care or DNACPR decisions can help the patient feel respected, and that their wishes are being heard. Figure 4.1 outlines the way that a patient-centred model of communication can help patients and clinicians agree on the desired outcome for the patient's health journey during stressful circumstances, and can be easily applied to the concepts and models that will be introduced within this chapter (Dean and Street 2014).

'GOALS OF CARE' AND DIFFICULT CONVERSATIONS

Moving forward, recommendations from NHS England (2021) suggest the implementation of 'Goals of Care' conversations. Specifically, these conversations are suggested for implementation in Acute Medical and Surgical Units for patients who are at risk of dying within the next 12 months. The conversations

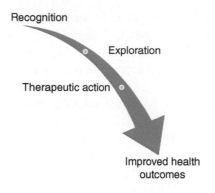

Source: Adapted from Dean and Street (2014).

FIGURE 4.1   Model of patient-centred communication. *Source*: Adapted from Dean and Street (2014).

TABLE 4.1   SPIKES communication framework.

S	Setting
P	Perception
I	Invitation or information
K	Knowledge
E	Empathy
S	Summarise or strategise

should be recorded in a care planning document and be focused on the values, priorities, goals, and treatment preferences of the patients. Over the coming years, there is a plan for widespread implementation of this model across different NHS settings but the key concepts of communication are applicable to other healthcare settings on a micro-scale already.

Breaking bad news, in particular, is a complex task within the field of communication (Kaplan 2010). There are multiple factors to be considered and in such cases the use of a model of communication can be useful. SPIKES (see Table 4.1) is a step-wise framework that allows the practitioner to demonstrate empathy and acknowledge the patient's and family's feelings. In addition, it allows for exploration of the patient's understanding (Kaplan 2010).

Following this step-wise approach to communication allows for appropriate settings to allow for open communication. Gauging the patient's and family's existing understanding of the situation will also give you the opportunity to establish appropriate language use – if the patient and family are using lay terminology, then you can make your communication appropriately. Invitation gives the opportunity to ask the patient and family how much information they would like. Knowledge gives the practitioner the opportunity to impart the relevant knowledge, using appropriate language as previously established. This knowledge should be provided with empathy and understanding. Following this, there is the opportunity to summarise the information provided into key points and advise the patient and carers of the next steps.

By using this tool, a clinician will have the opportunity to consider the information that needs to be relayed prior to the conversation taking place. In addition, thought must be given to strategy and plans going forward so that the patient and relatives understand the next steps.

Difficult conversations with patients are commonplace within the Acute, Emergency and Critical Care specialties. Following the COVID-19 pandemic, the CQC highlighted a number of concerns around DNACPR decisions and discussions. Within their recommendations following this, they have highlighted the importance of communicating such decisions in an accessible way that meets the needs of the patient (CQC 2022).

The General Medical Council (2022b) offers guidance on decision-making around attempting cardiopulmonary resuscitation (CPR). Within this guidance are suggestions for communication that include; considering patient wishes, with patient permission (where able), discussing this decision with relatives, and being clear to patients about the impacts and burden of CPR with a likely low level of success. Patients and their relatives/carers are often poorly informed or subject to unfounded assumptions about the impact of disability and quality of life following attempted CPR. Use of the SPIKES tool can give the clinician an understanding of the patient's and relatives' perceptions of CPR and allow the clinician to impart clear knowledge about the intervention and what the potential risks or benefits could be for that individual.

HUMAN FACTORS

It is not only the way in which one chooses to communicate that is important, however. As healthcare professionals, there are often multiple stresses and influences upon our practice at both technical and non-technical level, and the way a message can be conveyed or understood can be affected by the situation and environment in which we find ourselves. This is known as 'human factors' and, in turn, can create barriers to communication. It is estimated that each year in the NHS, there are 12 000 avoidable deaths and 24 000 serious incidents, and that by having an awareness of the role of human factors in healthcare, many of these could be avoided (Clinical Human Factors Group 2022). Human factors are concerned with the recognition and mitigation of errors through an understanding of human behaviour and its impact on teamwork, ability, workplace culture, and task management (NHSE 2013). Table 4.2 highlights some of the ways in which human factors can impact upon effective communication. Considerations such as societal differences, organisational culture, or sensory impairment can have significant impacts upon a person's ability to convey or receive information in a correct manner.

TABLE 4.2 Barriers to effective communication.

Sensory	Societal	Emotional	Organisational
Hearing	Age	Stress	Time
Sight	Gender	Worry	Hierarchy
Drugs	Culture	Anger	Stress
Noise	Language	Trust	Jargon
Light/darkness	Education	Pain	Handwriting

Source: Adapted from GMCCSI (2020).

Learning Event 1

Mrs. Smith is in the Intensive Care Unit (ICU). She is severely unwell with multi-organ failure following complications of chemotherapy for Non-Hodgkin's Lymphoma. Her family is asked to come in by the Intensive Care team for a discussion about the possible need to withdraw treatment. The ICU team had liaised prior to the family's arrival and concluded that Mrs. Smith was not making meaningful recovery and that despite maximum therapy, was continuing to deteriorate. As a result, the decision had been made that there would be withdrawal of treatment.

The ICU team held the discussion with the family in a separate room away from the patient's bedside. Mrs. Smith was unable to participate in the discussions due to being intubated and sedated. The family was informed of the decision to withdraw care due to the futility of treatment.

The family was fully understanding and appreciated that Mrs. Smith was not recovering and wished for her to have a peaceful death. Unfortunately, on returning to Mrs. Smith's room with the family, the Haematology team who were her primary team were there to see Mrs. Smith.

Unaware of the discussion with the family, they proceeded to inform Mrs. Smith's family that this particular cancer had a high rate of survival and that they were hopeful for the cancer to be treated with the right treatment regimen. The family was very upset and confused having expected Mrs. Smith to die, which she later did. This situation caused unnecessary trauma for the family.

What Went Wrong?

Lack of communication between the primary care team and the ICU team meant that there were two separate goals of therapy in place.

The family were given bad news and then provided with different information suggesting that she could make a recovery.

The haematology team considered the ability to cure the cancer but had not applied that to the patient, who was now in multi-organ failure.

The conversation with the haematology team occurred at the patient's bedside, this did not allow the family the chance to process this information effectively and raise any questions.

How Was This Resolved?

Later that day, the family had a further conversation with the ICU and haematology team after a multidisciplinary discussion where an agreement to withdraw treatment was reached.

The conversation took place in a private room allowing the family to ask questions about why Mrs. Smith could not survive this episode of care. They were later accepting of this decision.

What Can Be Learned From This?

Multidisciplinary discussion prior to breaking bad news is essential to avoid confusion for relatives.

Despite the suspected curability of disease, all assessments of this should be made on an individual basis according to the clinical condition of the patient. A holistic approach to recovery considers all aspects of a patient's meaningful recovery.

Conversations should take place in the appropriate environment, and the use of the SPIKES tool for communication could have established prior understanding from the family, thus avoiding any potential confusion or additional trauma.

Learning Event 2

Mr. West is transferred from the Emergency Department to the Intensive Care Unit after collapsing suddenly outside his place of work. His CT head showed a large intra-cerebral haemorrhage with mid-line shift and cerebral oedema. He is transferred to the ICU for intubation and ventilation for supportive care and consideration for organ donation, dependent upon wishes of patient and family. On arrival to the ICU, the family approach the nursing staff and request Mr. West's death certificate. The ICU staff are confused and make steps to clarify the family's understanding.

They were taken to a separate room by the ICU consultant and a member of the nursing team and asked to explain what their understanding was of Mr. West's condition. The family explained that they had been told that Mr. West was brain-stem dead and that this meant he was clinically dead and would not recover.

Review of the Emergency Department notes showed that the family was told that Mr. West had suffered a severe bleed on the brain and that he was likely brain-stem dead. The family explained that they had since researched this online and concluded that Mr. West had died.

What Went Wrong?

The family was misinformed by the Emergency Department team as they were given information based on an assumption that Mr. West's intra-cerebral haemorrhage had caused brain-stem death.

The family had used this information to deduce Mr. West's condition online.

Incorrect terminology was used. By saying the term 'brain-stem death' the family were incorrectly led to believe that their relative was legally dead.

Lack of communication between the Emergency Department and ICU meant that there was a lack of understanding around the onward plan of care for Mr. West.

How Was This Resolved?

Mr. West was reviewed in the ICU and his images and clinical condition was relayed to a local neuro-surgical centre. He was accepted for transfer of care the following morning. Following a decompressive craniectomy, he made a full recovery.

A discussion was undertaken with Mr. West's family to discover their understanding of events so far. Based upon this, the ICU Consultant was able to explain Mr. West's clinical condition and ongoing plan for care. It was explained that a diagnosis of brain-stem death must be made based on a rigorous and legally regulated process that can only occur a minimum of 24 hours after admission to the hospital.

The family was shocked but relieved to learn that Mr. West was not clinically dead and that there were options for ongoing care.

What Can Be Learned From This?

Terminology is very important. The public have access to further information and if incorrect terms are used, then they have access to potentially incorrect information.

Clear handover and communication between multidisciplinary teams are necessary to avoid confusion.

Asking relatives to relay their understanding (as per the SPIKES protocol) allows for the clinician to clarify or correct their understanding. In this way, it manages expectations for the family.

Case Study

You are working in Medical SDEC. Mr. Jones has attended for a follow up appointment. He was recently seen with acute onset shortness of breath and found to have a large unilateral pleural effusion. He had a pleural aspiration which showed this was a malignant effusion and a follow up HRCT Chest has demonstrated a new diagnosis of primary lung malignancy.

You are tasked with breaking the news to Mr. Jones who has attended with his wife.

Consider how you would break the bad news to Mr. Jones – you may wish to use the SPIKES framework to assist with this.

Consider:

- What considerations are needed with regards to the environment in which you break bad news?
- What questions can you use to gauge Mr. Jones' understanding of his investigations and treatment so far?
- What sort of language will you need to use in order to break bad news to the patient? Consider patient background and baseline understanding that they have offered you.
- How can you support Mr. Jones and his wife with their emotional response to breaking bad news?
- What plan is in place for Mr. Jones going forward? Are you able to advise him on the next steps in care planning and management?

CONSIDERATIONS FOR PAEDIATRIC AND YOUNG PERSONS POPULATIONS

Evidence has shown that there is a direct link between improved outcomes for patients when communication between patients, families, and clinicians is of a high quality. Furthermore, parents' experiences of communication can make all the difference in the level of satisfaction they experience when their child is critically unwell and it should aim to be informational and relational in nature, as well as nurture parental coping (Carnevale et al. 2016).

Given the complexity of communication where information is not always being given directly to the primary user of care services, and the involvement of family members in developing the care plan for their child, it is understandable that communication in paediatrics has many reported barriers, including clinicians feeling uncomfortable, lack of understanding, or a sense of guilt from family members, limited availability of time, strong emotional responses, and different priorities (Sisk et al. 2021).

Importantly, family members often desire to be involved in the decision-making processes for their loved ones with varying levels of control, particularly in circumstances where end-of-life care may become required (Johnson et al. 2011). Clinicians should manage this process with care, as often relatives' views can be misrepresented as the patient's own preferences, especially in conversations surrounding end-of-life and resuscitation, with the stress created by the situation guiding them towards any hope that recovery may happen, regardless of how futile (Arnold and Kellum 2003; Marks and Arkes 2008). Indeed, it is important for clinicians to be aware that often a patient's understanding of health stems from the experiences of those closest to them, who will often also be coping with stress (Bor et al. 2019).

Communication with the child themselves should also be a key concern for healthcare professionals. Clinicians should seek to be aware of their non-verbal language, listen carefully to the child, and gain trust through learning about their life and interests. This can help build a positive relationship with the patient (Desai and Pandya 2013). With younger children, it may be easier for them to use play to describe

1. Involve children and young people in discussions about their care.
2. Be honest and open with them and their parents, whilst respecting confidentiality.
3. Listen to and respect their views about their health, and respond to their concerns and preferences.
4. Explain things using language or other forms of communication they can understand.
5. Consider how you and they use non-verbal communication, and the surroundings in which you meet them.
6. Give them opportunities to ask questions, and answer these honestly and to the best of your ability.
7. Do all you can to make open and truthful discussion possible, taking into account that this can be helped or hindered by the involvement of parents or other people.
8. Give them the same time and respect you would give to adult patients.

FIGURE 4.2   GMC considerations for communicating with children. *Source*: GMC (2022a) / General Medical Council.

and understand about their health needs, such as using a teddy to point out anatomy or act as a medium to talk to, while with older children allowing them to express their views and preferences for their healthcare using simple, jargon-free language is helpful (Eleftheriadou et al. 2019).

The GMC has published guidance for communicating with children about their health (see Figure 4.2), which can help clinicians consider how best to structure these conversations in an open and non-threatening way (GMC 2022a).

MENTAL HEALTH CONSIDERATIONS

Within Acute, Emergency and Critical Care, there are many scenarios in which the ACP may need to consider their communication skills. Two examples of these include communicating with those who may not have the capacity to retain information, such as those with dementia, and people who are experiencing acute mental health crises. Within mental health care, the principles of person-centred and non-judgemental care remain crucial, and the way one communicates should reflect this in order to gain trust, build relationships and work towards mutually agreed outcomes for the benefit of patients. Advanced Clinical Practitioners should also be aware of physiological and developmental differences that can directly impact speech, language, and expression within the patient population, specifically in the domain of older people's mental health.

Within the acute setting, it is not unusual to encounter people with acute mental health crises. Often, acute care practitioners, rather than those specialising in mental health, can be the first contact for patients upon their presentation to the hospital, especially if this has led to a physical health issue arising from self-harm or overdoses. Current NICE guidelines (NICE 2021) call for patients who present to the emergency department following self-harm to be treated with compassion, respect, and dignity, and that assessment should cover more than merely physical health, assessing mental state and risk of suicide. Evidence has shown that patients often feel Emergency Department (ED) triage is a punitive measure, and therefore steps should be taken to ensure open communication with appropriate non-verbal language. 'We can talk' is a free online resource aimed at supporting acute care staff to think about the communication strategies used to support young people who present to hospital in crisis (see 'Further Reading').

CONSIDERATIONS FOR PERSONS WITH LEARNING DISABILITIES

Many people with learning difficulties face challenges with communication, through impaired processing skills, difficulties with expression, hearing difficulties, or being non-verbal. Evidence has shown that people with learning difficulties often experience discrimination in accessing healthcare due to poor communication and not knowing what to expect (Iacono et al. 2014).

When communicating with a person with learning difficulties, it can often be helpful to reflect on the setting and tools used. Holding a discussion in a quiet place where you will be undisturbed can help the patient feel comfortable. Ensure that your spoken language is slow, clear, and free from jargon while watching the body language of the other person to gain cues to how they may be feeling and clarify that they have understood the information they have been given (Mencap 2008).

Within UK healthcare practice, it is important that assessments are made around a person's mental capacity, with the clinician making an assessment of their wishes and ability to participate in shared decision-making. This can only be achieved through appropriate communication and ensuring that any reasonable adjustments have been accounted for (Noble 2019). It should also be noted that the default position is that all patients have the capacity to make a decision unless patients have clearly demonstrated, through assessment, that they are unable to understand or retain the information required to make a decision, and that they have the right to make what clinicians deem to be an 'unwise' decision and that this does not constitute a lack of mental capacity (NHS 2021). Reasonable adjustments to enable effective communication include ensuring access to written information, translation into sign language or Makaton, involving carers or other people known and trusted by the patient, ensuring extra time is available for the consultation, or being aware of any health passport the person may have to provide extra information to empower practitioners to communicate effectively (GMC 2022c).

Take Home Points
- Patient-centred communication is the process of partnering with one's patients to explore their needs and mutually agree on outcomes and priorities.
- Use of communication frameworks such as SPIKES can assist clinicians to guide their conversations and empower patients and their families to understand when bad news needs to be explained.
- Human factors is the way in which the environment, and cultural and social issues can affect communication, and clinicians should consider what barriers may exist to good communication.

REFERENCES

Arnold, R.M. and Kellum, J. (2003). Moral justifications for surrogate decision making in the intensive care unit: implications and limitations. *Critical Care Medicine* 31 (5) supplement: S347–S353.

Bennett, K.L. (2016). Use your words: healing communication with children and teens in healthcare settings. *Pediatric Nursing* 42 (4): 204–205.

Bhat, B.V. and Kingsley, M.K. (2020). Effective non-verbal communication. In: *Effective Medical Education: The A, B, C, D, E of it* (ed. S.C. Parija and B.V. Adkoli). Singapore: Springer.

Blanch-Hartigan, D., Ruben, M.A., Hall, J.A., and Schmid Mast, M. (2018). Measuring nonverbal behaviour in clinical interactions: a pragmatic guide. *Patient Education and Counselling* 101 (12): 2209–2218.

Bor, R., Lloyd, M., and Noble, L. (2019). Communication with a patient's family. In: *Clinical Communication Skills for Medicine*, 4e (ed. M. Lloyd, R. Bor, and L. Noble). Edinburgh: Elsevier.

Carnevale, F.A., Farrell, C., Cremer, R. et al. (2016). Communication in pediatric critical care: a proposal for an evidence-informed framework. *Journal of Child Health Care* 20 (1): 27–36.

CHFG. (2022). *Clinical Human Factors Group* [online]. Available from: https://www.chfg.org/ [accessed 20 June 2023].

Chichirez, C.M. and Purcărea, V.L. (2018). Interpersonal communication in healthcare. *Journal of Medicine and Life* 11 (2): 119–122.

CQC. (2022). *GP Mythbuster 105: Do Not Attempt Cardiopulmonary Resuscitation (DNACPR)* [online]. Available from: www.cqc.org.uk/guidance-providers/gps/gp-mythbuster-105-do-not-attempt-cardiopulmonary-resuscitation-dnacpr [accessed 20 June 2023].

Dean, M. and Street, R.L. (2014). A 3-stage model of patient-centred communication for addressing cancer patients' emotional stress. *Patient Education and Counseling* 94 (2): 143–148.

Deledda, G., Moretti, F., Rimondini, M., and Wimmermann, C. (2012). How patients want their doctor to communicate. A literature review on primary care patients' perspective. *Patient Education and Couselling* 90 (3): 297–306.

Desai, P.P. and Pandya, S.V. (2013). Communicating with children in healthcare settings. *Indian Journal of Paediatrics* 80 (12): 1028–1033.

Duggan, P. and Parrott, L. (2001). Physicians' nonverbal rapport building and patients' talk about the subjective component of illness. *Human Communications Research* 27 (2): 299–311.

Eleftheriadou, Z., Noble, L., and Bor, R. (2019). Communicating with children and young people. In: *Clinical Communication Skills for Medicine*, 4e (ed. M. Lloyd, R. Bor, and L. Noble). Edinburgh: Elsevier.

GMC. (2022a). *0-18 years: Guidance for All Doctors* [online]. *Communication*. Available from: gmc-uk.org [accessed 20 June 2023].

GMC. (2022b). *Cardiopulmonary Resuscitation (CPR)* [online]. Available from: https://www.gmc-uk.org/ethical-guidance/ethical-guidance-for-doctors/treatment-and-care-towards-the-end-of-life/cardiopulmonary-resuscitation-cpr [accessed 20 June 2023].

GMC. (2022c). *Learning Disabilities* [online]. Available from: https://www.gmc-uk.org/ethical-guidance/ethical-hub/learning-disabilities#Communication [accessed 20 June 2023].

Greater Manchester Critical Care Skills Institute (GMCCSI). (2020). *Acute Illness Management (Version 6)* [online]. Available from: Critical Care Skills Institute - MFT ODN (gmccmt.org.uk) [accessed 20 June 2023].

Health Education England (HEE). (2017). *Multi-professional Framework for Advanced Clinical Practice in England* [online]. Available from: https://www.hee.nhs.uk/sites/default/files/documents/multi-professionalframeworkforadvancedclinicalpracticeinengland.pdf [accessed 20 June 2023].

Health Education England (HEE). (2022). *Advanced Clinical Practice in Acute Medicine Curriculum Framework – Credentials* [online]. Available from: https://advanced-practice.hee.nhs.uk/our-work/credentials [accessed 20 June 2023].

Iacono, T., Bigby, C., Unsworth, C. et al. (2014). A systematic review of hospital experiences of people with intellectual disability. *BMC Health Services Research* 14 (1): 505–512.

Johnson, S.K., Bautista, C.A., Hong, S.Y. et al. (2011). An empirical study of surrogates' preferred level of control over value-laden life support decisions in intensive care units. *American Journal of Respiratory and Critical Care Medicine* 183 (7): 915–921.

Kaplan, M. (2010). SPIKES: a framework for breaking bad news to patients with cancer. *Clinical Journal of Oncology Nursing* 14 (4): 514–516.

Lloyd, C.E., Wilson, A., Holt, R.I.G. et al. on behalf of the Language Matters Group(2018). Language matters: a UK perspective. *Diabetic Medicine* 35 (12): 1635–1641.

Lloyd, M., Bor, R., and Noble, L. (2019). Core skills in clinical communication. In: *Clinical Communication Skills for Medicine*, 4e (ed. M. Lloyd, R. Bor, and L. Noble). Amsterdam: Elsevier.

Marks, M.A.Z. and Arkes, H.R. (2008). Patient and surrogate disagreement in end-of-life decisions: can surrogates accurately predict patients preferences? *Medical Decision Making* 28 (4): 524–531.

Mencap. (2008). *Communicating with People with a Learning Difficulty* [online]. Available from: www.mencap.org.uk/sites/default/files/2016-12/Communicating%20with%20people_updated%20%281%29.pdf [accessed 20 June 2023].

NHS. (2021). *Mental Capacity Act* [online]. Available from: https://www.nhs.uk/conditions/social-care-and-support-guide/making-decisions-for-someone-else/mental-capacity-act [accessed 20 June 2023].

NHS England (2013). *Human Factors in Healthcare. A Concordat from the National Quality Board* [online]. Available from: https://www.england.nhs.uk/wp-content/uploads/2013/11/nqb-hum-fact-concord.pdf [accessed 20 June 2023].

NHS England. (2021). *Improving Communication Between Health Care Professionals and Patients in the NHS in England – Findings of a Systematic Evidence Review and Recommendations for an Action Plan* [online]. Available from: https://www.england.nhs.uk/wp-content/uploads/2021/07/SQW-NHS-England-Improving-communications-report-30June.pdf [accessed 20 June 2023].

NICE (2021). *An A&E Self-Harm Follow Up by Compassionate Care Call (Pilot)* [online]. Available from: www.nice.org.uk/sharedlearning/an-a-e-self-harm-follow-up-by-compassionate-care-call-pilot [accessed 20 June 2023].

Noble, L. (2019). Diversity in communication – clinical communication skills for medicine. In: *Clinical Communication Skills for Medicine*, 4e (ed. M. Lloyd, R. Bor, and L. Noble). Amsterdam: Elsevier.

Rifkin, E. and Lazris, A. (2014). Shared decision making. In: *Interpreting Health Benefits and Risks, A Practical Guide to Facilitate Doctor–Patient Communication*. Cham: Springer.

Sisk, B.A., Friedrich, A.B., Kaye, E.C. et al. (2021). Multilevel barriers to communication in pediatric oncology: clinicians' perspectives. *Cancer* 127 (12): 2130–2138.

The Faculty of Intensive Care Medicine. (2018). *Curriculum for Training for Advanced Critical Care Practitioners – Syllabus. V1.1* [online]. Available from: www.ficm.ac.uk/media/6896 [accessed 20 June 2023].

The Intensive Care Society, Critical Care Networks – *National Nurse Leads and The National Outreach Forum*. (2022). *Advanced Critical Care Outreach Competencies* [online]. Available from: https://ics.ac.uk/asset/43B8C11B-4512-41D0-B97768FABA2C30B2 [accessed 20 June 2023].

The Royal College of Emergency Medicine. (2022). *Emergency Medicine Advanced Clinical Practitioner Curriculum 2022 (Adult)* [online]. Available from: https://rcem.ac.uk/wp-content/uploads/2022/09/ACP_Curriculum_Adult_Final_060922.pdf [accessed 20 June 2023].

FURTHER READING

National LGBT Health Education Center. (2016). *Providing Inclusive Services and Care for LGBT People. A Guide for Healthcare Staff* [online]. Available from: https://www.lgbtqiahealtheducation.org/wp-content/uploads/Providing-Inclusive-Services-and-Care-for-LGBT-People.pdf [accessed 20 June 2023].

We Can Talk [online]. *We Can Talk* [online]. Available from: http://www.wecantalk.online [accessed 20 June 2023].

CHAPTER 5

Advanced Clinical Decision-making and End-of-life Care

Rachel Allen-Ashcroft and Victoria Metaxa

Aim
The aim of this chapter is to critically develop the individual's knowledge and understanding of the multifaceted aspects of complex decision-making, to evaluate and critically reflect upon the legal, ethical, clinical, and holistic needs of individuals around end-of-life care.

LEARNING OUTCOMES

After reading this chapter the reader will:

1. Familiarise themselves with pertinent existing literature around complex decision-making, ethical reasoning, and end-of-life care.
2. Gain understanding of the intrinsic and extrinsic factors that influence advanced decision-making, including the use of decision-making tools.
3. Acquire practical skills on effective communication around end of life, putting the whole individual in the centre of advanced decision-making.
4. Navigate through landmark ethical principles, the relevant law, professional standards, and national guidelines to deliver patient-centred care around the end of life.
5. Develop and enhance skills of clinical reasoning, communication, and awareness of decision-making frameworks to enhance shared decision-making for individuals.

The Advanced Practitioner in Acute, Emergency and Critical Care, First Edition. Edited by Sadie Diamond-Fox, Barry Hill, Sonya Stone, Caroline McCrea, Natalie Gardner, and Angela Roberts.
© 2024 John Wiley & Sons Ltd. Published 2024 by John Wiley & Sons Ltd.

SELF-ASSESSMENT QUESTIONS

1. Medical knowledge and clinical experience obtained through the years are all that is needed enough to make the right clinical decisions. (true/<u>false</u>)
2. Being aware of one's own limitations (biases) and extrinsic factors that may influence decision-making (experiences, mood, emotions) ensure that the correct clinical decision will always be made. (true/<u>false</u>)
3. Dominating a family end-of-life conversation by talking most of the time ensures that the family understands all the information and thus is more satisfied. (true/<u>false</u>)
4. Inviting palliative care specialists or initiating palliative care interventions in high-risk dying patients shortens their lives and fills them with despair. (true/<u>false</u>)

INTRODUCTION

Advanced clinical decision-making and end-of-life care (EOLC) is complex whereby advanced decisions can only be made by the clinician within the parameters of their knowledge, competence, experience, and by engaging in deliberate practice (purposeful and systematic practice with appropriate supervision and feedback) in order to gain proficiency and develop skill acquisition (Ericsson et al. 1993). Clinicians are required to have a conscious awareness of the many ambient variables which may influence advanced decision-making and impact EOLC. Within this chapter, we will focus upon the key concepts and theories which underpin decision-making and highlight how frameworks and shared decision-making are central to these processes.

Multi-professional Framework for Advanced Clinical Practice (HEE 2017)

This chapter maps to the following statements within the MPF:

1. Clinical Practice:	1.1	1.2	1.3	1.4	1.5	1.6	1.7	1.8	1.9	1.10	1.11
2. Leadership and Management:	2.1	2.2	2.3	2.4	2.10	2.11					
3. Education:	3.1	3.2	3.5								
4. Research:	4.3	4.7									

Accreditation Considerations

This chapter maps to the following statements within the following national accreditation documents:

Curriculum for Training for Advanced Critical Care Practitioners Syllabus V1.1
(The Faculty of Intensive Care Medicine 2018)

2.6	2.9	3.1	3.2	3.3	3.4	3.5	3.6	3.7	3.8	3.10	3.11	3.12	3.13	3.15	3.17	3.19	4.7	

Advanced Critical Care Outreach Competencies
(The Intensive Care Society, Critical care Networks – National Nurse Leads and The National Outreach Forum 2022)

A1	A5	C1

Emergency Medicine Advanced Clinical Practitioner Curriculum 2022 – Adult (The Royal College of Emergency Medicine 2022)																	
CC1	CC2	CC3	CC5	CC6	CC7	CC9	CC11	CC12	CC13	CC17	CC18	CC21	CC24	CC1	CC2	CC3	CC5

Advanced Clinical Practice in Acute Medicine Curriculum Framework (Health Education England 2022)
• Generic CiPs: 6

ADVANCED DECISION-MAKING

Advanced decisions and developing deliberate practice are essential components to achieving expert professional practice status (Ericsson et al. 1993; Cooper and Frain 2017). The novice clinician may be unaware of what they don't yet know ('unknown unknowns'), therefore limiting their ability to consider all possibilities. As they gain more experience, through self-regulated learning and feedback from experts, they develop their clinical reasoning and become able to generate options, hypotheses, and decisions within their scope of practice. Clinical reasoning is described as 'skill, process, or outcome wherein clinicians observe, collect, and interpret data to diagnose and treat patients' (Daniel et al. 2019). It is an integral part of advanced decision-making in general and EOLC more specifically. The key factors and components in complex decision-making include information gathering, hypothesis generation, the formulation of a working diagnosis and differential diagnoses, and lastly, a final diagnosis (see Table 5.1).

Additional factors that influence effective decision-making include (Croskerry 2018):

- demographic profile of the clinician (e.g. culture, age, ethnicity, religion)
- thinking styles (lateral thinking, rationality, critical thinking, reflection, adaptiveness)
- cognitive load (sleep deprivation, stress, information overload, external distractions, environmental pressures)
- system factors (information technology, resources, nurse:patient ratio)
- presenting medical condition (signs, symptoms, comorbidities, potential associated stigma)
- patient/surrogates (presence of family, friends, advance directive).

The above factors are more pertinent in end-of-life decision-making, where ethical dilemmas can be approached in four steps (Harvey and Gardiner 2019):

1. Establish the facts of the decision in question
2. Decide what is in scope and out of scope
3. Specify the outcomes within the four principles of bioethics (Beauchamp 2003)
4. Balance the principles to give them action-guiding capacity.

TABLE 5.1   Key factors and components of clinical reasoning and complex decision making (Cooper and Frain 2017; Daniel et al. 2019; Diamond-Fox and Bone 2021; Kahneman 2017; Kohn 2014; Pellegrino 1979; Rees et al. 2020).

Components	Definition	Additional considerations/ theoretical applications
Information gathering	The process of gathering information to create or refine a hypothesis through active cognitive processes, focused physical examination, holistic history from all available sources, request of relevant investigations	Ensure an accurate and complete history is obtained. Relevant investigations are requested within the relevant clinical context
Hypothesis generation	A non-analytic and analytic process (fast and slow system), which the clinician uses for clinical reasoning. It can also include heuristics (shortcuts), hypothesis generation and use of an iterative process to make associations between existing knowledge and the presenting case	System 1 (thinking fast) • Pattern recognition • Intuition and heuristics • Highly influenced by context • Low scientific rigour • Driven by emotion. System 2 (thinking slow) • Based on hypothesis/deduction • Analytical considerations • High scientific rigour • Less influenced by emotion
Hypothesis modification	Consideration of all appropriate elements of the presenting case, enabling the clinician to refine the probabilities and re-think their initial hypothesis/diagnosis in a process of hypothesis modification	This process involves information processing and accessing stored knowledge; uses probability and causal reasoning; investigates and tests theories. The thinking process should be explicit and consider the potential for bias
Differential diagnosis	A list of diagnostic hypotheses, formed by the processes listed above, which require lateral thinking and overcoming fixation bias	This process depends on knowledge of the medical condition and previous experiences
Leading or working diagnosis	The working diagnosis is taken forward to be further refined by requesting specialist input and considering intrinsic and extrinsic factors that may influence the reasoning. An action/intervention/ treatment will be initiated in this stage, even if the clinician is not totally confident in their decision	Experts draw upon specific knowledge and experience to reach the final decision. Novices are in the process of developing these skills, hence tend to look at wider possibilities.

Harvey and Gardiner (2019) suggest the MORAL Balance mnemonic to assist decision-making:

- **M.** make sure of the facts, establish decisions, what is the certainty?
- **ORA**: what are the outcomes of relevance to the agents involved?
- **L**: populate and then level out the arguments (the four principles of medical ethics can be applied),
- **Balance**: the balancing box, identify key facts, what are the greatest conflicts? What are the agreements?

ADVANCED DECISION-MAKING IN COMPLEX ENVIRONMENTS

Making advanced decisions in complex environments, such as the emergency department or ICU cannot be based on evidence alone; the individuals' choices and values should be explored and respected (Sackett et al. 1996). In the present era of great technological achievements, embarking on a plethora of investigations and interventions is common, thus deciding 'what among the many things that can be done, ought to be done' is of utmost importance (Pellegrino 1979). Making decisions in such highly emotive and pressurised situations, is often 'being tyrannised by evidence and data' (Sackett et al. 1996), but also by the interesting concept of 'noise'. Kahneman et al. (2022) identify three types of noise: 'level noise', referring to the variability of judgements of an individual compared to the average; 'pattern noise', when decisions are unusually affected by a specific situation (e.g. death of a loved one); and 'occasion noise', when decision-making in similar situations differs due to numerous seemingly random factors (e.g. time of day, tiredness, hunger). Despite not being specific to clinicians, the impact of 'ambient factors' (i.e. noise) upon advanced decision-making and EOLC has been previously highlighted (Croskerry 2018). Experience renders clinicians more aware of intrinsic and extrinsic factors that affect clinical judgement and shifts decision-making to pattern recognition and heuristics instead of laborious hypothesis testing (Cooper and Frain 2017). Nonetheless, having a conscious awareness of the variables which may influence advanced decisions does not remove the risk entirely, and neither does reliance merely on heuristics (May 2017). An aid to assist clinical judgement in these complex medical environments, often in the face of uncertainty and other external factors, is the introduction of decision-support interventions (Rees et al. 2020). Often based on algorithms or artificial intelligence, they have demonstrated benefit to individuals, improved transparency of consultation and more efficient decision-making, regardless of clinical experience.

Case Study
A 55-year-old woman with advanced Hodgkin's lymphoma is referred to the outreach service. She is on palliative chemotherapy; the disease having progressed after an allogeneic stem cell transplant. On review, she has neutropenic septic shock, and the outreach team is asked about admission to the ICU. The Advanced Practitioner follows the stages of advanced decision-making: (i) gathers information by clinical examination/drug chart evaluation/discussion with haematology team, patient, family. (ii) Starts formulating a working diagnosis, in this scenario the most likely case being neutropenic sepsis. (iii) Concurrently considers the differential diagnoses, such as disease progression, and decides that their initial diagnosis of neutropenic sepsis should be amended (iv) reaches their decision to admit to the ICU or not, acknowledging the other factors that affect this decision (pessimism bias towards patients with malignancy, optimism bias by the parent team, availability of ICU bed, the patient's stated wishes).

END-OF-LIFE CARE

The goal of the ICU is to help patients, who face an acute threat to their lives, reverse critical illness, and restore its quality. Recent technological advances have made prolongation of life with invasive interventions possible, since approximately 80% of patients admitted to an ICU will survive to discharge (Capuzzo et al. 2014). However, despite the intensive organ support, some patients will continue to deteriorate, and the therapeutic goals will not be possible to achieve. In these cases, the care transitions from curative to comfort, and the focus shifts from restoration of health to palliative care provision. This transition sometimes poses significant ethical, legal, and practical challenges for the critical care clinicians, who may struggle with the complex decision-making around EOLC (Harvey and Gardiner 2019).

LEGAL AND ETHICAL CONSIDERATIONS

In law, patients have the right to refuse but not the right to demand treatments. The crucial question is that of capacity: for patients who have capacity to make decisions about their own care, healthcare professionals must provide them with sufficient information to make an informed decision about proposed treatments (MCA 2005). For those who have lost decision-making capacity (most ICU patients), decisions become more complex. Healthcare professionals should consider the patient's prior wishes and values, which can inform advance care planning. These can be written or verbal and include advance care plans, emergency care plans/treatment escalation plan (TEP) or even a Do Not Attempt Cardiopulmonary Resuscitation (DNACPR) decisions. Another example of such an advance document is the Recommended Summary Plan and Emergency Care Treatment (ReSPECT). Its central aim is to document patients' wishes not only relating to resuscitation but also for other life-sustaining treatment, which may be unwanted by the individual (Carley 2017).

OPEN AND HONEST CONVERSATIONS

Encouraging open and honest conversations about the patient's wishes regarding resuscitation and other aspects of emergency care helps clarifying the goals of care, minimising the risk of unnecessary treatments and harms (Perkins and Fritz 2019). Especially in critical care, where the patients are faced with acute, frequently unexpected, life-threatening conditions, the proposed model for approaching decisions relating to end-of-life transitions is shared decision-making between patients' families and the clinical team. Involving capacitous patients but also their families in decision-making around the end of life is paramount and can be achieved by open visiting in ICU, provision of family support (psychologists, social workers, chaplaincy, ethics consultations) (Davidson et al. 2017) and structured communication tools (Curtis 2008).

DECISIONS TO ESCALATE, LIMIT, OR WITHDRAW LIFE-SUSTAINING TREATMENT

Decisions to escalate, limit, or withdraw life-sustaining treatment are ethically and emotionally charged, with numerous studies showing that clinicians appear more comfortable withholding therapies than withdrawing them (Truog et al. 2008; Sprung et al. 2019). Despite claims from ethicists that there is

TABLE 5.2   Decision-making in complex scenarios and in EOLC decisions.

Ensure you have a shared understanding between the clinicians, patient, and those close to the patient of what the problems and issues are.

Discuss what the likely outcomes are. Try to help the patient identify which outcomes are most important to them and their family.

Be clear about what treatments are being proposed. If a treatment is not considered sufficiently beneficial to be offered, this will need communicating carefully and compassionately.

Agree on the proposed treatment plan and care you will be organising, for example, treatment on the ward or treatment in intensive care.

Include discussion of specific treatments that either require discussion (e.g. CPR) or are important to the patient.

no moral difference between the two practices, on a practical level, physicians continue to feel a sharp distinction, and the higher the importance of the intervention in sustaining life, the more hesitant the intensivists are to withdraw it (Metaxa 2021). Religious affiliation, culture, relevant legislation, and geographical location have all been shown to influence decision-making around EOLC (Sprung et al. 2003; Sprung et al. 2019). Shared decision-making around escalation of treatment facilitates the process, ensuring transparent communication with individuals and their family, and respect for their views and culture. NICE Critical Care Guidelines (NICE 2020) recommend a structure and approach to support complex clinical decision-making in these situations (see Table 5.2).

THE IMPORTANCE OF EFFECTIVE COMMUNICATION

During times of critical illness, most patients or their surrogates find themselves interacting with unfamiliar clinicians in a sterile environment at a time of great distress. Irrespective of the offered technological interventions, effective communication is key and should focus on patient and family understanding of the illness, prognosis, and treatment options, as well as their expectations and preferences for treatment and decision-making. Clear, candid discussions are linked with increased family satisfaction around EOLC, as is the respectful and empathetic listening: satisfaction with end-of-life meetings was higher when clinicians spoke less and listened more (Cook and Rocker 2014). The mnemonic 'VALUE' offers proposes five objectives for a proactive family conference: **V**alue and appreciate what family members say, **A**cknowledge the family members' emotions, **L**isten to their concerns, **U**nderstand who the patient was in active life by asking questions, and **E**licit questions from the family members (Curtis 2008). Nevertheless, communication does not resolve all differences, especially when patients or families insist on interventions clinicians consider inappropriate. In most circumstances, conflict can be resolved by sensitive negotiations, good listening, timely second opinions, and offer of external intervention (religious support, mediation, ethic consultation) (FICM 2019). It is paramount to focus on obtaining clarity about the goals of care, be transparent about what can be medically achieved and keep clear and contemporaneous documentation. Rarely, the only way to resolve the conflict is to apply to the courts (Court of Protection, Court of Appeal, Supreme Court, and European Court). In these cases, the challenge for clinicians is to continue to care for the patient and interact with the family, while legal proceedings are underway and the relationship between them is damaged.

PRACTICAL CONSIDERATIONS

After the decision to transition to comfort care, the interventions undertaken need to be evaluated. Several considerations exist: symptom assessment and management (pain, nausea, anxiety, delirium, dyspnoea, thirst); relief of existential and psychological burden; avoidance of inappropriate prolongation of dying (cessation of non-beneficial medication); meeting spiritual and/or religious needs; maintenance of meaningful relationships (FICM 2019). Involving the patient's family/friends by offering them direct involvement in all aspects of EOLC, is central at this stage. Removal of endotracheal tubes, tracheostomy decannulation, deactivation of cardiac devices, and stopping of vasoactive medications are practical considerations that should be individualised.

MEDICINES MANAGEMENT

Pharmacotherapy is considered the cornerstone of symptom control in EOLC, with opioids and benzodiazepines being commonly used agents, due to their ability to manage pain, anxiety, and dyspnoea. One of the main challenges in ensuring appropriate medication doses in the ICU is that many patients have impaired cognition or communication ability and may not be able to accurately report their level of discomfort (Sloss et al. 2022). A wide variation in medications and practices has been observed, with a progressive increase in drug dosing preceding the withdrawal of life support, a practice ethically justified by the Doctrine of Double Effect (Lindblad et al. 2014).

PALLIATIVE CARE IN CRITICAL ILLNESS

Critical care-based palliative care is a holistic approach to caring for critically ill patients. It focuses on improving the quality of dying and death by anticipating, preventing, and treating physical, psychological, spiritual, and existential suffering. Palliative care is not synonymous with EOLC, as it encompasses clear and sensitive communication with families, shared decision-making based on patients' values, and symptom management around the end of life. Critical care clinicians should be competent in primary palliative care skills, whereas specialist palliative care expertise can contribute when required, with good interdisciplinary collaboration. Such a mixed model will empower ICU staff in the day-to-day practice and help overcome the important barriers, such as insufficient palliative care specialist numbers and intensivist hesitancy.

Case Study

An 85-year-old man has arrived in the hospital in septic shock, after a perforated diverticulum. After a lengthy operation, he is admitted in the ICU in multi-organ failure. At day 3, he was still on noradrenaline 0.3 mg/kg/min, intubated with fiO$_2$ 0.45, and anuric, requiring renal replacement therapy. The ICU team organise a family meeting, with the patient's wife and two adult children, where they explain the current level of significant multi-organ support and the probability of him not surviving this ICU admission. The patient's third son attends the meeting via video link, as he lives far away. He is confrontational and refuses to accept the presented poor prognosis. After the meeting, the rest of the family explains that he has been estranged with his father for years, following a financial dispute. The patient's wife describes her husband as a 'proud man, who wouldn't want to be a burden on anyone'. However, she doesn't want to proceed with the withdrawal of treatment if the whole family is not in agreement. In the next few days, the ICU social worker contacts the wife and the estranged son and facilitates a visit. The ICU team continues to hold regular meetings, where a non-escalation (withholding of treatment) and a DNACPR decision are agreed upon. The patient's values (not wishing to live dependently), what can be achieved in the ICU (prolongation of life), but also what complications it entails (delirium, muscle wasting/frailty) continue to be discussed, stressing that all available treatment will not restore him to his previous good health. Two weeks after admission, since no significant improvement is observed, the vasopressors are discontinued, the endotracheal tube is removed, and the patient dies quickly in the presence of all his family.

Take Home Points

- When making shared decisions with individuals, the clinician should always consider 'what among the many things that can be done ought to be done?'
- Clinicians must have an awareness of intrinsic, extrinsic factors, and 'noise' (level noise, pattern noise, occasion noise), which may influence clinical reasoning and impact the decisions made.
- Ethical dilemmas can be approached in four steps: establishing the facts of the decision in question, deciding what is in and out of scope, specifying the outcomes within the four principles of bioethics, balancing the principles to give them action-guiding capacity.
- Legal, ethical, and practical considerations should be considered when providing EOLC. The patient's values and wishes should remain at the centre of the clinicians' decisions.

REFERENCES

Beauchamp, T.L. (2003). Methods and principles in biomedical ethics. *Journal of Medical Ethics* 29 (5): 269–274.

Capuzzo, M., Volta, C., Tassinati, T. et al. (2014). Working group on health economics of the European Society of Intensive Care Medicine. Hospital mortality of adults admitted to intensive care units in hospitals with and without intermediate care units: a multicentre European cohort study. *Critical Care* 18 (05): 551.

Carley, S. (2017). *Have a Bit of ReSPECT for End of Life Care*. St. Emlyn's, in *St. Emlyn's*, May 12 [online]. Available from: https://www.stemlynsblog.org/have-a-bit-of-respect-for-end-of-life-care-st-emlyns [accessed 20 June 2023].

Cook, D. and Rocker, G. (2014). Dying with dignity in the intensive care unit. *New England Journal of Medicine* 370 (26): 2506–2514.

Cooper, N. and Frain, J. (ed.) (2017). *ABC of Clinical Reasoning*. BMJ Publishing Group Limited, used under licence by Wiley.

Croskerry, P. (2018). Adaptive expertise in medical decision making. *Medical Teacher* 40 (8): 803–808.

Curtis, J.R. (2008). Caring for patients with critical illness and their families: the value of the integrated clinical team. *Respiratory Care* 53 (4): 480–487.

Daniel, M., Rencic, J., Durning, S.J. et al. (2019). Clinical reasoning assessment methods: a scoping review and practical guidance. *Academic Medicine* 94 (6): 902–912.

Davidson, J.E., Aslakson, R.A., Long, A.C. et al. (2017). Guidelines for family-centered care in the neonatal, pediatric, and adult ICU. *Critical Care Medicine* 45 (1): 103–128.

Diamond-Fox, S. and Bone, H. (2021). Advanced practice: critical thinking and clinical reasoning. *British Journal of Nursing* 30 (9): 526–532.

Ericsson, K.A., Krampe, R.T., and Tesch-Römer, C. (1993). The role of deliberate practice in the acquisition of expert performance. *Psychological Review* 100 (3): 363.

Harvey, D.J.R. and Gardiner, D. (2019). 'MORAL balance' decision-making in critical care. *BJA Education* 19 (3): 68.

Health Education England. (2022). *Advanced Clinical Practice in Acute Medicine Curriculum Framework – Credentials* [online]. Available from: https://advanced-practice.hee.nhs.uk/our-work/credentials [accessed 20 June 2023].

Health Education England. (2017). *Multi-professional framework for advanced clinical practice in England* [online]. Available from: https://www.hee.nhs.uk/sites/default/files/documents/multi-professionalframeworkforadvancedclinicalpracticeinengland.pdf [accessed 20 June 2023].

Kahneman, D. (2017). *Thinking, Fast and Slow*. UK: Penguin Books.

Kahneman, D., Sibony, O., and Sunstein, C.R. (2022). *Noise*. UK: Harper Collins.

Kohn, M.A. (2014). Understanding evidence-based diagnosis. *Diagnosis* 1 (1): 39–42.

Lindblad, A., Lynoe, N., and Juth, N. (2014). End-of-life decisions and the reinvented rule of double effect: a critical analysis. *Bioethics* 28 (7): 368–377.

May, N. (2017) *When Is a Door Not a Door? Bias, Heuristics and Metacognition* in St. Emlyn's, April 4 [online]. Available from: https://www.stemlynsblog.org/when-is-a-door-not-a-door [accessed 20 June 2023].

Mental Capacity Act. (2005). *Crown Copyright*; 2005, cited 15th December 2022 [online]. Available from: www.legislation.gov.uk/ukpga/2005/9/pdfs/ukpga_20050009_en.pdf

Metaxa, V. (2021. End-of-life issues in intensive care units. *Seminars in Respiratory and Critical Care Medicine*, 42(01), pp. 160–168. Thieme Medical Publishers, Inc.

NICE Critical Care Guidelines. (2020). *Clinical Decision Making* [online]. Available from: https://www.criticalcarenice.org.uk/clinical-guidelines [accessed 9 September 2022].

Pellegrino, E.D. (ed.) (1979). The anatomy of clinical judgments. In: *Clinical Judgment: A Critical Appraisal*, 169–194. Dordrecht: Springer.

Perkins, G.D. and Fritz, Z. (2019). Time to change from do-not-resuscitate orders to emergency care treatment plans. *JAMA Network Open* 2 (6): e195170–e195170.

Rees, S., Bassford, C., Dale, J. et al. (2020). Implementing an intervention to improve decision making around referral and admission to intensive care: results of feasibility testing in three NHS hospitals. *Journal of Evaluation in Clinical Practice* 26 (1): 56–65.

Sackett, D.L., Rosenberg, W.M., Gray, J.M. et al. (1996). Evidence based medicine: what it is and what it isn't. *BMJ* 312 (7023): 71–72.

Sloss, R., Mehta, R., and Metaxa, V. (2022). End-of-life and palliative care in a critical care setting: the crucial role of the critical care pharmacist. *Pharmacy (Basel)* 10 (5): 107.

Sprung, C.L., Cohen, S.L., Sjokvist, P. et al. (2003). End-of-life practices in European intensive care units: the Ethicus study. *JAMA* 290 (06): 790–797.

Sprung, C.L., Ricou, B., Hartog, C.S. et al. (2019). Changes in end-of-life practices in European intensive care units from 1999 to 2016. *Journal of the American Medical Association* 322 (17): 1692–1704.

The Faculty of Intensive Care Medicine. (2018). *Curriculum for Training for Advanced Critical Care Practitioners – Syllabus. V1.1* [online]. Available from: www.ficm.ac.uk/media/6896 [accessed 20 June 2023].

The Faculty of Intensive Care Medicine (FICM). (2019). *Care at the End of Life: A Guide to Best Practice, Discussion, and Decision-making in and Around Critical Care* [onlline]. Available from: https://www.ficm.ac.uk/sites/ficm/files/documents/2021-10/ficm-critical-condition_0.pdf [accessed 20 June 2023].

The Intensive Care Society, Critical Care Networks – National Nurse Leads & The National Outreach Forum. (2022). *Advanced Critical Care Outreach Competencies* [online]. Available from: https://ics.ac.uk/asset/43B8C11B-4512-41D0-B97768FABA2C30B2 [accessed 20 June 2023].

The Royal College of Emergency Medicine. (2022). *Emergency Medicine Advanced Clinical Practitioner Curriculum 2022 (Adult)* [online]. Available from: https://rcem.ac.uk/wp-content/uploads/2022/09/ACP_Curriculum_Adult_Final_060922.pdf [accessed 20 June 2023].

Truog, R.D., Campbell, M.L., Curtis, J.R. et al. (2008). Recommendations for end-of-life care in the intensive care unit: a consensus statement by the American College [corrected] of Critical Care Medicine. *Critical Care Medicine* 36 (3): 953–963.

FURTHER READING

FICM. (2019). *Care at the End of Life* [online]. Available from: www.ficm.ac.uk/standardssafety guidelinescriticalfutures/care-at-the-end-of-life [accessed 20 June 2023].

The Royal College of Emergence Medicine. (2020). *The RCEM End of Life Care Toolkit* [online]. Available from: https://rcem.ac.uk/wp-content/uploads/2021/10/RCEM_End_of_Life_Care_Toolkit_December_2020_v2.pdf [accessed 20 June 2023].

HISTORY TAKING AND PHYSICAL EXAMINATION SKILLS IN ACUTE, EMERGENCY, AND CRITICAL CARE

CHAPTER 6

Consultation Models and Diagnostic Reasoning

Sadie Diamond-Fox, Rebecca Connolly, Alexandra Gatehouse, John Wilkinson, Angela Roberts, Caroline McCrea, and Sonya Stone

Aim

The aim of this chapter is to provide a deeper understanding of the Consultation Models surrounding advanced practice and the underpinning processes and theories to ensure a comprehensive and effective clinical consultation is performed.

LEARNING OUTCOMES

After reading this chapter the reader will have a comprehensive knowledge of:

1. The multitude of consultation models that may be used to elicit a detailed medical history for diverse populations (including neurodiverse, non-verbal and LGBTQIA+ populations).
2. Evidence-based physical findings and their relation to common pathology.
3. The psychosocial considerations required to elicit an evidence-based diagnosis via the principles of History Taking and Physical Examination (HTPE).
4. Dual process theory and cognitive bias (including accuracies and inaccuracies), probabilistic reasoning, and the use of the contingency table.

The Advanced Practitioner in Acute, Emergency and Critical Care, First Edition. Edited by Sadie Diamond-Fox, Barry Hill, Sonya Stone, Caroline McCrea, Natalie Gardner, and Angela Roberts.

SELF-ASSESSMENT QUESTIONS

1. List the common conceptual frameworks that exist to guide clinicians through the patient consultation process.
2. Discuss the central importance of the clinical consultation in defining the potential outcomes for an episode of care, in particular in relation to equality, diversity, and inclusivity (EDI) considerations.
3. Discuss the multi-faceted construct that is clinical reasoning and how it relates to the consultation process.
4. List the components of a 2×2 contingency table.

INTRODUCTION

The knowledge obtained about the patient through a comprehensive history and physical examination informs diagnostic reasoning and, in turn, treatment options and clinical decisions. The process of conducting a patient consultation and performing a subsequent clinical assessment has historically been termed 'the most powerful, sensitive, and versatile instrument available to the physician' (Engel and Morgan 1973). Despite the rapid growth of healthcare technology, this remains the case today. A skilled practitioner has the potential to make a significant contribution to several fundamental outcomes, including patient satisfaction, patient concordance with prescribed therapies and interventions, and overall diagnostic accuracy. This can ultimately have measurable changes in health or quality of life that result from safe patient care. Evidence suggests that, by conducting a high-quality medical history alone, 60–80% of the relevant information to form a diagnosis can be ascertained (Peterson et al. 1992; Roshan and Rao 2000). The overall aim of a thorough clinical history and physical examination, is to identify symptoms and physical manifestations that represent a final common pathway of a wide range of pathologies, which may be highly suggestive or even pathognomonic of one such pathology, or multiple concurrent pathologies.

Various established consultation models exist to give structure to the consultation, with the aim of effectively, efficiently, and accurately collecting the required information from the patient while continuing to build rapport with them.

Multi-professional Framework (MPF) for Advanced Clinical Practice Guidance for Professional Development (HEE 2017)

This chapter maps to the following statements within the MPF:

1. Clinical Practice:	1.4	1.6
2. Leadership and Management:	2.1	

Accreditation Considerations

This chapter maps to the following statements within the following national accreditation documents:

Curriculum for Training for Advanced Critical Care Practitioners Syllabus V1.1 (The Faculty of Intensive Care Medicine 2018)			
2.2	3.1	3.2	4.2

Advanced Critical Care Outreach Competencies (The Intensive Care Society, Critical Care Networks – National Nurse Leads and The National Outreach Forum 2022)
A1

Emergency Medicine Advanced Clinical Practitioner Curriculum 2022 – Adult (The Royal College of Emergency Medicine 2022)			
SLO1 – 4	SLO7	SLO11	SLO12

Advanced Clinical Practice in Acute Medicine Curriculum Framework (Health Education England 2022)
Generic Clinical CiPs: 1

CLASSIFICATION OF CONSULTATION MODELS

To maximise the efficiency and efficacy of the consultation, several models or frameworks have been proposed over the decades. These can be task-oriented, clinician-centred, behaviour-centred, or patients-centred. Although most models have been developed for use within the primary care/GP setting, they are arguably also applicable to secondary care and tertiary care settings, with adaptation as necessary.

All consultation frameworks share the common task of obtaining a medical history; however, Mehay et al. (2012) classifies them as differing in three ways:

- **Concept versus implementation:** Conceptual frameworks have clear aims but lack integration of the process of implementation into practice. The more modern frameworks (2003 and onwards) include both aspects.

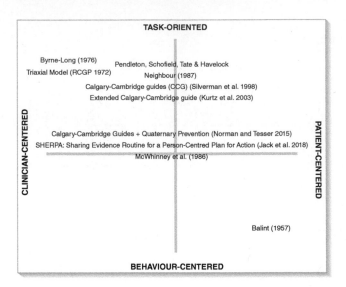

FIGURE 6.1   Consultation models and their differing emphasis on four common domains. *Source*: Adapted from Mehay et al. (2012).

- **Clinician versus patient-centredness:** Frameworks vary in their degree of focus on the consultation's agenda, process, and outcome in respect of the practitioner's perspective (biomedical/disease framework) versus the patient's perspective (illness framework). Although disease and illness usually co-exist, the same disease can lead to markedly different experiences of illness in different patient populations.
- **Task-oriented versus behavioural focus:** The degree to which frameworks focus on the tasks to be achieved in the consultation versus the range of behaviours required in the consultation.

Mehay et al. (2012) also propose a simple diagram which details the degree to which a selection of the existing frameworks differ, in terms of their focus on the three mentioned classifications. Figure 6.1 has been adapted from this original work to include more recent consultation frameworks.

CALGARY-CAMBRIDGE GUIDES TO THE MEDICAL INTERVIEW

The Calgary-Cambridge guides (CCG), which have evolved to become the enhanced Calgary Cambridge guides (eCCG), serve to give structure to the whole patient–practitioner interaction (see Table 6.1).

MNEMONICS

When using the eCCG there are a variety of mnemonics available to assist with the gathering of pertinent details and as a mental aid to ensure completeness of information (see Table 6.2).

TABLE 6.1 Enhanced Calgary-Cambridge consultation model.

Initiating the session

- Preparation
- Establishing rapport
- Identifying the reason(s) for consultation

Gathering information

Exploration of the patient's problems to discover the:

- *Biomedical perspective:*
  - Sequence of events
  - Symptom analysis
  - Relevant systems review

- *The patient's perspective:*
  - Patient's narrative
  - Question style: open to closed cone (see also Figure 6.2)
  - Attentive listening
  - Facilitative response
  - Picking up cues
  - Clarification
  - Time-framing
  - Internal summary
  - Appropriate use of language
  - Additional skills for understanding the patient's perspective

- *Background information – context:*
  - Past medical history
  - Drug and allergy history
  - Family history
  - Personal and social history
  - Review of systems

Physical examination

- Inspection
- Palpation
- Percussion
- Auscultation

Explanation and planning

- Providing the correct amount and type of information
- Aiding accurate recall and understanding
- Achieving a shared understanding: incorporating the patient's illness framework
- Planning: decision-making

Closing the session

- Ensuring appropriate point of closure
- Forward planning

Source: Adapted from Kurtz et al. (2003); Hill and Diamond-Fox (2022).

TABLE 6.2 Components of an adult health history and associated mnemonics.

Components of the adult health history	Data	Mnemonics
Identifying data/personal information	• Demographic data • Source of history (patient/carer/medical records) • Source of referral (if appropriate)	
Presenting complaint (PC)/ Principle symptoms (PS) (may be multiple)	• Major symptoms • Duration • Record each symptom using the patient's own terminology	O Onset of complaint P Progress of complaint E Exacerbating factors R Relieving factors A Associate symptoms T Timing E Episodes of being symptom-free S Relevant Systemic and general inquiry can be added here
History of presenting complaint (HPC)/ History of presenting illness (HPI)/ Present Illness (PI)	• Each presenting symptom should be explored in detail • Pulls in relevant portions of the ROS section • May include relevant medications, allergies, or social influences (alcohol, smoking, etc.) which may impact upon the PC. • Events should be presented in chronological order	OR S Start – When did it start? W Worse – What is making it worse? I Improve – What can improve it? P Pattern – When does it occur? E Evaluate – What is working? OR (for pain) S Site O Onset C Character/frequency R Radiation A Associations T Time course E Exacerbating/relieving factors S Severity

Past medical history (PMH)

- List childhood illnesses
- List adult illnesses (medical, surgical, obstetric/ gynaecological, and psychiatric) complete with date of initial diagnosis

Common illnesses with associated morbidity and mortality:

M	Myocardial Infarction
J	Jaundice
T	Tuberculosis
H	Hypertension
R	Rheumatic fever
E	Epilepsy
A	Asthma
D	Diabetes
S	Stroke
Ca	Cancer (and associated treatments)

Drug History (DH)

- Allergies and severity – ask specifically for PMH of Stevens-Johnson syndrome

D	Doctor – medications presented by a registered healthcare professional
R	Recreational – Tobacco, alcohol, illicit drugs, anabolic steroids
U	User – Over-the-counter purchases (Inc. alternative and homeopathic medicine)
G	Gynaecological – Contraceptives or hormone replacement
S	Sensitivities – Allergies and sensitivities to medications, including severity

Family History (FH)

- May be represented in diagram format
- Outlines age and health, or age and cause of death, siblings, parents, grandparents
- Consider a genetic cause or contribution to a patient's condition

FAMILY
Multiple affected siblings or individuals in multiple generations (lack of which does NOT rule out genetic causes)

G	Group of congenital anomalies – ≥2 may indicate the presence of a genetic-related syndrome
E	Extreme/Exceptional presentation – early onset cardiovascular disease, severe reactions to infections/metabolic stress, etc.
N	Neuro – Developmental delay or degeneration
E	Extreme/Exceptional pathology – pheochromocytoma, acoustic neuroma, medullary thyroid cancer, multiple colon polyps, neurofibromas, etc.

(Continued)

TABLE 6.2 (Continued)

Components of the adult health history	Data	Mnemonics
Social History (SH)	• Occupation and education • Overseas travel • Immunisations • Family of origin • Current household • Personal interests – hobbies, etc. • Lifestyle – activities of daily living, smoking, alcohol consumption, etc.	**S** Surprising lab results – in an otherwise apparently healthy individual W What do you do? – Note chemical, dust, animal, paint, and disease exposure H How do you do it? A Are you concerned about any exposure or experience? C Co-workers or others exposed? S Satisfied with your job?
Review of Symptoms (ROS)	Review of common symptoms associated with each body system, taking particularly note of any red flag symptoms	M Musculoskeletal – Bone and joint pain/ Muscular pain U Urinary – Volume of urine passed/Frequency/ Colour/Dysuria/Urgency/Incontinence N Neurological – Vision/Headache/Motor or sensory disturbance/Loss of consciousness/ Confusion C Cardiovascular – Chest pain/Palpitations/ Dyspnoea/Syncope/Orthopnoea/Peripheral oedema E Endocrine – Fatigue/Polyuria/Polydipsia/ Weight loss/Weight gain/Hair loss B Blood (and oncology) – Fever/Chills/Bruising/ Bleeding/Lumps/Bumps/Sweating/Previous clots A Alimentary – Appetite/Nausea/Vomiting/ Indigestion/Dysphagia/Weight loss/ Abdominal Pain/Bowel habit R Respiratory – Dyspnoea/Cough/Sputum/ Wheeze/Haemoptysis/Chest pain S Skin (and hair) – Hair loss/Growth/Skin eruptions/Rashes/Lesions/Ulcers

THE CONE TECHNIQUE

This established aid, described in the 'Three Function Approach to the Medical Interview' (Bird and Cohen-Cole 1990), guides the practitioner using open to gradually more closed questions (see Figure 6.2). This technique aims to collect information:

- thoroughly, reducing the risk of missing pertinent information using open questions
- efficiently, using closed questions
- while allowing the patient time to express the elements of their presentation which are significant to them.

THE PATIENT PERSPECTIVE OF CONSULTATION AND THE USE OF IDEAS, CONCERNS, AND EXPECTATIONS (ICE)

The Advanced Clinical Practitioner (ACP)–patient therapeutic relationship is one of the most unique and privileged relations a person can have with another human being and can be critical in treatment success. However, despite good intentions, patient-focused consultations can sometimes overlook patients, with the patient's perspective seldom taken into account. As such, the success of a medical consultation is the joint responsibility of both the patient and the clinician. This can pose specific challenges as ACPs are now faced with patients who use the internet for health-related information before or during the consultation – thus, patients are no longer passive recipients of health services; rather, they are active consumers and may have goals which may or may not align with those of the clinician.

Consultations with internet-informed patients allow patients and their clinician to collaborate in a mutual manner and increase their involvement in the decision-making process. The ACPs engaging in health consultations, therefore, must have the ability to evaluate the health-related information. Key research from patient perspectives highlights four key behaviours that should always form part of the consultation: listening attentively, taking the patient seriously, treating the patient as a person, and granting enough time. These key behaviours may be critical to rapport building and can easily fit within the initial relationship-building function of different medical consultation models.

While the consultation's primary aim is to collect information to formulate a differential diagnosis and management plan, the additional objectives are to build rapport, explore concerns, improve patient satisfaction, review the patient's agenda, and promote shared decision-making. Consideration of the acronym ICE throughout the consultation aims to achieve these objectives.

COMMUNICATION

Communication with patients is key to all aspects of clinical practice. Seminal NHS frameworks and policy drivers place effective communication at the core of providing a person-centred approach to health and care. Communication skills are consequently core strands of Advanced Practitioner (AP) training and ongoing professional development. Effective communication with patients can lead to improvement in both treatment quality and safety metrics; conversely, poor communication has been highlighted as one of the main concerns that lead to complaints to the Parliamentary and Health Service Ombudsman. This is a particular concern for patients from minority groups.

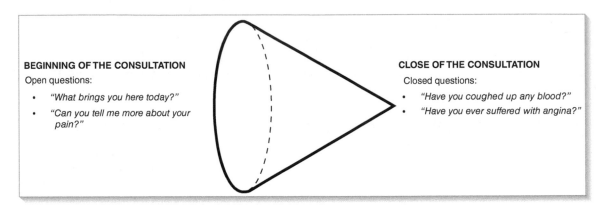

FIGURE 6.2   A pictorial representation of the open to closed cone described in the three function approach to the medical interview. *Source*: Adapted from Cohen et al. (1990); Hill and Diamond-Fox (2022).

KINESICS INTERVIEWING

A challenge when taking a medical history involves the distinction between truth and deception. Sometimes, patients may feel that in order to be taken seriously by their clinician or to expedite certain treatment protocols, they need to exaggerate their symptoms, or some may require treatment but may be unwilling/unable to give a salient history as to how their presentation came to be. Others may still be engaging in willing and conscious deception to achieve a predetermined consultation outcome (e.g. receipt of strong painkillers, or antibiotics that will then be given to someone else). Historical literature posits that the increased cognitive load instigated by deception can result in visible non-verbal cues; however, empirical evidence often fails to find significant relationships because individual non-verbal indicators are often too few and faint to accurately distinguish between truth-tellers and deceivers. Furthermore, the emotional stress and cognitive burden involved in those who are unwell and scared can muddy the waters further.

Understanding multiple kinesic behaviours during medical consultations may help the clinician understand patterns of deception which in turn may result in a more authentic patient experience. Studies have reliably shown that integration of interdependent verbal and non-verbal elements into a single message results in coherent meaning, and disruption of this (i.e. when engaging in cognitively taxing tasks like deception) can impair the quantity and quality of output (Burgoon et al. 2014). Of note is that eye contact is not a reliable indicator of truth or deception (Mann et al. 2012), but rather clusters of behaviours that, when taken holistically, can lead to understanding whether the patient is being deceptive for some reason.

Therefore, when engaging in a medical consultation, ask yourself whether the patient's non-verbal cues are consistent with their history. Is there discordance? Does the mother of a child with an injury keep looking to the father during history taking, seemingly for permission or confirmation? Does something 'not feel right'? Make a mental note as you engage in your consultation for exploration while maintaining metacognition that the complex emotions and feelings associated with healthcare and illness can result in patient cohorts behaving in ways that seem counter to what one would expect. Taking note of the non-verbal cues of the patient and their family/friends can help steer consultation direction, give key insights into the patient's cognitive status, and help the clinician in achieving effective therapeutic care.

EQUALITY, DIVERSITY, AND INCLUSIVITY CONSIDERATIONS

Patients from minority groups are at risk of substandard healthcare provision as a result of non-inclusive consultation practices. Practitioners should be sensitive to ensure language is inclusive. For example, members of the Lesbian, Gay, Bisexual, Transgender, Queer (questioning), Intersex, Asexual plus (LGBTQIA+) community face stigma and often feel afraid of revealing their sexual orientation or gender identity for fear of discrimination. Language should be non-gendered until the practitioner has clarified the patient's gender identity, similarly individuals should not be assumed heterosexual when referring to social or sexual history. Practitioners should be especially conscious of gendered language with non-binary (NB) or trans people; misgendering can be very distressing to patients and can be avoided by establishing the patient's preferred pronouns early in the consultation. When the consultation requires exploration of sexual history or genitalia, it is important to ensure this is approached sensitively and with an understanding of the psychological impact on the patient. It is important to only explore a person's sexual orientation or gender identity if it is pertinent to their presenting complaint and will add value to the consultation.

In order to develop effective clinician–patient relationships, consideration must be given to some of the fundamental principles of effective/therapeutic communication within the healthcare setting, such as patient health literacy, cultural understanding, and language barriers. However, there are other aspects that could potentially have an impact, such as those that have triggered the initial consultation.

Furthermore, for some clinicians, their personal socioreligious norms, attitudes, and experiences that shape their own schema may have implications for the care given to LGBT+ people. The diversity of workforce within the NHS is undoubtedly one of its greatest strengths: racial, religious, and cultural concordance between patient and clinician bodies contributes to a more effective therapeutic relationship and improved healthcare – put simply, we relate better to those with similar values and cultural frameworks. However, this diversity of religious and cultural expression may also present unique challenges for patients who are 'othered'; Judeo-Christian beliefs have been associated with 'deleterious anti-LGBT stigma and discrimination' (Scott et al. 2021) and religion-based sexual, heretical, and/or moral deviance has been associated with LGBT communities in many cultures. Thus, when clinicians from these cultures work in a clinician–patient relationship, they may bring with them (consciously or not) certain stigmas that may potentiate negative treatment of LGBT+ people.

Therefore, key to history-taking for patient populations that have been historically discriminated against or stigmatised is a collaborative and understanding approach – one that understands the challenges that are faced and a clinician that is willing to attempt to dismantle barriers and work in collaboration with the patient.

HISTORY-TAKING FOR NEURODIVERSE AND NON-VERBAL POPULATIONS

Neurodiverse populations challenge historical paradigms, where to be neurodiverse was thought of in terms of deficits focusing on impairments and limitations, or of people who are broken and need to be fixed. Neurodiversity is now rightly celebrated and rethought through the lens of human diversity with individuals possessing a complex combination of cognitive strengths and challenges. For example, difficulties in understanding social nuances, filtering competing sensory stimuli, and planning the tasks of daily living may be coupled with strengths in detailed thinking, memory, and complex pattern analysis (see Table 6.3).

TABLE 6.3   Specific challenges in taking a history of neurodiverse populations.

Verbal and non-verbal considerations	• May have difficulty with pragmatic language • May have difficulty expressing wants and needs • May not offer clarification when misunderstood • May speak with unusual volume, rhythm, and pitch • May have difficulty understanding nuances of sarcasms, idioms, and humour • Will often fail to make eye contact and understanding facial expressions or body language
Social interactions	• May have difficulty initiating conversations • May not respond when called by name or spoken directly to • May not take an interest in the feelings or preferences of others • May not respond to praise • May have an aversion to physical contact
Ritualised behaviour	• May have excessive resistance to change or unplanned events • May be inflexible in thinking

Thus, setting in history-taking may help obtain salient information to assist treatment. Ensure the consultation setting is low-stimulation, with as little change to the patient's routine as possible. Ask direct and simple questions that can easily be understood and are not open to interpretation.

Fields of Practice – Learning Disabilities

People with learning disabilities have increased prevalence of multi-morbidity at a younger age associated with poorer physical and mental health, and consequently premature mortality. Annual health checks were explicitly recommended to facilitate prompt detection and management of health conditions for anyone over the age of 14 on their general practitioners learning disability register. This resulted in increased investigations, recognition, and management of comorbid conditions, medication reviews, and specialist referrals in primary and secondary care.

Fields of Practice – Mental Health

An effective history, like in most specialities, is integral to help determine a possible aetiology, determine appropriate investigations, and form a clinical impression/diagnosis; however, the psychiatric history differs from a standard medical assessment slightly due to having a greater emphasis on the history component.

Furthermore, a large element of the examination is undertaken during the history component rather than a discrete set of procedures afterwards. As such, obtaining a collateral history may be necessary, and while a history may be taken from the patient alone, information from their friends, family, or from other healthcare professionals may offer additional important keys in establishing a clinical impression.

ORANGE FLAGS – PSYCHOLOGICAL CONSIDERATIONS

It is essential to establish a therapeutic alliance, as this forms the groundwork for history-taking because initially the patient will be making a decision as to your trustworthiness and as a corollary, instituting a therapeutic relationship is one of the key aims of the psychiatric interview. This is followed by eliciting the symptoms, history, and background information at the same time as examining the patient's mental state by means of the Mental State Examination (MSE), and concluding by providing information, reassurance, and advice to them.

HISTORY TAKING FOR ETHNIC MINORITY POPULATIONS

Effective history-taking and physical examination involve understanding the specific cultural nuances that exist with different patient populations and how different cultures consume and treat healthcare. This can sometimes lead to discordance in expectations or frustrations between clinicians, the patient, and the patient's wider network of friends and family.

Patients who do not speak English present a challenge due to the increased linguistic barrier, which can result in miscommunication and misinterpretation of expressing empathy or eliciting patients' feelings and expectations – it is recommended in these situations that telephone or in-person interpretation services are used, rather than a friend or family. This is to safeguard the clinician and ensure that the information given to the clinician and patient is a direct translation of each other, and not a facsimile provided by someone who is not an independent participant in the medical consultation.

TRIGGERS TO CONSULTATION

The primary trigger for a consultation can be extremely varied, considering the trigger for a consultation can be a powerful tool in setting up and directing the consultation appropriately.

Triggers may include:

- Interpersonal crisis
- Interference with social or personal relations
- Sanctioning or pressure from family or friends
- Interference with work or physical activity
- Reaching the limit of tolerance with symptoms.

CONSULTATIONS WITH AN ALTERNATIVE AGENDA

A typical agenda for a medical consultation is to gain information to assist with creating a differential diagnosis. Not all interactions between patient and practitioner attempt to achieve this agenda. It is undeniable that therapeutic communication is complex, however several constructs have been proposed to aid the clinician/practitioner in working with patients as partners. Examples of these alternative agendas and communication tools to approach them are detailed in Table 6.4.

TABLE 6.4   Alternative agendas and suggested communication tools.

Breaking bad news	
A	Anxiety – acknowledge
K	Knowledge – what do they already know?
I	Information – how much information do they want? Keep it simple, avoid overload
S	Sympathy + emotional management
S	Support – ask what would help
S	Support + ask what would help
S	Summarise strategy and key points

Dealing with an angry patient	
A	Avoid confrontation
F	Facilitate discussion
V	Ventilate feelings
E	Explore reasons
R	Refer/investigate

Conflict situations	
D	Disagree
A	Agree
N	Negotiate a compromise
C	Counsel
E	Educate
R	Refer to third party

Ethical considerations	
A	Autonomy (patient) – be fair (Justice)
B	Beneficence
C + C	Consent + confidentiality
D	Do not lie
E	Everybody else (society versus individual) – virtue, duty, utility, and rights

Source: Adapted from Mehay et al. (2012); Hill and Diamond-Fox (2022).

Field of Practice – Paediatrics

The Paediatric Assessment Triangle can be used as a rapid tool that can help clinicians evaluate a child's clinical status and need for rapid intervention (Ma et al. 2021).

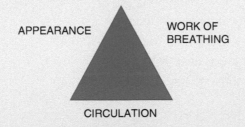

Appearance	The **TICLS** mnemonic can be used here: **T (Tone)** – How is the patient's tone? Is the patient floppy or obtunded? **I (Interactivity)** – Is the patient interacting with their environment or caregiver? **C (Consolability)** – Can the child be consoled by their caregivers? **L (Look/gaze)** – Is the patient tracking things appropriately with their eyes, or is it non-focused and/or dysconjugated? **S (Speech)** – Is there stridor? Hoarse cry? Barking cough? Absent sound?

Work of breathing	**Abnormal airway sounds:** snoring, muffled/hoarse speech, stridor, grunting, wheezing
	Abnormal positioning: sniffing position, tripoding, prefers seated posture
	Retractions: supraclavicular, intercostal, substernal, head bobbing
	Flaring: flaring of the nares on inspiration
Circulation	**Pallor:** white/pale skin or mucous membranes
	Mottling: patchy skin discolouration due to variable vasoconstriction
	Cyanosis: Blue discolouration of the skin or mucous membranes

---

GREEN FLAGS – SOCIAL CONSIDERATIONS

Physical manifestations of disease can be as a result of social, behavioural, and cultural factors. These factors have clear implications for health and disease outcomes. The AP should ensure that the social history is given due care and attention within the consultation.

CLINICAL REASONING AND THE CONSULTATION

Clinical reasoning is a multi-faceted and complex construct (see Figure 6.3), the understanding of which has emerged from multiple fields outside of healthcare literature, primarily the psychological and behavioural sciences. Clinical reasoning does not present us with a simple 'yes/no' answer to the presence or absence of a disease; rather, it challenges the probability of the presence or absence; thus, it is not a black-and-white process.

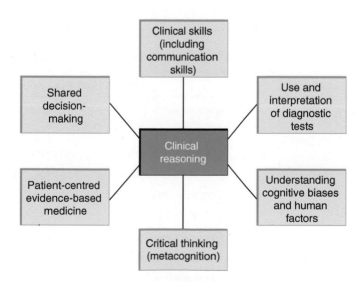

FIGURE 6.3   The elements involved in clinical reasoning, underpinned by a knowledge of basic and clinical sciences. *Source*: Frain et al. (2016) / John Wiley & Sons.

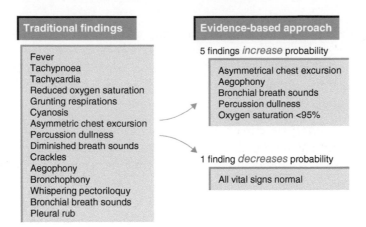

FIGURE 6.4 Traditional findings versus evidence-based method of diagnosis. A textbook presents 15 traditional physical findings of pneumonia (left), along with the assumption that each finding has similar diagnostic weight. The EBD method (right), which is based upon studies of actual patients, shows that five findings accurately increase the probability of pneumonia, and only one decreases it. *Source*: Frain et al. (2016) / John Wiley & Sons.

The application of clinical reasoning is central to advanced practice roles; not only is it embedded within credentialing frameworks, but it is also essential as complex patient caseloads with undifferentiated and undiagnosed diseases are now a regular feature in healthcare practice. It is also vital for improving evidence-based diagnosis and subsequent effective care planning, moving the clinician away from the traditional findings method (see Figure 6.4).

Clinical reasoning may be defined as 'a complex ability, requiring both declarative and procedural knowledge, such as physical examination and communication skills' (Rencic et al. 2020). A plethora of literature exists surrounding this topic, with a recent systematic review identifying 625 papers, spanning 47 years, across the health professions (Young et al. 2020).

A diverse range of terms are used to refer to clinical reasoning within the healthcare literature (see Table 6.5), which can make defining their influence on their use within clinical practice and educational

TABLE 6.5 The diverse range of terms used to refer to clinical reasoning within the healthcare literature.

Category	Sub-categories	Terms identified in this review:	
Reasoning skills		Clinical skills	Critical thinking
		Cognitive skill	Reasoning
		Critical reasoning	Reasoning skills
Reasoning performance	Expert reasoning	Adaptive expertise	Expert reasoning
		Cognitive expertise	Expertise
		Diagnostic expertise	Medical expertise
	Reasoning competence	Clinical competence	Diagnostic acumen
		Clinical performance	Diagnostic performance
		Competency	

TABLE 6.5   (Continued)

Category	Sub-categories	Terms identified in this review:	
Reasoning processes (components)	Cognitive	Analytic reasoning	Inductive and deductive reasoning
		Analytical thinking	Intuition
		Backward forward reasoning	Intuitive reasoning
		Backward reasoning	Medical information processing
		Bayesian probabilistic thinking	Pattern matching
		Cognitive processes	Pattern recognition
		Heuristics	'Street diagnosis' or 'in the blink of the eye'
		Hypothetico-deductive reasoning	
	Metacognitive	Metacognition	Self-monitoring
		Reflective thinking skills	
Outcome of reasoning	Errors/failures of reasoning	Cognitive bias	Medical error
		Error prevention	Premature closure
		Judgement errors	Reasoning errors
	Outcome/aim	Choice of treatment	Differential diagnosis
		Classification	Management plan
		Clinical management decisions	
		Diagnosis	
	Quality of outcome	Accuracy	Diagnostic success
		Diagnostic accuracy	
		Diagnostic and management quality	
Context of reasoning		Dialectical reasoning	Shared understanding
		Informed decision-making	Situation awareness
		Participatory decision-making	Situational judgement
		Shared decision-making	
Purpose/goal of reasoning	Different goals of reasoning	Diagnostic justification	
	Outcome-focused goal of reasoning	Case management	Patient management
		Diagnostic reasoning	Therapeutic reasoning
		Diagnostic thinking	Treatment decision making

Source: Adapted from Young et al. (2020); Hill and Diamond-Fox (2022); Hill and Mitchell (2022).

arenas somewhat challenging. The concept of clinical reasoning has changed dramatically over the past four decades. What was once thought to be a process-dependent task is now considered to present a more dynamic state of practice, which is affected by 'complex, non-linear interactions between the clinician, patient, and the environment' (Rencic et al. 2020).

COGNITIVE AND META-COGNITIVE PROCESSES

Multiple themes surrounding the cognitive and meta-cognitive processes that underpin clinical reasoning have been identified (see Table 6.5). Central to these processes is the practice of critical thinking. Much like the definition of clinical reasoning, there is also diversity with regard to definitions and conceptualisation of critical thinking in the healthcare setting. Critical thinking has been described as 'purposeful reflective judgement' that consists of six discrete cognitive skills: analysis, inference, interpretation, explanation, synthesis, and self–regulation (Facione 2020).

Critical thinking positively correlates with academic success, professionalism, clinical decision-making, wider reasoning, and problem-solving capabilities (Papathanasiou et al. 2014). Patient outcomes and safety have been directly linked to critical thinking skills. There are nine discrete cognitive steps that may be applied to the process of critical thinking, which integrates both cognitive and meta-cognitive processes (Harasym et al. 2008):

1. Gather relevant information
2. Formulate clearly defined questions and problems
3. Evaluate relevant information
4. Utilise and interpret abstract ideas effectively
5. Infer well-reasoned conclusions and solutions
6. Pilot outcomes against relevant criteria and standards
7. Use alternative thought processes if needed
8. Consider all assumptions, implications, and practical consequences
9. Communicate effectively with others to solve complex problems.

There are a number of widely used strategies to develop critical thinking and evidence-based diagnosis. These include simulated problem-based learning platforms, high-fidelity simulation scenarios, case-based discussion forums, reflective journals as part of continuing professional development (CPD) portfolios and journal clubs.

DUAL PROCESS THEORY AND COGNITIVE BIAS IN DIAGNOSTIC REASONING

A lack of understanding of the interrelationship between critical thinking and clinical reasoning can result in cognitive bias, which can in turn lead to diagnostic errors. Embedded within an understanding of how diagnostic errors occur is dual process theory; system 1 and system 2 thinking (see Table 6.6).

Although much of the literature in this area regards dual process theory as a valid representation of clinical reasoning, the exact causes of diagnostic errors remain unclear and require further research (Norman et al. 2017). The most effective way in which to teach and also learn critical thinking skills in healthcare settings remains unclear; however, a five-step strategy has been proposed based on well-known

TABLE 6.6   The characteristics of dual process theory.

	Characteristics
System 1 ('default interventionist')	• Rapid • Intuitive • Heuristic • Based on cognitive shortcuts • Utilises knowledge-lean strategies based on pattern recognition
System 2	• Slow • Analytical • Conscious • Effortful • Decontextualised process • Employs the principles of metacognition – self-reflection and self-regulation

Source: Adapted from Hill and Diamond-Fox (2022); Hill and Mitchell (2022).

educational theory and principles, that they have found to be effective for teaching and learning critical thinking within the 'high-octane' and high-stakes 'environment' of the intensive care unit (see Table 6.7) (Hayes et al. 2017). This is arguably a setting that does not always present an ideal environment for learning given its fast pace and constant sensory stimulation. However, it may be argued that if a model has proven to be effective in this setting, it could be extrapolated to other busy clinical environments and may even provide a useful aide memoire for self-assessment and reflective practices.

INTEGRATING THE CLINICAL REASONING PROCESS INTO THE CLINICAL CONSULTATION

The clinical consultation has been described as 'the practical embodiment of the clinical reasoning process by which data are gathered, considered, challenged, and integrated to form a diagnosis that can lead to appropriate management' (Linn et al. 2012). The application of the previously mentioned psychological and behavioural science theories is intertwined throughout the clinical consultation via the following discrete processes:

1. The clinical history generates an initial hypothesis regarding diagnosis, and said hypothesis is then tested through skilled and specific questioning.
2. The clinician formulates a primary diagnosis and differential diagnoses in order of likelihood.
3. Physical examination is carried out, aimed at gathering further data necessary to confirm or refute the hypotheses.
4. A selection of appropriate investigations, using an evidence-based approach, may be ordered to gather additional data.
5. The clinician (in partnership with the patient) then implements a targeted and rationalised management plan, based on best-available clinical evidence.

Table 6.8 details a useful framework of how the above methods can be applied to the process of undertaking the clinical consultation process.

TABLE 6.7   Five steps to improve teaching and learning critical thinking skills in healthcare settings.

	Explanation	Relevant psychological and educational theory
Step 1: Make the 'thinking process' explicit	• The teacher/facilitator/mentor (T/F/M) probes/questions the thought process used to arrive at a diagnosis and subsequent management plan • The learner is encouraged to discuss their thought process (metacognition) and to explore their initial thoughts (system 1) and subsequent analysis of their initial diagnosis and management plan (system 2)	• The revised Bloom's taxonomy contains six levels of the cognitive domain: 1. Remember 2. Understand 3. Apply 4. Analyse 5. Evaluate 6. Metacognition
Step 2: Discuss cognitive biases and de-biasing strategies	• The T/F/M explores potential cognitive biases (metacognition) that may be influencing the diagnosis and management plan and encourages the learner to consider alternative diagnoses	• Availability bias • Confirmation bias • Anchoring bias • Framing effect • Diagnostic momentum • Premature closure • Metacognition • Dual process theory

Step 3: Model and teach inductive reasoning	• The T/F/M encourages an inductive reasoning versus hypothetico-deductive strategy. The latter relies on memory and pattern recognition, which may be more subject to cognitive biases.
	• The learner may be encouraged to utilise a mechanism or concept map:
	  • Mechanism map; a visual representation of how pathophysiology of disease may lead to the clinical symptoms
	  • Concept map; graphically represent relationships between multiple concepts such as pathophysiology and presenting symptoms
		• Metacognition
		• Dual process theory
		• Problem-based learning

Step 4: Use questions to stimulate critical thinking	• The T/F/M utilised questions to engage and inspire the learner to think critically	• Metacognition • Dual process theory • Problem-based learning

Step 5: Assess the learners' critical thinking skills	• The T/F/M encourages the learner to utilise a framework in order to guide reflection, based on the milestones of critical thinking:
	  • Challenged thinker
	  • Unreflective thinker
	  • Beginning critical thinker
	  • Practicing critical thinker
	  • Advanced critical thinker
		Milestones of critical thinking

Source: Adapted from Hayes et al. (2017).

TABLE 6.8 The clinical reasoning process within a consultation.

Presenting complaint	Allow the patient to describe their presenting symptom(s)
Consider three or more hypotheses relating to diagnosis	Consider the following: • The patient's presenting symptom(s) and basic demographics (age, gender) • Key features of each of the three hypotheses • Distinguishing features of each of the hypotheses
Refine the diagnosis	• Formulate a primary hypothesis • Formulate a differential diagnosis or diagnoses
Physical examination	• Consider what findings are expected given the hypothesis and look for them • Relevant positives and negatives should refine the hypothesis
Relevant investigations	• Consider diagnostic testing if required • Will the investigation confirm or alter your hypothesis? If not, is it necessary?

Source: Adapted from Ross et al. (2016).

EVIDENCE-BASED DIAGNOSIS

Using the principles underlying critical thinking and clinical reasoning, there is potential to make a significant contribution to diagnostic accuracy, treatment options, and overall patient outcomes. Clinical reasoning and evidence-based diagnosis go together. Much like consultation and clinical assessment, the process of the application of clinical reasoning and evidence-based diagnosis was once seen as solely the duty of a doctor; however, the non-medical prescriber (NMP) role crosses those traditional boundaries. A recent systematic review of health professionals' understanding of diagnostic information and the accuracy metrics of specific diagnostics tests demonstrated that confusion often surrounds this subject due to its complexity (Whiting et al. 2015).

As explored earlier in the chapter, the principles of clinical reasoning are embedded within the practices of formulating an evidence-based diagnosis.

Evidence-based diagnosis quantifies the probability of the presence of a disease using diagnostic tests. Three pertinent questions to consider in this respect are (Kohn 2014):

1. How likely is the patient to have a particular disease?
2. How good is this test for the disease in question?
3. Is the test worth performing to guide treatment?

Evidence-based diagnosis gives a statistically discriminatory weighting to update the probability of a disease to either support or refute the working and differential diagnoses, which can then determine the appropriate course of further diagnostic testing and treatments.

BAYES' THEOREM

As with clinical reasoning, evidence-based diagnosis does not present us with a simple 'yes/no' answer when questioning the presence or absence of a disease; rather, it challenges the probability of the presence or absence, thus it is not a black-and-white process. The processes underlying clinical reasoning are complex and require an array of underpinning knowledge of not only the clinical sciences, but also psychological and behavioural science theories.

In order to practice evidence-based diagnosis effectively, we need to apply the process of formal probabilistic reasoning. Such reasoning requires use of Bayes' theorem, a technique used to calculate the conditional probability of events using a simple mathematical formula. Conditional probability is the probability of an event happening, given that it has some relationship to one or more other events. For example, the probability of getting a car parking space, prior to commencing a clinical shift in an inner-city hospital car park, is connected to the start time of your shift, whether said car park is shared with patients' visitors, and whether you have a car parking staff. Baye's theorem is applied within the clinical sciences to assess diagnostic accuracy using a 2×2 contingency table.

2×2 CONTINGENCY TABLE

The construction of a two-by-two contingency table (2×2 square) (see Figure 6.5) allows the accuracy of pertinent points of a patient's history-taking exercise, a finding/sign on a physical examination, or a test result to be weighted. Calculation of several statistical weightings can then be determined from this construct (see Table 6.9).

There are various online statistical calculators that can aid in the above calculations, such as the British Medical Journal Best Practice statistical calculators, which may used as a guide (`https://best-practice.bmj.com/info/toolkit/ebm-toolbox/statistics-calculators`).

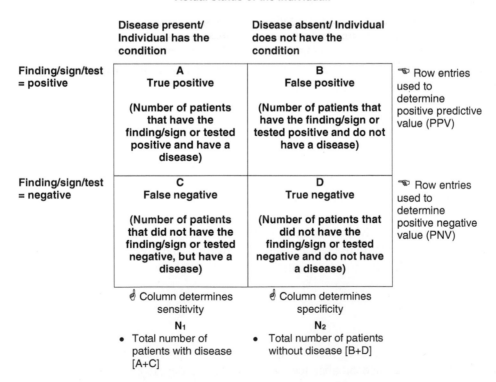

Actual status of the individual:

	Disease present/ Individual has the condition	Disease absent/ Individual does not have the condition	
Finding/sign/test = positive	**A** True positive (Number of patients that have the finding/sign or tested positive and have a disease)	**B** False positive (Number of patients that have the finding/sign or tested positive and do not have a disease)	☞ Row entries used to determine positive predictive value (PPV)
Finding/sign/test = negative	**C** False negative (Number of patients that did not have the finding/sign or tested negative, but have a disease)	**D** True negative (Number of patients that did not have the finding/sign or tested negative and do not have a disease)	☞ Row entries used to determine positive negative value (PNV)
	✎ Column determines sensitivity	✎ Column determines specificity	
	N₁ • Total number of patients with disease [A+C]	N₂ • Total number of patients without disease [B+D]	

FIGURE 6.5   A two-by-two square.

TABLE 6.9   Statistical terms pertaining to evidence-based diagnosis.

Term	Meaning
True positive	• Column A • People with the target condition who have a positive test result
True negative	• Column D • People without the target condition who have a negative test result
False positive	• Column B • People without the target condition who have a positive test result
False negative	• Colum C • People with the target condition who have a negative test result
Sensitivity	• Proportion of patients with the diagnosis who have the physical sign or a positive test result • Calculation: A ÷ (A + C)
Specificity	• Proportion of patients without the diagnosis who lack the physical sign or have a negative test result • Calculation: D ÷ (B + D)
Positive predictive value	• Proportion of patients with disease who have a physical sign divided by the proportion of patients without disease who also have the same sign • Calculation: A ÷ (A + B)
Negative predictive value	• Proportion of patients with disease lacking a physical sign divided by the proportion of patients without disease also lacking the sign • Calculation: D ÷ (C + D)
Likelihood ratio (LR)	• Finding/sign/test results sensitivity divided by the false-positive rate • A test of no value has an LR of 1. Therefore, the test would have no impact on the patient's odds of disease
Positive likelihood ratio	• Proportion of patients with disease who have a positive finding/sign/test, divided by proportion of patients without disease who have a positive finding/sign/test Calculation: (A ÷ N1) ÷ (B ÷ N2), or sensitivity ÷ (1 − specificity) • The more positive an LR (the further above 1), the more the finding/sign/test result raises a patient's probability of disease • Thresholds ≥4 are often considered to be significant when focusing a clinician's interest on the most pertinent positive findings, clinical signs or tests
Negative likelihood ratio	• Proportion of patients with disease who have a negative finding/sign/test result, divided by the proportion of patients without disease who have a positive finding/sign/test • Calculation: (C ÷ N1) ÷ (D ÷ N1) or (1 − sensitivity) ÷ specificity • The more negative an LR (the closer to 0), the more the finding/sign/test result lowers a patient's probability of disease • Thresholds <0.4 are often considered to be significant when focusing clinician's interest on the most pertinent negative findings, clinical signs or tests
Prevalence	• Equal to the pre-test probability
Post-test probability	• The probability of the presence of a condition after a diagnostic test is performed
Pre-test probability	• The probability of the presence of a condition prior to a diagnostic test is performed
Pre-test odds	• Pre-test odds = pre-test probability/(1 − pre-test probability)

THE INACCURACIES OF DIAGNOSTIC ACCURACY

Diagnostic accuracy refers to how positive or negative findings change the probability of the presence of disease. Unfortunately, on occasion, bias and variability in the reporting of research concerning diagnostic testing have been reported in studies, particularly in studies within which a new or alternative test is being evaluated against a clinical reference or 'gold' standard. This has been reported to be due to researchers omitting vital reporting information such as those detailed within the Standards for the Reporting of Diagnostic Accuracy Studies (STARD) statement (Bossuyt et al. 2015; Equator Network 2021).

Examination – Chest Pain and Dyspnoea

A 54-year-old female patient is admitted to the emergency department.
    PC: Chest pain and Dyspnoea
    HPC: arthroscopy of the left knee one week ago

- 24-hour history of worsening chest pain and shortness of breath

    PMHx: Smoker, angina, osteoarthritis

On Examination:

(A) Own

(B) Self-ventilating on 15 l/min oxygen via non-rebreather mask. Oxygen saturations 90%, Bilateral chest expansion, Bilateral air entry, no added sounds on auscultation.

(C) Sinus tachycardia 120 bpm, ECG shows Sinus tachycardia with incomplete right bundle branch block, Warm well perfused, BP 110/64 mmHg. Capillary refill time <2 seconds.

(D) GCS 15/15. Full power to all limbs.

(E) Abdomen soft non-tender. Calves soft non-tender. Left knee slightly hot to touch. Apyrexial, White cell count (WCC) = 14, C-reactive protein (CRP) = 120

Differentials:

- Pulmonary embolism (PE)
- Acute coronary syndrome (ACS)
- Community acquired pneumonia

Diagnostic reasoning for PE:
Pulmonary embolism is difficult to diagnose with a single test. History and examination findings should be taken into context prior to performing diagnostic tests.
    Wells' Criteria (Wells et al. 2001) for Pulmonary Embolism objectifies the risk of PE. The criteria should only be applied after a history and physical examination suggest that venous thromboembolism is a diagnostic possibility. The two-level PE Wells' score is then applied (NICE 2020). Wells' criteria has

a reported sensitivity of 72% and specificity of 62% in hospitalised patients. The addition of D-dimer to Wells' criteria improves sensitivity to 99% and decreases specificity to 11% (Bass et al. 2017).

The pulmonary embolism rule-out criteria (PERC) rule for PE (Kline et al. 2004) is used in the setting of a low-risk patient and may help avoid further testing. PERC is only valid in clinical settings with a low prevalence of PE (pre-test probability <15%) (Penaloza et al. 2012).

Diagnostic Tests:

D-dimer

- Sensitive, but not specific
- Negative D-dimer largely reduces the probability of PE (LR = 0.12 [0.07–0.21])
- Positive D-dimer increases probability of suspected PE (LR = 1.16 [1.07–1.31])

ECG

- Right ventricular (RV) strain pattern present is not sensitive (11.1%), but is specific (97.4%) (Thomson et al. 2019)
- The most common ECG abnormality reported in patients with PE is sinus tachycardia.

Examination – Dyspnoea

A 65-year-old male patient is admitted to the emergency department.

PC: Dyspnoea

HPC: Worsening shortness of breath over the past two months

- Increased ankle swelling
- Intermittent chest pain

PMHx: Recent anterior STEMI, hypertension, type two diabetes

On Examination:

(A) Own

(B) 4 l/min oxygen via nasal cannula, oxygen saturations 94%, respiratory rate 26 bpm, bilateral crackles to all zones on auscultation. Chest x-ray shows bilateral widespread opacification with a small right pleural effusion.

(C) Sinus rhythm 98 bpm, ECG shows pathological Q waves, Warm well perfused, BP 160/78 mmHg, moderate pitting peripheral oedema up to knees.

(D) GCS 15/15 no focal neurology, no reports of chest pain at present

(E) Abdomen soft non-tender, no change in bowel habits. Not yet catheterised but reports drop in urine output in the last 48 hours. Inflammatory markers slightly raised WCC = 11.4, CRP = 88, Troponin = 46, BNP = 3268.

(continued)

(continued)

Differentials:

- Decompensated heart failure secondary to recent STEMI
- Community acquired pneumonia
- Further ACS

Diagnostic reasoning:

Natriuretic Peptides (NPs): plasma concentration of NPs can be used as an initial diagnostic test

- Patients with normal plasma NP concentrations are unlikely to have Heart Failure (HF)
- Negative predictive values are similar in both acute and non-acute settings (0.94–0.98)
- Positive predictive values are lower in both the settings (0.66–0.67)
- Can be used to rule out HF but not to establish the diagnosis

(Maisel et al. 2008; Roberts et al. 2015; ESC 2016)

Chest x-ray: Most useful in ruling out other causes of patient's symptoms

- Limited use in diagnostic workup in non-acute settings
- Important to note that significant LV dysfunction can be present without seeing cardiomegaly

(Hawkins et al. 2009)

CLINICAL INVESTIGATION

STARD Statement

The STARD checklist was developed to improve the quality of reporting of diagnostic accuracy studies. It contains 30 essential items that should be included in every report of a diagnostic accuracy study. It may also be used to report other studies which evaluate the performance of tests, such as studies which report prognostication data. The STARD research team have become part of an international initiative (EQUATOR) that seeks to improve the value or published health research. Multiple toolkits from writing your own research to guidance on reporting clinical trials and evaluation data can be found on their website: https://www.equator-network.org.

CLINICAL INVESTIGATION

Clinical Scoring Systems

Evidence-based literature supports the practice of determining clinical pre-test probability of certain diseases prior to proceeding with a diagnostic test. There are numerous validated pre-test clinical scoring systems and clinical prediction tools that can be used in this context and accessed via various online platforms such as MDCalc (https://www.mdcalc.com/#all). Such clinical prediction tools include:

- 4Ts score for heparin-induced thrombocytopenia (HIT)
- ABCD^2 score for transient ischaemic attack (TIA)
- CHADS$_2$ score for atrial fibrillation stroke risk
- Aortic Dissection Detection Risk Score (ADD-RS).

Take Home Points
- A comprehensive health consultation should be well structured with a clear focus, allowing the clinician and patient to equally share information.
- The clinician should be sensitive to individuals' needs and ensure communication and approach are adapted accordingly, being particularly mindful of the additional needs of minority groups.
- Successful clinical decision-making, and diagnostics depend on a clinician's awareness of potential cognitive biases. Meta-cognitive de-biasing strategies may assist clinicians in overcoming the common pitfalls associated with unconscious cognitive biases.
- The pre-test probability, sensitivity and specificity, and test reliability are key concepts the competent practitioner should master to maximise the value of any diagnostic test or screening tool, while remaining mindful of disease prevalence, individual lifestyle, and other confounding factors.

REFERENCES

Balint, M. (1957). The doctor, his patient, and the illness. *The American Journal of the Medical Sciences*. 234: 609. https://doi.org/10.1097/00000441-195711000-00016

Bass, A.R., Fields, K.G., Goto, R. et al. (2017). Clinical decision rules for pulmonary embolism in hospitalized patients: a systematic literature review and meta-analysis. *Thrombosis and Haemostasis* 117 (11): 2176–2185. https://doi.org/10.1160/th17-06-0395. PMID: 29044295.

Bird, J. and Cohen-Cole, S.A. (1990). The three-function model of the medical interview. An educational device. *Advances in Psychosomic Medicine* 20 (1): 65–88.

Bossuyt, P.M., Reitsma, J.B., Bruns, D.E. et al. (2015). An updated list of essential items for reporting diagnostic accuracy studies. *BMJ* 351 (5527): 1–8.

Burgoon, J.K., Proudfoot, J.G., Schuetzler, R. et al. (2014). Patterns of Nonverbal Behavior Associated with Truth and Deception: Illustrations from Three Experiments. *Journal of Nonverbal Behavior* 38: 325–354. https://doi.org/10.1007/s10919-014-0181-5

Byrne, P.S.B., Long, E.L., and Great Britain Department of Health and Social Security (1976). *Doctors Talking to Patients: A Study of the Verbal Behaviour of General Practitioners Consulting in Their Surgeries.* London: H.M.S.O.

Engel, G.L. and Morgan, W.L. (1973). *Interviewing the Patient.* London WB Saunders.

Equator Network. (2021). *STARD 2015: An Updated List of Essential Items for Reporting Diagnostic Accuracy Studies* [online]. Available from: https://www.equator-network.org/reporting-guidelines/stard/ [accessed 20 June 2023].

ESC (2016). ESC guidelines for the diagnosis and treatment of acute and chronic heart failure. *European Heart Journal* 37 (27): 2129–2200.

Facione, P. (2020). *Critical Thinking: What It Is and Why It Counts* [online]. Available from: https://tinyurl.com/ybz73bnx [accessed 2 February 2022].

Frain, J. and Cooper, N. (2016). ABC of Clinical reasoning. John Wiley & Sons.

Harasym, P.H., Tsai, T.C., and Hemmati, P. (2008). Current trends in developing medical students' critical thinking abilities. *The Kaohsiung Journal of Medical Sciences* 24 (7): 341–355.

Hawkins, N.M., Petrie, M.C., Jhund, P.S. et al. (2009). Heart failure and chronic obstructive pulmonary disease: diagnostic pitfalls and epidemiology. *European Journal of Heart Failure* 11 (2): 130–139.

Hayes, M.M., Chatterjee, S., and Schwartzstein, R.M. (2017). Critical thinking in critical care: five strategies to improve teaching and learning in the intensive care unit. *Annuals American Thoracic Society* 14 (4): 569–575.

Health Education England (HEE). (2017). *Multi-professional Framework for Advanced Clinical Practice in England* [online]. Available from: `https://www.hee.nhs.uk/sites/default/files/documents/multi-professionalframeworkforadvancedclinicalpracticeinengland.pdf` [accessed 20 June 2023].

Health Education England (HEE). (2022). *Advanced Clinical Practice in Acute Medicine Curriculum Framework – Credentials* [online]. Available from: `https://advanced-practice.hee.nhs.uk/our-work/credentials` [accessed 20 June 2023].

Hill, B. and Diamond-Fox, S. (2022). *Advanced Clinical Practice at a Glance.* Wiley.

Hill, B. and Mitchell, A. (2022). *Independent and Supplementary Prescribing at a Glance.* Wiley.

Jack, E., Maskrey, N., and Byng, R. (2018). SHERPA: a new model for clinical decision making in patients with multimorbidity. *Lancet* 392 (10156): 1397–1399. https://doi.org/10.1016/S0140-6736(18)31371-0. PMID: 30343853.

Kline, J.A., Mitchell, A.M., Kabrhel, C. et al. (2004). Clinical criteria to prevent unnecessary diagnostic testing in emergency department patients with suspected pulmonary embolism. *Journal of Thrombosis and Haemostasis* 2 (8): 1247–1255. `https://doi.org/10.1111/j.1538-7836.2004.00790.x`. PMID: 15304025.

Kohn, M.A. (2014). Understanding evidence-based diagnosis. *Diagnosis (Berlin)* 1 (1): 39–42.

Kurtz, S., Silverman, J., Benson, J., and Draper, J. (2003). Marrying content and process in clinical method teaching. Enhancing the Calgary–Cambridge Guides. *Academic Medicine* 78 (8): 802–809 https://doi.org/10.1097/00001888-200308000-00011. PMID: 12915371

Linn, A., Khaw, C., Kildea, H., and Tonkin, A. (2012). Clinical reasoning—a guide to improving teaching and practice. *Australian Family Physician* 41 (1–2): 18–20.

Ma, X., Liu, Y., Du, M. et al. (2021). The accuracy of the pediatric assessment triangle in assessing triage of critically ill patients in emergency pediatric department. *International Emergency Nursing* 58: 101041.

Maisel, A., Mueller, C., Adams, K. et al. (2008). State of the art: using natriuretic peptide levels in clinical practice. *European Journal of Heart Failure* 10: 824–839.

Mann, S., Vrij, A., Leal, S. et al (2012). Windows to the Soul? Deliberate Eye Contact as a Cue to Deceit. *Journal of Nonverbal Behavior* 36: 205–215. https://doi.org/10.1007/s10919-012-0132-y

McWhinney, I.R., Levenstein, J.H., McCracken, E.C. et al. (1986). The patient-centred clinical method. 1. A model for the doctor-patient interaction in family medicine. *Family Practice* 3: 24–30.

Mehay, R., Beaumont, R., Draper, J. et al. (2012). Revisiting models of the consultation (online-only content, `https://tinyurl.com/yaxqupm3`). In: *The Essential Handbook for GP Training and Education* (ed. R. Mehay). London: Radcliffe Publishing.

National Institute of Clinical Excellence. (2020). *Venous Thromboembolic Disease: Diagnosis, Management and Thrombophilia Testing: Evidence Reviews for D-Dimer Testing in the Diagnosis of Deep Vein Thrombosis and Pulmonary Embolism* [online]. Available from: `www.nice.org.uk/guidance/ng158/evidence/a--ddimer-testing-in-the-diagnosis-of-deep-vein-thrombosis-and-pulmonary-embolism-pdf-8710588334` [accessed 3 March 2022].

Neighbour, R. (1987). *The Inner Consultation: How to Develop an Effective and Intuitive Consulting Style.* Roger Neighbour.

Norman, A.H. and Tesser, C.D. (2015). Quaternary prevention: the basis for its operationalization in the doctor-patient relationship (original in Portuguese). *Revista Brasileira de Medicina de Família e Comunidade* 10 (35): 1–10. https://doi.org/10.5712/rbmfc10(35)1011

Norman, G.R., Monteiro, S.D., Sherbino, J. et al. (2017). The causes of errors in clinical reasoning: cognitive biases, knowledge deficits and dual process thinking. *Academic Medicine* 92 (1): 23–30.

Papathanasiou, I.V., Kleisiaris, C.F., Fradelos, E.C. et al. (2014). Critical thinking: the development of an essential skill for nursing students. *Acta Informatica Medica* 22 (4): 283–286.

Penaloza, A., Verschuren, F., Dambrine, S. et al. (2012). Performance of the pulmonary embolism rule-out criteria (the PERC rule) combined with low clinical probability in high prevalence population. *Thrombosis Research* 129 (5): e189–e193. `https://doi.org/10.1016/j.thromres.2012.02.016`. Epub 2012 Mar 15. PMID: 22424852.

Pendleton, D., Schofield, T., and Tate, P. (1984). *The Consultation: An Approach to Learning and Teaching.* Oxford: Oxford University Press.

Peterson, M.C., Holbrook, J.H., von Vales, D. et al. (1992). Contributions of the history, physical examination, and laboratory investigation in making medical diagnosis. *The Western Journal of Medicine* 156 (2): 163–165.

Rencic, J., Lambert, W.T., Schuwirth, L., and Durning, S.J. (2020). Clinical reasoning performance assessment: using situated cognition theory as a conceptual framework. *Diagnosis* 7 (3): 177–179.

Roberts, E., Ludman, A.J., Dworzynski, K. et al. (2015). The diagnostic accuracy of the natriuretic peptides in heart failure: systematic review and diagnostic meta-analysis in the acute care setting. *BMJ* 350 (1): 1–17.

Roshan, M. and Rao, A.P. (2000). A study on relative contributions of the history, physical examination and investigations in making medical diagnosis. *Journal of Associate Physicians India* 48 (8): 771–775.

Ross, D., Schipper, S., and Westbury, C. (2016). Examining critical thinking skills in family medicine residents. *Family Medicine* 48 (2): 121–126.

Scott, D., Pereira, N.M., Harrison, S.E. et al. (2021). "In the Bible Belt:" The role of religion in HIV care and prevention for transgender people in the United States South. *Health Place.* 70:102613. https://doi.org/10.1016/j.healthplace.2021.102613. Epub 2021 Jun 27. PMID: 34186379; PMCID: PMC8922555.

Silverman, J.D., Kurtz, S.M., Draper, J. (1998). *Skills for Communicating with Patients.* Oxford: Radcliffe Medical Press.

The Faculty of Intensive Care Medicine. (2018). *Curriculum for Training for Advanced Critical Care Practitioners – Syllabus. V1.1* [online]. Available from: `www.ficm.ac.uk/media/6896` [accessed 20 June 2023].

The Intensive Care Society, Critical Care Networks – *National Nurse Leads and The National Outreach Forum.* (2022). *Advanced Critical Care Outreach Competencies* [online]. Available from: `https://ics.ac.uk/asset/43B8C11B-4512-41D0-B97768FABA2C30B2` [accessed 20 June 2023].

The Royal College of Emergency Medicine. (2022). *Emergency Medicine Advanced Clinical Practitioner Curriculum 2022 (Adult)* [online]. Available from: `https://rcem.ac.uk/wp-content/uploads/2022/09/ACP_Curriculum_Adult_Final_060922.pdf` [accessed 20 June 2023].

Thomson, D., Kourounis, G., Trenear, R. et al. (2019). ECG in suspected pulmonary embolism. *Post Graduate Medical Journal* 95 (1119): 12–17.

Wells, P.S., Anderson, D.R., Rodger, M. et al. (2001). Excluding pulmonary embolism at the bedside without diagnostic imaging: management of patients with suspected pulmonary embolism presenting to the emergency department by using a simple clinical model and d-dimer. *Annals of Internal Medicine* 135 (2): 98–107. `https://doi.org/10.7326/0003-4819-135-2-200107170-00010`. PMID: 11453709.

Whiting, P.F., Davenport, C., Jameson, C. et al. (2015). How well do health professionals interpret diagnostic information? A systematic review. *BMJ* 5 (7): 1–8.

Young, M.E., Thomas, A., Lubarsky, S. et al. (2020). Mapping clinical reasoning literature across the health professions: a scoping review. *BMC Medical Education* 20 (107): 1–11.

FURTHER READING

Bickley, L. (2020). *Bates' Guide to Physical Examination and History Taking.* Wolters Kluwer.

McGee, S. (2021). *Evidence Based Physical Diagnosis*, 5e. Elsevier.

CHAPTER 7

Respiratory Presentations

Andrew Lee, Rebecca Chamoto, Rebecca Kurylec, Kirsty Laing, Kathryn Thomas, Emma Toplis, Padma Parthasarathy, and Rebecca Stacey

Aim

The aim of this chapter is to provide the reader with comprehensive knowledge in relation to patients who present with respiratory disorders in the context of advanced clinical practice.

LEARNING OUTCOMES

After reading this chapter the reader will have:

1. A thorough knowledge of history taking skills within the context of patients who present with respiratory disorders.
2. A comprehensive understanding of the types of respiratory failure that lead to acute and emergency presentations.
3. An advanced understanding of common acute and emergency care respiratory disorders inclusive of asthma, chronic obstructive pulmonary disease (COPD), pneumonia, pulmonary embolism (PE), and lung cancer.
4. An enhanced insight of the evidence base that underpins advanced practice in respiratory care.

SELF-ASSESSMENT QUESTIONS

1. What are respiratory emergencies?
2. Explain some of the adjuvant, neo-adjuvant, and palliative treatments available.
3. What investigations are considered essential when assessing patients who present to acute care services with respiratory presentations?
4. Discuss the key considerations that inform a diagnosis and differential of which aides a clinical assessment.

The Advanced Practitioner in Acute, Emergency and Critical Care, First Edition. Edited by Sadie Diamond-Fox, Barry Hill, Sonya Stone, Caroline McCrea, Natalie Gardner, and Angela Roberts.
© 2024 John Wiley & Sons Ltd. Published 2024 by John Wiley & Sons Ltd.

INTRODUCTION

In recent years, mounting pressure on NHS healthcare delivery has been challenged by the deficit in workforce and the disparity between supply and demand. Advanced Clinical Practitioners (ACPs) have been recognised as part of the solution in developing alternative ways to meet healthcare needs. The NHS Long-Term People Plan (2019) also advocates that advanced practice roles such as these can fill in the gaps in the medical workforce, improve clinical continuity, and provide mentoring and training for less experienced staff. In recent years, the respiratory specialty has seen a growing number of these high-level practitioners recruited to meet the respiratory care demand.

Multi-professional Framework (MPF) for Advanced Clinical Practice Guidance for Professional Development (HEE 2017)

This chapter maps to the following statements within the MPF:

1. Clinical Practice:	1.2	1.3	1.4	1.6	1.7	1.10	1.11
2. Leadership and Management:	2.7	2.9					
3. Education:	3.1	3.2					
4. Research:	4.1						

Accreditation Considerations

This chapter maps to the following statements within the following national accreditation documents:

Curriculum for Training for Advanced Critical Care Practitioners Syllabus V1.1
(The Faculty of Intensive Care Medicine 2018)

2.1	2.6	3.2	4.1	4.2	4.3

Advanced Critical Care Outreach Competencies
(The Intensive Care Society, Critical Care Networks – National Nurse Leads and The National Outreach Forum 2022)

A3	A4

Emergency Medicine Advanced Clinical Practitioner Curriculum 2022 – Adult
(The Royal College of Emergency Medicine 2022)

SLO3	RP5	RP5	ResP:1–4	ResC: 1,3,6,7,8,10

Advanced Clinical Practice in Acute Medicine Curriculum Framework
(Health Education England 2022)

Generic Clinical CiPs: 1, 2, 3, 4, 5, 6,
Specialty Clinical CiPs: 5
Presentations and Conditions of Acute Medicine by System/Specialty: Respiratory medicine

RESPIRATORY HISTORY-TAKING

Respiratory diseases result in a large proportion of emergency admissions to secondary care. A search of the hospital episodes statistics dashboard identified 132 751 emergency admissions for respiratory presentations between May 2021 and May 2022 (NHS Digital 2022). There has been a remarkable rise in the number of hospital admissions over the last decade, further adding to the pressures within the healthcare system that we see today. With an ageing co-morbid population, there has been a 104.7% increase in hospital admissions in the 10 years (1999–2019) for respiratory conditions (see Figure 7.1).

Signs and Symptoms

The signs and symptoms of respiratory disease are numerous, and telling them apart from other systems and illnesses can be tricky. Figure 7.2 demonstrates the wide range of symptoms that patients may present to the hospital with and further highlights the importance of taking a detailed history.

Subjective Data Gathering

The following questions will help in narrowing down the differential diagnosis when used in conjunction with the presenting signs and symptoms. By utilising this enhanced questioning, it may even provide a cause for the patients presenting complaint. The following factors are considered as equally important when taking a focussed respiratory history.

SOCIAL HISTORY

Recent Foreign Travel

Has the patient travelled abroad anywhere, and was there any air conditioning in the room they were staying in? Have they used a hot tub recently? This is essential information if a patient presents with pneumonia, as the bacteria in question could be *Legionella*.

Employment

There are careers that may predispose patients to presenting with respiratory disease such as:

- Farmers
- Miners
- Asbestos exposure i.e. gas engineers with exposure to lagging. They can also have exposure through washing overalls that have asbestos fibres on them.

Smoking History

This is essential when taking a respiratory history and quantifying the volume of smoking is also important. The term pack year history is used as a standardised way of informing the amount an individual has smoked. Calculating this is a straightforward approach as 1 pack = 20 cigarettes. For example: 10 cigarettes

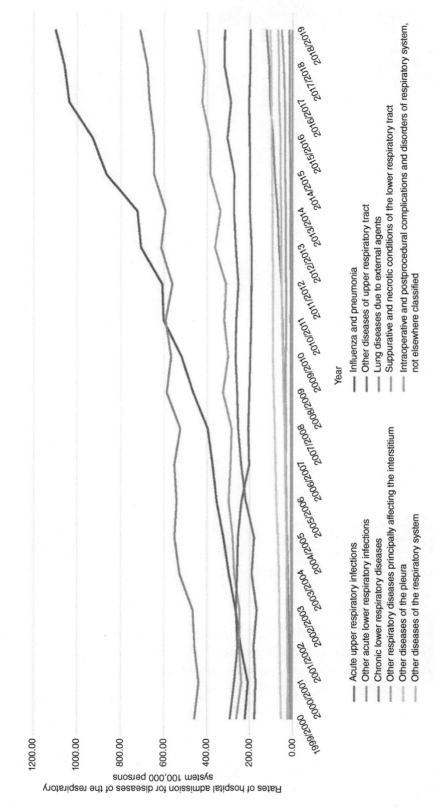

FIGURE 7.1 Hospital admissions in the 10years (1999–2019) for respiratory conditions. *Source:* Naser et al. (2021) / Springer Nature/ Public Domain. Available from: https://bmcpulmmed.biomedcentral.com/articles/10.1186/s12890-021-01736-8/figures/1.

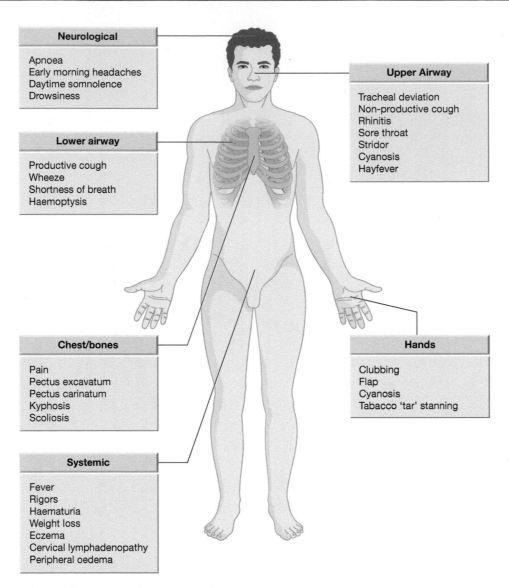

FIGURE 7.2   Signs and symptoms of respiratory illness.

a day over 40 years would give a pack year of 20. For those who smoke roll ups, 25 g or 1 oz of tobacco is the equivalent of 50 cigarettes. This is equivariant to approximately 7 cigarettes a day. It is also important to establish if the patient smokes illicit drugs such as Cannabis or Heroin.

Performance Status

Establishing functional status is important for decision-making for either escalation of care or potential cancer treatment. There are two scales used routinely which is the Modified Medical Research Council (mMRC) Dyspnoea Scale (see Table 7.1) and the Eastern Cooperative Oncology Group (ECOG) performance status (see Table 7.2).

TABLE 7.1   mMRC dyspnoea scale.

Grade	Severity of dyspnoea
0	No breathlessness except on strenuous exertion
1	Shortness of breath when hurrying on the level or up a slight hill
2	Walks slower than people of the same age on the flat due to shortness of breath or has to stop when walking at own pace on the level
3	Stops after walking around 100 m due to shortness of breath
4	Too breathless to leave the house or breathless when washing and dressing

TABLE 7.2   ECOG performance status.

Grade	Performance status
0	Fully active, able to carry on all pre-disease performance without restriction
1	Restricted in physically strenuous activity but ambulatory and able to carry out work of a light or sedentary nature, e.g. light house work, office work
2	Ambulatory and capable of all selfcare but unable to carry out any work activities; up and about more than 50% of waking hours
3	Capable of only limited selfcare; confined to bed or chair more than 50% of waking hours
4	Completely disabled; cannot carry on any selfcare; totally confined to bed or chair

Source: Adapted from Oken et al. (1982).

MEDICATION HISTORY

Along with the patient's usual list of medications, it should be considered what acute or disease-specific medications have been prescribed, such as:

- Recent courses of antibiotics or steroids.
- How many courses of steroids have they needed in the past 12 months?
- Number of Salbutamol inhalers needed each month?
- Use of nebulisers while at home.
- Long-term or ambulatory use of oxygen at home.

Clarify with the Patient their Vaccine Status Checking for

- COVID-19 – initial doses plus any boosters
- Annual Influenza
- Pneumococcal

FAMILY HISTORY

It is important to note if any direct family members have a history of a primary respiratory condition:

- COPD
- Asthma
- Lung cancer
- Pulmonary embolism or any venous thromboembolism (VTE)
- Alpha 1 anti-trypsin
- Pulmonary tuberculosis

OTHER QUESTIONS TO CONSIDER

- Recent microbiology results such as sputum cultures – this will help with antimicrobial steward-ship and will target antibiotic therapy to the microbiology for that patient. Particularly important for bronchiectasis and cystic fibrosis.
- Do they keep pets at home? Making sure to be specific as there is increased risk of hypersensitivity pneumonitis through close contact with birds.
- Do they have any allergies or hay fever? Have they ever suffered with eczema or other signs of atopy? This may point towards an asthma diagnosis.
- For known asthmatics, have they had previous admission to the hospital for their asthma and if so have they been admitted to ICU and intubated before? What is their best peak expiratory flow rate (PEFR)?
- Finally, it is important to note the number of hospital admissions within the past 12 months that, may point towards overall deteriorating health or that the patient may need increased support from community-based teams to support them with managing their condition.

ASTHMA

Asthma is a common chronic respiratory condition which affects both adults and children. It is characterised by airway hyper responsiveness.

The two key distinguishing features of asthma are:

- Episodic airflow obstruction caused by smooth muscle constriction of the bronchi, airway wall oedema, inflammation, and mucous gland hypersecretion resulting in dyspnoea, chest tightness, wheeze, and cough particularly at night.
- Air flow obstruction is partially or fully reversible either spontaneously or by treatment.

Epidemiology

According to British Lung Foundation (BLF), around 8 million people are diagnosed with asthma in the UK, with a prevalence of 12% making asthma as the most common lung condition in the UK (BLF 2023). Asthma accounts for 60 000 hospital admissions and 200 000 bed days a year. Asthma affects more women than men.

Despite the aetiology of asthma remaining unclear, there are a range of environmental and innate factors such as genetic, atopy, exposure to allergens, and occupational sensitising agents that are considered important risk factors for asthma. Some of the common precipitating factors of asthma are shown in Table 7.3.

The phenotyping of asthma is becoming increasingly important due to its heterogenicity and attempts to promote a patient-centred, individualised approach to treatment. Some of the common asthma phenotypes are shown in Box 7.1.

Clinical Features

Symptoms of asthma can be non-specific, and it is important to consider and exclude alternative diagnoses. Some of the conditions that can mimic asthma are highlighted in Table 7.4

TABLE 7.3   The common precipitating factors of asthma.

Common precipitating factors	Asthma triggers
Infection	Respiratory viral illnesses such as RSV or Influenza Sinusitis Bronchitis or Bronchiolitis
Inhaled allergens	Pollens, weeds, grasses, tree House dusts Feathers Animal danders Furniture stuffing Fungal spores
Irritant inhalers	Paint Gasoline Tobacco smoke Industrial chemicals Industrial dye Cold air Air pollutants
Trigger mechanisms	Laughter Exercise Psychological stress Drugs such as NSAIDS or Aspirin

Box 7.1   Some of the Common Asthma Phenotypes

Early onset of allergic asthma

Late onset of eosinophilic asthma

Late onset of non-eosinophilic asthma

Cough-variant asthma

Obesity-related asthma

Asthma with persistent airflow obstruction

Perennial asthma

Exacerbation-prone asthma

Exercise-induced asthma

Aspirin-induced asthma

Occupational asthma

Neutrophilic asthma

Seasonal asthma

TABLE 7.4   Differential diagnosis of asthma.

Differential diagnosis of asthma	
Localised pathology	Foreign body aspiration Endobronchial tumour Vocal cord dysfunction Induced laryngeal obstruction
Diffuse airway pathology	COPD Bronchiectasis Bronchiolitis Interstitial lung disease (asbestosis, pneumoconiosis, fibrosing alveolitis, sarcoidosis, vasculitis)
Other pathologies	Gastro-oesophageal reflux Congestive cardiac failure Pulmonary eosinophilia Dysfunctional breathing Intolerance to angiotensin-converting enzyme (ACE) inhibitors Hyperventilation syndrome

Common clinical features of asthma are episodic shortness of breath, wheeze, chest tightness and/or cough; typically these symptoms are:

- Variable
- Intermittent
- Worse at night
- Associated with specific triggers such as pollens or animal dander
- Non-specific triggers such as cold air, perfumes or bleaches, due to airway hypersensitivity.

Physical Examination

Physical examination is usually normal in stable asthma patients but becomes abnormal during exacerbations. The common signs of asthma exacerbation are:

- Severe life-threatening asthma patients may present with no wheeze or silent chest, tachycardia, cyanosis, fatigue, confusion, and agitation, which will require immediate intensive care management
- Generalised expiratory wheeze which commonly reflects airflow limitation
- Cough could be productive or non-productive
- Expiratory rhonchi throughout the chest on auscultation may be heard
- Use of accessory muscle or poor diaphragmatic excursion
- Prolonged expiratory phase
- Patients may present with hypertension along with tachycardia due to catecholamine release.

Diagnosis

The diagnosis of asthma is often challenging due to its heterogenicity and absence of consistent gold-standard diagnostic criteria. Usually, asthma diagnosis is made when:

- Patients present with episodic symptoms of wheeze, breathlessness, chest tightness, and cough
- Wheeze confirmed by healthcare professional on auscultation
- Evidence of diurnal variability (symptoms worse at night or early morning)
- History of atopy (personal history of eczema or hay fever or a family history of asthma and/or atopic conditions)
- Variability in peak expiratory flow (PEF) measurements (>20% diurnal variability on more than three days per week in a week of peak flow monitoring)
- Spirometry with bronchodilator reversibility – with obstructive spirometry (FEV1/FVC ratio less than 70%) showing an improvement in FEV1 of 12% or more along with an increase in volume of 200 ml or more post–bronchodilator, is considered a positive test
- Measurement of Fractional exhaled nitric oxide (FeNO) test – FeNO level of 40 parts per billion (ppb) or more is considered a positive test. However, overall sensitivity of this test is low. Therefore, this test is not advised outside the specialist centres.

BTS/SIGN has proposed the following algorithm for asthma diagnosis (see Figure 7.3).

Management

The aim of asthma treatment is to manage symptoms and to prevent asthma exacerbation. Management of asthma can be divided into acute and long-term management. Table 7.5 summarises the acute management for all asthma exacerbations that could be encountered in emergency care settings.

The long-term management of asthma focuses on controlling the disease, improving quality of life, therefore reducing hospital admissions and preventing asthma-related deaths.

The control of disease is defined as:

- Absence of daytime symptoms
- No nocturnal awakening
- No exacerbations
- Not using rescue medications
- No exercise or activity limitations due to asthma
- Normal lung function (FEV1 and/or PEF > 80% predicted or best)
- Minimal side effects from asthma medications

The effective long-term asthma management requires a partnership between the patient and healthcare professionals. Chronic asthma management includes both pharmacological and non-pharmacological measures. Asthma self-management programme includes a written personalised action plan and education. Periodic reviews on asthma control, medication compliance and inhaler technique, support for smoking cessation, and interventions are some of the non-pharmacological measures to improve asthma control.

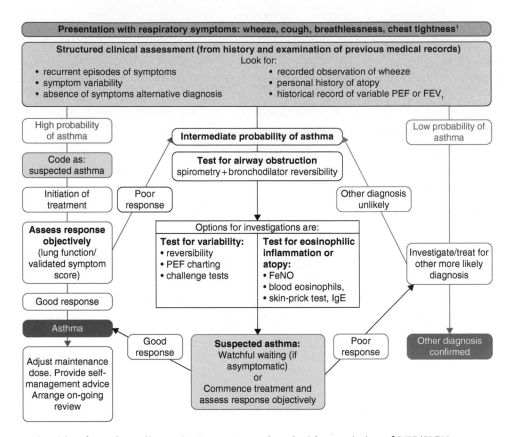

FIGURE 7.3   Algorithm for asthma diagnosis. *Source*: Reproduced with permission of BTS/SIGN.

TABLE 7.5   Management of acute asthma.

Step 1: Diagnosis

*Likely asthma – typical symptoms of wheeze, breathlessness, cough, nocturnal and early morning symptoms, family history of asthma or atopy, low PEFR, raised eosinophils. Go to Step 2.

*Possibly not asthma – No wheeze on examination, normal PEFR (when symptomatic), heavy smoker for prolonged period, voice disturbance, cardiac disease, productive cough. Consider other diagnosis.

Step 2: Assessment

Document clinical examination including RR, SaO_2, HR
Request ECG to rule out arrythmias.
Chest x-ray not routinely required unless consolidation or pneumothorax suspected. CXR is indicated for patients with life-threatening features or those who fail to improve with initial treatment.

PEF during admission _____ Peak flow Best/predicted _____ % of PEF of best _____

Step 3: Severity and management

| Moderate exacerbation | PEF 50–75% of best or predicted. No features of severe asthma | Controlled oxygen to maintain SaO_2 94–98% Nebulised salbutamol Prednisolone 40–50 mg stat, then until recovery (minimum of five days) |

TABLE 7.5   (Continued)

Severe exacerbation	Any one of: PEF 33–50% of best or predicted. Cannot complete a sentence in one breath. Heart rate ≥ 110/min Respiratory rate ≥ 25/min	In addition to above Discharge if PEF is > 75% best or predicted one hour after initial treatment Admit if severe asthma attack persisting after initial treatment Consider back-to-back continuous salbutamol nebuliser Nebulised ipratropium bromide 500 µg stat Nebuliser should be driven by oxygen
Life-threatening or near-fatal asthma	PEF < 30% of best or predicted. SaO2 < 92% on RA or ABG pO_2 < 8 kPa ABG CO_2 normal or high (>4.6 kPa) Cyanosis, poor respiratory effort near, or fully silent chest Exhaustion, confusion, arrythmias, or hypotension	In addition to above Consider single dose of IV magnesium sulphate (1.2–2 g infusion over 20 minutes) after discussion with senior medical staff Request ITU review

The well-established BTS/SIGN (2019) asthma guidelines provide a stepwise approach to pharmacological management of asthma (see Figure 7.4).

When starting inhaled corticosteroids (ICS), the dose should be adjusted based on the initial severity to achieve early control, then the dose needs to be adjusted (increased or decreased) based on the response. The success of inhaled treatment is dependent on the interaction between patient, drug, and device. Therefore, the inhaler technique should be checked during each contact with healthcare professionals.

Despite the long-term treatment, patients with asthma can develop mild exacerbations that would warrant follow up by the general practitioner (GP) following discharge from an emergency department. The discharge criteria for asthma patients are detailed in Table 7.6, and it is essential that if the patient has required admission to the hospital, they should be followed up by a respiratory or specialist asthma team.

Referral to a specialist service and/or additional investigations are recommended if the diagnosis is unclear, suspected occupational asthma, poor response to asthma treatment, patients with severe/life-threatening asthma attack, unexplained clinical findings such as fever, myalgia, weight loss, abnormal voice, dysphagia, stridor, crackles and clubbing, persistent breathlessness, chronic cough, chronic sputum production, unexplained restrictive spirometry, and abnormal chest x-ray (CXR) findings.

CHRONIC OBSTRUCTIVE PULMONARY DISEASE (COPD)

Chronic Obstructive Pulmonary Disease (COPD) is a preventable and chronic disease of the airways and lung parenchyma, the cardinal characteristics are gradual and consistent onset of breathlessness, productive cough, and recurrent chest infections associated with winter months. COPD exacerbations are responsible for the second highest rate of emergency admissions in the UK and 52.5% of COPD deaths occur in hospitals (OHID 2022).

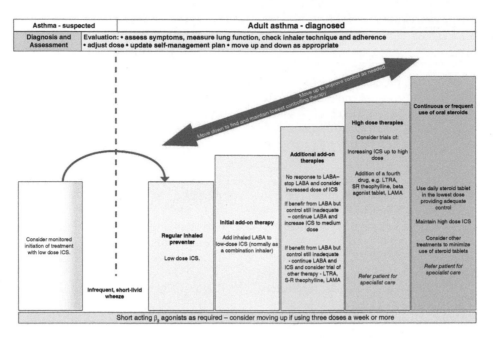

FIGURE 7.4   Pharmacological management of asthma. *Source*: Reproduced with permission from BTS/SIGN.

TABLE 7.6   Discharge criteria for a patient with asthma.

Discharge criteria
When patients are treated for severe or life-threatening asthma in secondary care, they can be discharged when their peak flow is >75% without nebuliser.
Five days course of steroids or longer course if eosinophilic.
Patients need to be referred to asthma specialist nurse.
When a patient is discharged from secondary care after being treated for an asthma exacerbation, the patient's primary care practice should be informed within 24 hours of discharge.
Patients should be given personalised asthma action plan.
Patients who had life-threatening/near-fatal asthma exacerbation should be under specialist care follow-up indefinitely.
Patients treated for a severe asthma exacerbation should be under respiratory specialist follow-up for at least one year.

Pathophysiology

Historically, there have been three overlapping pathophysiological phenotypes, with a recent addition of the term 'eosinophilic COPD'. Chronic Bronchitis affects predominantly the patency and architecture of the airways and typically features excessive sputum and recurrent chest infections. Emphysema primarily affects the parenchyma and airways by reducing compliance, damaging the alveoli and capillary interface causing air trapping. Both eosinophilic COPD and chronic asthma are characterised by a raised eosinophil count and are more responsive to tailored maintenance inhaled steroids where there is evidence of two exacerbations or more and/or at least one hospitalisation within the last year (GOLD 2022). More often, all of these features may exist within one individual of varying degrees which change as part of a continuum of the disease process. Aetiological susceptibilities include a minimum of 20 pack year smoking, exposure to airborne pollutants, genetic predisposition, and abnormal lung development. In COPD's later stages of disease progression, treatment modalities such as long-term oxygen therapy (LTOT) and non-invasive ventilation (NIV) are used to manage chronic and acute type 1 and type 2 respiratory failures, respectively.

Exacerbation – Characteristics and Risk Factors

An exacerbation of COPD can be described as an acute worsening of symptoms often requiring additional pharmacological support and can be further defined as infective or non-infective. The main exacerbation risk factors are bacterial and viral infections, air pollutants, gastro-oesophageal reflux (GORD), and swallowing dysfunction. Viruses are estimated to account for 22–50% of infective exacerbations. The most common bacterial pathogens identified are *Haemophilus Influenzae*, *Streptococcus Pneumoniae*, and *Moraxella Catarrhalis*. (GOLD 2022). Antibiotics should be given in accordance with local guidelines and with clinical symptoms of bacterial infection present. For example, a change in colour of sputum from the patient's normal or coughing up green sputum is usually clear. When presenting to secondary care the most common signs and symptoms of an exacerbation are shortness of breath and wheeze. Initial management would include bronchodilators and steroids given as close to presentation as possible. A nebulised solution of salbutamol should be administered to aid in rapid absorption locally within the airways and aim to prevent any further deterioration. Treatment should be tailored to the presenting complaint when considering an infective or non-infective exacerbation, with good antimicrobial stewardship playing an important role in the patient's long-term health outcomes.

Any patient presenting with worsening of their chronic symptoms should have a blood gas analysis performed as this will help rapidly identify those patients who have developed acute hypercapnic respiratory failure and may need NIV if optimal medical management is not successful. Optimal medical management is defined as back-to-back nebulised salbutamol and/or ipratropium nebulisers and steroids, administered either orally or intravenously, as soon as possible after presentation and reviewed after one hour of treatment to identify if the patient has improved. If after an hour of optimal medical management, the patient remains in hypercapnic respiratory failure, then NIV should be commenced according to local guidelines. Indications for NIV in hypercapnic respiratory failure are detailed later in this chapter.

Exacerbations may also be triggered by co-existing co-morbidities and patients with severe COPD are more likely to have right-sided heart failure known as Cor pulmonale. This is due to hyperinflation in the lungs causing increased pulmonary artery pressure leading to right ventricular dilatation. Lifestyle advice can be as important as any pharmacological intervention. Very brief smoking advice should be given at each presentation, and patients should be encouraged and assisted to stop smoking. Nicotine replacement therapy in conjunction with a referral to specialist stop-smoking services will vastly improve the likelihood of achieving smoking cessation. Patients whose symptoms are leading to a reduction in their ability to undertake activities of daily livings (ADL's) and a reduction in their exercise tolerance should be offered pulmonary rehabilitation which is organised by local community respiratory teams.

Clinical Investigations

Vital Signs

Monitoring vital signs once admitted is essential to notice any deterioration in the patient's condition. If the patient is known to have chronic hypercapnic respiratory failure, a reduction in target saturations should be recorded on the oxygen prescription chart and controlled oxygen titrated appropriately. This could help prevent the patient from further deterioration or needing NIV to correct over oxygenation.

Chest X-ray

This will provide valuable information on potential causes of the exacerbation. It will also be useful for any differential diagnoses such as pneumonia, pneumothorax, or pleural effusion. It is essential to take a thorough approach to CXR interpretation and compare to previous imaging if available. Patients with severe COPD may develop bullae, which, if large enough, may be confused with a pneumothorax, and in these cases, a chest drain insertion may prove fatal.

Biomarkers

Routine blood tests should be performed according to the presenting complaint and this will provide evidence to inform decision-making around antibiotics or other treatment. Interpretation should occur in context of the patient history including medication history. Recent course of steroids or long-term steroid use can give a raised white cell count that may not be because of an infective aetiology.

Blood Gas Analysis

As a screening test a venous blood gas (VBG) can be performed, this will identify if the patient has evidence of chronic hypercapnic respiratory failure or if there is evidence of an acute decompensation. If the patient is acidotic on a VBG, then an arterial blood gas analysis (ABG) should be performed to confirm or rule out acute decompensation.

Discharging

When considering discharging patients from a non-specialist area, it is important to consider the following:

- Provide very brief stop-smoking advice where appropriate and refer to outpatient stop-smoking services
- Refer to local community COPD team for COPD diagnosis, if this is a first presentation, or long-term management
- Refer to community pulmonary rehabilitation team.

RESPIRATORY FAILURE

Respiratory failure is a potentially life-threatening condition, so timely identification and management are important. In the first instance, it is important to consider whether the patient has acute, chronic, or acute-on-chronic respiratory failure. Gathering a past medical history from the patient or, if they are unable to communicate, from a relative or friend is paramount. There are two types of respiratory failure, hypoxic and hypercapnic.

Type 1 Respiratory Failure (Hypoxic)

This is an oxygenation issue secondary to ventilation perfusion mismatch resulting in the patient becoming hypoxic. This is defined as a $PaO2 < 8\,kpa$ on an ABG. Several pathologies can cause hypoxic respiratory failure resulting in oxygen not reaching the circulatory system; for example, pneumonia, pulmonary oedema, pulmonary embolism (PE), asthma, emphysema, pulmonary fibrosis, or acute respiratory distress syndrome (ARDS).

Type 2 Respiratory Failure (Hypercapnic)

This is a ventilation issue that causes inadequate removal of carbon dioxide through normal exhalation. It is characterised by hypercapnia which is defined as a $PaCO2 > 6.0\,kpa$ on an ABG. Hypercapnic respiratory failure can be caused by diseases such as COPD, asthma, end-stage pulmonary fibrosis, reduced respiratory drive from sedative drugs, neuromuscular disease such as motor neurone disease, Guillain-Barre syndrome, or a thoracic wall deformity such as kyphoscoliosis.

Signs and Symptoms of Respiratory Failure

The signs the patient will be exhibiting will depend on which type of respiratory failure and what the underlying cause is. Patients with chronic lung disease may show signs that will help identify the cause of their respiratory failure, such as high body mass index with obesity hypoventilation syndrome although this may not always be the case. Common signs and symptoms of respiratory failure can be seen in Table 7.7.

Investigations

Arterial blood gas: This is crucial in identifying what type of respiratory failure the patient is presenting with. Even if you have established from the past medical history that the patient has an underlying respiratory condition a blood gas will help monitor any subsequent response to treatment and identify how far off their baseline the patient is. Examples of ABG showing respiratory failure can be seen in Table 7.8.

Chest X-ray

This is helpful in identifying any potential causes of the respiratory failure and ruling out any contraindications for NIV that may affect further treatment, for example, pneumothorax. Further, Computed Tomography (CT) imaging may be necessary but referral to a respiratory specialist and stability of the patient's condition should take priority.

TABLE 7.7   Signs and symptoms of respiratory failure.

Signs of Type 1 respiratory failure	Signs of Type 2 respiratory failure
• Tachypnoea • Cyanosis • Agitation • Tachycardia	• Dyspnoea • Hypoventilation • Reduced conscious level • Confusion • Bounding radial pulse • CO_2 retention flap (asterixis)

TABLE 7.8 Examples of ABG showing respiratory failure.

Example of T1RF	Example of T2RF
pH – normal/high	pH – low
PaO_2 – low	PaO_2 – low
pCO_2 – normal/low	$PaCO_2$ – high
HCO_3 – normal	HCO_3 – raised (if chronic and is a marker of chronicity)

Vital Signs

Most importantly, oxygen saturations but also blood pressure, heart rate, respiratory rate, and temperature.

Biomarkers

Blood tests include urea and electrolytes, full blood count, liver function tests and C – reactive protein. This is not an exhaustive list, and other factors pertinent to the presenting complaint should also be considered.

Management of Type 1 Respiratory Failure

Oxygen therapy should be commenced and titrated to achieve the target oxygen saturations according to the prescription. The amount of oxygen required may determine the most appropriate mode of delivery and aid in decision-making around escalation of care and destination for the patient, such as a level one or two area. The treatment of the underlying cause is paramount in correcting the hypoxaemia, as oxygen is a supportive measure, for example antibiotics for pneumonia, anticoagulation for pulmonary embolus (PE), and diuretics for pulmonary oedema.

Management of Type 2 Respiratory Failure

Commence controlled oxygen therapy to keep saturations within a reduced target of 88–92%. If there is hypoxia and hypercapnia, then the hypoxia should not go untreated, but the patient needs to be closely monitored. A repeat blood gas analysis should be undertaken 30 minutes after commencing oxygen therapy and any time the oxygen is titrated. The danger is that the patient receives too much oxygen, which dampens their respiratory drive and makes the hypercapnia worse.

An appropriate management plan will consider the ceiling of care a patient should receive. If oxygen therapy for a patient in T2RF causes a patient's acidosis to get worse, for example, then NIV may be required. To initiate NIV, it is encouraged that early conversations with seniors or the respiratory team will support decisions in this treatment pathway. Prior to commencing NIV, it is essential that an ABG is obtained rather than a venous sample; this is important to monitor response to treatment. Contraindications to NIV should be excluded and the settings used should be commenced according to local guidelines. Settings should be titrated as tolerated and assessed at regular intervals to determine clinical response.

COMMUNITY ACQUIRED PNEUMONIA (CAP)

Pneumonia can be caused by many different organisms including bacteria, viruses, and fungi. The most common organism associated with the development of pneumonia is the *Streptococcus pneumoniae* bacteria. Other common organisms that can cause pneumonia include *Haemophilus influenzae*, *Legionella pneumophilia*, and *Staphylococcus aureus*.

Certain groups of people are more at risk of developing pneumonia than others:

- Extremes of age – elderly and babies/young children
- Those with other co-morbidities such as asthma, cystic fibrosis
- Immunocompromised patients – cancer, immunosuppression medication, Human Immunodeficiency Virus (HIV), Acquired Immunodeficiency Syndrome (AIDS)
- Smokers

Altered Pathophysiology

Pneumonia is a respiratory tract infection in which the alveoli become filled with fluid and exudate, and therefore impair gaseous exchange. Community acquired pneumonia is defined as pneumonia acquired outside of a hospital or healthcare setting, most commonly caused by bacterial or viral pathogens (BMJ 2021). These pathogens cause inflammation or consolidation in the lungs. There are several types of pneumonia which include:

- **Bacterial pneumonia**
- **Viral pneumonia including COVID-19 pneumonia** – associated with viruses such as the influenza virus and respiratory syncytial virus (RSV).
- **Aspiration pneumonia** – small amounts of stomach contents can be aspirated into the lungs in those who have been unconscious or drowsy, and in those with dysphagia.
- **Hospital acquired pneumonia (HAP)** – diagnostic criteria and guidelines vary but is associated with pneumonia that develops during an inpatient stay in a healthcare facility. HAP develops within 48 hours following admission to the hospital or within 7 days of discharge. Antibiotic choice is governed by the pathogens which cause healthcare associated pneumonia.
- ***Pneumocystis jirovecii* pneumonia (PJP)** – pneumonia caused by the fungal organism *Pneumocystis jirovecii* in those immunocompromised patients. This may be a first presentation of HIV.

Diagnosis of CAP

Pneumonia is diagnosed based on clinical signs and symptoms and investigation results. The most common signs and symptoms seen in a patient with pneumonia can be seen in Table 7.9. NICE advises that all patients admitted to the hospital with suspected pneumonia have a diagnosis and treatment commenced within four hours of presentation.

TABLE 7.9   Signs and symptoms of CAP.

- Shortness of breath
- Pleuritic chest pain
- Hypoxia
- Fever
- Cough
- Purulent sputum

Investigations

- **Full set of observations** – most importantly the respiratory rate, and oxygen saturations to look for evidence of hypoxia.
- **Chest x-ray** – all patients admitted to the hospital should have a CXR if they have signs or symptoms of infection. This will show any areas of consolidation in the lung and confirm diagnosis.
- **Blood tests** – U&Es (assess for dehydration and calculate CURB 65 score), CRP (establish a baseline and will be elevated in infection), and FBC (elevated white cell count can indicate infection).
- Microbiological investigations should be performed on those with a moderate or severe CAP (BTS 2015) – in hospital sputum cultures, blood cultures, and urine antigens should be sent.
- **Sputum culture** – send sputum cultures in all patients who are productive to identify any causative organisms.
- **Pneumococcal and *Legionella* urinary antigens** – should be sent in those with moderate or severe pneumonia.
- **Arterial blood gas** – in those with hypoxia/oxygen requirement to assess for evidence of respiratory failure requiring further treatment and careful oxygen titration.
- **HIV test** – recommended in those <65 years.

Treatments

The CURB 65 score is used to categorise risk of mortality into low, moderate, or high based on the criteria in Table 7.10. These criteria can be used in primary care to assess need for hospital treatment (excluding urea) or in hospital to assess risk of mortality and guide treatment decisions (NICE 2022). Antibiotic guidelines will vary from trust to trust – therefore please consult your own trusted CAP antibiotic policy. Remember antibiotic stewardship – start with broad spectrum antibiotics based on severity according to local guidelines then focus according to microbiological results.

TABLE 7.10   CURB 65 criteria to assess risk of mortality in hospital.

CURB 65 criteria to assess risk of mortality in hospital (one point allocated to each feature)

Confusion – AMT 8 or less or new confusion
Urea – elevated level >7 mmol/l
Respiratory rate – ≥30
Blood pressure – systolic <90 mmHg or diastolic <60 mmHg
65 years or more age

Score 0–1 – low risk (<3% mortality risk)
2 – intermediate risk (3–15% mortality risk)
3–5 – high risk (>15% mortality risk)
(Lim et al. 2003)

Complications

All inpatients who fail to improve with maximal treatment should be reassessed for any evidence of complications. Further investigations such as CT, thoracentesis, and discussion with microbiology and/or thoracic surgeons may be required depending on the complication identified. Table 7.11 identifies some complications associated with pneumonia.

Follow Up and Clinical Review

Patients can be discharged from hospital when they are clinically stable. NICE criteria for safe discharge from hospital should be followed (see Table 7.12). Patients should be informed that it may take up to six months for their symptoms to fully resolve and for them to feel back to normal (NICE 2022). A follow up CXR should be organised six weeks after discharge for those patients in hospital, who have a confirmed diagnosis of CAP and have persistent symptoms or high risk of malignancy (especially smokers, age > 50 years) whether admitted to the hospital or not (BTS 2015). However, all patients should receive clinical review with their hospital or GP after six weeks. Some hospital trusts have a respiratory infections team with dedicated specialist nurses who will provide the patients with written information, supported discharge, and organise follow up imaging. Further investigations such as imaging or bronchoscopy may be required if there are persistent symptoms or non-resolving CXR changes.

TABLE 7.11 Complications of CAP.

Complications of CAP

- **Parapneumonic effusion** – may require ultrasound guided diagnostic/therapeutic drainage.
- **Empyema** – may require chest drain insertion and/or prolonged course of antibiotics. If no improvement/ signs of deterioration, then discussion with thoracic surgeons regarding any surgical intervention that may be required.
- **Type 1 respiratory failure** – may require ventilator support in a high dependency or intensive care setting. Usually in those with severe pneumonia.
- **Pleurisy** – should be relieved with treatment of the pneumonia and analgesia.
- **Lung abscess** – prolonged antibiotic course will be required.

TABLE 7.12 NICE criteria for safe discharge from hospital.

Safe discharge from hospital

Not to be discharged if the patient has had two of the following within the last 48 hours.
- Pyrexia > 37.5
- Respiratory rate > 24
- Tachycardia > 100
- Systolic blood pressure < 90 mmHg
- Oxygen saturations <90% on air
- Abnormal mental status
- Inability to eat without assistance

PULMONARY EMBOLISM

A pulmonary embolism (PE) is a blockage of one or multiple pulmonary arteries in your lungs. Pulmonary embolism is one of the most common acute cardiovascular presentations alongside myocardial infarction and stroke. While no exact epidemiological data is available, the incidence is estimated to be 60 per 100 000. Symptoms are variable from asymptomatic, incidental findings to sudden cardiovascular collapse and death, and is a major cause of morbidity and mortality in healthcare.

Altered Pathophysiology

Around 70% of PE are generated in the deep venous system of the lower limbs and pelvis. Clots ascend the inferior vena cava to the right heart and obstruct the pulmonary vasculature. Platelet aggregation around venous valve sinuses, activation of the clotting cascade, and the influence of Virchow's triad (see Figure 7.5) result in thrombus formation. The haemodynamic effects of a PE depend upon thrombus size, area of obstruction, and pre-existing cardiac function. Clinical characteristics can be seen in Table 7.13.

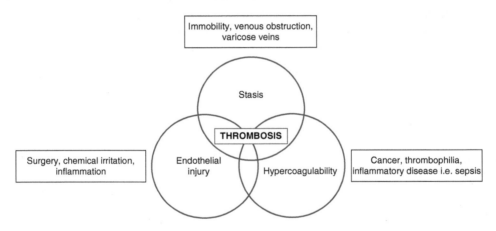

FIGURE 7.5   Virchow's Triad.

TABLE 7.13   Clinical characteristics of PE.

Feature	PE Confirmed (%)
Dyspnoea	50
Pleuritic chest pain	39
Cough	23
Sub-sternal chest pain	15
Fever	10
Haemoptysis	8
Syncope	6
Signs of DVT	24

TABLE 7.14   Risk factors for PE.

Strong risk factors (odds ratio > 10)
Lower limb fracture
Hospitalisation for heart failure or atrial fibrillation/flutter (within three months)
Hip or knee replacement
Major trauma
MI (within three months)
Previous VTE
Acute spinal cord injury
Puerperium

Moderate risk factors (odds ratio 2–9)
Arthroscopic knee surgery
Auto-immune diseases
Blood transfusion
Central venous lines
Congestive heart or respiratory failure
Erythropoiesis stimulating agents
HRT (depends on formulation)
In vitro fertilisation
Infection (specifically pneumonia, UTI, and HIV)
Inflammatory bowel disease
Cancer (highest risk in metastatic disease)
Oral contraceptive therapy
Paralytic stroke
Pregnancy
Superficial vein thrombosis
Thrombophilia

Weak risk factors (odds ratio < 2)
Bed rest >3 days
Diabetes mellitus
Hypertension
Immobility due to sitting (e.g. prolonged car or air travel)
Increasing age
Laparoscopic surgery (e.g. cholecystectomy)
Obesity
Varicose veins

There are several risk factors which increase the risk for developing a PE (see Table 7.14). This is not an exhaustive list and clinical judgement should be used when considering PE as a differential diagnosis.

Diagnosis

Diagnosis of PE can be challenging, and initial evaluation should include comprehensive history and examination coupled with pre-test probability assessment. The Pulmonary Embolism Rule-out Criteria (PERC) is utilised by clinicians to avoid further testing for PE in patients deemed low risk. The PERC rule (see Table 7.15) is a 'rule-out' tool – all variables must receive a 'no' to be negative. When used correctly, the PERC score is as accurate for ruling out PE as D-dimer.

TABLE 7.15   The PERC rule.

PERC rule for pulmonary embolism	
Age > 50	Yes/No
HR > or equal to 100	Yes/No
O$_2$ saturation on room air < 95%	Yes/No
Prior history of DVT/PE	Yes/No
Recent trauma or surgery	Yes/No
Haemoptysis	Yes/No
Exogenous oestrogen	Yes/No
Unilateral leg swelling	Yes/No

TABLE 7.16   Wells score.

Criteria	Points
Clinical signs/symptoms of DVT	3
PE is the most likely diagnosis	3
Tachycardia (>100 bpm)	1.5
Immobilisation/surgery in previous four weeks	1.5
Prior DVT/PE	1.5
Haemoptysis	1
Active malignancy	1
Low risk < 2 points **intermediate risk** 2–6 points **high risk** > 6 points	
PE Unlikely 0–4 points **PE likely > 4 points**	

Wells' Score

The score is simple to use and provides clear limits for the predicted probability of PE to support ratio-nalisation of Computerised Tomography Pulmonary Artery (CTPA) (see Table 7.16).

Investigations

Chest X-Ray

Often normal findings, it is not diagnostic of PE; however, linear wedge-shaped shadows, small pleural effusions, and localised patchiness of vasculature may be visible. CXR is a useful test in the evaluation and exclusion of alternative diagnosis the may account for the presenting complaint.

Electrocardiogram (ECG)

Electrocardiogram is neither sensitive nor specific enough to diagnose or exclude PE with around 18% patients having a completely normal ECG. Changes seen are related to dilation and pressure on right atrium/right ventricle, right ventricular ischaemia, and increased stimulation of sympathetic nervous system secondary to hypoxia, pain, and anxiety. Findings may include sinus tachycardia, right axis deviation, right Bundle branch block (RBBB), or S1Q3T3. The most common finding on ECG is sinus tachycardia with S1Q3T3 being very rare.

Biomarkers

Troponin

Elevated levels of troponin I and T are found in over 30% of patients with acute PE. Meta-analysis has shown that elevated troponin concentrations are associated with an increased risk of mortality, which becomes important to assess when considering management via an ambulatory pathway.

D-Dimer

D-dimer are breakdown products from fibrinolysis and are raised in several circumstances. They are only useful for exclusion of PE in patients already deemed to be at low risk, and used in conjunction with pre-test clinical probability assessment and clinical evaluation. D-dimer levels are sensitive for PE diagnosis and have a high negative predictive value, but low specificity, being elevated in conditions such as malignancy, sepsis, and pregnancy.

Computerised Tomography Pulmonary Artery (CTPA)

Gold standard modality of choice, CTPA has a sensitivity of 83% and specificity of 96% for PE diagnosis. Counselling of radiation must occur with patients undergoing imaging modality.

V/Q Scan

Ventilation/perfusion single photon emission computed tomography (V/Q SPECT) scan may be offered as an alternative in some cases. V/Q scan is only useful in patients who do not have an alternative pathology that will affect ventilation or perfusion, as the imaging is unable to differentiate alternative causes of V/Q mismatch, such as pneumonia.

Management

Classification of PE severity (see Table 7.17) dictates place of management and observation. Low-risk patients can be managed ambulatory if circumstances allow with all other cases managed as inpatients. In haemodynamic instability and those patients in the intermediate/high-risk category should have a minimum period of 48 hours with cardiac monitoring in a level 1 environment. Those in the intermediate/low-risk category are safe to be observed on a medical or respiratory ward.

TABLE 7.17   PE severity risk.

Early mortality risk		Indicators of risk			
		Haemodynamic instability	Clinical parameters and PESI 3–4	RV dysfunction on TTE/CTPA	Elevated cardiac troponin levels
High		+	+	+	+
Intermediate	High	–	+	+	+
	Low	–	+	One (or none) positive	
Low		–	–	–	– (assessment optional)

Clinical Guidelines

NICE guidelines recommend CTPA is performed within one hour in suspected massive PE, and within 24 hours in non-massive PE. Patients with suspected PE and a raised troponin should have a CTPA within four hours. Leg ultrasound may be performed as the initial investigation, where there are signs and symptoms of both deep vein thrombosis (DVT) and PE. If imaging is not being performed immediately, give interim anticoagulation and, if possible, choose an anticoagulant that can be continued if PE is confirmed. Imaging should be performed within 24 hours to avoid the need for prolonged unnecessary anticoagulation. PE should be treated with anticoagulation for a minimum of three months. Patients with no identifiable risk factors for venous thromboembolism should be considered for lifelong anticoagulation after balancing risk of recurrence against bleeding risk. Choice of coagulation can be seen in Table 7.18.

TABLE 7.18   Choice of coagulation.

DOACS – 1st choice	LMWH/heparin	Warfarin
• Inhibit Factor Xa, Reduces thrombin production	• Activate antithrombin which accelerates the inactivation of coagulation enzymes	• Competitively inhibits vitamin K epoxide reductase complex 1 (VKORC1),
• 1st line treatment in VTE • Predictable pharmacokinetics and dynamics • Baseline bloods needed to assess if appropriate	• Used in GI malignancy • 1st line in pregnancy • Used in severe hepatic impairment	• Good INR control • Antiphospholipid • Mechanical valve • CrCL < 30 ml/min • Recurrent VTE on DOAC

Bleeding risk must be assessed on a case by case basis
Check Hb and renal function

Discharge Criteria

Dependent on severity, the length of stay will vary from ambulatory management to a prolonged inpatient stay if complications develop. Follow up in designated PE clinic at three months to assess symptoms and ongoing management is essential and will vary depending on what provisions are available locally.

LUNG CANCER

Lung cancer remains the biggest cause for cancer-related death in the western world, with 85–90% of these cases related to smoking. Survival from lung cancer is largely affected by the staging of extent of the disease at diagnosis; therefore, early detection is imperative. Symptoms can be non-specific such as anorexia and weight loss or more specific such as chronic cough or haemoptysis and related to localised tumour effect or metastatic disease effect. Treatment options are guided by staging, type of lung cancer, and performance status (see Section 7.2). Treatment options can include traditional chemotherapy and radiotherapy through to immunotherapy depending on genotyping of malignancy. There are several risk factors for lung cancer which can be seen in Table 7.19.

Patients can present with signs and symptoms that are both specific and non-specific to lung cancer. This can make diagnosing lung cancer difficult as symptoms can overlap with other pathologies and may help to explain why patients present at a later stage. The key symptoms that should make a clinician consider lung cancer as a diagnosis are persistent cough which is present in around 50% of the cases, haemoptysis around 35%, shortness of breath and inspiratory wheeze or stridor that could represent large airway obstruction. A list of other signs and symptoms to consider are in Figure 7.6.

Signs and symptoms concerning a lung malignancy (see Figure 7.6) should initially be investigated with a CXR. However, this only has a detection rate of between 77% and 80%. A CXR alone cannot exclude a malignancy if no abnormality is detected, and symptoms are highly suggestive. The next stage is CT of the chest, abdomen, and pelvis. This will determine the extent of disease and sites for tissue or cytological biopsy. Tissue or cytological diagnosis along with radiological findings is used to confirm staging of disease (see Tables 7.20 and 7.21). Staging in conjunction with performance status is essential to determine what treatment options are available for patients. These decisions are typically guided by the lung cancer multidisciplinary team. Investigations and rationale can be seen in Table 7.20.

TABLE 7.19   Risk factors for lung cancer.

Occupational	Environmental	Genetics	Pre-disposing medical conditions
Radiation exposure	Air pollution	Previous family history of lung cancer	Pulmonary fibrosis
Asbestos exposure such as mines, mills, shipyard workers	Smoking and second-hand smoke	Previous history of lung cancer	Emphysema
Silica exposure	Heavy metal/arsenic exposure	Previous history of cancer that could metastasize to the lungs	HIV

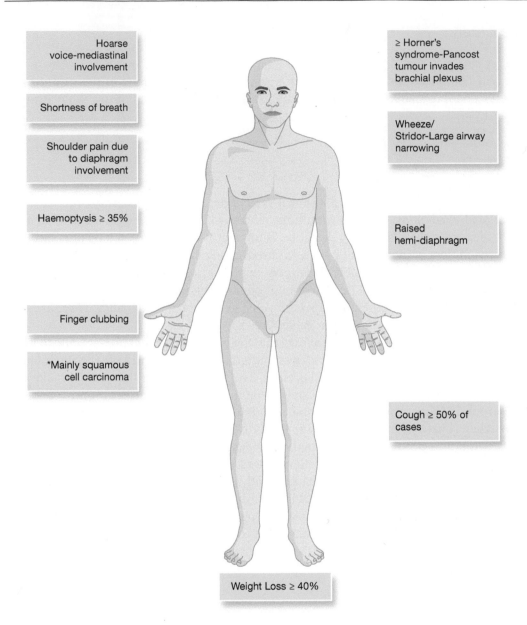

FIGURE 7.6   Signs and symptoms of both specific and non-specific to lung cancer.

Initial Acute Management

The initial management of findings in an emergent setting will depend on how stable the patient is, availability of initial investigations, and what ambulatory pathways are available.

The most common finding for lung cancer prompting admission to the hospital is a unilateral pleural effusion. In most cases, a pleural effusion alone will not be enough to make a patient hypoxic, but they may be breathless depending on the volume of the effusion. For most cases, a patient with a unilateral effusion can be managed as an outpatient with investigations such as diagnostic and/or therapeutic aspiration. This may lead to more invasive investigations such as bronchoscopy or medical thoracoscopy.

TABLE 7.20   Investigations and rationale.

Investigation	Rationale
CT neck, chest, abdomen, and pelvis with contrast	Initial investigation to assess stage of disease and assess appropriate site for biopsy to confirm tissue diagnosis
PET CT	Shows metabolically active sites and can pick up metastasis and further potential sites for biopsy to aid tissue diagnosis
Endobronchial Ultrasound (EBUS)/EUS	Ultrasound is used to examine the airways and take biopsies of abnormal tissue within the airways
Pleural tap/aspiration	Sample of pleural fluid is removed and sent for diagnosis. If symptomatic, a larger volume up to 1500 ml can be removed.
Fine needle aspiration/deep core biopsy	Small needle is inserted into mass or fluid to get a sample of cells
Radiological guided biopsy	Sample of cells is taken under guidance of CT

TABLE 7.21   Classification of lung cancer.

Lung cancers are classified into two main groups	Common sub-type	Presentation
Non-small cell lung cancer 80% of lung cancer	Squamous cell lung cancer including Pancoast tumour	• Potential mass on CXR • Can cavitate and look like lung abscess • Consider hypercalcaemia
	Adenocarcinoma	• Not always smoking related • Can occur in scar tissue or fibrosis • Can cause pleural effusions
	Mesothelioma	• Unilateral disease • Pleural thickening • Unilateral pleural effusion
Small cell lung cancer 15% of lung cancer	Neuroendocrine tumours	• Aggressive and usually metastatic at the time of presentation • Metastasizes to liver, bones, bone marrow, brain, adrenals • SIADH with hyponatraemia (~10% of patients) • Rapidly progressive with median survival six weeks, if extensive disease and left untreated

When patients present with haemoptysis, the preferred investigation is CT, the type of CT will depend largely on the amount of haemoptysis present. More commonly, a CTPA will be performed which is useful to rule out PE as a cause for haemoptysis. In large volume haemoptysis, a CT of the thoracic aorta could be considered to try and isolate a bleeding point amenable to embolisation. The amount to define a large volume is difficult to judge and the term 'life threatening' haemoptysis is starting to be used. A volume of around 100 ml in 24 hours should be used as this is the most common amount in the literature that could pose a risk to a patient's life (Ibrahim 2008).

Classification of Lung Cancer

Tissue or cytological diagnosis will determine classification of lung cancer (see Table 7.15). This is broadly divided into two main categories: non-small cell and small cell malignancy. Details of typical radiological and biochemical findings are listed in the table.

Treatments

Initial acute treatment should address the presenting complaint and focus on symptomatic relief. For those who present with large volume haemoptysis, tranexamic acid can be used as a holding measure while awaiting imaging and definitive treatment plan.

Long-term treatment options for lung cancer can include chemotherapy, radiotherapy, surgery, and immunotherapy, which is dependent on genotyping. This is considered in context of performance status and type of lung cancer identified. Performance status greater than three can limit radical treatment options and focus can be for best supportive care rather than curative, such as palliative radiotherapy if severe pain at sites of bony metastases. A move towards and enhanced supportive care with early palliative care involvement has shown an improvement in mean survival following non-curative lung cancer diagnosis.

Take Home Points
- Advanced practitioners must have expert knowledge and the ability to lead on the care of patients presenting with acute respiratory illness.
- Effective history-taking and physical examination skills are paramount for patient safety and offer improved differential diagnosis
- Evidence-based practice using tools, clinical guidelines, and contemporary research encourages clinicians to deliver modern, safe, and effective respiratory treatment and management for acutely unwell patients.

REFERENCES

BLF. (2023) *Asthama Statistics* [online]. Available from: https://statistics.blf.org.uk/asthma [accessed 21 June 2023].

BMJ Best Practice. (2021). *Overview of Pneumonia* [online]. Available from: https://bestpractice.bmj.com [accessed 21 June 2023].

British Thoracic Society (BTS). (updated 2015). *Annotated BTS Guideline for the Management of CAP in Adults (2009) Summary of Recommendations* [online]. Available from: http://www.brit-thoracic.org.uk [accessed 21 June 2023].

Global Initiative for Chronic Obstructive Lung Disease (GOLD) (2022). *Global Strategy for Prevention, Diagnosis and Management of COPD* [online]. Available from: https://goldcopd.org/2022-gold-reports/# [accessed 21 June 2023].

Health Education England (HEE). (2022). *Advanced Clinical Practice in Acute Medicine Curriculum Framework – Credentials* [online]. Available from: https://advanced-practice.hee.nhs.uk/our-work/credentials [accessed 20 June 2023].

Health Education England (HEE). (2017). *Multi-professional Framework for Advanced Clinical Practice in England* [online]. Available from: `https://www.hee.nhs.uk/sites/default/files/documents/multi-professionalframeworkforadvancedclinicalpracticeinengland.pdf` [accessed 20 June 2023].

Ibrahim, W.H. (2008). Massive haemoptysis: the definition should be revised. *European Respiratory Journal* 2008 (32): 1131.

Lim, W.S., Van der Eerden, M.M., Laing, R. et al. (2003). Defining community-acquired pneumonia severity on presentation to hospital: an international derivation and validation study. *Thorax* 58: 377–382.

Naser, A.Y. et al. (2021). Hospital admission trends due to respiratory diseases in England and Wales between 1999 and 2019: an ecologic study. *BMC Pulmonary Medicine* 21: 356. `https://doi.org/10.1186/s12890-021-01736-8`.

NHS Digital. (2022). *Provisional Monthly Hospital Episode Statistics for Admitted Patient Care, Outpatient and Accident and Emergency Data* [online]. Available from: `https://digital.nhs.uk/data-and-information/publications/statistical/provisional-monthly-hospital-episode-statistics-for-admitted-patient-care-outpatient-and-accident-and-emergency-data/april-2022---may-2022` [accessed 21 June 2023].

Oken, M.M., Creech, R.H., Tormey, D.C. et al. (1982). Toxicity and response criteria of the Eastern Cooperative Oncology Group. *American Journal of Clinical Oncology* 5 (6): 649–655. PMID: 7165009.

The Faculty of Intensive Care Medicine. (2018). *Curriculum for Training for Advanced Critical Care Practitioners – Syllabus. V1.1* [online]. Available from: `www.ficm.ac.uk/media/6896` [accessed 20 June 2023].

The Intensive Care Society, Critical Care Networks – *National Nurse Leads and The National Outreach Forum*. (2022). *Advanced Critical Care Outreach Competencies* [online]. Available from: `https://ics.ac.uk/asset/43B8C11B-4512-41D0-B97768FABA2C30B2` [accessed 20 June 2023].

The Royal College of Emergency Medicine. (2022). *Emergency Medicine Advanced Clinical Practitioner Curriculum 2022 (Adult)* [online]. Available from: `https://rcem.ac.uk/wp-content/uploads/2022/09/ACP_Curriculum_Adult_Final_060922.pdf` [accessed 20 June 2023].

FURTHER READING

NICE Quality standards [online]. Available from: `www.nice.org.uk/search?q=respiratory+&ndt=Guidance&ndt=Quality+standards` [accessed 21 June 2023].

CHAPTER 8

Cardiac Presentations

Rachel Wong

Aim

This chapter aims to enable the Advanced Practitioner (AP) to critically develop their clinical reasoning and diagnostic skills when assessing and managing patients presenting with acute cardiac emergencies.

LEARNING OUTCOMES

After reading this chapter the reader will have a comprehensive knowledge of:

1. Cardiac anatomy and physiology.
2. The application of understanding of cardiac physiology when making a diagnosis.
3. The knowledge and skills needed to undertake a detailed, focused cardiac history and clinical assessment.
4. The evidence base for the use and interpretation of clinical investigations when assessing patients presenting with cardiac conditions.
5. Decision-making skills around pharmacological interventions for patients with acute cardiac emergencies.
6. The application of advanced cardiac clinical diagnostic and management skills to patient scenarios.

SELF-ASSESSMENT QUESTIONS

1. Which ventricle is most susceptible to ischaemia and why?
2. Name three modifiable risk factors for cardiovascular disease.

The Advanced Practitioner in Acute, Emergency and Critical Care, First Edition. Edited by Sadie Diamond-Fox, Barry Hill, Sonya Stone, Caroline McCrea, Natalie Gardner, and Angela Roberts.
© 2024 John Wiley & Sons Ltd. Published 2024 by John Wiley & Sons Ltd.

3. Which diuretic is commonly used in heart failure? What is its mechanism of action?
4. List three ECG findings in a patient presenting with an Acute Coronary Syndrome.

INTRODUCTION

Ischaemic heart disease is the leading cause of death worldwide, responsible for 16% of the world's total deaths (WHO 2020). It is of paramount importance that the ACP can diagnose and promote health-seeking behaviours to prevent and manage this disease.

This chapter will provide an overview of the clinical assessment and examination of the patient presenting with an acute cardiac emergency. This will be aligned with national and international guidelines to allow the reader to uphold professional and best standards of practice.

We will review cardiac anatomy and physiology and explore the application of this knowledge when assessing and diagnosing cardiac conditions, to enable the ACP to develop the necessary skills and knowledge to undertake a focused cardiac history and examination. The reader will critically explore and justify the use of clinical investigations and pharmacological interventions to assist with making a competent diagnosis and management plan for patients with acute cardiac emergencies.

This chapter will enable the reader to evaluate and reflect upon their cardiac assessment skills through exploration of clinical case scenarios from patients presenting with a variety of cardiac conditions.

Multi-professional Framework (MPF) for Advanced Clinical Practice Guidance for Professional Development (HEE 2017)

This chapter maps to the following statements within the MPF:

1. Clinical Practice:	1.1	1.2	1.3	1.4	1.5	1.6	1.7	1.8	1.9	1.10	1.11
2. Leadership and Management:	2.1	2.2	2.3	2.4	2.7	2.8					
3. Education:	3.1	3.2	3.6								
4. Research:	4.3										

Accreditation Considerations

This chapter maps to the following statements within the following national accreditation documents:

Curriculum for Training for Advanced Critical Care Practitioners Syllabus V1.1
(The Faculty of Intensive Care Medicine 2018)

2.1	2.2	2.3	2.6	2.7	4.1	4.2	4.3	4.4

Advanced Critical Care Outreach Competencies
(The Intensive Care Society, Critical Care Networks – National Nurse Leads and The National Outreach Forum 2022)

A3	A4

Emergency Medicine Advanced Clinical Practitioner Curriculum 2022 – Adult (The Royal College of Emergency Medicine 2022)						
SLO3	SLO6	RP3	CP1-3	CC1-CC8	CC11-CC13	

Advanced Clinical Practice in Acute Medicine Curriculum Framework
(Health Education England 2022)

- Generic clinical CiPs: 1, 2, 4
- Specialty Clinical CiPs: 3, 4
- Presentations and Conditions for ACPs in Acute Medicine: Cardiology, Clinical pharmacology

THE CARDIOVASCULAR SYSTEM

Anatomy

The heart is situated in the centre of the thorax, to the left of the midline, and between the lungs. This vital muscular organ pumps blood around the two main circulatory systems, the pulmonary and systemic circulations. It is divided into four chambers, two atria and two ventricles, which can be further subdivided into their right and left sides. The atrioventricular valves, tricuspid on the right and mitral on the left, divide the atria and ventricles to ensure that blood flows in one direction. A defect in the structure and function of any one of these components can lead to a detrimental failure of the cardiovascular system. The heart, major structures, and blood flow can be seen in Figure 8.1. Structures of arteries, veins and capillaries in Figure 8.2, and the circulatory system in Figure 8.3.

Pulmonary Circulation

Deoxygenated blood drains from the upper body, through the superior vena cava, and from the lower body, through the inferior vena cava, into the right atrium and then to the right ventricle. The right ventricle ejects blood past the pulmonary valve into the pulmonary artery and onward to the pulmonary circulation. Carbon dioxide is released, and oxygen absorbed as it travels through the lungs. This results in the return of oxygenated blood through the pulmonary veins to the left atrium.

Systemic Circulation

Oxygenated blood travels through the left atrium to the left ventricle. Here it is ejected past the aortic valve, into the aorta, supplying oxygen-rich blood to all other organs of the body. Once oxygen is utilised, carbon dioxide waste enters the bloodstream to be returned to the pulmonary circulation. As the left heart is responsible for pumping blood through most of the circulation, it has a much thicker muscular wall than the right ventricle.

Coronary Circulation

The coronary arteries originate from the aortic root and supply oxygenated blood to the myocardium. Myocardial infarction results from a blockage to one or more coronary arteries leading to damage of

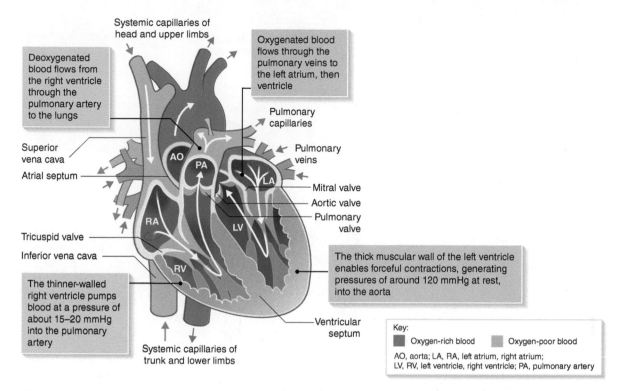

FIGURE 8.1   The heart, major structures and blood flow. *Source*: Dutton and Finch (2018) / John Wiley & Sons.

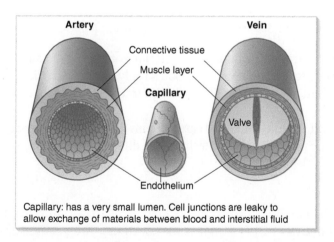

FIGURE 8.2   Structures of arteries, veins, and capillaries. *Source*: Dutton and Finch (2018) / John Wiley & Sons.

the underlying muscle due to a lack of oxygen supply. In order to determine the location of a blockage, it is important to understand the structures and myocardial territories supplied by each coronary artery.

Left coronary artery – arises from the left posterior aortic sinus and splits into the left anterior descending artery (LAD) and left circumflex artery (LCx). The LAD supplies the anterior wall of the left ventricle and the LCx supplies the lateral and posterior walls. The muscular wall of the left ventricle is susceptible to ischaemia; as the LAD is responsible for the majority of the blood supply to the left heart, an infarct here carries the highest associated morbidity and mortality.

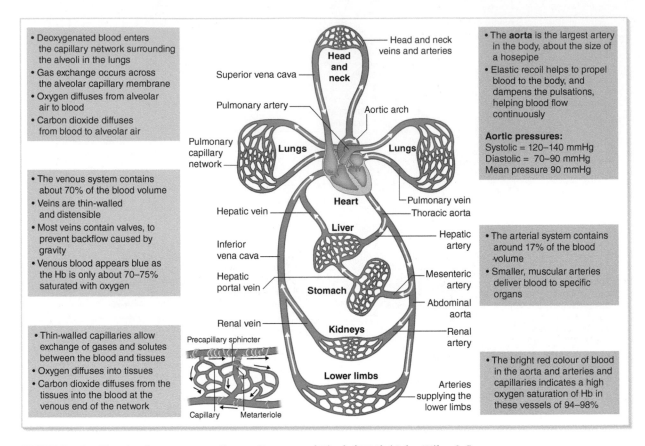

- Deoxygenated blood enters the capillary network surrounding the alveoli in the lungs
- Gas exchange occurs across the alveolar capillary membrane
- Oxygen diffuses from alveolar air to blood
- Carbon dioxide diffuses from blood to alveolar air

- The venous system contains about 70% of the blood volume
- Veins are thin-walled and distensible
- Most veins contain valves, to prevent backflow caused by gravity
- Venous blood appears blue as the Hb is only about 70–75% saturated with oxygen

- Thin-walled capillaries allow exchange of gases and solutes between the blood and tissues
- Oxygen diffuses into tissues
- Carbon dioxide diffuses from the tissues into the blood at the venous end of the network

- The **aorta** is the largest artery in the body, about the size of a hosepipe
- Elastic recoil helps to propel blood to the body, and dampens the pulsations, helping blood flow continuously

Aortic pressures:
Systolic = 120–140 mmHg
Diastolic = 70–90 mmHg
Mean pressure 90 mmHg

- The arterial system contains around 17% of the blood volume
- Smaller, muscular arteries deliver blood to specific organs

- The bright red colour of blood in the aorta and arteries and capillaries indicates a high oxygen saturation of Hb in these vessels of 94–98%

Head and neck veins and arteries
Head and neck
Superior vena cava
Pulmonary artery
Aortic arch
Pulmonary capillary network
Lungs
Lungs
Heart
Pulmonary vein
Hepatic vein
Thoracic aorta
Liver
Hepatic artery
Inferior vena cava
Hepatic portal vein
Mesenteric artery
Stomach
Abdominal aorta
Renal vein
Kidneys
Renal artery
Precapillary sphincter
Lower limbs
Arteries supplying the lower limbs
Capillary   Metarteriole

FIGURE 8.3   The circulatory system. *Source*: Dutton and Finch (2018) / John Wiley & Sons.

Right coronary artery – arises from the right anterior aortic sinus to supply blood to the right heart and posterior wall. It is also responsible for the blood supply to the sinoatrial node in 60% of individuals, and atrioventricular node in 80% of individuals. An infarct here may therefore result in rhythm disturbances or heart block.

Cardiac veins – the great, middle, and small cardiac veins drain deoxygenated blood through the coronary sinus into the right atrium. Smaller Thebesian veins drain directly into their corresponding chambers.

Physiology

Cardiac output (CO) is the amount of blood ejected by the heart per minute and is the product of heart rate (HR) and stroke volume (SV). This is approximately 5 l in a 70 kg patient as demonstrated below.

$$CO = HR \times SV$$
$$4900 \, ml/min = 70 \, bpm \times 70 \, ml$$

Key:
  HR = approx. 70 bpm
  SV = EDV – ESV or approx. 1 ml/kg ~70 ml
  bpm = beats per minute
  SV = SV = Its value is obtained by subtracting end-systolic volume (ESV) from end-diastolic volume (EDV) for a given ventricle.

Mean arterial pressure (MAP) is determined by the CO and resistance to blood flow within the systemic circulation. MAP can be derived from the following equations:

$$MAP = Diastolic\ Pressure + 1/3\ Pulse\ Pressure$$

$$MAP = CO \times SVR$$

Key:
    Pulse Pressure = Systolic – Diastolic
    SVR = Systemic Vascular Resistance

Conduction System of the Heart

For ejection to take place, electrical impulses are generated to facilitate the rhythmic contraction of the cardiac muscle cells (see Figure 8.4). Impulses originate in the sinoatrial node situated in the right atrium. This natural pacemaker sets a heart rate dependent on physiological needs. The impulses travel through the atria to the atrioventricular node, causing them to contract and force blood into the ventricles. The atrioventricular node institutes a brief delay to allow sufficient time for ventricular filling. Once both ventricles are filled, the impulses travel along the bundle of His, left and right bundle branches, and Purkinje fibres to stimulate ventricular muscle contraction, and thus the ejection of blood from the heart. Any delay or disruption to this conduction process can lead to varying degrees of heart block. To prevent cardiac arrest, a ventricular escape rhythm with a rate of 20–40 bpm may be seen in the event of conduction failure.

History

Combined with a generic history, the cardiovascular review should elicit salient cardiac symptoms, including chest pain (see Table 8.1), dyspnoea (see Table 8.2), orthopnoea, paroxysmal nocturnal dyspnoea, oedema, palpitations, dizziness, and syncope.

The comprehensive ACP should also recognise the principal risk factors associated with an increased risk of cardiovascular disease (see Table 8.3). When modifiable risk factors are identified, there exists the potential for us to promote lifestyle-modification advice, such as referral to smoking cessation clinics, providing weight-loss activities, and information regarding healthier dieting, as prevention is always

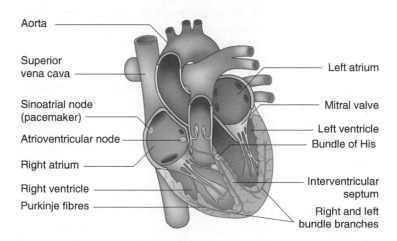

FIGURE 8.4   Conduction system of the heart. *Source*: Dutton and Finch (2018) / John Wiley & Sons.

TABLE 8.1   Causes of red flag: chest pain.

Red flag: chest pain	
Site	**MI**: central chest, epigastric **Dissection**: chest, retrosternal or back **PE**: chest, ribs
Onset	Typically sudden
Character	**MI**: crushing, dull, pressure **Dissection**: sharp, tearing **PE**: pleuritic, sharp
Radiation	**MI**: neck, jaw, left arm **Dissection**: interscapular, back, abdomen
Associated symptoms	**MI**: dyspnoea, nausea, sweating **Dissection**: features of MI and tamponade **PE**: cough, dyspnoea, tachypnoea, haemoptysis, palpitations
Timing	**MI**: may be acute, intermittent/remitting, or prolonged **Dissection**: acute and constant **PE**: intermittent, pleuritic, recent DVT
Exacerbating/relieving factors	**MI**: exercise, cold/relieved by GTN **PE**: recent travel, immobility, oral contraceptive pill
Severity	Severe 10/10

TABLE 8.2   Causes of red flag: shortness of breath.

Red flag: shortness of breath		
Dyspnoea		Non-specific symptom with multiple causes
Heart failure	Orthopnoea	Breathlessness associated with lying flat 'How many pillows do you sleep with at night?'
	Paroxysmal nocturnal dyspnoea	Breathlessness during sleep causing patient to wake up gasping
	Oedema association	Assess distribution: Peripheral oedema (right heart failure) Pulmonary oedema (left heart failure) Combination of both

better than cure. Comorbidities associated with an increased risk of the development of cardiovascular disease, should prompt the question as to whether they are on the appropriate therapy for their condition, in order to reduce any impact of disease.

Specific Patient Groups

Knowledge of groups with distinct presenting features will ensure the experienced ACP takes a thorough history, allowing them to navigate the unique complexities associated with these individuals (see Table 8.4). These patients may require referral to targeted cardiac rehabilitation and psychological support following the diagnosis of a cardiac event.

TABLE 8.3   Risk factors in CVD.

Modifiable risk factors for cardiovascular disease (NICE 2014b)
Smoking
Obesity
Hypercholesterolaemia
Unhealthy diet
Alcohol
Inactivity

Non-modifiable risk factors for cardiovascular disease (Piepoli et al. 2016)
Age >50
Gender M > F
Family history
Ethnic background

Comorbidities associated with increased risk of cardiovascular disease (PHE 2017)
Hypertension
Previous angina/MI/CABG
Diabetes mellitus
Chronic kidney disease
Atrial fibrillation
RA/SLE
Serious mental health problems

TABLE 8.4   Special cardiac considerations in diverse groups.

Population	Consideration
Obstetrics	The advanced clinical assessment and management of cardiac disease in the obstetric population often warrants early specialist involvement. Cardiac emergencies occurring during pregnancy include: • Exacerbation of pre-existing disease • Spontaneous coronary artery dissection (SCAD) – most common in the 3rd trimester, >50% mortality (Krishnamurthy et al. 2004) • Peripartum cardiomyopathy – occurs in late pregnancy and early postpartum period causing dilated cardiomyopathy with systolic dysfunction, often recovers (Honigberg and Givertz 2019)
Mental Health Conditions	Independent risk factor for cardiovascular disease. • Increased stress response and cardiac reactivity due to underlying condition which may also encourage the adoption of behaviours such as smoking, drug abuse, excessive alcohol intake or reduced medication compliance and concordance. • Antipsychotic medication is associated with diabetes, obesity, and cardiac disease (CDC 2020) • Takotsubo cardiomyopathy – severe dysfunction of the left ventricle typically in response to profound stress. • Drug overdose – cocaine-induced myocardial infarction; tricyclic antidepressant induced arrhythmias.

(Continued)

TABLE 8.4 (Continued)

Population	Consideration
Child Health	Congenital heart disorders and previous cardiac surgery should act as a prompt to seek specialist advice. Patients may be predisposed to atypical presentations of common emergencies, i.e. infective endocarditis in structural heart defects.
Ethnic Minority Groups	Ethnic differences in cardiovascular disease risk. Promote respect and dignity when communicating with patient, ensuring translator services and appropriate support available.
LGBTQIA+	Evidence of 'disparities across several cardiovascular risk factors compared with their cisgender heterosexual peers' (Caceres et al. 2020)

Cardiovascular Examination

Source: Hill and Diamond Fox (2022) / John Wiley & Sons.

TABLE 8.5   Inspection findings.

	Inspection
General	Unwell, pale, clammy, breathless, GTN, pain
Eyes	Xanthelasma, pallor, corneal arcus, Roth spots (fundoscopy)
Neck	Elevated JVP, distended neck veins
Chest	Scars, PPM/ICD
Hands	Clubbing, splinter haemorrhages, Osler's nodes, Janeway lesions, xanthomata

TABLE 8.6   Palpation findings.

	Palpation
Capillary refill time	<3 seconds
Pulses	Radial: rate, rhythm, collapsing pulse Brachial, carotid, femoral: character, volume Assess for radio-radial and radio-femoral delay in the instance of dissection, aneurysm, or coarctation of the aorta
Blood pressure	Systolic, diastolic, mean, and pulse pressure
Chest	Apex beat – 5th intercostal space midclavicular line
	Parasternal heave – right ventricular hypertrophy
	Thrills – palpable murmur
Hepatojugular reflux	Compression of the liver causing distension of neck veins indicating right heart dysfunction
Sacrum and ankles	Pitting oedema

A focused clinical examination should elicit the relevant cardiac signs to support a clinical diagnosis. Tables 8.5–8.7 outline the key cardiovascular examination findings using the physical assessment techniques of inspection, palpation, and auscultation. Figure 8.5 demonstrates the four main auscultation points of the heart.

Clinical Investigations

In order to support or refute a differential diagnosis from the history and examination, the ACP must develop an understanding of the clinical investigations available and their comparative merits and limitations.

Electrocardiogram (ECG)

Cardiac diseases can manifest themselves in the patients presenting with a vague collection of symptoms, including chest pain, dyspnoea, palpitations, dizziness, or syncope. Second to a thorough history and examination, the ECG is a rapid non-invasive bedside test offering excellent diagnostic capabilities in the detection of myocardial ischaemia, arrhythmias, conduction abnormalities, and ventricular strain, such as in heart failure.

TABLE 8.7   Auscultation findings.

	Auscultation
General	Mechanical 'click' of prosthetic valve.
Aortic region	2nd intercostal space to the right of the sternum
Pulmonary region	2nd intercostal space to the left of the sternum
Tricuspid region	4th intercostal space to the left of the sternum
Mitral region	5th intercostal space, midclavicular line
Special manoeuvres	Aortic stenosis – ejection systolic murmur radiating to carotids
	Aortic regurgitation – early-diastolic murmur at left sternal edge, sitting forward on expiration
	Mitral regurgitation – pan-systolic murmur radiating to axilla
	Mitral stenosis – rolling left to accentuate mid-diastolic murmur on expiration
	Carotid bruits – stenosis
Lung bases	Large pleural effusions associated with heart failure

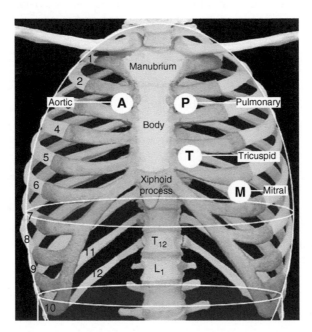

FIGURE 8.5   Heart sound auscultation points. *Source*: Casha et al. (2015) / John Wiley & Sons.

A 12-lead ECG is a recording of the electrical impulses generated in the heart. The electrodes are placed at defined points on the limbs and chest wall in order to identify the precise location of the cardiac problem. Chest lead and limb lead placement can be seen in Figures 8.6 and 8.7.

A good understanding of the ECG is key in enabling the ACP to differentiate between different cardiac diagnoses. A systematic approach to ECG interpretation will ensure no pathology is missed. The individual ACP should develop their own process for ECG interpretation; a useful method is to consider each deflection of the ECG waveform in turn: the P, Q, R, S, and T waves. See Figure 8.8 and Table 8.8.

A normal 12-lead ECG can be seen in Figure 8.9.

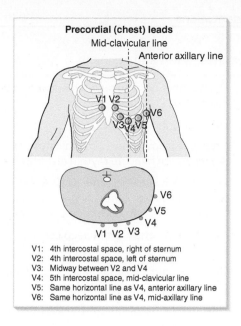

FIGURE 8.6   Chest leads.

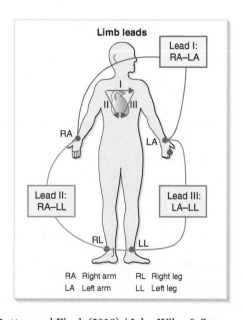

FIGURE 8.7   Limb leads. *Source*: Dutton and Finch (2018) / John Wiley & Sons.

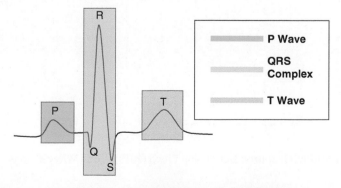

FIGURE 8.8   ECG waveform. *Source*: Srivastva and Singh (2019) / John Wiley & Sons.

TABLE 8.8   ECG features, waves and segments.

Rate	300/number of large squares between consecutive R waves Normal: 60–100 bpm
Rhythm	Regular or irregular
P	Presence followed by QRS indicates normal sinus rhythm Absence can indicate rhythm disturbance: AF/CHB
PR interval	Normal: 3–5 small squares (0.12–0.2 s) Short PR: fast AV conduction – accessory pathway (WPW) Prolonged PR: AV conduction delay – heart block
Q	>0.04 s wide and >2 mm deep can indicate previous infarction
QRS complex	Normal: <3 small squares (<0.12 s) Broad: ventricular arrhythmia or conduction defect
QT interval	Normal: Females 0.36–0.46 s/Males 0.35–0.45 s Prolonged QT can lead to Torsades de Pointes/VT
ST segment	Infarction: elevation > 1 mm Ischaemia: depression > 0.5 mm
T	Normal: aVR and V1 inversion Abnormal: inversion in any other lead Hyperkalaemia: 'tall-tented T waves'
Axis	Normal: positive lead I and II Left axis deviation: positive lead I, negative lead II (MI, conduction defect) Right axis deviation: negative lead I, positive lead II (MI, PE, right ventricular hypertrophy)
Bundle branch block	Ventricular conduction defects

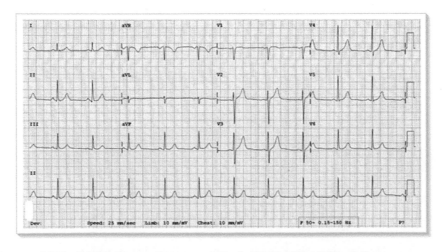

FIGURE 8.9   A normal 12-lead ECG. *Source*: Dutton and Finch (2018) / John Wiley & Sons.

RED FLAG: ECGs

Altered heart rhythms detected in 12-lead ECG recordings indicate red flags. A selection of altered heart rhythms can be seen in Figure 8.10 (sinus tachycardia), Figure 8.11 (ventricular arrhythmias), and Figure 8.12 (atrioventricular rhythms).

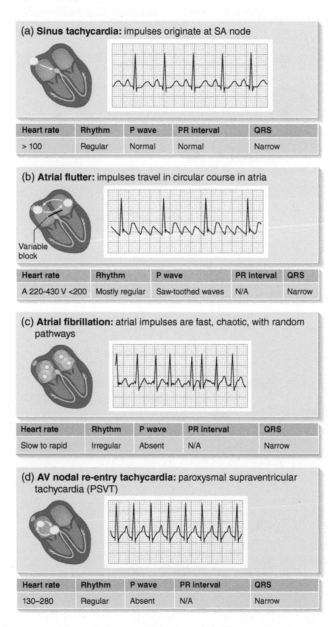

(a) Sinus tachycardia: impulses originate at SA node

Heart rate	Rhythm	P wave	PR interval	QRS
> 100	Regular	Normal	Normal	Narrow

(b) Atrial flutter: impulses travel in circular course in atria

Variable block

Heart rate	Rhythm	P wave	PR interval	QRS
A 220-430 V <200	Mostly regular	Saw-toothed waves	N/A	Narrow

(c) Atrial fibrillation: atrial impulses are fast, chaotic, with random pathways

Heart rate	Rhythm	P wave	PR interval	QRS
Slow to rapid	Irregular	Absent	N/A	Narrow

(d) AV nodal re-entry tachycardia: paroxysmal supraventricular tachycardia (PSVT)

Heart rate	Rhythm	P wave	PR interval	QRS
130–280	Regular	Absent	N/A	Narrow

FIGURE 8.10   Sinus tachycardia. *Source*: Dutton and Finch (2018) / John Wiley & Sons.

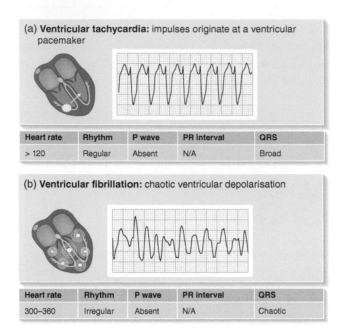

FIGURE 8.11 Ventricular arrhythmias. *Source*: Dutton and Finch (2018) / John Wiley & Sons.

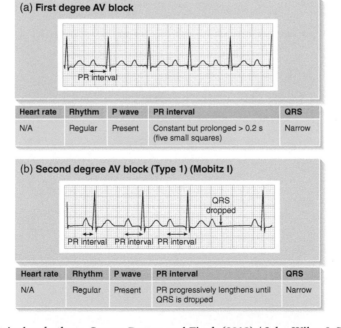

FIGURE 8.12 Atrioventricular rhythms. *Source*: Dutton and Finch (2018) / John Wiley & Sons.

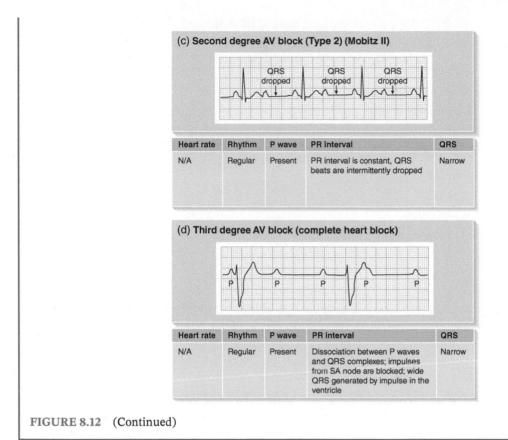

(c) Second degree AV block (Type 2) (Mobitz II)

Heart rate	Rhythm	P wave	PR interval	QRS
N/A	Regular	Present	PR interval is constant, QRS beats are intermittently dropped	Narrow

(d) Third degree AV block (complete heart block)

Heart rate	Rhythm	P wave	PR interval	QRS
N/A	Regular	Present	Dissociation between P waves and QRS complexes; impulses from SA node are blocked; wide QRS generated by impulse in the ventricle	Narrow

FIGURE 8.12   (Continued)

Exercise ECG

Myocardial ischaemia occasionally only becomes apparent when the heart undergoes exercise or becomes 'stressed'. An exercise ECG or 'exercise tolerance' test can be conducted, where the patient performs graduated exercise on a treadmill or bicycle, with continuous 12-lead ECG and blood pressure monitoring, to demonstrate inducible ischaemia or other ECG changes. An ECG is no longer a recommended exercise to diagnose coronary artery disease, as CT coronary angiography is more efficient. Exercise ECG may still have a role in people with confirmed coronary artery disease, to differentiate between cardiac and non-cardiac chest pain. Cardiopulmonary exercise testing (CPET) is a particular form of exercise tolerance test carried out to assess cardiopulmonary fitness in patients undergoing major surgery. CPET incorporates ECG monitoring under exercise conditions to assess cardiac function and limitations (Chambers and Wisely 2019).

Ambulatory ECG

A resting ECG may not detect any abnormality if a patient suffers from transient or paroxysmal rhythm disturbances as these may have resolved at the time of presentation. A Holter monitor is a portable ECG device which allows prolonged cardiac monitoring for periods of up to seven days. These may run continuously or may be activated by the patient during symptomatic episodes. In cases where arrhythmias occur less frequently, but are associated with a higher embolic risk of stroke, an implantable cardiac monitor may be inserted for extended monitoring (NICE 2020).

TABLE 8.9 Routine blood tests to be requested in conjunction with cardiac-specific assays.

Full blood count
Urea and electrolytes
Liver function tests
Thyroid function tests
Iron studies
Glucose
HbA1c
Fasting lipids

Laboratory Tests

This section covers the notable cardiac blood assays, but it is also important to consider other risk factors or prognostic markers for cardiac disease when requesting routine blood tests (see Table 8.9).

Creatine Kinase (CK)

Creatine Kinase is present in multiple tissues as a group of three isoenzymes, characterised by two polypeptide chains: CK-MM, CK-MB, and CK-BB (GP Notebook 2021b). Cardiac and skeletal muscles have a very high CK content, which can rise within the plasma following damage by conditions such as myocardial infarction, myocarditis, and rhabdomyolysis. Elevated plasma CK levels can also be found in numerous non-neuromuscular conditions, such as endocrine, connective tissue, and malignant disease, along with the use of certain medications such as statins (Moghadam-Kia et al. 2016). Cardiac muscle is ordinarily the only tissue containing CK-MB concentrations of over 5%; however, exceptions exist in athletes or patients with muscle disorders. The ratio of total CK to CK-MB has been used historically to detect the presence of myocardial damage following myocardial infarction (GP Notebook 2021a). While this test is highly sensitive, it has a low specificity for myocardial infarction as it can be influenced by the multiple processes mentioned above; therefore its use has largely been replaced in favour of troponin measurement.

Troponin

The troponin complex (see Figure 8.13) comprises the troponin I, C, and T subunits, which along with tropomysin, actin, and myosin, form the fundamental components of cardiac and skeletal muscle contraction (Takeda et al. 2003). Cardiac troponin I and cardiac troponin T are cardiac-specific proteins which differ in form to those found in skeletal muscle. These are released into the bloodstream following cardiac muscle damage and can be detected to signify a myocardial infarction has occurred. High-sensitivity troponin assays are now able to detect lower levels of troponin within four hours from the onset of symptoms (NICE 2019). Renal disease, severe infections, and heart failure may cause a false positive result, and caution should be taken when interpreting results in these populations. The trend of rising or falling troponin levels always carries more significance than a single elevated value alone.

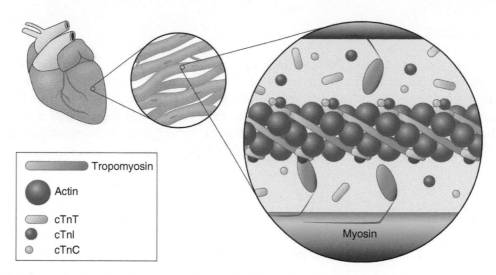

FIGURE 8.13   Troponin Complex. *Source*: Langhorn and Willesen (2016) / John Wiley & Sons.

B-type Natriuretic Peptide (BNP) and N-terminal Pro-BNP (NT-proBNP)

The prohormone pro-BNP is secreted in response to myocardial wall stretch and is processed to form the active BNP and inactive NT proBNP fragments (Farnsworth 2019). Conditions, such as heart failure, where the heart becomes enlarged due to increased pressure, result in a proportional increase in the plasma concentrations of both BNP and NT-proBNP. These can be measured using biochemical assays, with distinct plasma thresholds, to assist in the diagnosis and prognosis of acute and chronic heart failure. Both fragments demonstrate a similar sensitivity and specificity for the clinical evaluation of heart failure, where a normal result is useful in excluding the diagnosis and very high levels are associated with increased mortality. The degree of elevation can also be compared when assessing a patient's response to therapy or intervention (see Table 8.10).

CARDIAC IMAGING

We will now explore the common imaging modalities available for the investigation of acute cardiac emergencies.

TABLE 8.10   BNP and NT-proBNP as a diagnostic tool for heart failure.

BNP and NT-proBNP as a diagnostic tool for heart failure (NICE 2014a, NICE 2022)	
Plasma BNP < 100 ng/l Plasma NT-proBNP < 300 ng/l	Diagnosis of heart failure less likely Review alternative causes for symptoms
NT-proBNP 400–2000 ng/l	Referral for specialist assessment and transthoracic echocardiography within six weeks
NT-proBNP > 2000 ng/l	Poor prognosis Referral for specialist assessment and transthoracic echocardiography within two weeks

Chest X-ray (CXR)

In the acute, emergency and critical care settings a plain film CXR offers a rapid snapshot of the intra-thoracic cavity. The CXR enables a crude assessment of the heart with limited detail; however, it can often provide vital clues to best direct our patient management. Pulmonary oedema (see Figure 8.14a), cardiomegaly (see Figure 8.14b) and pleural effusions may point us toward a diagnosis of congestive cardiac failure, whereas evidence of previous cardiothoracic surgery and intracardiac devices can highlight the requirement for more specialist intervention (see Figure 8.14c).

Echocardiography

Echocardiography, either transthoracic or transoesophageal, remains the principal investigation for most patients with suspected or established cardiac disease. Transthoracic echocardiography is the preferred standard as it is portable, non-invasive, and non-ionising. It offers real-time assessment of

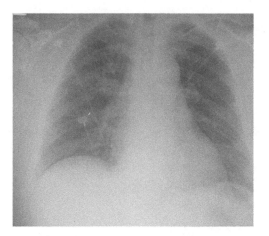

FIGURE 8.14a   CXR pulmonary oedema. *Source*: Chaudhry et al. (2021) / John Wiley & Sons.

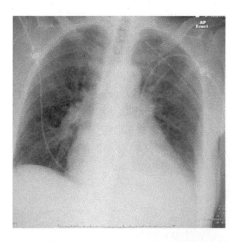

FIGURE 8.14b   CXR cardiomegaly. *Source*: Baker et al. (2013) / John Wiley & Sons.

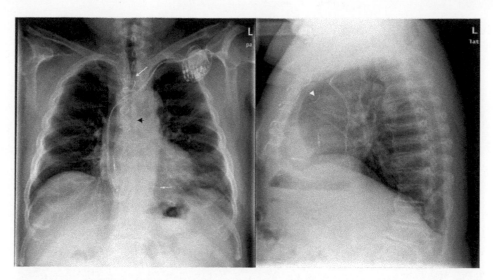

FIGURE 8.14c   CXR pacemaker/ICD and sternotomy wires in PA and lateral views. *Source*: Mokhtar et al. (2020) / John Wiley & Sons.

the heart by quantifying biventricular function and can detect structural abnormalities such as hypertrophic cardiomyopathy, valvular pathology, and endocarditis. This subject will be explored further in Chapter 16: Principles of Point of Care Ultrasound (POCUS). Stress echocardiography, where the stressor may be physiological (exercise) or pharmacological (dobutamine), elicits echocardiographic signs that may not be present at rest, in a similar way to which exercise ECG identifies stress-inducible ischaemia.

Computed Tomography Coronary Angiography (CTCA)

The high risks associated with invasive transcatheter coronary angiography have propelled the use of CTCA as the first-line imaging modality for the assessment of coronary artery disease (NICE 2012). Concerns over high radiation doses have been mitigated through advances in CT technology, which permit the entire scan to be obtained during a single breath hold (Wilkinson et al. 2017). Despite both a high sensitivity and specificity for diagnosing coronary artery disease in low-intermediate risk populations, it is the high negative predictive value of CTCA that makes it an extremely effective modality in excluding coronary artery disease (Soon and Wong 2012). Due to CT image degradation in the presence of heavy coronary artery calcification, such as in extensive disease states, CTCA becomes less effective and second-line modalities should be considered. Figures 8.15a, b demonstrate how the CT images are restacked to form reconstructed images of the coronary arteries. Figure 8.15c highlights how well these reconstructed images correlate with the coronary angiogram findings.

Cardiac Magnetic Resonance Imaging (MRI)

Cardiac MRI is a non-invasive imaging modality, referenced as the gold standard for accurate assessment of ventricular size, structure, and function (Simpson et al. 2018; Kilner et al. 2010; NICE 2018). MRI generates images with far superior resolution than traditional techniques, allowing detailed characterisation

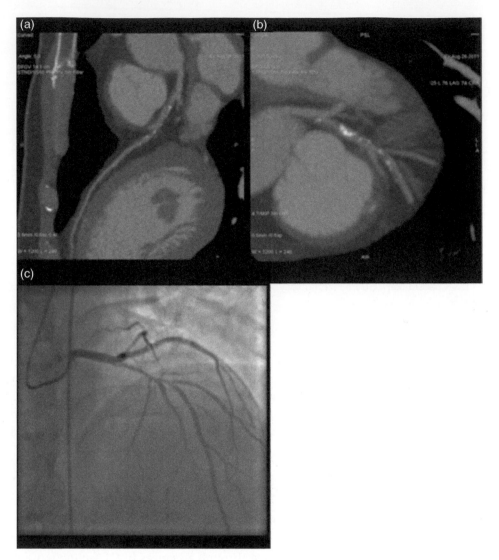

FIGURE 8.15   (a and b) Curved multiplanar reconstruction of CTCA correlates well with the finding of invasive coronary angiography (c) showing a severe stenosis in the mid-left anterior descending artery. *Source*: Soon and Wong (2012) / John Wiley & Sons.

of several complex structural and functional cardiac abnormalities, such as congenital heart disease, cardiomyopathies, valvular heart disease, and intra-cardiac tumours. Although expensive, the high associated cost may be offset by its radiation-free safety profile and its reproducible accuracy, lending itself as the first-line imaging modality to populations requiring long-term cardiac follow-up (Wilkinson et al. 2017).

Caution – the ACP should always check the compatibility of older pacemakers and implantable car-dioverter defibrillators, and consider other non-MRI compatible substances, when requesting a cardiac MRI. Figure 8.16 illustrates the clarity in which cardiac MRI can be utilised to accurately assess ventric-ular dimensions in (a) a normal heart and (b) a patient with pulmonary hypertension.

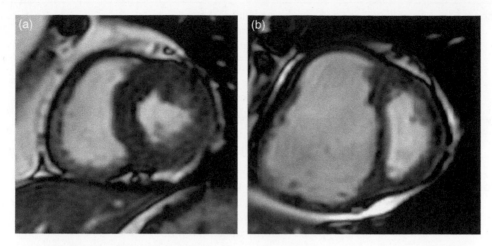

FIGURE 8.16   Cardiac MRI short-axis view depicting (a) normal heart and (b) pulmonary hypertension. *Source*: Saunders et al. (2022) / John Wiley & Sons.

Myocardial Perfusion Imaging

Nuclear imaging is a technique involving the injection of small amounts of radioisotope, at rest and after induction of physiological or pharmacological 'stress', to evaluate the function and perfusion of the myocardium via the coronary arteries (NICE 2003). It is particularly useful for detecting stress-induced regional wall motion abnormalities and viable myocardium following myocardial infarction.

Cardiac Catheterisation

It is an invasive diagnostic and interventional procedure where a catheter is inserted via a large vein or the radial or femoral artery, to access the heart and coronary circulation. This enables visualisation of the heart, valves, and vessels to assess pressures, oxygenation saturations, structure, and function. There is a high associated risk, however it remains the gold standard modality for performing percutaneous coronary intervention following STEMI, using balloon angioplasty and stenting to open blocked coronary arteries. Valvuloplasty, closure of septal defects, ablative therapy, and valvular implantation are some of the many therapeutic indications for right and left heart catheterisation.

Pharmacological Principles

The ACP should be aware of the existence of both preventive and pharmacological treatment strategies in the management of cardiovascular disease.

- **Primary prevention:** aims to prevent disease before it happens – through lifestyle and behavioural change.
- **Secondary prevention:** aims to reduce the impact of disease once it happens – through early diagnosis and treatment, often with medication.
- **Tertiary prevention:** aims to reduce the impact of chronic disease – through education and rehabilitation.

Table 8.11 outlines a few examples of drugs that are commonly used in the management of acute cardiac emergencies.

TABLE 8.11 Commonly used cardiac drugs in AECC.

ACE-inhibitors	Indication: Hypertension, heart failure, post-MI Action: Inhibit the conversion of angiotensin I to angiotensin II Caution: First-dose hypotension, monitor renal function
Adenosine	Indication: Paroxysmal supraventricular tachycardias Action: Short-acting SA and AV node depression Caution: Asthma, heart block, accessory pathway
Amiodarone	Indication: Atrial and ventricular tachyarrhythmias Action: Class III anti-arrhythmic – prolongs cardiac action potential Caution: Thyroid and liver dysfunction, pulmonary fibrosis, CNS toxicity and visual disturbance, heart block
Anticoagulants	Indication: Prevention of venous thrombus formation or extension Action: Xa inhibition (direct-acting oral anticoagulants), vitamin K antagonism (warfarin), thrombin inhibition (dabigatran, bivalirudin), antithrombin III binding (heparin) Caution: Haemorrhage, heparin-induced thrombocytopaenia
Antiplatelets	Indication: Secondary prevention post-MI and stent insertion Action: Decrease arterial platelet aggregation and inhibit thrombus formation – COX inhibition (aspirin), ADP antagonism (clopidogrel, ticagrelor, prasugrel), glycoprotein IIb/IIIa antagonism (tirofiban) Caution: GI-bleeding, haemorrhage
β-blockers	Indication: Hypertension, angina, MI, arrhythmias, heart failure Action: β-adrenoreceptor antagonism – negative inotropy and chronotropy Caution: Asthma/COPD, heart block
Calcium antagonists	Dihydropyridines (amlodipine, nifedipine, felodipine) Indication: Hypertension, angina Action: Reduce entry of Ca^{2+} in smooth muscle resulting in peripheral vasodilatation Caution: ankle oedema, heart failure Non-dihydropyridines (verapamil, diltiazem) Indication: Hypertension, angina, arrhythmias Action: Reduce SA and AV node conduction – negative inotropy and chronotropy Caution: Profound bradycardia with β-blockers, heart block
Digoxin	Indication: AF, flutter, heart failure Action: NA^+/K^+-ATPase inhibition reduces intracellular K^+ slowing AV conduction and increases availability of Ca^{2+} resulting in weak positive inotropy Caution: Toxicity – hypokalaemia, elderly, renal failure
Diuretics	Indication: Relieve oedema in heart failure, hypertension Action: Inhibit chloride reabsorption (loop diuretics – furosemide, bumetanide), inhibit sodium reabsorption (thiazides – bendroflumethiazide, indapamide, metolazone), block sodium channels (potassium-sparing diuretics – amiloride), aldosterone antagonism (potassium-sparing mineralocorticoid receptor antagonists – spironolactone, eplerenone) Caution: Renal failure, electrolyte disturbance
Isoprenaline	Indication: Bradycardia, heart block Action: β-adrenoreceptor agonism – positive inotropy and chronotropy Caution: Tachyarrhythmias, angina
Statins	Indication: Hypercholesterolaemia and hypertriglyceridaemia Action: Inhibit enzyme HMG-COA reductase responsible for cholesterol synthesis Caution: Muscle pain, rhabdomyolysis, liver dysfunction
Vasodilators	Indication: Angina, heart failure, hypertension Action: vasodilatation of arteries and veins (examples: GTN – sublingual or intravenous, hydralazine, prazosin) Caution: Hypotension, (hydralazine: lupus-like syndrome)

Clinical Case Scenarios

The case scenarios in Tables 8.12–8.15 demonstrate how the acquired knowledge in this chapter can be applied to clinical practice.

TABLE 8.12   Acute coronary syndromes.

1. Acute Coronary Syndromes (ACS)

Presentation:

A 50-year-old male presents to A&E with a history of sudden onset central crushing chest pain radiating to his left arm. Pain is associated with nausea and vomiting. The patient appears pale and diaphoretic. He has a history of hypertension, a strong family history of ischaemic heart disease and is a current smoker.

Key features:

- Central 'crushing' or 'heavy' chest pain
- Pain radiating to jaw or left arm
- Shortness of breath
- Palpitations

- Nausea and vomiting
- Diaphoresis
- Preceding angina
- Identify risk factors

Examination:

Capillary refill time and pulse normal
No radio-radial or radio-femoral delay
JVP mildly elevated
Heart sounds normal
No peripheral oedema

Baseline Observations:

Respiratory rate 25
Oxygen saturations (room air) 94%
Heart rate 94
BP 162/88
Temp 36.2°C

Investigations:

1. 12-lead ECG: Positive ECG findings suggestive of ACS include ST elevation, ST depression, T wave inversion, LBBB and pathological Q waves (see Figure 8.17).

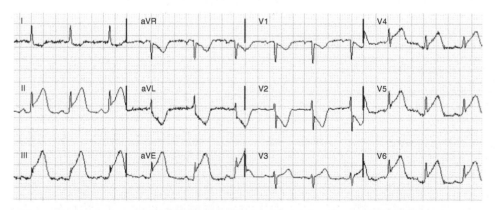

FIGURE 8.17   ECG with inferior and lateral ST elevation-ACS. There is ST elevation in the leads II, III, aVF, and V_4–V_6. Leads I and aVL show reciprocal ST depression. *Source*: Birnbaum et al. (2014) / John Wiley & Sons.

2. Cardiac markers: Troponin and CK-MB elevated

(Continued)

TABLE 8.12   (Continued)

3. Blood tests: elevated WCC and CRP, hyperglycaemia, hypertriglyceridaemia
4. CXR: normal
5. ABG: normal
6. ECHO: mildly reduced left ventricular ejection fraction with regional wall motion abnormalities of the inferior and lateral walls – consistent with ECG findings. Valvular defects, ventricular aneurysm, rupture and pericardial effusions are also associated with ACS.

Differential diagnosis:
Cardiac – ACS, aortic dissection, pericarditis, myocarditis, Takotsubo cardiomyopathy
Respiratory – pulmonary embolism, pneumothorax, community acquired pneumonia
Other – pancreatitis, oesophageal spasm, costochondritis, anxiety

Types of ACS:
Caused by rupture of atherosclerotic plaque which leads to platelet aggregation and thrombus formation within a coronary artery. This leads to myocardial ischaemia followed by infarction (death).

1. Unstable angina: non-occlusive thrombus causing ischaemia but not infarction, normal ECG, normal troponin
2. Non-ST-elevation myocardial infarction (NSTEMI): partial occlusion, ST depression and T wave inversion, mild-moderate troponin and CK-MB rise
3. ST-elevation myocardial infarction (STEMI): total occlusion, ST elevation, marked troponin and CK-MB rise

Management:
Immediate:

- ABCDE and serial ECGs
- Aspirin 300 mg: prevents platelet aggregation and reduces thrombus formation (ticagrelor and clopidogrel are newer alternatives)
- Analgesia: morphine to reduce pain and anxiety + anti-emetic
- Oxygen: maintain saturations >94%
- GTN (sublingual or intravenous): increases blood flow to the myocardium

Primary percutaneous coronary intervention (PCI):

- STEMI presenting within 12 hours from onset of symptoms
- Revascularisation within 120 minutes improves outcomes and cardiac function
- Thrombolysis if PCI not available within 120 minutes
- High-risk NSTEMI should be considered for inpatient angiography

CTCA:

- Consider in unstable angina if no previous history of coronary artery disease

Coronary artery bypass grafts:

- Surgery if coronary artery disease not amenable to PCI

TABLE 8.13   Heart failure.

2. Heart failure

Presentation:
A 74-year-old female presents to A&E with a six-week history of fatigue, cough, and worsening shortness of breath on exertion. She has associated palpitations, swollen ankles, and reduced exercise tolerance. She is on medication for diabetes and stopped smoking following her coronary artery bypass graft surgery seven years ago.

Key features:

- Dyspnoea
- PND
- Orthopnoea
- Cough/wheeze
- Peripheral oedema
- Poor exercise tolerance
- History of cardiovascular disease and risk factors

TABLE 8.13   (Continued)

Examination:
Capillary refill time prolonged
JVP elevated
Coarse respiratory crackles
Heart sounds 'Gallop rhythm'
Pitting peripheral oedema up to sacrum

Baseline Observations:
Respiratory rate 32
Oxygen saturations (room air) 89%
Heart rate 148
BP 85/67
Temp 35.8°C

Investigations:

1. 12-lead ECG (see Figure 8.18):

FIGURE 8.18   ECG with broad-complex tachycardia, LBBB pattern. *Source*: Duncan et al. (2012) / John Wiley & Sons.

2. Cardiac markers: BNP and NT-proBNP elevated
3. Blood tests: leucocytosis, reduced e-GFR
4. CXR: pulmonary oedema (cardiomegaly and pleural effusions may also be present) (see Figure 8.19)

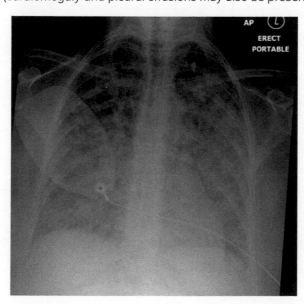

FIGURE 8.19   CXR of pulmonary oedema. *Source*: Duncan et al. (2012) / John Wiley & Sons.

5. ABG: type 1 respiratory failure, lactate 3.2
6. ECHO: severely impaired left ventricular systolic function with moderate mitral regurgitation

TABLE 8.13   (Continued)

Differential diagnosis:
The Framingham Heart Criteria can aid with the diagnosis of heart failure.
Cardiac – congestive heart failure, valvular disease, cardiomyopathies
Respiratory – COPD (exacerbation), pulmonary fibrosis, pneumonia, pulmonary hypertension
Other – nephrotic syndrome, thyrotoxicosis, liver disease

Heart failure definition:
Cardiac output is insufficient to meet the body's metabolic requirements. Demonstrated by high lactate and other organ dysfunction: liver, kidney, brain.

New York classification of heart failure (NYHA):
I – Presence of cardiac disease with no limitation of physical activity.
II – Slight limitation of physical activity.
III – Marked limitation of physical activity.
IV – Symptoms at rest.

Management:
Immediate:

- ABCDE
- High-flow oxygen via non-rebreather mask: O_2 saturations >94%
- Early-escalation for senior support
- Heart rate and arrhythmia control: digoxin, amiodarone, DCCV
- Intravenous furosemide ± GTN (caution with hypotension – may need inotropes)
- Urinary catheterisation

Establish the underlying cause and treat:

- Cardiac catheterisation
- Cardiac MRI
- Myocardial perfusion imaging

Secondary and tertiary prevention:

- Modifiable factors: lifestyle education, optimising medication, rehabilitation
- Pharmacological 'Best Medical Therapy': ACE-I, β-blockers, diuretics

If medical management fails, consider cardiac resynchronisation therapy, ventricular assist devices, and even heart transplantation.

TABLE 8.14   Supraventricular tachycardia.

3. Supraventricular tachycardia (SVT)

Presentation:
A 20-year-old female, studying for her final examinations, presents to A&E with sudden onset breathlessness and palpitations. She is otherwise fit and well but has had a similar self-terminating episode in the past, which was associated with dizziness.

Key features:

- Palpitations
- Dizziness
- Presyncope/syncope
- Breathlessness
- Exacerbating factors: caffeine, stress, tiredness, alcohol

TABLE 8.14   (Continued)

Examination:	**Baseline observations:**
Anxious ++	Respiratory rate 22
Pale	Oxygen saturations (room air) 96%
Diaphoretic	Heart rate 185
Cool peripheries	BP 100/67
	Temperature 37°C

Investigations:

1. 12-lead ECG (see Figure 8.20):

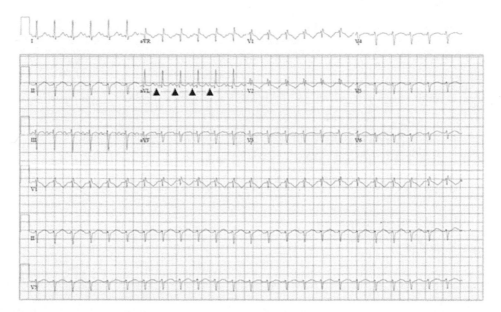

FIGURE 8.20   ECG with supraventricular tachycardia. Arrow heads point to P waves. *Source*: Kaspar et al. (2018) / John Wiley & Sons.

2. Blood tests: check electrolytes, thyroid function

Differential diagnosis:
Regular rhythm: sinus tachycardia, focal atrial tachycardia, atrial flutter, atrioventricular re-entry tachycardia, junctional tachycardia, ventricular tachycardias
Irregular rhythm: sinus arrhythmia, atrial fibrillation, atrial flutter with variable block, ventricular fibrillation, polymorphic ventricular tachycardia

Management:
Immediate:

- ABCDE
- IV access and consider fluid bolus if hypotensive
- Continuous ECG monitoring

Vagal manoeuvres:

- Carotid sinus massage
- Valsalva/reverse Valsalva – exhaling/inhaling through a syringe

(Continued)

TABLE 8.14   (Continued)

Medication:

- Adenosine – warn patient of 'a sense of impending doom'
- Verapamil as alternative
- Amiodarone in refractory arrhythmias
- Propranolol 'Pill-in-the-Pocket' drug strategy

Synchronised DC cardioversion:

- If haemodynamically unstable
- If not responding to pharmacological management
- Will need general anaesthetic/sedation

Echocardiogram

- While SVTs are often benign, an echocardiogram should be performed as an outpatient to exclude structural heart disease

Cardiac catheterisation

- Electrophysiological studies
  - Characterisation of Wolff-Parkinson-White syndrome and accessory pathways
- Catheter ablation to reduce future incidence of arrhythmias

TABLE 8.15   Infective endocarditis.

4. Infective endocarditis (IE)

Presentation:
A 38-year-old male presents to A&E with a two-week history of fever, myalgia, malaise, and shortness of breath. He had a renal transplant as a child.

Key features:

- Fever + new murmur = IE
- Non-specific symptoms: mimics other diseases
- Risk factors: diabetes, IVDU, poor dentition, immunosuppression, structural heart disease, prosthetic valves

Examination:
Splinter haemorrhages
Janeway lesions/Osler's nodes
Clubbing
Splenomegaly
New murmur in aortic region

Baseline observations:
Respiratory rate 28
Oxygen saturations (room air) 95%
Heart rate 102
BP 115/42
Temp 38.6°C

Investigations:

1. 12-lead ECG: normal
2. Blood tests: raised inflammatory markers, anaemia, renal function normal
3. Blood cultures: Three sets at different times from different sites during temperature spike
   Common organisms: *Streptococcus viridans* and *Staphylococcus aureus*
4. CXR: cardiomegaly
5. ABG: normal

TABLE 8.15   (Continued)

6. Echocardiogram (see Figure 8.21):

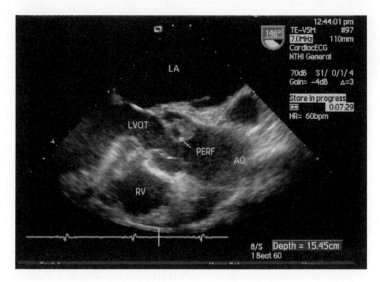

FIGURE 8.21   Transoesophageal echocardiogram of aortic valve vegetation and perforation. *Source*: Ivanovic et al. (2022) / John Wiley & Sons.

7. CT: evaluation of splenomegaly and emboli

Diagnosis of infective endocarditis:
Modified Duke criteria
Pathological criteria

- Microorganism in vegetation
- Pathological lesion

Major criteria

- Positive blood culture (typical organism for IE from two separate cultures)
- Endocardium involved

Minor criteria

- Predisposing heart condition or IVDU
- Fever
- Vascular phenomena
- Immunological phenomena
- Microbiological evidence

Diagnosis Criteria: 1 Pathological, 2 Major, 1 Major and 3 Minor, or 5 Minor

Management:

- Liaise with microbiology for antibiotic regime (Gram +ve and Gram −ve organism cover)
- Liaise with cardiology for echocardiogram
- Surgery: valve destruction, prosthetic valves, heart failure

Take Home Points
- A detailed understanding of the intricacies of cardiac anatomy and physiology provides a sound basis from which the ACP can develop their clinical skill.
- Where 80% of diagnoses are made from the history alone, consideration of the underlying pathological processes involved, ensures a comprehensive assessment and targeted investigative strategy.
- Comparing the strengths and limitations of individual investigations and therapies, will promote the ACP's adherence to the NICE ethos of 'balancing the best care with value for money across the NHS and social care, to deliver for both individuals and society as a whole' (NICE 2023).

REFERENCES

Baker, K., Mitchell, G., Thompson, A.G., and Stieler, G. (2013). Comparison of a basic lung scanning protocol against formally reported chest x-ray in the diagnosis of pulmonary oedema. *Australasian Journal of Ultrasound in Medicine* 16 (4): 183–189.

Birnbaum, Y., Wilson, J.M., Fiol, M. et al. (2014). ECG diagnosis and classification of acute coronary syndromes. *Annals of Noninvasive Electrocardiology* 19 (1): 4–14.

Caceres, B.A., Streed, C.G. Jr., Corliss, H.L. et al. (2020). Assessing and addressing cardiovascular health in LGBTQ adults: a scientific statement from the American Heart Association. *Circulation* 142 (19): e321–e332.

Casha, A.R., Camilleri, L., Manché, A. et al. (2015). External rib structure can be predicted using mathematical models: an anatomical study with application to understanding fractures and intercostal muscle function. *Clinical Anatomy* 28 (4): 512–519.

Centres for Disease Control and Prevention (CDC). (2020). *Heart Disease and Mental Health Disorders* [online]. Available from: https://www.cdc.gov/heartdisease/mentalhealth.htm#:~:text=People%20experiencing%20depression%2C%20anxiety%2C%20stress,and%20heightened%20levels%20of%20cortisol.2023 [accessed 21 June 2023].

Chambers, D.J. and Wisely, N.A. (2019). Cardiopulmonary exercise testing—a beginner's guide to the nine-panel plot. *BJA Education* 19 (5): 158–164.

Chaudhry, H., Nimmala, S., Papudesi, B.N. et al. (2021). Negative pressure pulmonary oedema due to rigors and chills associated with liver abscess. *Respirology Case Reports* 9 (9): e0826.

Duncan, E., Rao, K., and Sporton, S. (2012). Recurrent acute pulmonary oedema and cardiac arrest secondary to intermittent electrical dyssynchrony: a role for cardiac resynchronization despite preserved left ventricular function. *European Journal of Heart Failure* 14 (4): 445–448.

Dutton, H. and Finch, J. (2018). *Acute and Critical Care Nursing: At a Glance (Nursing and Healthcare)*. Wiley Blackwell.

Farnsworth, C. (2019). *BNP or NT-proBNP*: AACC [online]. Available from: https://www.aacc.org/science-and-research/scientific-shorts/2019/bnp-or-nt-probnp2023 [accessed 21 June 2023].

GP notebook (2021a). *CK in Myocardial Disease* [online]. Available from: https://gpnotebook.com/simplepage.cfm?ID=2033516569&linkID=11264 [accessed 21 June 2023].

GP notebook (2021b). *Creatine Kinase* [online]. Available from: https://gpnotebook.com/simplepage.cfm?ID=1436155929 [accessed 21 June 2023].

Health Education England (HEE). (2017). *Multi-professional Framework for Advanced Clinical Practice in England* [online]. Available from: https://www.hee.nhs.uk/sites/default/files/documents/multi-professionalframeworkforadvancedclinicalpracticeinengland.pdf [accessed 20 June 2023].

Health Education England (HEE). (2022). *Advanced Clinical Practice in Acute Medicine Curriculum Framework – Credentials* [online]. Available from: `https://advanced-practice.hee.nhs.uk/our-work/credentials` [accessed 20 June 2023].

Hill, B. and Diamond-Fox, S. (2022). *Advanced Clinical Practice at a glance.* Wiley Blackwell.

Honigberg, M.C. and Givertz, M.M. (2019). Peripartum cardiomyopathy. *BMJ* 364: k5287.

Ivanovic, B., Popovic, J., Dukic, D. et al. (2022). The role of imaging in infective endocarditis. *Journal of Clinical Ultrasound* 50 (8): 1060–1065.

Kaspar, G., Sanam, K., Gundlapalli, S., and Shah, D. (2018). Successful fluoroless radiofrequency catheter ablation of supraventricular tachycardia during pregnancy. *Clinical Case Reports* 6 (7): 1334–1337.

Kilner, P.J., Geva, T., and Kaemmerer, H. (2010). Recommendations for cardiovascular magnetic resonance in adults with congenital heart disease from the respective working groups of the European Society of Cardiology. *European Heart Journal* 31 (7): 794–805.

Krishnamurthy, M., Desai, R., and Patel, H. (2004). Spontaneous coronary artery dissection in the postpartum period: association with antiphospholipid antibody. *Heart* 90 (9): e53.

Langhorn, R. and Willesen, J.L. (2016). Cardiac troponins in dogs and cats. *Journal of Veterinary Internal Medicine* 30: 36–50.

Moghadam-Kia, S., Oddis, C.V., and Aggarwal, R. (2016). Approach to asymptomatic creatine kinase elevation. *Cleveland Clinic Journal of Medicine* 83 (1): 37–42.

Mokhtar, A.T., Baghaffar, A., Ramer, S.A., and Fraser, J.D. (2020). Migrated fractured sternal wire in proximity to the main pulmonary artery: case report and review. *Journal of Cardiac Surgery* 35 (3): 692–695.

National Institute for Health and Care Excellence (NICE). (2003). *Myocardial Perfusion Scintigraphy for the Diagnosis and Management of Angina and Myocardial Infarction* [online]. Available from: `https://www.nice.org.uk/guidance/ta73/chapter/3-The-technology2023` [accessed 21 June 2023].

National Institute for Health and Care Excellence (NICE). (2014a). *Acute Heart Failure: Diagnosis and Management* [online]. Available from: `https://www.nice.org.uk/guidance/cg187/chapter/1-Recommendations#diagnosis-assessment-and-monitoring` [accessed 21 June 2023].

National Institute for Health and Care Excellence (NICE). (2018). *Individual Research Recommendation Details* [online]. Available from: `https://www.nice.org.uk/researchrecommendation/what-is-the-optimal-imaging-technique-for-the-diagnosis-of-heart-failure` [accessed 21 June 2023].

National Institute for Health and Care Excellence (NICE). (2019). *High-sensitivity Troponin for the Early Rule Out of Acute Myocardial Infarction* [online]. Available from: `https://www.nice.org.uk/guidance/dg40/documents/final-scope-2` [accessed 21 June 2023].

National Institute for Health and Care Excellence (NICE). (2020). *Implantable Cardiac Monitors to Detect Atrial Fibrillation After Cryptogenic Stroke* [online]. Available from: `https://www.nice.org.uk/guidance/dg41/chapter/1-Recommendations2023` [accessed 21 June 2023].

National Institute for Health and Care Excellence (NICE). (2022). *How Should I Assess a Person with Suspected Chronic Heart Failure?* [online]:. Available from: `https://cks.nice.org.uk/topics/heart-failure-chronic/diagnosis/how-to-assess/2023` [accessed 21 June 2023].

National Institute for Health and Excellence (NICE). (2014b). *Cardiovascular Disease: Risk Assessment and Reduction, Including Lipid Modification* [online]. Available from: `https://www.nice.org.uk/guidance/cg181` [accessed 21 June 2023].

National Institute for Health and Excellence (NICE). (2023). *About* [online]. Available from: `https://www.nice.org.uk/about` [accessed 21 June 2023].

National Institute of Health and Care Excellence (NICE). (2012). *CT Coronary Angiography* [online]. Available from: Shared learning | Recent-onset chest pain of suspected cardiac origin: assessment and diagnosis | Guidance | NICE Recent-onset chest pain of suspected cardiac origin: assessment and diagnosis Clinical guideline [CG95] [accessed 21 June 2023]. Updated in 2016.

PHE. (2017). *NHS Health Check Best Practice Guidance* [online]. Available from: england.nhs.uk [accessed 21 June 2023].

Piepoli, M.F., Hoes, A.W., Agewall, S. et al. (2016). 2016 European Guidelines on cardiovascular disease prevention in clinical practice: the sixth joint task force of the european society of cardiology and other societies on cardiovascular disease prevention in clinical practice (constituted by representatives of 10 societies and by invited experts) developed with the special contribution of the European Association for Cardiovascular Prevention & Rehabilitation (EACPR). *European Heart Journal* 37 (29): 2315–2381.

Saunders, L.C., Hughes, P.J.C., Alabed, S. et al. (2022). Integrated cardiopulmonary MRI assessment of pulmonary hypertension. *Journal of Magnetic Resonance Imaging* 55 (3): 633–652.

Simpson, R., Schwartz, M.L., Prakash, A. et al. (2018). Comparing echocardiography and cardiac magnetic resonance measures of ejection fraction: implications for HFMRF research. *Heart* 104 (Suppl 5): A3–A3.

Soon, K. and Wong, C. (2012). Coronary computed tomography angiography: a new wave of cardiac imaging. *Internal Medicine Journal* 42 (S5): 22–29.

Srivastva, R. and Singh, Y.N. (2019). ECG analysis for human recognition using non-fiducial methods. *IET Biometrics* 8 (5): 295–305.

Takeda, S. et al. (2003). Structure of the core domain of human cardiac troponin in the Ca^{2+}-saturated form. *Nature* 424 (6944): 35–41.

The Faculty of Intensive Care Medicine. (2018). *Curriculum for Training for Advanced Critical Care Practitioners – Syllabus. V1.1* [online]. Available from: www.ficm.ac.uk/media/6896 [accessed 20 June 2023].

The Intensive Care Society, Critical Care Networks – *National Nurse Leads and The National Outreach Forum*. (2022). *Advanced Critical Care Outreach Competencies* [online]. Available from: https://ics.ac.uk/asset/43B8C11B-4512-41D0-B97768FABA2C30B2 [accessed 20 June 2023].

The Royal College of Emergency Medicine. (2022). *Emergency Medicine Advanced Clinical Practitioner Curriculum 2022 (Adult)* [online]. Available from: https://rcem.ac.uk/wp-content/uploads/2022/09/ACP_Curriculum_Adult_Final_060922.pdf [accessed 20 June 2023].

Wilkinson, I., Raine, T., Wiles, K. et al. (2017). *Oxford Handbook of Clinical Medicine*, 10e. Oxford University Press.

World Health Organisation (WHO). (2020). *The Top 10 Causes of Death* [online]. Available from: https://www.who.int/news-room/fact-sheets/detail/the-top-10-causes-of-death [accessed 21 June 2023].

CHAPTER 9

Neurological and Endocrine Presentations

Rebecca Connolly and Sonya Stone

Aim

The aim of this chapter is to provide the reader with a comprehensive knowledge of common presentations in relation to the neurological and endocrinological systems in the context of advanced practice.

LEARNING OUTCOMES

After reading this chapter the reader will have:

1. Advanced knowledge of common neurological and endocrinological presentations to acute and critical care settings, including: stroke, diabetic ketoacidosis, hyperosmolar hyperglycaemic state, and hyperthyroidism.
2. Detailed insight into common clinical investigations including: CT head scan, MRI brain, and endocrine function testing.
3. Comprehensive insight into pharmacological considerations in neurological and endocrinological medicines including corticosteroids, Gonadotropin-releasing Hormone (GnRH) agonists, and radioactive iodine.
4. An advanced understanding of the evidence base underpinning decision-making in relation to the neurological and endocrinological systems.

The Advanced Practitioner in Acute, Emergency and Critical Care, First Edition. Edited by Sadie Diamond-Fox, Barry Hill, Sonya Stone, Caroline McCrea, Natalie Gardner, and Angela Roberts.
© 2024 John Wiley & Sons Ltd. Published 2024 by John Wiley & Sons Ltd.

SELF-ASSESSMENT QUESTIONS

1. Which useful mnemonic might help you assess a patient presenting with a headache?
2. What are the three main foci of pathogenesis of diabetic ketoacidosis (DKA)?
3. How might you classify seizures?
4. How might a patient with thyrotoxicosis present?

Multi-professional Framework (MPF) for Advanced Clinical Practice Guidance for Professional Development (HEE 2017)

This chapter maps to the following statements within the MPF:

1. Clinical Practice:	1.1	1.2	1.3	1.4	1.5	1.6	1.7	1.8	1.11
2. Leadership and Management:	2.1	2.3	2.7	2.9					
3. Education:	3.1,	3.2							
4. Research:	4.3	4.4							

Accreditation Considerations

This chapter maps to the following statements within the following national accreditation documents:

Curriculum for Training for Advanced Critical Care Practitioners Syllabus V1.1
(The Faculty of Intensive Care Medicine 2018):

2.1	2.2	2.3	2.5	2.6	2.7	2.11	3.1	3.2	3.3	3.5	3.6	3.7	3.8	3.11	3.13	3.19	3.21	4.1	4.2	4.3	4.4	4.12	4.13

Advanced Critical Care Outreach Competencies
(The Intensive Care Society, Critical Care Networks – National Nurse Leads and The National Outreach Forum 2022):

A1	A4

Emergency Medicine Advanced Clinical Practitioner Curriculum 2022 – Adult
(The Royal College of Emergency Medicine 2022):

RP8	CP3	EnP2	EnP3	EnC2	EnC4	EnC6	NeuP1	NeuP2	NeuP3	NeuP4	NeuP5	NeuP7	NeuP8	NeuC6	NeuC9	NeuC11	PhP1	PhC1	TP1

Acute Med:

Generic Clinical CiPs:	1	2	3	4
Specialty Clinical CiPs:	3	4		

INTRODUCTION

The neurological and endocrine systems are complex and often very challenging to assess, diagnose, and manage. The plethora of potential presentations is beyond the scope of this chapter, but common, life-threatening presentations will be covered with a focus on pathophysiology, diagnostics, and management. It is important to remember that acute, emergency, and critical care patients with neurological and endocrine disorders often require immediate treatment but that specialist advice and management from neurology, neurosurgical, and/or endocrinology teams is often required.

This chapter will give an overview of clinical investigations employed to assess the neurological and endocrinological systems, and will offer diagnostic reasoning data to demonstrate the value of tests in particular pathology. Pharmacological principles are explored through commonly used medications, and patient-specific considerations are explained. Case studies are utilised to demonstrate patient presentations and to enable the reader to critically reflect upon their own practice in managing these complex patient groups.

NEUROLOGICAL AND ENDOCRINOLOGICAL HISTORY-TAKING

In addition to routine history-taking practices, focussed questioning relating to 'red flags' in the neurological and endocrine systems will enable the practitioner to differentiate signs and symptoms to develop potential diagnoses. Examples might include, but are not limited to:

- **Neurological** – Headaches, limb weakness (unilateral versus bilateral, upper versus lower), paraesthesia, visual or hearing disturbances, aphasia/dysphasia/dysphagia, dyscoordination, confusion, and cognitive impairment.
- **Endocrinological** – Recent weight loss/gain, unusual hair distribution, sleep disturbance, tachycardia, or palpitations, hormonal considerations including the use of hormone replacement therapies, the presence of autoimmune disorders.

In this chapter, we will explore common presentations and consider their presentations, highlighting signs and symptoms that may indicate specific pathology in the neurological and endocrine systems.

NEUROLOGICAL PRESENTATIONS

Stroke

Pathophysiology and Diagnosis

A stroke occurs because of disruptions in cerebral perfusion, either due to an 'ischaemic' or 'haemorrhagic' event. Being able to discern the difference through examination alone is seldom possible, and prompt CT scanning is fundamental to diagnosis. Further, scanning may be needed to help inform most appropriate treatment approach (see the Clinical Investigations section for types of haemorrhage and how they manifest on CT images).

National Institutes of Health Stroke Scale (NIHSS)

The NIHSS assesses stroke severity and neurological impairment and considers 15 items (see Table 9.1). The tool has been shown to be a good predictor of both short- and long-term outcomes of stroke patients (National Institutes of Health, National Institute of Neurological Disorders and Stroke).

TABLE 9.1   The NIHSS tool.

Category	Scale
1a. Level of consciousness	0 = **Alert** 1 = **Not alert**. Rouses to minor stimulation. 2 = **Not alert**. Requires repeated stimulation or painful stimulus. 3 = **Unresponsive**. Postures are unresponsive, flaccid, and are flexic.
1b. LOC questions Ask month and age. (Patients unable to speak because of endotracheal intubation, trauma, dysarthria, language barrier, or any other problem that is NOT aphasia are given 1a.)	0 = **Answers** both questions correctly. 1 = **Answers** 1 question correctly. 2 = **Answers** no questions correctly.
1c. LOC commands Ask patient to open and close eyes and to squeeze hands.	0 = **Performs** both tasks correctly. 1 = **Performs** one task correctly. 2 = **Performs** neither task correctly.
2. Best gaze Only horizontal ocular movement is assessed	0 = **Normal** 1 = **Partial gaze palsy** (can be overcome with oculocephalic reflex) 2 = **Forced deviation** (cannot be overcome)
3. Visual fields	0 = **No visual field loss** 1 = **Partial hemianopia** 2 = **Complete hemianopia** 3 = **Bilateral hemianopia**
4. Facial palsy Ask the patient to show their teeth or rise their eyebrows and close their eyes	0 = **Normal** symmetrical movements 1 = **Minor paralysis** (asymmetry on smiling) 2 = **Partial paralysis** (total or near total paralysis of lower face) 3 = **Complete paralysis** of one or both sides of the face
5. Motor (arm) • **5a Left arm** • **5b Right arm**	0 = **No drift** 1 = **Drift** 2 = **Some effort against gravity** 3 = **No effort against gravity** 4 = **No movement**
6. Motor (leg) • **6a Left leg** • **6b Right leg**	0 = **No drift** 1 = **Drift** 2 = **Some effort against gravity** 3 = **No effort against gravity** 4 = **No movement**
7. Limb ataxia Finger-nose-finger and heel-shin tests performed on both sides. Aimed at finding unilateral cerebellar lesion	0 = **Absent** 1 = **Present in one limb** 2 = **Present in two limbs**

TABLE 9.1   (Continued)

Category	Scale
8. Sensory Sharp and dull test using pinprick or noxious stimulus test.	0 = **Normal** 1 = **Mild to moderate sensory loss** 2 = **Severe to total sensory loss**
9. Best language	0 = **No aphasia** 1 = **Mild to moderate aphasia** 2 = **Severe aphasia** 3 = **Mute or global aphasia**
10. Dysarthria	0 = **Normal** 1 = **Mild to moderate dysarthria** 2 = **Severe dysarthria**
11. Extinction and Inattention	0 = **No abnormality** 1 = **Visual, tactile, auditory, spatial, or personal inattention** 2 = **Profound hemi-inattention or extinction to more than one modality**

Source: Adapted from http://Stroke.nih.gov.uk.

Treatment Options

Immediate treatment considerations include neuroprotective measures, which are often complex and not fully understood: Maintain euvolaemia judiciously – hypovolaemia decreases cerebral perfusion pressure (CPP), worsening cerebral ischaemia and potentiates further thromboses, while hypervolaemia worsens cerebral oedema.

1. Maintain euglycaemia and normothermia
2. If ventilated, maintain norm/hyperoxia and normocapnia
3. Swallowing assessment

Ischaemic Strokes

1. Immediate revascularisation of the affected vessel is vital to preserve brain tissue and prevent further damage.
2. Patients with an onset time of <4 hours may be suitable for intravenous thrombolysis.
3. Those outside of a four-hour onset window may be treated with intra-arterial thrombolysis or mechanical thrombectomy (these patients usually require additional imaging prior).

Haemorrhagic Strokes

Haemorrhagic strokes are normally treated with supportive measures and/or neurosurgical options. Depending on severity, this may include management in a critical care environment with sedation, ventilation, and intracranial pressure (ICP) monitoring and management.

Surgical options for stroke may include decompressive craniectomy, which should be considered within 48 hours in those with infarction in the territory of the middle cerebral artery (MCA), with an NIHSS score >15, a decreased level of consciousness, and signs of infarct of at least 50% of the MCA territory with or without additional infarction in the posterior (PCA) or anterior (ACA) territories

$$CPP = MAP - ICP$$

FIGURE 9.1   Equation for cerebral perfusion pressure where MAP is mean arterial pressure and ICP is intracranial pressure.

(NICE 2019). In those patients who qualify for, and undergo decompressive craniectomy, there has been a statistically significant reduction in one-year mortality (risk ratio [RR] 0.52). The primary goal in neurological management is to prevent secondary brain injury by maintaining adequate CPP. The equation for CPP is in Figure 9.1.

SEIZURES AND STATUS EPILEPTICUS

Pathophysiology and Diagnosis

Seizures are classified according to the origin of onset and the presence or absence of patient awareness during the episode. Broadly, there are three main types of seizure; focussed, generalised, and onset unknown. Sub-types of seizures enable better descriptors of seizure activity; examples include focal aware, focal impaired, generalised onset, tonic clonic, atonic, myoclonic, and absence seizures.

Status epilepticus is diagnosed clinically by an unremitting generalised seizure lasting >5 minutes, or multiple seizures without an interictal return to a baseline level of consciousness.

Treatment Options

Immediate treatment of any seizure includes an A–E approach:

1. Support the patient's airway through positioning or adjuncts as appropriate.
2. High-flow oxygen.
3. Obtain early IV access for blood sampling (FBC, U&E, Ca^{2+}, Mg, Coag, and LFTs $\pm$ HCG in the patient who can bear children) and early administration of medications (especially in status epilepticus). Alternative routes of administration should be considered (i.e. buccal, IM, or rectal) if access will be delayed.
4. Early VBG to assess glucose, pH and electrolytes.
5. Serum anti-epileptic medication levels in known epileptics.

Status Epilepticus

1. Be aware of the underlying causes of status epilepticus, including hypoglycaemia, eclampsia, and alcohol withdrawal, which may need to be treated with additional medication.
2. 4 mg IV lorazepam.
3. Administer a second dose of 4 mg IV lorazepam after 10 minutes if there is ongoing seizure activity.
4. If after the second dose of benzodiazepine the seizure has not stopped, administer IV second-line treatment (according to local guidelines):
   a. Levetiracetam
   b. Phenytoin
   c. Sodium Valproate

5. If the patient has a uterus and is of child bearing age, sodium valproate should not be used due to its teratogenic effects.

6. If the patient fails to respond to second-line treatment consider critical care support.

MENINGITIS AND ENCEPHALITIS

Pathophysiology and Diagnosis

Viral infections of the central nervous system (CNS) may result in aseptic meningitis and/or encephalitis with the presence or absence of normal brain function being an important distinguishing feature.

Generally, patients with meningitis tend to retain normal cerebral function, whereas those with encephalitis present with an altered status, or other brain abnormalities may be found. Be careful however, as sometimes the lines can be blurred: seizures and post ictal states can be seen with meningitis alone. Signs and symptoms of meningeal irritation are normally not found in pure encephalitis but can accompany meningoencephalitis.

Diagnostic tools include:

- CT imaging – Easily available, CTs are often the first imaging modality used, and can be used to rule out conditions, such as space occupying lesions.
- Magnetic Resonance Imaging (MRI) is useful to ascertain demyelination.
- Lumbar Punctures (LPs) are of limited value in distinguishing between aseptic meningitis and encephalitis, but can be used to ascertain inflammation of the CNS. LP should be avoided in those with reduced levels of consciousness where there is concern of raised ICP or in those with a coagulopathy.
- In addition to CSF analysis, other tools such as PCR testing for HSVs, HIV should be considered.

Treatment Options

Treatment options are largely empiric, with usual antiviral pharmacologic agents such as Acyclovir IV being initiated. Local guidelines may differ, and discussions with clinical pharmacy, infectious diseases, and microbiology colleagues are advised.

ENDOCRINE PRESENTATIONS

Diabetic Ketoacidosis (DKA) and Hyperosmolar Hyperglycaemic State (HHS)

Pathophysiology and Diagnosis

DKA

Three main foci of pathogenesis:

- **Osmotic diuresis**: insulin deficiency → hyperglycaemia → hyperosmolality → osmotic diuresis and loss of electrolytes → hypovolaemia

- **HAGMA[1]**: insulin deficiency → ↑ lipolysis → ↑ free fatty acids (acetoacetic acid and beta-hydroxybutyric acid) → hepatic ketone production → ketosis → bicarb consumption as a buffer → HAGMA
- **Intracellular K+ deficit**: insulin deficiency → hyperosmolality → K+ shifts out of cells and lack of insulin to promote K+ uptake → intracellular K+ depletion → total body K+ deficit

Diagnosis is made when all three of the following criteria are met:

1. Raised blood glucose >11 mmol/l *or* known diabetic
2. Capillary ketones >3 mmol/l *or* urinary ketones >2+
3. Venous pH <7.35 *or* venous HCO_3^- <15 mmol/l

Always consider level 1 or critical care input. Consider a euglycaemic DKA in an unwell patient taking sodium-glucose co-transporter-2 inhibitors (SGLT-2i) as the increasing use of these medications has resulted in reports of increased euDKA phenomena.

HHS

As above, but with small amounts of insulin preventing DKA. Characterised by marked dehydration due to hyperglycaemia and osmotic diuresis. HHS can be either the initial presentation of diabetes mellitus → inadequate insulin replacement (i.e. non-compliance with treatment) or ↑ insulin demand (i.e. illness, surgery, stress). Remember that HHS is more insidious, whereas DKA is rapid.

HHS is characterised by:

- symptoms of marked dehydration (and loss of electrolytes) due to the predominating hyperglycaemia and osmotic diuresis
- Severe hyperglycaemia → ↑ serum osmolality → osmotic diuresis → dehydration

Treatment Options

1. **Immediate**:
   a. 1000 ml 0.9% NaCl over 1hour, if systolic >90 mmHg (if systolic <90 mmHg then consider repeated 500 ml boluses over 10 minutes)
2. **Start IV insulin infusion**:
   a. Common orthodoxy treatment is 50 units of human soluble (ACTRAPID) insulin added to 49.5 ml 0.9% NaCl → 1 unit/ml solution at a rate of 0.1 units/kg/h and you are aiming for:
   b. Blood glucose fall of >3 mmol/l/h or until <14 mmol/l
   c. Capillary ketones fall of >0.5 mmol/l/h
   d. Venous HCO_3^- rise of >33 mmol/l/h
3. **Continue the patient's long-acting insulin**
4. **IV fluid:**
   a. 1000 ml 0.9% NaCl over 1hour
   b. 1000 ml 0.9% NaCl over 2hours (consider KCl)
   c. 1000 ml 0.9% NaCl over 2hours (consider KCl)

---

[1] HAGMA = High Anion Gap Metabolic Acidosis (CATMUDPILES is a useful mnemonic to think about why a person may have a HAGMA, if the cause is unclear).

    d. 1000 ml 0.9% NaCl over 4 hours

    e. Continue 0.9% NaCl (+KCl) as needed, to restore circulating volume

5. When glucose <14 mmol/l, continue 0.9% NaCl (±KCl) and add 10% glucose over 125 ml/h. Adjust the rate in 50 ml increments to maintain glucose in the range of 8–14 mmol/l

6. **Potassium:**

    a. Do not add KCl prior to the second bag of fluid unless $K^+ < 3.5$ (use VBG for rapid interpretation – do not wait for serum results)

    b. If K^+ is <5.4 then add 40 mmol/l of 0.9% NaCl

Remember to measure Na^+ levels and serum osmolality.

Hyperthyroidism

Pathophysiology and Diagnosis

Most cases of hyperthyroidism are attributable to autoimmune thyrotoxicosis (Graves' Disease), with a small proportion caused by toxic multinodular goitre or thyroid adenoma. Cases of transient thyrotoxicosis caused by thyroiditis are fairly common and can be related to toxins including drugs. Additionally, thyrotoxicosis may occur because of other endocrine pathology such as tumours of the pituitary gland, although this type of presentation is rare.

There are several common clinical features of thyrotoxicosis caused by thyroid hormone excess. Graves' disease shares these common features, but additionally, patients may present with additional signs associated with autoimmunity (Figure 9.2).

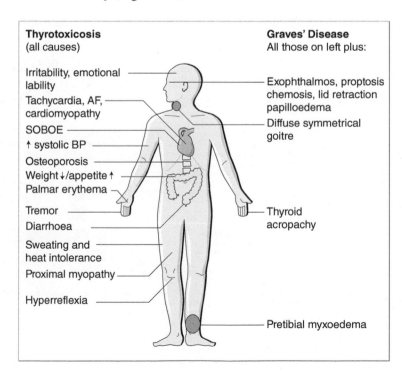

FIGURE 9.2 Clinical features of thyrotoxicosis and the additional features of graves' disease. *Source*: Greenstein et al. (2011) / John Wiley & Sons.

Treatment Options

Treatment depends on theaetiology. Pharmacological management with antithyroid drugs being first-line, in combination with additional therapies, including radioactive iodine, and surgical management when indicated, including hemi and total thyroidectomy.

Ongoing monitoring and treatment should include regular thyroid function tests (TFTs) (Thyroid Stimulating Hormone (TSH), Free T4 (FT4), and Free T3 (FT3)), usually every six weeks for the first six months until TSH is normal, and then every three to six months. For those patients undergoing hemi or total thyroidectomy, levothyroxine or other thyroid replacement medication should be offered and TSH and FT4 offered at two months, six months, and then yearly.

Neurological Examination

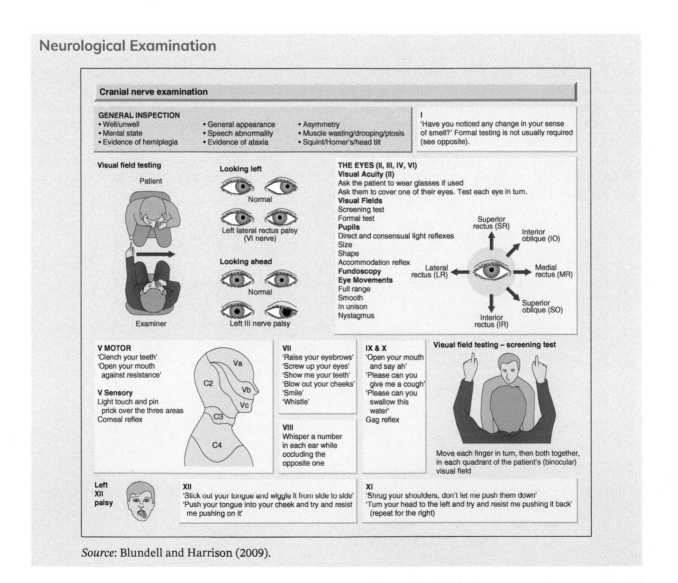

Source: Blundell and Harrison (2009).

CLINICAL INVESTIGATIONS

Neurological Imaging

1. **Computed Tomography (CT): Head**

   Non-contrast Computed Tomography (NCCT) c for investigation of acute stroke. However, research suggests that while NCCT has sensitivity up to 89% for acute intracranial haemorrhage, sensitivity for ischaemic strokes may be as low as 12% in infarctions less than 3 hours old, rising to only 16% after 12 hours. Despite this, image manipulation techniques performed by radiology can assist in the detection of ischaemia.

   Computed tomography angiography (CTA) is fundamental in identification of culprit vascular lesions (sensitivity 83%, specificity 95%), and additionally, is excellent in identifying acute ischaemic stroke (sensitivity 93%, specificity 100%).

   Scanning protocols may vary from institution to institution, but the scan in adults is normally performed with 5 mm cuts from the skull base to the vertex, and remains a sensitive investigation for intracranial haemorrhage, oedema, and mass effect (Sjoholm and Ross 2008). While formal reports must always be used from which clinical decisions and dispositions are made, a useful mnemonic for evaluating a head CT (developed by Dr. Andrew Perron, a United States Emergency Medicine physician) is: **Blood Can Be Very Bad**.

B(LOOD) Is for Blood

- Acute bleed will appear bright white (once it clots), and at around one week becomes isodense. At around two weeks it becomes hypodense.
- Basic categories are: epidural, subdural, intraparenchymal/intracerebral, intraventricular, and subarachnoid

Epidural haematoma (EDH) (also known as extradural) is formed between inner surface of the skull and outer layer of the dura. It is usually associated with trauma ± skull fracture. The bleeding is normally arterial, most frequently from a torn middle meningeal artery (Figure 9.3).

They are usually biconvex (looking somewhat like an egg: EGGstradural) and do not cross suture lines.

They have a low mortality (<20%), if treated prior to unconsciousness.

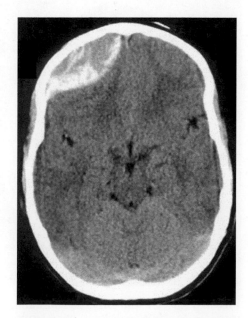

FIGURE 9.3 CT scan showing left-sided EDH. *Source*: Jpogi / Wikimedia Commons / CC BY-SA 3.0.

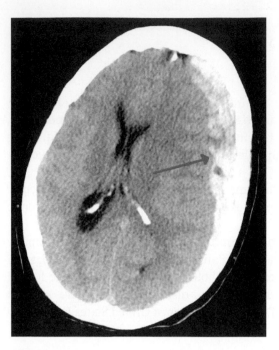

FIGURE 9.4   CT scan image demonstrating right sided SDH. *Source*: James Heilman, MD / Wikimedia Commons / CC BY-SA 3.0.

Subdural haematoma/haemorrhage (SDH) is formed by blood accumulating in the subdural space – the potential space between the dura and arachnoid mater. They can happen in any age group but clinical presentations in the elderly, in particular, can be very vague and may be thought to be a new dementia (Figure 9.4).

They are usually falx or sickle shaped, cross suture lines, but do not cross the midline.

Acute SDH is a marker of severe head injury with high mortality, but chronic SDHs are usually a slow venous bleed and are normally well tolerated.

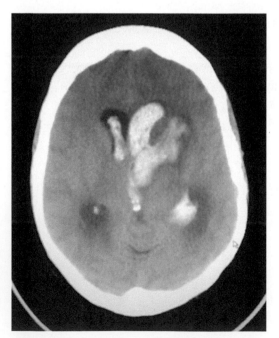

FIGURE 9.5   CT scan image demonstrating an IPH with ventricular extension. *Source*: Glitzy queen00 / Wikimedia Commons / Public Domain.

Intraparenchymal/Intracerebral   haemorrhage (IPH) is either primary (i.e. with no underlying lesion) or secondary (i.e. some other lesion complicated by haemorrhage). Non-traumatic lesions due to hypertensive disease are typically seen in elderly patients and occur most frequently in the basal ganglia region (Figure 9.5).

There can also often be surrounding hypodense oedema with other complications, such as extension of the haemorrhage into other compartments.

Intraventricular haemorrhage (IVH) means that the blood is within the cerebral ventricular system and is associated with significant morbidity.

Primary IVHs have blood in the ventricles with no (or very little) parenchymal blood. Secondary IVHs have a large extra ventricular component with secondary extension into the ventricles. It may also be from a subarachnoid haemorrhage (SAH) with ventricular rupture (e.g. PICA aneurysms) (Figure 9.6).

Hydrocephalus may result regardless of aetiology.

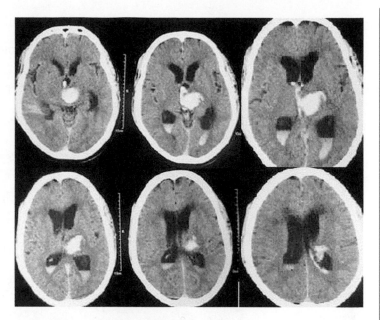

FIGURE 9.6   CT scan image demonstrating IVH. *Source*: Yadav YR / Wikimedia Commons / CC BY 2.0.

Subarachnoid haemorrhage (SAH) is recognised by the presence of blood in the subarachnoid space (cisterns/cortical gyral surface), and while no cause is found in ~10% of cases, the most common causes of SAH are aneurysms (70–80%).

Patients typically present with a thunderclap headache, and although MRI is thought to be most sensitive, non-contrast head CTs are often performed first within the emergency setting. The sensitivity is strongly influenced by the amount of blood and time since the haemorrhage (Figure 9.7).

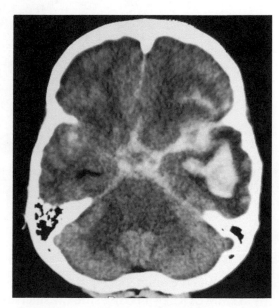

FIGURE 9.7   Non-contrast CT head demonstrating SAH.

C(AN) Is for Cisterns

- Two key questions to answer regarding the four key cisterns are: is there blood, and are the cisterns open?
- Check the Suprasellar, Circummensencephalic, Quadrigeminal, and Sylvian cisterns (Figure 9.8).

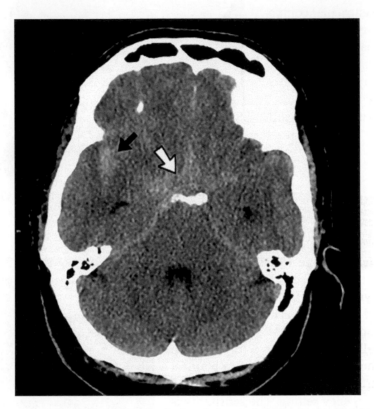

FIGURE 9.8   This image shows hyperdense SAH in the basal cisterns (white arrow) and right-sided sylvian fissure (black arrow). Note the hypodensity in the adjacent parenchyma that represents secondary oedema.

B(E) Is for Brain

- Examine the brain for (Figure 9.9).
- SYMMETRY by making sure the sulci and gyri appear the same on both sides and checking for unilateral or bilateral sulci effacement.
- GREY–WHITE differentiation: the earliest sign of a stroke is the loss of grey–white interface. Compare side to side.
- SHIFT – the falx should be midline with ventricles the same on both sides.
- HYPER/HYPODENSITY

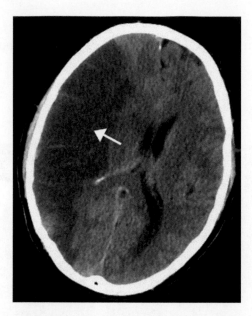

FIGURE 9.9 This image shows a prior left-sided ischaemic stroke due to an MCA territory infarct. Changes on a CT may not be visible early on. *Source*: Lucien Monfils / Wikimedia Commons / CC BY-SA 3.0.

V(ERY) Is for Ventricles/Vessels

- Examine III, IV, and lateral ventricles for dilation or compression/shift (Figure 9.10).

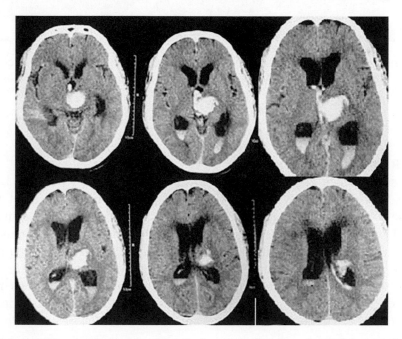

FIGURE 9.10 This image shows a pre-operative CT scan of a patient showing a thalamic haemorrhage with associated hydrocephalus and blood in the third and both lateral ventricles. *Source*: Yadav YR / Wikimedia Commons / CC BY 2.0.

B(AD) Is for Bone

- Bone has the highest density on CT and is therefore whitest in appearance. Check for any fractures (Figure 9.11).

(a)   (b)

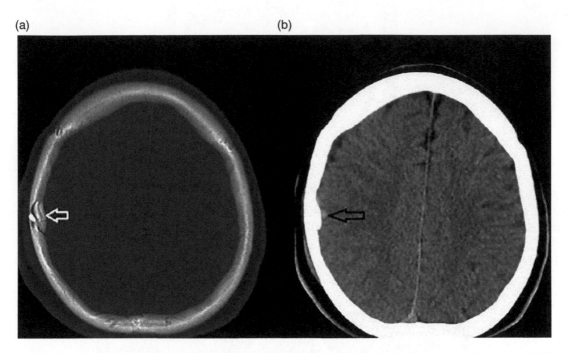

FIGURE 9.11   This image shows a young man with shotgun injury. Bone window (a) reveals a depressed skull fracture (arrow in a). Note the hyperdense pellet embedded near the fracture. Parenchymal window (b) shows a contusion (arrow in b) in the adjacent parenchyma. *Source*: Reza Akhavan/iEM.

2. **Magnetic Resonance Imaging (MRI): Head**
   Unlike CT scans which employ ionising radiation, MRIs employ electromagnetic fields and radio waves to visualise bodily structures and processes, and is therefore not related to associated adverse effects. They are particularly suitable for soft tissue structures and nervous tissue, although CT remains the modality of choice within the emergency setting and for the evaluation of bone structures. A good underpinning knowledge of anatomy is essential because MRIs produce a very clear view of structures (Figures 9.12 to 9.14).

   MRI is used in the investigation and diagnosis of a number of conditions including Parkinson's Disease (see Figure 9.16 'swallow tail sign'), Multiple Sclerosis (sensitivity 94%, specificity 83%), and Alzheimer's disease through the evaluation of volume loss with a diagnostic accuracy up to 87%.

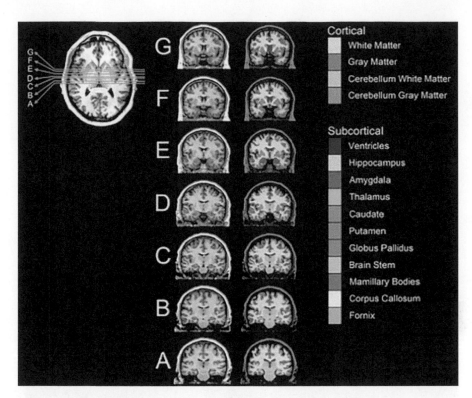

FIGURE 9.12 Coronal MRI structures.

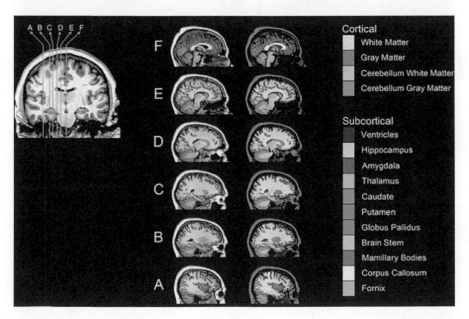

FIGURE 9.13 Sagittal MRI brain slices.

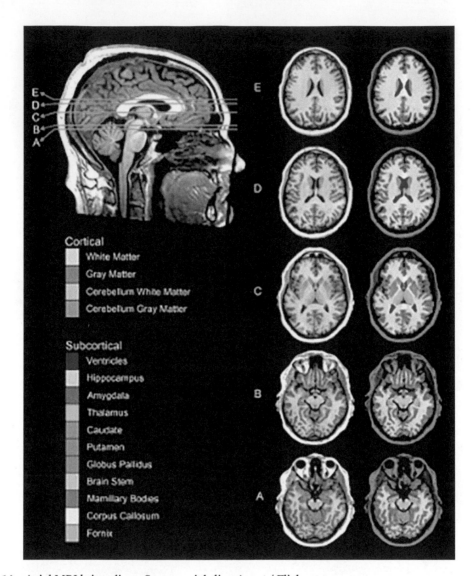

FIGURE 9.14   Axial MRI brian slices. *Source*: axial slices4 port / Flickr.

MRI Structures (Figures 9.12 to 9.14)

Eye of the Tiger Sign

Bilateral abnormal low signal on MRI scan caused by abnormal accumulation of iron in the globus pallidus. This can sometimes be helpful due to its association with pantothenate kinase-associated neurodegeneration. Caution must be taken, however, as it can also be seen in other conditions, including atypical parkinsonism and organophosphate poisoning. It may be normal for some individuals (Figure 9.15).

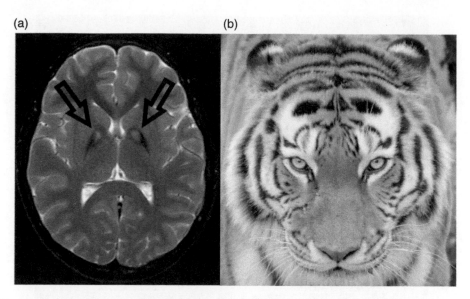

FIGURE 9.15 (a) Iron deposits in the Globus Pallidus (black arrows). (b) Comparison made with image of tiger. *Source*: (a) I, Enro 2002 / Wikimedia Commons / CC BY-SA 3.0. (b) 9143 images / Pixabay.

Swallow Tail Sign

The 'swallow tail sign' describes a normal axial image of the substantia nigra on MRI. The absence of this sign has been found to have a >90% diagnostic accuracy for Parkinson's Disease (sensitivity 79–100%, specificity 85–100%) and Lewy Body Dementia. It is also reported that patients with multiple sclerosis may also have an abnormal swallow tail sign on MRI (Figures 9.16 and 9.17).

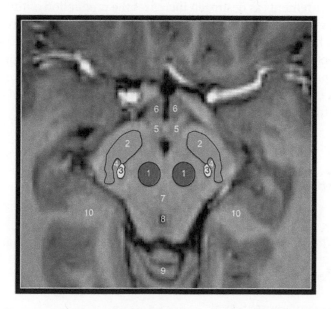

FIGURE 9.16 Illustrates the normal swallow tail sign of the substantia nigra (2). Note to publisher: *Source*: Image taken from Wiley online Claudia E. / https://onlinelibrary.wiley.com/doi/10.1111/jon.12775 / last accessed February 22, 2023.

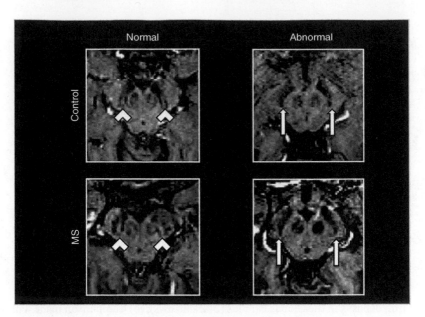

FIGURE 9.17   Representative examples of normal (arrowheads) and abnormal (arrows) swallow tail signs in controls (top row) and multiple sclerosis (MS) patients (bottom row). *Source*: NEW.

Thyroid Function Tests (TFTs)

Measurement and interpretation of TFTs needs careful consideration. The majority (99%) of thyroid hormones are protein bound at any one time, and therefore results of T3 and T4 assays are largely affected by any physiological condition affecting protein binding; for example, pregnant people may show high total T4 measurements as oestrogen increases the production of thyroxine binding globulin. To mitigate against spurious results, assays of TSH, FT3, and FT4 are widely recommended as they are less affected by protein binding.

In patients with suspected thyroid disease, TSH is a reliable assay (sensitivity 98%, specificity 92%). The application of the principles of negative feedback allows for interpretation of TSH along with FT3 and FT4. For example, in hyperthyroidism, TSH is low, because FT3 and FT4 are high. Conversely, in primary hypothyroidism, TSH is elevated and FT4 is low.

Fields of Practice – Paediatrics

Febrile Convulsions

A febrile seizure is the most common neurologic disorder of infants and young people, and defined as a single generalised seizure lasting <15 minutes in one 24-hour period with the following criteria:

- Associated with a temperature >38°C
- >6 months and <5 years of age
- Absence of CNS infection or any systemic metabolic abnormality (that may induce convulsions)
- No prior history of febrile seizures

Risk factors include recent immunisation and/or viral infection (bacterial infections have a lower association with febrile seizures).

Useful diagnostic approaches include identifying the cause of the fever, so include a physical examination and urinalysis, and consider a full blood panel $\pm$ toxicology screen in cases where the source is unclear or if the patient is unwell. Complex febrile seizures (accounting approx. 25% of all febrile seizures) require specific investigations such as imaging, lumbar puncture, or EEGs.

Fields of Practice – Mental Health

While the pathogenesis of mental pathology is complex and not yet fully understood, there may be a symbiotic relationship between a patient's biological, social, and psychological factors which pervade multiple health outcomes. Thus, understanding neurobiological pathogenesis of various conditions that are linked with mental illness is helpful, but it is just as important to remember that even bidirectional correlation does not necessarily equal causation.

For example, in the field of addiction some evidence suggests that a Taq1A polymorphism of the dopamine D2 receptor DRD2 gene may predispose an individual to a greater risk of addiction, but the importance of social and psychological behaviours and influences must also be considered fully when thinking about treatment and targeted medicine.

Fields of Practice – Learning Disabilities

As with the neurobiological aetiology of neurological and endocrinological dysfunction potentiating certain mental health presentations, so too does the pathophysiology of learning disabilities. Remembering that the patient is an individual with neurodiverse features and treating accordingly will allow for holistic and patient-centred care.

Learning Events (Reflection)

- The aetiology of neurological and endocrinological presentations is usually multifaceted and is associated with a constellation of symptoms. Consider presentations to your clinical area and reflect upon cases demonstrating the interaction of these complex systems.
- How will your history-taking change to ensure you are asking salient system-specific questions when assessing neurological and/or endocrinological presentations?

Pharmacological Principles

Corticosteroids

- Steroids are used in several conditions that could present with neurological or endocrine presentations, and they are a class of steroid hormones that includes glucocorticoids and mineralocorticoids:
  - Humans synthesise endogenous glucocorticoids from cholesterol in the adrenal cortex and are very important for immunosuppressant and metabolic processes. Interestingly, increased levels of cortisol (a glucocorticoid) are shown to increase abdominal visceral fat
  - Endogenous mineralocorticoids are important for regulation of the renin-angiotensin system

- Synthetic steroids have several short- and long-term pharmacodynamics effects:
  - Acute anti-inflammatory properties due to decreased vasodilation and capillary permeability
  - Long-term effects result in neutrophilic leucocytosis, decreased production of prostaglandins, suppression of B and T cells, inhibition of histamine release from mast cells (which is why it is given in allergic reactions)
  - Mineralocorticoids can include increased potassium excretion
  - They can also increase muscle mass and strength

Gonadotropin-releasing Hormone (GnRH) Agonists

- Works by increasing pituitary gland stimulation of GnRH, which results in a shutdown of the GnRH receptors. This in turn results in a decrease in FH and FSH secretion, which has the end effect of halting testosterone production in the testicles, and oestradiol production in the ovaries.
- Because of the initial increased release of pituitary gonadotropins, patients with testicles may suffer a transient increase in testosterone levels ('flare-up' symptoms). This is an important point to discuss in those for whom a GnRH agonist is prescribed as a result of prostate cancer (known as tumour flare).
- The transient effects are then followed by complete suppression of the hypothalamic-pituitary-gonadal axis.
- Common indications include male-to-female gender medicine, uterine leiomyoma, precocious puberty, endometriosis, breast/prostate cancers.

Oral Oestrogen

- When bioidentical works in the same way as the naturally circulating hormone.
- Is prescribed as an adjunct for numerous conditions, including but not limited to vulvovaginal atrophy or conditions associated with reduced oestrogen.
- Estradiol is metabolised to estrone, and both are converted to estriol, which is later excreted in the urine.
- Estradiol may cause an increased risk of cardiovascular disease and DVT because Oestrogen induces a hypercoagulable state. Further, Oestrogen also causes increased levels of angiotensin, which causes sodium retention and can result in hypertension.

Radioactive Iodine

- May be offered as first-line treatment in thyrotoxicosis caused by Graves' disease or toxic multi-nodular goitre.
- Taken orally and rapidly absorbed by the thyroid. The radiation collects in thyroid tissue and results in cell death thereby reducing the functional capacity of the thyroid gland in producing thyroxine.
- Those who are pregnant, or breastfeeding must not be treated with radioactive iodine, and those with a uterus should refrain from pregnancy for 12 months following treatment due to increased risk of neonatal hypothyroidism and goitre. Sperm is thought to be affected for six months and therefore precautions to mitigate against pregnancy should be used.

RED FLAGS – PATHOLOGICAL CONSIDERATIONS

Headache

A useful mnemonic to utilise when examining the patient with a headache is **SNOOP10**, which covers many red flags

- **Systemic symptoms** (e.g. fever, meningism, malaise) as this may indicate intracranial infections, non-vascular intracranial disorders, carcinoid or pheochromocytoma, and SAH (blood can irritate the meninges, manifesting with signs of meningitis)
- **Neoplasm** as this may indicate metastases
- **Neurological deficit** (e.g. altered status or seizures)
- **Onset is sudden** which is an SAH until proven otherwise
- **Older age at onset** (>50 years) – a new or progressive headache in a patient aged >50 may indicate a tumour or haemorrhage and should always be treated as a high-risk headache
- **Pattern changes of normal headache or recent onset** as this may indicate neoplasm
- **Positional headache** as this may indicate intracranial hypertension/hypotension
- **Precipitated by sneezing, coughing,** *or* exercise as this may indicate posterior fossa malformations or Chiari malformation
- **Progressive headache** and atypical features
- **Pregnancy or postpartum period** as this may be a feature of conditions such as pre-eclampsia, eclampsia, pituitary apoplexy, and cerebral sinus thrombosis
- **Pain in the eye** with autonomic features and visual defects as this may indicate conditions of the posterior fossa, or pituitary region
- **Post-traumatic** onset as may indicate a subdural haematoma
- **Pathology of the immune system** (e.g. HIV) as being immunocompromised increases the risk of meningoencephalitis
- **Papilloedema** as this is a sign of increased ICP
- **Painkiller** overuse as may indicate overuse headache of adverse drug effects

Idiopathic Facial Nerve Palsy (or Bell's Palsy) (versus Stroke)

- Usually has a viral aetiology (normally HSV) but can be secondary to facial trauma, malignant otitis externa, GBS, sarcoidosis.
- Be aware that Bell's Palsy can coexist secondary to stroke.
- Affects Cranial Nerve VII – the facial nerve. This is a mixed nerve.
- The risk is three times greater in pregnancy, especially in the third trimester.
- The key for clinicians is to establish whether the palsy is central or peripheral.
- The muscles responsible for eyelid and forehead movement are innervated by fibres from both sides, however, in central nerve palsy there is a unilateral UPPER MOTOR NEURON lesion within the corticobulbar tract, but the muscles of the eyelid and forehead are still supplied from the other side, so function is preserved. In peripheral facial nerve palsy, however, there is a unilateral LOWER MOTOR NEURON lesion, which results in paralysis of the ipsilateral eyelid and forehead muscles because no other input reaches them. Mouth drooping is present in both.

- In addition, with peripheral facial nerve palsy there may be an ophthalmic reflexive movement of the eye upwards and outwards, when the eyelid is actively closed. You may find that the patient is also unable to close their eye due to paralysis of the orbicular oculi muscle.
- When an acute central cause is suspected, be highly suspicious for an ischaemic stroke.
- Consider a tumour in patients with gradual onset, or slowly progressive neurological symptoms.

ORANGE FLAGS – PSYCHOLOGICAL CONSIDERATIONS

Dementia – Psychological, Physiological, or Both?

Around 7.1% of UK adults over the age of 65 are diagnosed with dementia and while the pathophysiology is still not fully understood, evidence does suggest a symbiosis of mind, body, and spirit mediated through neurological damage. The most common constellation of processes falls under an Alzheimer's umbrella, followed by vascular, Lewy body, and then frontotemporal lobe dementia.

Alzheimer's Dementia

- Key genetic factors include:
  - Amyloid precursor protein (people with Trisomy 21, or Down Syndrome have an increased risk of Alzheimer's because the APP gene is located on chromosome 21)
  - Presenilin-1 (linked to around 50% of familial cases)
  - Presenilin-2 (rare)
  - ApoE
- Key pathophysiological processes include:
  - Extracellular neurotoxic neuritic plaques within the brain grey matter are deposited from Aβ peptide formation
  - Development of intracellular Neurofibrillatory Tangles which are produced from increased phosphorylation of the tau protein. The tangle are also neurotoxic, and the number of tangles has a correlation with cognitive impairment
  - Reduced cholinergic function

Vascular Dementia

- Usually presents as a result of chronic prolonged and severe cerebral ischaemia of any aetiology
- Can be subdivided into Small and Large Vessel Disease
  - Small vessel: predominantly caused by lipohyalinosis, which causes infarcts or chronic ischaemia in the subcortical white matter or within the lacunes
  - Large vessel: predominantly caused by atherosclerosis which causes progressive damage to neural networks

Lewy Body Dementia

- Dementia which is caused by the deposition of alpha-synuclein proteins in cerebral neurons and is characterised by visual hallucinations and parkinsonian symptoms
- Patients will present with not only classical dementia symptoms, but also with other symptoms such as extrapyramidal motor dysfunction, visual hallucinations, and frequent falls

Frontotemporal Lobe Dementia

- A dementia characterised by degeneration of the frontal, insular, and/or temporal cortices as a result of tau protein mutation (note the difference from hyperphosphorylation of the tau protein which is present in Alzheimer's Dementia)
- This has a hereditary component, with an autosomal dominance resulting in around 10–20% of cases being as such
- Classical features include
  - Corticobasal syndrome (akinetic movement issues)
  - Posterior cortical atrophy – blurred vision
  - Semantic
  - Progressive non-fluent aphasia, so things like apraxia
  - Behavioural variant, which presents with changes in personality

Case Studies

Case Study 1: Transgender Presentation

A 25-year-old transgender female patient presents feeling generally unwell, complaining of palpitations, nausea, hot flushes, and abdominal discomfort. She has no history of temperature, no altered sensorium, no claudication, and no haemoptysis. She mentions a mild chest discomfort, but no shortness of breath or intrascapulae pain.

She has been under her own GP for a number of months in relation to her gender dysphoria, and has been referred to a local Gender Dysphoria Clinic, but due to extended wait times, she tells you that she has been sourcing her own medication from the internet and had been self-medicating with 100 mg Spironolactone for its anti-androgen properties, and oral oestrogen tablets, taking 8 mg in divided doses through the day.

She was referred by her GP to an Endocrinologist who prescribed Decapeptyl SR 11.25 mg every 12 weeks, and she had this administered by the practice nurse three days ago. The endocrinologist has also switched her oestrogen to a 150 mcg/24 h patch preparation.

1. Based on this history, what concerns do you have?
2. What further investigations do you need?
3. What differentials have you considered with this patient?

You then ask for a full set of investigations, and are presented with the following:

- Venous Blood Gas shows a pH of 7.37, pCO_2 5 kPa, BE 0, HCO_3^- 15, Na 130, K^+ 6.2
- ECG shows a sinus rhythm with normal axis and intervals, but with tented T-waves
- FBC, LFT, CRP is all normal. She has a slight left-sided neutrophilia and serum potassium is 6. All other values are normal. You are unable to request hormonal levels such as serum testosterone, oestradiol, FSH, LH, Prolactin.

Your physical exam is unremarkable.

1. Has this information changed your concerns?
2. What are your priorities?
3. What has happened with this patient?

Transgender Case Study, Discussion Points

This patient is presenting with hyperkalaemia, likely secondary to Spironolactone use, and this needs immediate management and monitoring, with a consideration of Pulmonary Embolism due to oral oestrogen which has been self-managed. Hot flushes may be related to a flare up of testosterone related to recent Decapeptyl, which should settle, although her endocrinologist could have considered prescribing a safe alternative to Spironolactone (such as Bicalutamide) for a week post Decapeptyl injection to help mitigate any of potential exacerbations.

Case Study 2: Tachycardia

A 31-year-old female presents with episodic tachycardia at rest, worse at night. They report no associated chest pain or shortness of breath, but describe palpitations and a feeling that their 'heart is racing'. Over the last 24 hours, these episodes have increased, and their GP has sent them to the Emergency Department for investigation.

- What are your initial differential diagnoses?
- What system specific questions will you ask to guide your decision-making?

Their initial ECG shows sinus tachycardia, all other vital signs are normal. Physical examination is unremarkable.

- What other diagnostic tests would you consider at this point?

During the consultation, the patient reports palpitations and a repeat ECG shows a supraventricular tachycardia (SVT) with a rate of 180 bpm.

- What immediate management strategies would you consider?

Laboratory results show a normal FBC, U&E, CRP, and Troponin. However, TSH is unrecordable and FT4 is very high.

- What is the diagnosis?
- What medications should be prescribed and what considerations should be made before doing so?
- What referrals does the patient require?

Take Home Points
- Advanced practitioners must have the expert knowledge required to recognise and manage the complexities of neurological and endocrinological presentations.
- Recognition of the nuances of history-taking and clinical examination in these systems is paramount to ensuring patient safety and the development of differential diagnoses.

- The utilisation of clinical decision-making tools and clinical reasoning techniques will ensure the advanced practitioner delivers safe and efficient care to these patient groups.
- Collegiate working with specialist teams is paramount to the successful delivery of effective care in these complex patients.
- Maintaining an up-to-date working knowledge of contemporary medicine is essential to ensure patient presentations are managed effectively. This includes knowledge of diverse presentations and the implications on wider groups such as the LGBTQIA+ community, paediatrics, and the BAME community.

REFERENCES

Blundell, A. and Harrison, R. (2009). *OSCEs at a Glance.* Wiley.

Greenstein, B. and Wood, D.F. (2011). *The Endocrine System at a Glance.* Wiley.

Health Education England (HEE). (2017). *Multi-professional Framework for Advanced Clinical Practice in England* [online]. Available from https://www.hee.nhs.uk/sites/default/files/documents/multi-profe ssionalframeworkforadvancedclinicalpracticeinengland.pdf [accessed 20 June 2023].

National Institute for Health and Care Excellence (NICE). (2019). *Thyroid Disease: Assessment and Management (NG145).* [online]. Available from: https://www.nice.org.uk/guidance/ng145/resources/ thyroid-disease-assessment-and-management-pdf-66141781496773 [accessed 21 June 2023].

Sjoholm, L.O. and Ross, S.E. (2008). The use of computed tomography in initial trauma evaluation. In: *Current Therapy of Trauma and Surgical Critical Care*, 136–138. Available from: https://doi.org/10.1016/ B978-0-323-04418-9.50025-4 [accessed 21 June 2023].

The Faculty of Intensive Care Medicine. (2018). *Curriculum for Training for Advanced Critical Care Practitioners – Syllabus. V1.1* [online]. Available from: www.ficm.ac.uk/media/6896 [accessed 20 June 2023].

The Intensive Care Society, Critical Care Networks – National Nurse Leads and The National Outreach Forum. (2022). *Advanced Critical Care Outreach Competencies* [online]. Available from: https://ics.ac.uk/ asset/43B8C11B-4512-41D0-B97768FABA2C30B2 [accessed 20 June 2023].

The Royal College of Emergency Medicine. (2022). *Emergency Medicine Advanced Clinical Practitioner Curriculum 2022 (Adult)* [online]. Available from: https://rcem.ac.uk/wp-content/ uploads/2022/09/ACP_Curriculum_Adult_Final_060922.pdf [accessed 20 June 2023].

FURTHER READING

Hill, R. and Diamond-Fox, J. (2022). *ACP at a Glance.* Wiley.

Peate, I., Diamond-Fox, J., and Hill, R. (2023). *The Advanced Practitioner.* Wiley.

CHAPTER 10

AECC Renal and Genitourinary Presentations

Rachel Allen-Ashcroft and Sonya Stone

Aim

The aim of this chapter is to critically develop the individual's knowledge, understanding, and clinical application of renal and genitourinary presentations. This includes the differentiation between normal and abnormal findings in acute and chronic presentations, consideration of key clinical features, laboratory investigations, altered physiology, pharmacological principles, and considerations of the wider specialist subject areas.

LEARNING OUTCOMES

After reading this chapter the reader will be able to:

1. Synthesise the information presented in this chapter and consider how this may apply to the management of individuals with renal and genitourinary presentations, including appropriate requests for clinical investigations to inform a clinical diagnosis relating to renal and genitourinary presentations.
2. Evaluate the issues surrounding comprehensive assessment, including the clinical reasoning examination of individuals with acute and complex renal and genitourinary presentations.
3. Critically reflect on and evaluate the key decision-making skills required when managing complex and emergency scenarios.
4. Develop and enhance skills of prioritisation, negotiation, and communication when providing holistic care.

The Advanced Practitioner in Acute, Emergency and Critical Care, First Edition. Edited by Sadie Diamond-Fox, Barry Hill, Sonya Stone, Caroline McCrea, Natalie Gardner, and Angela Roberts.
© 2024 John Wiley & Sons Ltd. Published 2024 by John Wiley & Sons Ltd.

SELF-ASSESSMENT QUESTIONS

1. Which equations are used to assess eGFR?
2. What are the considerations for prescribing to patients with renal impairment?
3. What factors affect the value of Creatinine?
4. What are the red flag signs for urosepsis?

INTRODUCTION

In this chapter, we will review renal and genitourinary presentations, important clinical investigations, and diagnostic tests, which inform clinical diagnosis, and explore red, orange, and green flags. Clinical reasoning and diagnostic accuracy will be explored.

Multi-professional Framework for Advanced Clinical Practice (HEE 2017)

This chapter maps to the following statements within the MPF:

1. Clinical Practice:	1.1	1.2	1.3	1.4	1.5	1.6	1.7	1.8	1.9	1.10	1.11	2.10	2.11
2. Leadership and Management:	2.3	2.4											
3. Education:	3.1	3.2											
4. Research:	4.3	4.7											

Accreditation Considerations

This chapter maps to the following statements within the following national accreditation documents:

Curriculum for Training for Advanced Critical Care Practitioners Syllabus V1.1
(The Faculty of Intensive Care Medicine 2018)

FICM	2.2	2.5	2.6	3.2	3.3	3.5	3.6	3.7	3.10

Advanced Critical Care Outreach Competencies
(The Intensive Care Society, Critical Care Networks – National Nurse Leads and The National Outreach Forum 2022)

A1	A4

Emergency Medicine Advanced Clinical Practitioner Curriculum 2022 – Adult (The Royal College of Emergency Medicine 2022)									
	CC1	CC2	CC5	CC6	CC7	CC11	CC12	CC16	
CAP14	CAP26	CAP27	CAP34	CAP36	CAP38	PAP2	PAP6	PAP7	

Advanced Clinical Practice in Acute Medicine Curriculum Framework (Health Education England 2022)								
CiP1	CiP4	ClinCiP1	ClinCiP2	ClinCiP3	ClinCiP4	ClinCiP5	SpecClin CiP3	Spec ClinCiP4

RENAL FAILURE

Acute Kidney Injury (AKI)

Acute Kidney Injury is characterised by a decrease in renal function over hours or days and tends to be reversible over days or weeks. AKI is a common and often overlooked condition which is associated with poor clinical outcomes including an increased risk of developing chronic kidney disease (CKD). An increased incidence of AKI is seen in conditions including heart failure, liver failure, CKD, and sepsis. The existence of an AKI in conjunction with these diagnoses can provide a marker of disease severity. AKI manifests as oliguria and is usually otherwise asymptomatic until severe.

AKI should be considered according to aetiology as detailed in Table 10.1.

The Kidney Diseases Improving Global Outcomes International group (KDIGO 2012) allows a diagnosis of AKI to be made if the criteria in Table 10.2 are met. AKI can then be staged according to severity, as detailed in Table 10.3.

TABLE 10.1   The aetiology of AKI.

Aetiology	Common causes
Pre-renal	• Hypovolaemia (reduced cardiac output, renal artery obstruction) • Reduced perfusion
Intrinsic	• Acute tubular necrosis (ATN) • Acute interstitial nephritis • Acute glomerulonephritis (GN)
Post-renal	• Post-renal obstruction

TABLE 10.2   AKI diagnostic criteria.

An increase in Serum Creatinine (SCr) by >3 mg/dl (>26.5 mmol/l) within 48 hours; **or**

An increase in SCr to >1.5 times baseline which has occurred within the prior 7 days: **or**

A urine volume < 0.5 ml/kg/hr. for 6 hours

Source: Adapted from KDIGO (2012).

TABLE 10.3   AKI staging criteria.

Stage	Serum Creatinine	Urine output
1	1.5–1.9 times baseline OR ≥0.3 mg/dl (≥26.5 µmol/l) increase	<0.5 ml/kg/h for 6–12 h
2	2.0–2.9 times baseline	<0.5 ml/kg/h for ≥12 h
3	3.0 times baseline OR Increase in Serum Creatinine to ≥4.0 md/dl (353.6 µmol/l) OR Initiation of renal replacement therapy OR, in patients <18 years, decrease in eGFR to <35 ml/min per 1.73 m²	<0.3 ml/kg/h for ≥24 h OR Anuria for ≥12 h

Source: Adapted from KDIGO (2012).

Chronic Kidney Disease (CKD)

Chronic Kidney Disease is defined as abnormalities of renal function for three months or more, based on eGFR <60 ml/min/1.73 m² on two occasions more than 90 days apart (UK Kidney Association 2023). It is a chronic progressive condition that is mostly irreversible, it effects >10% of the population worldwide but increased prevalence is seen in certain populations including individuals who have diabetes mellitus and hypertension. Common causes include diabetes, cardiovascular disease, AKI leading to chronic kidney disease, structural renal tract disease, multisystem disease, family history of kidney disease, and childhood kidney disease.

Early-stage CKD is primarily asymptomatic and is usually detected when other testing or monitoring is undertaken related to the primary diagnosis. CKD can be classified according to the criteria given in Figure 10.1.

Clinical signs of CKD are associated with hyperureamia and are potentially extensive. Table 10.4 demonstrates the multisystem signs and symptoms of CKD.

Interconnected Syndrome of Acute and Chronic Renal Failure

While AKI and CKD exist independently, there is often a degree of crossover due to the shared risk factors and disease modifiers. The existence of AKI in a usually well patient can result in the development of CKD. Conversely, CKD is an important risk factor for the development of AKI. A diagnosis of AKI, CKD, or acute-on-chronic renal failure increases mortality, and the risk of interconnected disease including cardiovascular disease.

Classification of chronic kidney disease using GFR and ACR categories

GFR and ACR categories and risk of adverse outcomes		ACR categories (mg/mmol), description and range		
		<3 Normal to mildly increased	3–30 Moderately increased	>30 Severely increased
		A1	A2	A3
≥90 Normal and high	G1	No CKD in the absence of markers of kidney damage		
60–89 Mild reduction related to normal range for a young adult	G2			
45–59 Mild–moderate reduction	G3a[1]			
30–44 Moderate–severe reduction	G3b			
15–29 Severe reduction	G4			
<15 Kidney failure	G5			

GFR categories (ml/min/1.73m^2), description and range

Increasing risk

Increasing risk

[1]Consider using eGFRcystatinC for people with CKD G3aA1 (see recommendations 1.1.14 and 1.1.15)

Abbreviations: ACR, albumin: creatinine ratio; CKD, chronic kidney disease; GFR, glomerular filtration rate

Adapted with permission from Kidney Disease; Improving Global Outcomes (KDIGO) CKD Work Group (2013) KDIGO 2012 clinical practice guideline for the evaluation and management of chronic kidney disease. Kidney International (Suppl. 3): 1–150

FIGURE 10.1   CKD classifications. *Source*: UK Kidney Association (2023) / https://ukkidney.org/health-professionals/information-resources/uk-eckd-guide/ckd-stages last accessed March 01, 2023.

TABLE 10.4   A demonstration of multisystem signs and symptoms of CKD.

System	Sign (symptom)
Cardiovascular	Uraemic pericarditis (palpitations, chest pain) Peripheral vascular disease (cold extremities, numbness) Heart failure (shortness of breath, palpitations)
Haematological	Anaemia (pallor, fatigue, malaise, shortness of breath) Platelet abnormality (epistaxis, bruising)
Skin	Hyperpigmentation (pruritis)
Central nervous system	Coma, seizure, tremor (irritability, restlessness, insomnia)
Renal	Nocturia Polyuria Oedema
Musculoskeletal	Renal bone disease Vitamin D deficiency
Endocrine	Infertility (erectile dysfunction, amenorrhea)

Physical Examination in Renal Impairment

Physical examination is key to understanding the multisystem effects of renal failure (see Figure 10.2).

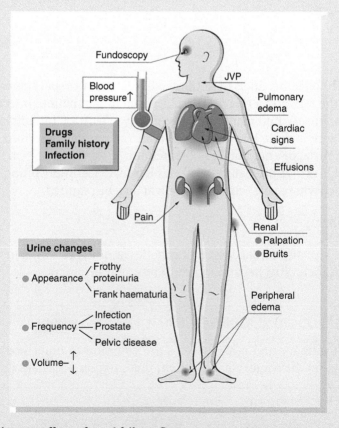

FIGURE 10.2   The multisystem effects of renal failure. *Source*: https://www.ataglanceseries.com/renalsystem/flashcards/flashcard9.asp last accessed February 27, 2023.

TABLE 10.5   UTI sites, signs, and symptoms.

Site of infection	Signs and symptoms
Bladder (cystitis)	Urinary frequency Dysuria Urgency Haematuria Suprapubic pain
Kidney (pyelonephritis)	Fever Rigors Vomiting Loin pain Oliguria
Prostate (prostatitis)	Flu-like symptoms Lower back pain Swollen, tender prostate

Urinary Tract Infection (UTI)

A UTI is diagnosed in the presence of >100 000 colony forming units/ml in the urine. The site of a UTI needs careful consideration of the presenting signs and symptoms (see Table 10.5). The site will affect treatment plans and ongoing management. Inaccurate or delayed diagnosis of UTI may result in urosepsis, which can result in death.

RENAL CALCULI

Renal calculi form in the collecting ducts from the accumulation of crystal aggregates. The calculi can be deposited anywhere in the renal tract and result in localised inflammation, infection, and obstruction.

Renal calculi are often asymptomatic until secondary effects of inflammation, infection, and/or obstruction are seen. These include loin pain, renal colic (commonly described as 'loin to groin' pain), haematuria, pyrexia, oliguria, or anuria in full obstruction.

Management should involve specialist (renal, urology) advice/intervention, treatment of resultant infection, catheterisation (where able). Surgical removal may be required.

Polycystic Renal Disease

Polycystic renal disease is an autosomal dominant genetic condition resulting in multiple renal cysts and extrarenal abnormalities including, hepatic and cardiovascular disorders.

RED FLAGS – PATHOLOGICAL CONSIDERATIONS

Red flags of the genitourinary and renal systems are common to other body systems and should, therefore, be considered in the context of the patient presentation. Red flags include:

Oliguria	Hyperkalaemia	Hyperuraemia	Abdominal pain
Metabolic acidosis	Testicular pain	Recurrent viral/bacterial infections	Altered mental state

Urosepsis Red Flags	Haematuria Red Flags
Hypovolaemia	Pyrexia or hypothermia
Oliguria	Trauma
Pyrexia	Severe abdominal pain
Increased respiratory rate	Flank pain
Acute confusion	Altered mental state
Raised lactate	Anaemia
Renal dysfunction	Prostatic bleeding
Prostate pain	Unintentional weight loss
Coagulopathy	

Signs and symptoms include loin pain, haematuria (due to cystic haemorrhage), cyst infection, urinary tract stone development, abdominal pain, hypertension.

To investigate polycystic renal disease, imaging of the renal system is required, this usually includes ultrasound and CT scan in the first instance. Specific blood tests including Anti-neutrophil cytoplasmic antibody (ANCA), immunofluorescence, and complement may also be requested by renal specialists. Treatment of this disease usually culminates in the requirement of renal replacement and transplant.

Glomerular Nephropathy (GN) – Nephrotic versus Nephritic Syndrome

Glomerular Nephropathy is largely classified into proliferative (nephritic) and non-proliferative (nephrotic). The aetiology of the disease allows for easier classification (see Figure 10.3) and the presenting signs and symptoms result from the underlying pathology (see Figure 10.4).

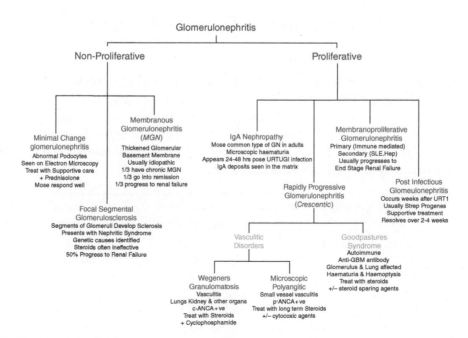

FIGURE 10.3   Glomerular nephritis.

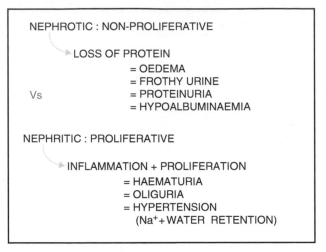

FIGURE 10.4   Neprotic versus nephritic syndromes.

CLINICAL INVESTIGATIONS

Blood Tests

The investigations specific to genitourinary or renal presentations are, Full Blood Count (FBC), Urea, Creatinine, Electrolytes (U&E), Venous/Arterial Blood Gas (V/ABG), and urinalysis.

Urea

The excretion of urea by the kidneys is a vital part of metabolism. Urea is ultimately the excretable form of nitrogen, a waste product of protein metabolism. Nitrogen is converted to ammonia, and quickly to urea in the liver, as a less toxic, excretable form.

$$H + N = \underbrace{NH_3}_{\text{Ammonia}} + CO_2 = \underbrace{CH_4N_2O}_{\text{Urea}}$$

Additionally, urea is important in the reabsorption of water and electrolytes in the nephron. Urea is absorbed in the collecting ducts of the nephrons, thus raising the osmolarity in the interstitium surrounding the descending limb of the loop of Henle, resulting in water resorption.

Urea can be a useful biomarker in renal function, specifically excretory function. It may also provide an indication of the efficacy of the liver to undertake its role in the formation of urea.

Urea levels are heavily affected by additional factors which include;

Age	High protein diet	Medication	Acute renal dysfunction	Viral illness	Prostate cancer
Gastrointestinal bleeding	Recent myocardial infarction	Severe burns	Obstructive renal pathology	Congestive cardiac failure	Dehydration

Results should be examined and interpreted in the context of the patient and any underlying pathology that may be pertinent to the presentation.

Serum Creatinine

Serum Creatinine (SCr) is a common biomarker of renal function. It is used to estimate the glomerular filtration rate and is an endogenous marker for the assessment of renal function, specifically related to the kidneys' ability to undertake creatinine clearance. SCr and urine output continue to remain the best biomarkers for AKI. SCr allows calculation of Creatinine Clearance (CrCl) using the Cockcroft-Gault equation, to measure renal function in CKD; current guidance for estimating glomerular filtration rate based on CrCl using CKD EPI Formula is the gold standard.

The synthesis of Creatinine is complex and involves many organ systems. Creatinine is the product of creatine and creatine phosphate metabolism. It is a nitrogenous organic acid that is generated predominantly in the kidney and liver, and at a reduced rate in the pancreas, using three amino acids, glycine, arginine, and methionine. Despite this marker being a central measure of renal function, the use of SCr should be interpreted with caution as factors such as an individual's muscle mass (high and low), diet, critical illness, medications, existing chronic conditions, and age can influence the result.

Interpretation of SCr

Pregnancy

Due to the physiological changes that occur in pregnancy, from the fifth week of gestation, there is a significant increase in hyperfiltration. The use of SCr to estimate eGFR is thought to underestimate in the first trimester of pregnancy; however, AKI can occur at any time of gestation, and consideration should be given to the trimester and presenting clinical features. There are no standard diagnostic criteria for AKI in pregnancy, as such up to 40% of pregnancy-associated AKI may be missed.

The Elderly

Due to relatively lower muscle mass, the interpretation of SCr in the elderly population may be difficult. It is important to consider altered baseline, and changes to normal reference ranges. Incidence of patients with severe renal impairment, but with SCr within the normal reference range, are common in this group. Sensitivity is thought to be as low as 12%, and specificity of 99%, this leads to under investigation and under recognition in this vulnerable population. A more accurate measure may be CrCl.

Further Specific Investigations

The complexity of renal and GU pathology may require further, more specialised testing and investigation (see Table 10.6), these should be arranged in conjunction with specialist renal advice.

Point of care testing, including arterial or venous blood gases and urinalysis can be useful in managing acute renal and GU presentations, providing rapid access to important biomarkers of pathology including pH, acid-base balance, lactate, and electrolyte levels.

TABLE 10.6   Specialist tests and investigations.

Renal immunology screen	Cytoglobulin
Complement C3/C4	Anti-GMB
C3 Nephritic factor	Rheumatoid factor and immunoglobulins
Anti-neutrophil cytoplasmic antibody (ANCA)	Hepatitis B surface antigen
Hepatitis C antibody	HIV antibody

SERUM ELECTROLYTES AND RENAL INSUFFICIENCY

Potassium

Potassium is an intracellular cation; its main role is to maintain resting membrane potentials. In acute or chronic renal impairment, potassium dysregulation can result in hypo or hyperkalaemia, which should be treated urgently to avoid potentially catastrophic symptoms (see Pharmacological Principles section later in the chapter). Potassium homeostasis is predominantly regulated by the renal system (see Figure 10.5), and is influenced by hormonal action, specifically aldosterone, which stimulates the retention of sodium by increased excretion and loss of Potassium by the kidney.

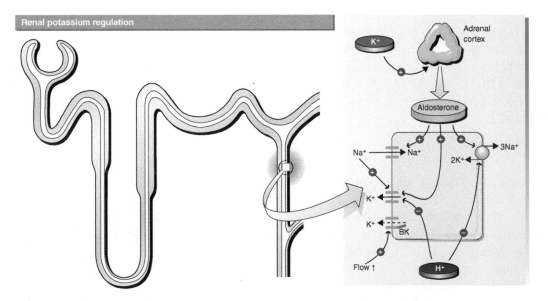

FIGURE 10.5   Renal potassium regulation. *Source*: O'Callaghan (2016) / John Wiley & Sons.

Sodium

The movement of sodium is vital to maintaining the electrical potential across cell membranes, more specifically sodium and potassium. ATPase actively transports sodium out of cells in exchange for potassium; this acts to maintain the electrochemical gradient between the intra- and extracellular compartments. Sodium is the main cation found in extracellular fluid; this cation is the central chemical element linked to water homoeostasis; variations in the extracellular water volume will initiate a change in sodium level. A significant change of osmolality activates various physiological systems such as the arginine vasopressin, or anti-diuretic hormone system. The equilibrium of this system is necessary to ensure adequate balance, where Sodium levels rise may be seen in conjunction with water loss, alongside a rise in urea. The reverse of this may be noted in patients who have significant losses, water retention, end stage liver disease, haematological disease, and with the use of certain medication such as diuretics and anti-depressants.

Chloride

Chloride is an anion, it plays a key role in the regulation, in both the intracellular and extracellular acid-base regulation. A decrease in bicarbonate ions triggers an increase in chloride ions to maintain electroneutrality; this may consequently contribute to hyperchloremic metabolic acidosis. Some of the main causes of hyperchloremia are dehydration, volume losses, hypernatraemia, and some medications. Additionally, the use of Normal Saline solution (0.9% NaCl), contains super physiological amounts of chloride, this can, without careful review, contribute to hyperchloraemia. Where individuals have received 0.9% NaCl during fluid resuscitation as opposed to a physiologically balanced solution, during the immediate salvage phase of shock, they can be more susceptible to hyperchloremia in the post-resuscitation phase.

The renal system is fundamental in the management of acid-base balance, specifically the regulation of chloride ions (see Figure 10.6).

Electrolyte Imbalance and the Anion Gap

The maintenance of acid base balance within normal physiological limits is essential to maintain the adequate functioning of all body systems. When there is an imbalance, calculating the anion gap may guide the clinician to assess the severity of derangement and enable diagnosis. A blood gas will provide clues as to the primary and secondary causes that may be present in examination findings. When evaluating the primary acid base disorder, by estimating the gap between positively charged ions (cations) and negatively charged (anions), there may be an indication of underlying pathology. More specifically, the evaluation of Chloride (Cl^-) and bicarbonate (HCO_3^-) which are the main anions, and Sodium the main cation, will enable the diagnosis of metabolic acidosis with a normal or high anion gap. The anion gap is an indicator of potentially life-threatening conditions relating to metabolic acidosis. Where there is a metabolic acidosis with a normal anion gap, usually relating to loss of bicarbonate and retention of chloride ions, which leads to a hyperchloremic metabolic acidosis. The determination of the gap is dependent upon the serum albumin and serum phosphate concentration levels; it is necessary that the interpretation of the gap is adjusted to reflect the serum albumin as outlined in Figure 10.7. Common causes of normal anion gap metabolic acidosis

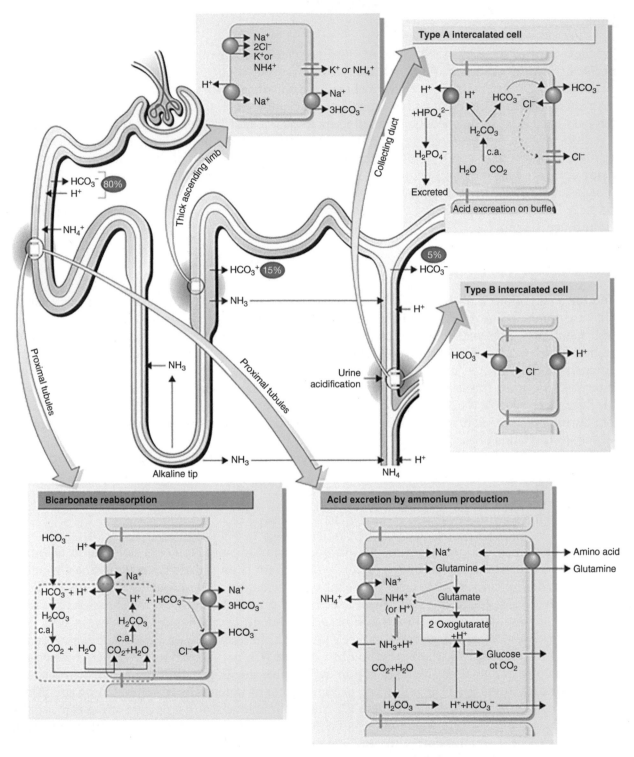

FIGURE 10.6   Renal acid-base handling. *Source*: https://www.ataglanceseries.com/renalsystem/flashcards/flashcard29.asp [accessed 27 February 2023].

$$\text{Anion Gap (AG)} = Na^+ - (Cl^- + HCO_3^-)$$
$$\text{Albumin corrected Anion Gap} = AG + [2.5 \times (4 - Albumin)]$$

FIGURE 10.7   Anion gap equations.

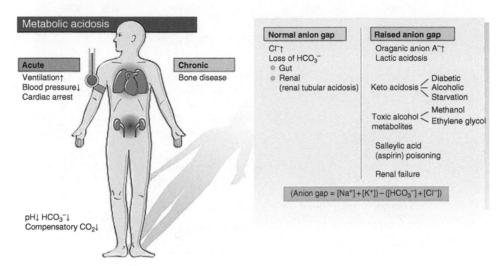

FIGURE 10.8   HAGMA/NAGMA. *Source*: https://www.ataglanceseries.com/renalsystem/flashcards/flashcard31.asp [last accessed 27 February 2023].

(NAGMA) and high anion gap metabolic acidosis (HAGMA) are illustrated in Figure 10.8. The validity of using the anion gap calculation may be less helpful in cases where there is lactic acidosis, where the Positive Predictive Value (PPV) can be as low as 50% when the anion gap is ≥ 12 mmol/l for elevated lactate ≥ 4.0 mmol/l.

Pharmacological Principles

When presented with an individual who has an AKI or CKD, it is essential to establish a comprehensive history, to consider interconnected syndromes, and to ensure a drug history is taken. Around two-thirds of drugs are excreted by the kidneys, therefore the potential for substances to accumulate in individuals with an AKI, and or with CKD is significant. It is essential to review and undertake careful dose adjustment, making allowance for renal dysfunction, especially in CKD, as drugs can accumulate. Understanding how changes to physiology affect the pharmacokinetics is essential to ensure safe and effective pharmacological treatment. Key pharmacokinetic considerations can be found in Figure 10.9. Key considerations for prescribing in renal impairment can be found in Table 10.7, and are categorised according to patient specific, drug specific, and monitoring considerations.

Electrolyte Replacement

Common electrolyte derangements are hyper/hypokalaemia, hyper/hypomagnesemia, hyper/hypophosphatemia, and hyper/hypocalcaemia. The aetiology of electrolyte derangement should be assessed to ensure a safe approach to replacement. Underlying causes should be treated initially where

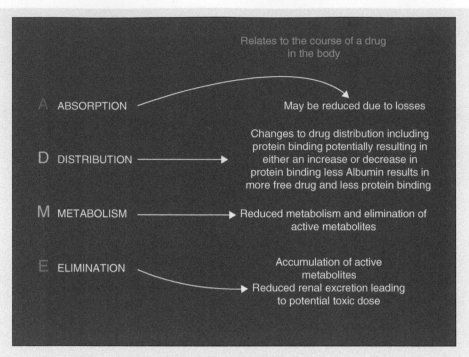

FIGURE 10.9   Pharmacokinetics in renal impairment. *Source*: Author.

TABLE 10.7   Key prescribing considerations in renal presentations.

Patient specific	Drug specific	Monitoring considerations
Renal function – often required daily in AKI	Dose – may require alteration or consideration of daily dosing	Renal function
Weight – often required daily in AKI	Dosing interval and frequencies	Drug levels (e.g. nephrotoxic antibiotics, lithium)
Age	Alternative therapies	Fluid status
Dialysis requirement/prescription	Prescription end-date	Protein (albumin) level
Nutritional status – consider monitoring albumin levels	Pharmacological interactions	

Ensure prescribing is multidisciplinary – this should include specialty pharmacists and medical teams.

possible, and where the cause is a medication then dose alteration or cessation should be considered in the first instance. Underlying pathology aside from AKI or CKD should be considered and investigated appropriately.

Biochemical data should be reviewed, alongside previous test results, to assess the urgency of treatment against patient outcomes. Local guidance for specific electrolyte replacement should be consulted prior to electrolyte replacement. Replacement protocols usually focus on the severity of derangement and then offer algorithms for its replacement. Route of replacement is also an important factor as if prescribing electrolyte replacement orally, it is important that you consider the impact of first pass metabolism, and the drug formulation.

Sodium

The replacement of Sodium should be of sufficient pace to correct potentially serious signs, such as reduced consciousness, seizures, or signs of increased intracranial pressure. However, a sodium level that has fallen over a longer period should be replaced with caution to avoid large fluid shifts and to reduce the risk of severe complications such as cerebral oedema. Caution should be given to reversing the manifestations of hypotonicity, as replacing too fast may increase the risk of the development of osmotic demyelination. Despite there being no UK wide consensus, most guidance suggest an initial replacement of 1–2 mmol/l per hour in the initial few hours, with no more that 10–12 mmol/l in a 24-hour period. A syndrome of inappropriate ADH secretion (SIADH) should be considered in presentations of hyponatraemia, and a serum osmolality should be requested to aid in decision-making. In most cases where there is severe hyponatremia, the treatment is to replace with caution using a combination of sodium-containing fluid.

Potassium

Potassium regulation has been discussed earlier in this chapter; however, an additional consideration should be given to where there is potassium depletion, there may be interdependency with magnesium deficiency, this can be seen more specifically with loop diuretics. This interdependency of magnesium is particularly important in cardiac myocytes, where individuals may be at risk of desensitisation when magnesium levels are low. Surgical patients are also at risk of intestinal losses, therefore prompt treatment and management is required to reduce an individual's risk. Consideration should be given to the route of replacement and the pace of replacement. If replaced with dispersible preparations, this may contain large amounts of sodium, and the individual may not be able to absorb the oral preparation. Where replacing potassium in intravenous fluids or in more concentrated forms via central access routes, regular hourly monitoring using ABG/VBG may be required to evaluate the values. Rapid replacement in individuals with renal impairment may increase the risk of arrhythmia and/or death. Signs and symptoms of hyper and hypokalaemia can be seen in Figure 10.10.

Calcium

Hypocalcaemia may be seen in individuals who have Vitamin D deficiency, those individuals with hyperphosphatemia, those who have malignancy, and some prescribed certain groups of drugs (i.e. cytotoxics). In severe cases of hypocalcaemia where serum calcium is <1.9 mmol/l, this should be treated as an emergency with intravenous replacement initiated against local protocols. The rate of replacement is also an important factor, as if replaced rapidly via central vein access, there may be an increased risk of cardiac arrhythmia. Magnesium levels should be considered for joint replacement. Mild hypocalcaemia can be treated with oral calcium supplements, this may need to be supplemented in some cases with Vitamin D if deficiency is suspected.

Phosphate

In end stage renal disease (ESRD), phosphate metabolism is altered. As renal function declines the interactions between the kidney, gut, and bone become increasingly dysregulated, leading to a hyperphosphataemia. This interaction is regulated by parathyroid hormone, Vitamin D, and fibroblast growth factor 23. Where there is a decline in renal function, phosphate is not excreted as efficiently and can accumulate. Other causes of hypophosphatemia are mainly linked to extra renal causes, such as losses related to the gastrointestinal tract, reduced dietary intake, redistribution into cells, and in continuous renal replacement therapy. Replacement of phosphate can be via the oral route, and in more severe cases intravenously.

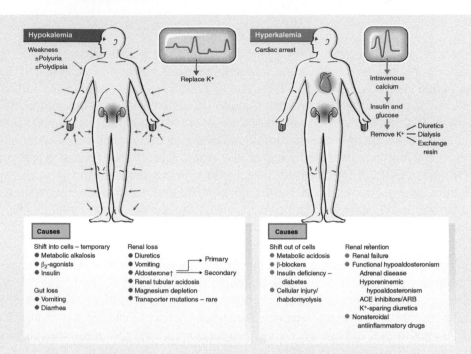

FIGURE 10.10   Hyper and hypokalaemia. *Source*: Adapted from O'Callaghan (2016).

Fields of Practice – Mental Health

Lithium and Renal Toxicity

Lithium has been used for many years as a first-line treatment for the management of type 1 Bi-polar disorder, and in the treatment of depressive disorders and mania. Lithium has a considerable impact on renal function, and due to potential toxicity has been decreasing in its use. The monitoring of lithium levels is essential to ensuring safety and accuracy and to avoid toxicity. The lithium dose is usually adjusted to achieve a plasma level of 0.4–1 mmol/l.

Lithium positioning can trigger several complications. The acute ingestion and or chronic accumulation can result in the following manifestations:

Body system	Signs and symptoms
CNS	Confusion, coma, cerebellar signs, seizure
GI	Nausea, vomiting, bloating
CVS	Syncope
Renal	Polyuria, polydipsia, renal insufficiency
Neuromuscular	Peripheral neuropathy, myopathy
Endocrine	Hypothermia, hyperthermia

Any persistent neurological signs and symptoms should trigger consideration of Syndrome of Irreversible Lithium Intoxication (SILENT), resulting in damage to the cerebellum, brain stem dysfunction, and extrapyramidal symptoms. It is important to establish the underlying causes of lithium toxicity, including infection, volume losses, GI losses, drug interactions especially relating to ACE inhibitors, Alpha Receptor Blockers, non-steroidal anti-inflammatory drugs and COX-2 inhibitors, accidental and intentional overdose.

Depression, Suicide, and CKD

Depression and suicide are prevalent conditions with individuals diagnosed with CKD. The increased risk of suicide, depression and anhedonia may be seen individuals with end-stage renal disease when first commencing dialysis. Such individuals have been identified as posing the greatest risk of committing suicide due to the impact and progression of the disease. In patients with CKD, it is estimated that 20% of individuals suffer from major depressive mood disorder, which increases when combined with other chronic conditions. Contributing factors include dramatic lifestyle changes, and lack of independence. An increased risk of suicide is seen in individuals who came from poorer socioeconomic backgrounds, and individuals who experienced issues such as material deprivation, and unemployment. As CKD progresses there can be an increase in symptom burden, such as fatigue, anorexia, sexual dysfunction, pain, sleep disturbance, and lack of independence, all which can contribute to a reduction of quality of life and a worsening depressive state. The presence of depressive symptoms is linked to poorer outcomes in patients who require dialysis.

Field of Practice – Paediatrics and Learning Disabilities

Paediatric Autism Spectrum Disorders (ASD) and Kidney Disease

There is a recognised association between paediatric kidney disease and neurodevelopmental impairments. Individuals with ASD have a higher mortality rate compared to the general population, and links can be made between ASD and pathological ageing, 25% being linked to chronic kidney disease. Some of the genetic conditions associated with ASD and renal or GU impairment can be found in the table below.

Kidney disorder group	Condition and genetics
Congenital anomalies of kidneys and urinary tract	Bardel–Biedl syndrome **BBS**
	Brachio-oto-renal syndrome **EYA1**
	CHARGE **CHD7**
	Cornelia de Lange **NIPBL**
	Di George syndrome 22q11.2
	Down syndrome **Trisomy 21**

(Continued)

Kidney disorder group	Condition and genetics
	FOXP1 syndrome **FOXP1**
	Fragile X **FMR1**
	Fraser syndrome **GRIP1**
	Gabriele-de-Vries syndrome **YY1**
	HDR syndrome **GATA3**
	Jacobsen syndrome **ETS1**
	Kleefstra syndrome **EHMT1**
	Phelan-McDermid syndrome 22q13.3 including **SHANK3**
	Rubinstein Taybi syndrome **CREBBP**
	Smith Lemi-Opitz **DHCR7**
	Smith Magenis syndrome **RAI1**
	Sotos syndrome **NSD1**
	Williams syndrome 7q11.23
	Wolf-Hirshhorn syndrome 4p-
Tubular disease	Familial hyperkalemic hypertension **CUL3** WNK kinases implicated in ASD
	Pseudohypoaldosteronism, type 1 **SLC12A**
	Renal tubular acidosis **CA2**
	Hyperaldosteronism **CACNA1D**
	Lowe syndrome **OCRL**
Cystic disease	RCAD (HNF1beta nephropathy HNF1B) (if17q12 deletion encompassing **HNF1b**)
	Tuberous sclerosis complex **TSC1, TSC2**
	Nephronophthisis **NPHP1, NPHP6**
	Orofaciodigital syndrome **OFD1**
Cancer	PTEN hamartoma tumour syndrome **PTEN**
	WAGR **PRRG4**
Other	Rett syndrome **MECP2**
	Wilson's disease **ATP7B**
	Neurofibromatosis **NF1**

Source: Clothier and Absoud (2021) / Springer Nature / CC BY 4.0.

As a clinician, when reviewing individuals who present with signs and symptoms of renal or GU disease and have a diagnosis of ASD, a high index of suspicion should be taken when investigating renal function. The usual assessment tools should be used to guide clinical decision-making, whether this be to screen for AKI and/or CKD.

Examination: GUS Examination

GUS examination in males

- Inspection of anus and perineum

  Examination (with or without specimen collection for smears and cultures) of genitalia including:
- Scrotum (e.g. lesions, cysts, rashes)
- Epididymites (e.g. size, symmetry, masses)
- Testes (e.g. size, symmetry, masses)
- Urethral meatus (e.g. size, location, lesions, discharge)
- Penis (e.g. lesions, presence or absence of foreskin, foreskin retractability, plaque, masses, scarring, deformities)

  Digital rectal examination including:
- Prostate gland (e.g. size, symmetry, nodularity, tenderness)
- Seminal vesicles (e.g. symmetry, tenderness, masses, enlargement)
- Sphincter tone, presence of haemorrhoids, rectal masses

GUS examination in females

- Inspection and palpation of breasts (e.g. masses or lumps, tenderness, symmetry, nipple discharge)
- Digital rectal examination including sphincter tone, presence of haemorrhoids, rectal masses

  Pelvic examination (with or without specimen collection for smears and cultures) including:
- External genitalia (e.g. general appearance, hair distribution, lesions)
- Urethral meatus (e.g. size, location, lesions, prolapse)
- Bladder (e.g. fullness, masses, tenderness)
- Vagina (e.g. general appearance, oestrogen effect, discharge, lesions, pelvic support, cystocoele, rectocoele)
- Cervix (e.g. general appearance, lesions, discharge)
- Uterus (e.g. contour, position, mobility, tenderness, consistency, descent or support)
- Adnexa/parametria (e.g. masses, tenderness, organomegaly, nodularity)
- Anus and perineum

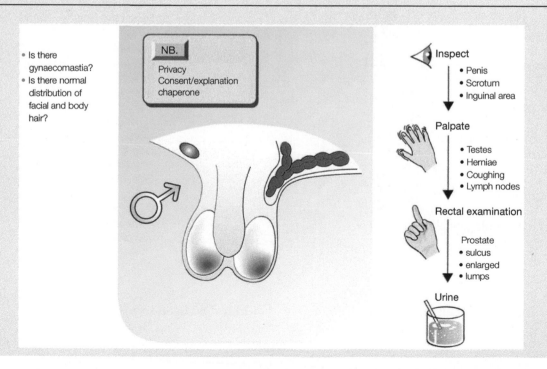

History
- Menstruation
- Bleeding
- Discharge

Sexual history
- Contraception
- Urinary symptoms
- Obstetric history

NB.
Privacy
Consent/explanation
Chaperone

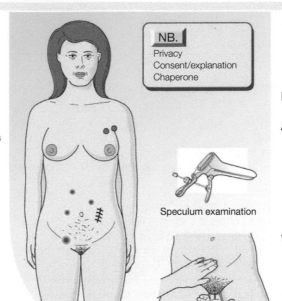

Speculum examination

Examination
- Well/unwell
- Anaemia
- Discharge

Breast examination

Abdominal examination
- Scars
- Masses
- Distension
- Striae
- Body hair
- Herniae

Vaginal examination

Inspection

Digital bimanual examination

History
Last menstrual period
Menstrual cycle

Any:
Bleeding
Anaemia
Hypertension
Diabetes
Infection
Vomiting
Thromboses

Past obstetric history
Gravidity
Parity
Mode of delivery
Complications

Past gynaecological history

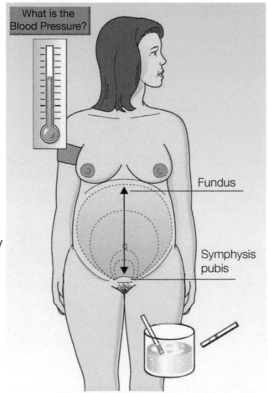

What is the Blood Pressure?

Fundus

Symphysis pubis

Examination
Well/unwell
Anaemia
Fever
Blood pressure
Breast examination

Oedema
Cardiovascular examination
Respiratory examination
Urinalysis

Uterine swelling
Measure symphysis pubis–fundal height
Tenderness
Fetal parts:
- Lie
- Liquor volume
- Presentation
- Engagement
- Fetal heart

SAFETY NOTE this method outlined below would not be used in pregnancy

---

Learning Event

1. Acute on chronic renal failure – what are the important considerations of this interlinked syndrome?

The Impact of Unequal Care for LGBTQIA+ Individuals

LGBTQIA+ individuals despite legislative changes continue to experience discrimination and exclusion when accessing healthcare. When providing care to LGBTQIA+ patients, there are many complex factors to consider. Individuals who have received gender affirming treatment may present with complications of gender affirming surgery, adverse effects of gender affirming hormone therapy, AKI/CKD due to the adverse effects of gender affirming drugs. Care should always be taken to consider the complexities of presentations in the transgender community and ensure the risk of pathology is considered; for example, a transgender woman may present with prostatitis, this needs to be approached with care and recognition of the dysphoria that may result.

The impact upon an LGBTQIA+ individual may be so great that it can adversely affect the management of their conditions. Impacting factors may include the omission of treatment, non-attendance of appointments, and late presentations due to fear and or lack of a safe and welcoming environment for patients. Consideration should be given to gender-affirming treatments and procedures, to ensure safe, effective, and holistic care is provided. When considering genitourinary conditions, gay and bisexual men have been shown to have an increased risk of the development of liver and kidney diseases, and transgender adults are linked to having more complex comorbidities, which may have a higher demand for treatment and interventions compared to cisgender adults.

It is indicated that gender-diverse people have a higher incidence of cardiovascular disease including hypertension compared with cisgender people. Hypertension is a known risk factor for the development of CKD and thus individuals receiving gender-affirming therapy are likely to experience increased cardiovascular disease, hypertension, and renal disease.

When assessing for the presence of an AKI and or progression of CKD, using verified algorithm tools, it is essential to ensure appropriate decision-making. Consideration should be given to the validity of the equations where the formulae have variables for biological sex, there is potential for error or discrepancy when prescribing and/or estimating renal function in the transgender population. This increases the risk of over or underdosing of drugs for transgender patients. Within the UK, there remains a lack of clear consensus guidance surrounding transgender individuals and the use of clinical algorithms to evaluate GFR. However, the primary consideration should be open, respectful, and empathetic communication to establish an accurate clinical history.

ORANGE FLAGS – PSYCHOLOGICAL CONSIDERATIONS

Psychosocial Health in Renal Disease – The Psychosocial Care Manifesto

Kidney Care UK (2022a & b) has published a manifesto as part of a working group to address the key issues that individuals living with CKD face and the psychosocial issues they face due to the increased burden and relationship between CKD and mental health issues. The below provides the 10 key health priorities.

Every kidney patient should have their psychosocial care needs assessed using validated methods.

Every kidney patient should be provided with appropriate psychosocial care that fully supports their level of need, as part of their standard NHS care.

Psychosocial care interventions should increase with a person's level of need.

Psychosocial care needs should be integrated into kidney patient care plans (which are produced by a patient's hospital kidney team).

New NHS Integrated Care Systems should ensure different parts of the system are better joined-up to support the psychosocial care needs of people with kidney disease, as well as their physical health.

Renal multidisciplinary teams (MDTs) should integrate renal specialist psychology, counselling, social work, and psychiatry to ensure kidney patients have access to all the support they need to help them manage their condition and the complex interactions between mental and physical health.

Staffing levels should be monitored to support access and equality to psychosocial care.

All renal staff should receive training in the mental health needs of patients so that they are able to act as 'first responders' and know who and where to refer patients. Mental health staff should receive training about renal disease screening and management for their patients with severe mental illness and dementia.

Minimum national standards of psychosocial care should be introduced and monitored so all patients receive equal access to the care they need, no matter where they are in the country.

A dashboard should be created to monitor the success of psychosocial care services in improving kidney patient's health.

Source: https://www.kidneycareuk.org/about-kidney-health/living-kidney-disease/mental-health/manifesto/ [last accessed 27 February 2023].

GREEN FLAGS

Racial and Ethnic Disparities and Renal Disease

Within the Black Asian and minority ethnic (BAME) groups there continues to remain significant health inequalities relating to renal disease; more specifically it is five times more common in these groups of individuals. Individuals who are from South Asian and Black backgrounds are approximately three to five times more likely to start dialysis than people who are white. South Asian and Black ethnicity is associated with the more severe form of CKD (stages 4, 5), in particular, eGFR is suggested to demonstrate a faster decline in function within the Bangladeshi community. Much more is needed to address the key health inequalities below:

Genetics and genetic abnormalities	Environmental factors	Psychosocial factors
Diet and health	Education and life opportunities	Physical and mental health
Health literacy	Access to healthcare	

Case Study 1

A 65-year-old female presents to ED with increased shortness of breath (SOB) worsening over the last 24 hours. Unable to speak in full sentences. The patient describes flecks of haemoptysis within the sputum. Loss of appetite, pain in the chest worse on inspiration. Recent admission following STEMI four weeks ago. The following observations and information are noted down in the ED triage records: Temp. 38.9, BP 80/58, HR 132 bpm, RR 29 breaths/minute, SaO_2 89% in room air, central capillary refill time 6 seconds. Can't remember when she last passed urine, GCS 14/15 (E:4 M:4 V:6).

Key laboratory results are: WCC 16×10^9/l, CRP 124, Urea 12.2, Creatinine 130.

- What are your initial considerations? Please approach using an ABCDE framework.
- You need to take a clinical history. What are the pertinent questions you will ask? What are the considerations you may make at this point?
- What is your differential diagnosis based on these findings.
- Discuss with a colleague, your initial management plan.

Case Study 2

A 70-year-old male, presented to ED following a GP with bloody diarrhoea; initial impressions are that the individual appears pale, can speak in full sentences. The patient describes blood in their faeces and abdominal pain. This started when he was away this weekend and ate some mussels and shellfish raw from a bayside restaurant. The diarrhoea started shortly after and then has become worse over the last 48 hours. The observations causing concern include:

Temp. 39.7, HR 128 bpm, very dark concentrated urine. Further investigations demonstrate a lactate of 4.0 mmol, Hb 70 g/l, platelets 26×10^9/l, Increased ESR and WCC 20×10^9/l, urea 26 mmol/l, creatinine 328 mmol/l

- What are your initial considerations? Please approach using an ABCDE framework.
- You need to take a patient history. What are the pertinent questions you will ask? What are the considerations you may make at this point?
- What is your differential diagnosis based on these findings?
- Discuss with a colleague, your initial management plan.
- What special tests might you need to consider for this patient?
- Which specialities might you need to discuss this presentation with?

Tip: Consider the presence of the classic triad: Microangiopathic haemolytic uraemia, thrombocytopenia, and AKI.

Take Home Points
- It is essential to take a comprehensive and holistic history and to understand and consider biochemical data including context of trends.
- Have a high index of suspicion for AKI, and where an individual has CKD to consider the interdependency of the interlinked syndromes, and those groups who may have significantly higher risk factors linked to high mortality.
- Consider the impact on the pharmacokinetics of drugs when making prescribing decisions in this complex patient group.
- Liaise with and involve specialist teams early.
- Be considerate of the diversity of patient groups and consider the impact of renal and GU presentations in the wider context of the patient's life.

REFERENCES

Clothier, J. and Absoud, M. (2021). Autism spectrum disorder and kidney disease. *Pediatric Nephrology* 36 (10): 2987–2995.

Health Education England (HEE). (2017). *Multi-professional Framework for Advanced Clinical Practice in England* [online]. Available from: https://www.hee.nhs.uk/sites/default/files/documents/multi-professionalframeworkforadvancedclinicalpracticeinengland.pdf [accessed 20 June 2023].

Health Education England (HEE). (2022). *Advanced Clinical Practice in Acute Medicine Curriculum Framework – Credentials* [online]. Available from: https://advanced-practice.hee.nhs.uk/our-work/credentials [accessed 20 June 2023].

Kidney Care UK. 2022a. *Caring for People with Kidney Disease, Psychosocial Health – A Manifesto for Action* [online]. Available from: https://www.kidneycareuk.org/about-kidney-health/living-kidney-disease/mental-health/manifesto [accessed 21 June 2023].

Kidney Care UK and National Psychosocial Working Group. (2022b). *Psychosocial Health – a Manifesto for Action* [online]. Available from: https://www.kidneycareuk.org/about-kidney-health/living-kidney-disease/mental-health/manifesto/#:~:text=Renal%20multidisciplinary%20teams%20%28MDTs%29%20should%20integrate%20renal%20specialist,mental%20and%20physical%20health.%20Psychosocial%20care%20workforce%20needs [accessed 21 June 2023].

Kidney Disease: Improving Global Outcomes (KDIGO) Acute Kidney Injury Work Group (2012). KDIGO clinical practice guideline for acute kidney injury. *Kidney International* Suppl. 2 (1): 1–138.

O'Callaghan, C.A. (2016). *The Renal System at a Glance*. Wiley-Blackwell.

The Faculty of Intensive Care Medicine. (2018). *Curriculum for Training for Advanced Critical Care Practitioners – Syllabus. V1.1* [online]. Available from: www.ficm.ac.uk/media/6896 [accessed 20 June 2023].

The Intensive Care Society, Critical Care Networks – National Nurse Leads and The National Outreach Forum. (2022). *Advanced Critical Care Outreach Competencies* [online]. Available from: https://ics.ac.uk/asset/43B8C11B-4512-41D0-B97768FABA2C30B2 [accessed 20 June 2023].

The Royal College of Emergency Medicine. (2022). *Emergency Medicine Advanced Clinical Practitioner Curriculum 2022 (Adult)* [online]. Available from: https://rcem.ac.uk/wp-content/uploads/2022/09/ACP_Curriculum_Adult_Final_060922.pdf [accessed 20 June 2023].

UK Kidney Association. (2023). *CKD Stages* [online]. Available from: https://ukkidney.org/health-professionals/information-resources/uk-eckd-guide/ckd-stages [accessed 21 June 2023].

FURTHER READING

Hill, R. and Diamond-Fox, J. (2022). *ACP at a Glance*. Wiley.

Kidney Research UK. (2019). *Report. Kidney Health Inequalities in the United Kingdom, Reflecting on the Past, Reducing in the Future* [online]. Available from: https://kidneyresearchuk.org/wp-content/uploads/2019/02/Health_Inequalities_Report_Complete_FINAL_Web_20181017.pdf [accessed 21 June 2023].

NHSE. (2016). *Think Kidneys, Guidelines for Medicines Optimisation in Patients with Acute Kidney Injury* [online]. Available from: https://www.thinkkidneys.nhs.uk/aki/wp-content/uploads/sites/2/2016/07/Medicines-optimisation-toolkit-for-AKI-MAY17.pdf [accessed 21 June 2023].

NICE. (2013). *Acute Kidney Injury: Prevention, Detection and Management of Acute Kidney Injury up to the Point of Renal all Replacement Therapy*. In: NICE Clinical Guideline 169. National Institute for Health and Care Excellence.

NICE. (2019). *Acute Kidney Injury: Prevention Detection and Management* [online]. Available from: www.nice.org.uk/guidance/ng148/resources/acute-kidney-injury-prevention-detection-and-management-pdf-66141786535621 [accessed 21 June 2023].

NICE. (2021). *Chronic Kidney Disease: Assessment and Management. (NG203)* [online]. Available from: https://www.nice.org.uk/guidance/ng203 [accessed 21 June 2023].

NICE. (2022). *Assessment and Diagnosis of Chronic Kidney Disease* [online]. Available from: https://www.nice.org.uk/guidance/ng203 [accessed 21 June 2023].

Peate, I., Diamond-Fox, J., and Hill, R. (2023). *The Advanced Practitioner*. Wiley.

CHAPTER 11

Gastrointestinal and Hepato-Pancreato-Biliary

Angela Roberts

Aim

The aim of this chapter is to postulate and expand the underpinning knowledge of the advanced practitioner in relation to the patient with gastrointestinal (GI) and/or Hepato-Pancreato-Biliary (HPB) disorders.

LEARNING OUTCOMES

After reading this chapter the reader will:

1. Have comprehensive knowledge of the history-taking skills of patients who present with GI and/or HPB disorders and diseases.
2. Have a thorough knowledge of the common types of acute and emergency care presentations.
3. Discuss key diagnostics and investigations to support a diagnosis or differential.
4. Augment the understanding of evidence-based treatments and guidelines in advanced practice within the emergency and critical care settings.

SELF-ASSESSMENT QUESTIONS

1. What are the components of the Kings College criteria for Acute Liver Failure (ALF)?
2. Which investigations (including biomarkers) would measure the synthetic function of the liver?
3. Are you able to list the common causes of acute pancreatitis?

INTRODUCTION

Gastrointestinal (GI) and Hepatobiliary (HPB) dysfunction and complications are frequently seen in a large prevalence of patients irrespective of their presenting complaint; iatrogenic, spontaneous, or self-induced. Organ dysfunction is an event in the critically ill affecting up to 70% of patients during their ICU stay, and with consideration of the pathophysiology of the GI and HPB system this has a huge impact. This can contribute to consequences such as prolonged critical care stay, surgical interventions, and increased mortality rates.

This chapter will collate some issues seen within GI and HPB dysfunction, diseases, and phenomena seen across emergency and critical care. There is a plethora of GI and HPB conditions and it is beyond the scope of this chapter to discuss all possible conditions and presentations, therefore, the focus will be on matters pertinent to acute, emergency and/or critical care.

Multi-professional Framework (MPF) for Advanced Clinical Practice Guidance for Professional Development (HEE 2017)

This chapter maps to the following statements within the MPF:

1. Clinical Practice:	1.1	1.2	1.3	1.4	1.5	1.6	1.7
2. Leadership and Management:	2.1	2.2	2.3	2.9			
3. Education:	3.2	3.3	3.4				
4. Research:	4.1						

Accreditation Considerations

This chapter maps to the following statements within the following national accreditation documents:

Curriculum for Training for Advanced Critical Care Practitioners Syllabus V1.1
(The Faculty of Intensive Care Medicine 2018):

2.2	2.4	2.5	2.6	3.1	3.2	3.3	3.5	3.6	3.7	3.9	3.10	3.11

Advanced Critical Care Outreach Competencies
(The Intensive Care Society, Critical Care Networks – National Nurse Leads and The National Outreach Forum 2022):

A1	A4

Emergency Medicine Advanced Clinical Practitioner Curriculum 2022 – Adult
(The Royal College of Emergency Medicine 2022):

GP1–10	GC1 = 8	SuP1–7	SuC2	4	12

Advanced Clinical Practice in Acute Medicine Curriculum Framework
(Health Education England 2022):

Presentations and Conditions of Acute Medicine by System/Specialty: Gastroenterology and hepatology

The symptoms and presentations of GI and HPB diseases and conditions can be broad and overlap with other symptoms and illnesses. Systemically patients may also present with anorexia, weight loss, nausea, fatigue, pruritus, confusion, and pyrexia.

Figures 11.1 and 11.2 demonstrate some of the common presenting symptoms and their association with GI and HPB disorders.

Case Study

As the bleep holder you attend a medical emergency for an 82 year old lady who had an elective right total hip arthroplasty three days ago. On arrival, she is in the bathroom on the floor semi-conscious complaining of feeling nauseous after having her bowels opened. You note haematochezia in the toilet.

- Initial observations: BP 74/43, HR 101 (irregular), CRT 3 seconds. She looked pale and clammy.
- Pertinent PMH: Hypertension.
   1. What are your initial concerns and approach?
   2. What questions are pertinent in a clinical history to gain diagnosis and differential diagnosis?
   3. What key laboratory tests would you initially order?
   4. What would your management plan be after diagnosis?

It is important to note that individuals respond and explain pain to healthcare professionals in many ways; some may endure pain, whereas to others the same pain can be debilitating, and they may not be able to proceed with their usual daily tasks. Therefore, it is important that history-taking is done holistically to understand how the pain is uniquely affecting that individual.

There are many acronyms and mnemonics which can aid a comprehensive history-taking, but it is important as the advanced practitioner to 'tailor make' the appropriate tool to ensure the signs and symptoms are ascertained. Such mnemonics and acronyms to be aware of include SOCRATES and OPQRST.

Case Study

A 29-year-old man presents to the ED with severe dull epigastric pain radiating into his back, and has been nauseated for the last 24 hours so had minimal diet and fluid intake.

- Initial observations noted are: HR 128 bpm, BP 83/60, RR 27 breaths/minute, CRT 4 seconds.
- Pertinent PMH: Bi-Polar disorder, Non-smoker, Non-alcohol drinker.
   1. What are your initial concerns and approach?
   2. What questions are pertinent in a clinical history to gain diagnosis and differential diagnosis?
   3. What key laboratory tests would you initially order?
   4. What would your management plan be after diagnosis?

Mouth

- **Angular cheilitis** and **Apthous ulceration** secondary to chron's disease, Iron, B12 and/or folate deficiencies,
- **Haematemesis** secondary to mallory-weiss tear, oesophageal rupture, peptic ulcer disease, oesophagitis, gastritis and duodenitis, varices, portal hypertensive gastropathy (PHG), angiodysplasia, dieulafoy lesion, gastric antral valvular ectasia, aortoenteric fistulas, post-surgical bleeds, upper GI tumors, haemobilia, haemosuccus pancreaticus
- **Vomiting** secondary to mechanical gastrointestinal obstruction or manipulation, gastrointestinal pseudo-obstructions, gastric neuromuscular disorders, toxins, uraemia, Idiopathic nausea and vomiting, eating disorders, malignancy, ischaemic gastroparesis, peritoneal irritation, adrenal insufficiency, type 1 and type 2 diabetes, electrolyte disorders, central nervous system (CNS) disorders, acute coronary syndrome, gastrointestinal infections.
- **Puetz-Jeghers syndrome** associated with increased risk of GI adenocarcinoma
- **Fetor hepaticus** secondary to hyperammonemia associated with severe parenchymal liver disease.

Lymph nodes

- **Mesenteric lymphadenitis** secondary to infection
- **Left axillary lymphadenopathy** secondary to gastric carcinoma

Oesophagus

- **Dysphagia** and **Odynophagia** secondary to oropharyngeal infection/ inflammation, oral cavity structural abnormalities, oropharyngeal structural abnormalities, oropharyngeal neuromuscular abnormalities, oesophageal structural abnormalities, oesophageal motor abnormalities
- **Dyspepsia** secondary to duodenal ulcer, gastric ulcer, oesophageal or gastric cancer, oesopha-

Abdomen

- Please refer to Figure 11.2

Systemic and cutaneous signs

- **Jaundice/icterus** secondary to haemolysis, impaired bilirubin conjugation (e.g. Gilbert's syndrome), viral hepatitides A, B, C, D, and E, HIV infection, parasitic infections, leptospirosis, acute alcoholic hepatitis, prolonged alcohol intoxication or as a manifestation of advanced cirrhosis, Drug induced liver injury, hepatocellular and cholangio neoplasia (carcimoma, lymphoma, colorectal metastases), autoimmune hepatitis, primary biliary cholangitis, primary sclerosing cholangitis, wilson's disease, hereditary, haemochromatosis, alpha-1 antitrypsin deficiency, choledocholithiasis, postoperative stricture, ascending cholangitis, pregnancy, and end-stage liver disease
- **Nail bed clubbing** secondary to gastric sarcoidosis, primary biliary cholangitis, achalasia, ulcerative oesophagitis, coeliac disease, ulcerative colitis, crohn's disease, tropical sprue
- **Lecuonychia** (Terry's nails) secondary to hypoalbuminaemia in chronic liver disease
- **Acanthosis nigricans** associated with increased risk of GI carcinoma
- **Gardeners Triad** (osteomas, polyposis coli, and mesenchymal tumours of the skin and soft tissue), associated with gastrointestinal polyps and adenocarcinoma.
- **Telengectasia** associated with Carcenoid syndrome which is characterised by GI & HPB symptoms such as hepatomegaly and watery diarrhoea
- **Dystrophic nails** associated with cronkhite-canda syndrome which is characterised by GI & HPB symptoms such as diarrhoea, pancreatic insufficiency
- **Palmar erythema** secondary to chronic liver disease
- **Bronze skin pigmentation** one of three of the triad of signs associated with haemochromatosis, the other two being; liver cirrhosis and diabetes mellitus.
- **Spider naevi** associated with liver cirrhosis, alcoholic hepatitis, and hepatopulmonary syndrome. Their presence increases likelihood of oesophageal varices and are indicative of the extent of hepatic fibrosis.
- **Leukoplakia** may occur in the mouth, larynx and anus.

FIGURE 11.1 Common presenting symptoms and their association with GI and HPB disorders. *Source:* Sadie Diamond-Fox.

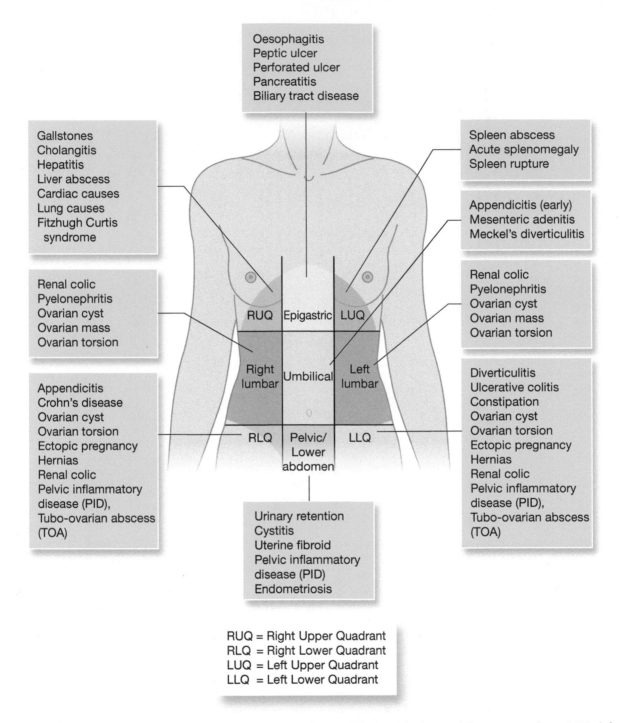

FIGURE 11.2 Abdominal quadrants and the potential or differential diagnosis. (RUQ–right upper quadrant, LUQ–left upper quadrant, LLQ–left lower quadrant, RLQ–right lower quadrant). *Source*: Adapted from Tintinalli et al. (2020).

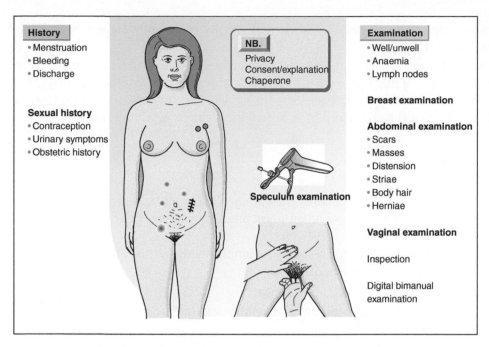

FIGURE 11.3   Process for performing an abdominal examination. *Source*: Gleadle (2012) / John Wiley & Sons.

Figure 11.3 presents the process for performing a comprehensive abdominal examination. This includes the liver, spleen, kidneys, aorta, hernia, and genitalia and aids diagnosis and/or differentials.

Fields of Practice – Learning Disabilities

Chronic upper gastrointestinal (UGI) dysmotility problems for patients with learning disabilities include dysphagia (60%), pulmonary aspiration (41%), malnutrition (33%), gastroesophageal reflux (GERD) (32%), and gastritis (32%). Uncoordinated swallowing can lead to inadequate nutrition and caloric intake. Infection with *Helicobacter pylori* is higher in people with developmental disabilities who live in group homes than in the general population. This can lead to peptic ulcer disease (PUD) and potentially gastric adenocarcinoma (Curtis et al. 2021).

Fields of Practice – Paediatrics

There are nine standards in the Paediatric Gastroenterology, Hepatology & Nutrition (2017). To reduce variation in care, to improve quality of life and health outcomes and to ensure impartial services. It emphasises the need for:

- Clinical network for all trusts and boards across the UK.
- Access for all hospitals to specialists by telephone with adequate capacity to transfer to a tertiary centre 24 hours a day, 7 days a week.
- Transition to adult care is agreed by all parties involved, the child, paediatric team, and adult specialty.

- In an age-appropriate facility, children with suspected inflammatory bowel disease are seen within four weeks.
- Children requiring specialist dietary treatment have a named paediatrician and a specialist dietician. If parenteral nutrition is required, a paediatric dietitian, parenteral nutrition pharmacist, and children's clinical nurse specialist with knowledge and experience in nutrition support is required. They must be reviewed in an in-patient setting at least once a week.

Jaundice

There is an abundance of causes of patients presenting with jaundice. Therefore, it is simpler to differentiate the causes. There are three causes of jaundice; pre-hepatic, hepatic, and post-hepatic.

1. Pre-hepatic causes of jaundice result in unconjugated hyperbilirubinaemia, which is not water soluble, so cannot enter the bloodstream.
   - Conjugation disorders i.e. Gilberts disease
   - Haemolysis e.g. malaria, haemolytic anaemia, sickle cell
   - Drugs i.e. Rifampicin, amoxicillin/clavulanic acid, cimetidine, chlorpromazine, anabolic steroids
2. Hepatic dysfunction results in a conjugated hyperbilirubinaemia.
   - Viruses i.e. hepatitis, CMV, EBV
   - Liver mass i.e. abscess or malignancy
   - Autoimmune hepatitis
   - Alpha-1 antitrypsin deficiency
   - Budd-Chiari
   - Wilsons disease
   - Cirrhosis
   - Drugs i.e. paracetamol overdose, valproate, statins, halothane.
3. Post-hepatic jaundice results from impaired excretion of conjugated bilirubin. Conjugated bilirubin is water soluble, making the urine darker in colour, less bilirubin reaches the gut so acholic faeces are the result.
   - Malignancy i.e. pancreatic cancer
   - Primary biliary cirrhosis or Primary sclerosing cholangitis
   - Bile duct obstruction
   - Drugs e.g. amoxicillin/clavulanic acid, flucloxacillin.

ACUTE PANCREATITIS

Pancreatitis is a disease which is one of the most common causes of hospitalisation among GI disorders. It is the acute inflammation of the pancreas which has varying severities ranging from mild, requiring conservative treatment, to severe which can then lead to high mortality rates if not treated in a responsive and appropriate manner. This is predominantly due to systemic inflammatory response syndrome (SIRS) and organ failure within the initial two-week period, after this mortality is due to complications and sepsis.

The Revised Atlanta classification system (Thoeni, 2012) highlights local and systemic determinants to grade the severity (mild, moderate, severe/critical). It states that at least two of the following criteria must be present to be classed as severe/critical:

- Abdominal pain consistent with acute pancreatitis
- Characteristic evidence via imaging – ultrasound scan (USS), computed tomography (CT) scan and/or Magnetic Resonance Imaging (MRI)
- Serum amylase or lipase >3 times the upper limit of normal.

The classification also divides acute pancreatitis into two types:

1. Interstitial oedematous pancreatitis
2. Necrotising pancreatitis, which is further subdivided into:
   - Parenchymal necrosis
   - Peripancreatic necrosis
   - Combined type (peripancreatic and parenchymal necrosis). This is the most common.

Acute pancreatitis is a prevalent reason for patients presenting with acute abdominal pain in the AECC setting. Approximately, in the UK, 56 cases per 100 000 people per year is the incidence (NICE 2020). The main causes include gallstones, alcohol, and complications associated with kidney or respiratory failure, or post-surgical or spontaneous fluid collections. Table 11.1 shows the more in-depth causes of acute pancreatitis.

Chronic pancreatitis prevalence, although potentially underestimated, in Western Europe is 5 cases per 100 000 annually. It is more prevalent in males than females (7:1) with an average age onset between 36 and 55 years (NICE 2020). Alcohol use causes 70–80% of presentations. Other causes

TABLE 11.1   Causes of acute pancreatitis.

Mechanical	Gallstones, biliary sludge, ascariasis, ampullary, or peri-ampullary cancer, duodenal stricture obstruction	Trauma	Blunt abdominal, iatrogenic e.g. ERCP
Toxic	Ethanol, methanol, venom (scorpion or snake bites)	Metabolic	Hyperlipidaemia, hypercalcaemia
Infection	Virus; Coxsackie, Hepatitis B, HIV, HSV Bacteria; *Mycoplasma, Legionella, Leptospira* Fungi; *Aspergillus* Parasites; *Toxoplasma, Cryptosporidium*	Drugs	HIV therapy; didanosine, pentamidine Antibiotics; metronidazole, tetracycline Diuretics; thiazides, furosemide Immunosuppressive; azathioprine Neuropsychiatric; valproate Anti-inflammatory drugs; salicylates
Congenital	Anatomical defects	Vascular	Ischaemia, vasculitis
Miscellaneous	Hypothermia, pregnancy, post-renal transplant	Genetic	Alpha-1-antitrypsin deficiency

Source: Adapted from Langrish (2007).

TABLE 11.2   Clinical features of pancreatitis.

Symptom	Occurrence frequency (%)
Abdominal pain radiating to the back	95
Anorexia	85
Nausea, vomiting	75
Decreased sound of intestinal peristalsis	60
Pyrexia	60
Muscular defence	50
Shock	15
Jaundice	15
Heamatemasis	10

Source: Adapted from Kiriyama et al. (2010).

include cigarette smoking, hypercalcaemia, hyperlipidaemia, or autoimmune disease, idiopathic causes or hereditary factors. Clinical features and investigations are described in Tables 11.2 and 11.3.

Initial Management

The initial management of acute pancreatitis should be conducted with a systematic A-I approach utilising key investigations regularly, such as ABGs, FBC, U&Es, coagulation, etc. Severe cases should be treated in ICU or HDU setting. Most hospitals have their own guidelines for the management of acute pancreatitis, however, below are some of the key management strategies to focus on during early detection of organ dysfunction and infection to prevent the development of organ failure.

TABLE 11.3   Investigations in acute pancreatitis.

Investigation	Results	Sensitivity	Specificity	Differential
Serum lipase	>3× upper limit of normal. More than two-thirds of patients with acute pancreatitis with normal amylase will have elevated lipase. Lipase rises within 4–8 hours and remains elevated for 8–14 days.	100%	99%	May be elevated in other conditions such as Hepatitis C, IBD, DKA, and renal failure
Serum amylase	>1000 IU/ml	61%	100%	
Abdominal CT	Gallstone pancreatitis	52%	100%	
Abdominal USS	Gallstone pancreatitis	72%	98%	

Source: Yadav et al. (2002), Wang et al. (1988).

Fluid Resuscitation

Pancreatic ducts are disrupted during acute pancreatitis which exudates serine proteases into, initially, the peritoneum and then plasma. Kinin, coagulation, and cytokine cascades are activated inducing systemic inflammatory response and hypovoleamia follows. If fluid response and/or vasopressor support are inadequate, tissue ischemia, regional hypo-perfusion and end-organ damage will occur. NICE current guidelines recommend goal-directed therapy for fluid management.

Arterial Monitoring

Arterial monitoring is essential to aid fluid resuscitation. In conjunction with oxygen saturation levels and hourly fluid output (via a urinary catheter measurement), this may facilitate early recognition of renal and cardiac dysfunction.

Adequate Analgesia

Severe abdominal pain is a predominant symptom, and effective analgesia is essential. If pain control is inadequate, hypo or hyper ventilation can occur, leading to further respiratory complications such as ARDS, which have marked negative effects on arterial blood results (pH, acid-base balance), which can lead to an abundance of other complications. Analgesia should be either IV or via a PCA route – usually opiate based. When gut absorption has been demonstrated IV can be changed to oral analgesics.

Nutrition

Patients should be 'nil by mouth' and a nasogastric (NG) tube should be placed (beyond the ligament of Treitz) when vomiting and ileus are present. Enteral Nutrition (EN) can then be commenced 72 hours after and titrated to relevant feeding regimes as tolerated, this will also provide gut protection and limit bacterial translocation. A proton pump inhibitor should be prescribed for gastric protection. If pancreatitis is related to excessive alcohol, then IV Pabrinex should be prescribed. IV Pabrinex provides additional Vitamins B and C to correct deficiencies that may have occurred in alcoholism, infections, or postoperatively.

Antibiotics

In acute severe pancreatitis with no clear evidence of infection, antibiotics are not required. Indications to commence antibiotics include cholangitis or signs of sepsis, proven bacterial infection, suspected infected pancreatic necrosis or a concurrent bacterial infection of another source (e.g. pneumonia). Antibiotics should be prescribed as per local micro guide guidance and discussions with the microbiologist.

Removal of Cause

Following referral to the Gastroenterologist, ERCP should be performed if there is biliary pancreatitis with concurrent cholangitis (urgent) and biliary pancreatitis with obstructive jaundice. Cholangitis is an inflammation of the bile duct system. The bile duct system carries bile from your liver and gallbladder into the first part of your small intestine (the duodenum). In most cases, cholangitis is caused by a bacterial infection, and often happens suddenly. But in some cases, it may be long-term (chronic).

Aftercare

The most important aftercare in acute pancreatitis is the prevention of recurrence. This should be done by minimising the risk via alcohol or smoking cessation, reviewing medications which can cause pancreatitis and referring patients to the relevant teams for post-critical care after-care.

Acute Liver Failure

Acute liver failure (ALF) is characterised by coagulopathy and hepatic encephalopathy within 26 weeks of being diagnosed with liver disease. It is associated with multi-organ failure and high mortality rate if not treated with appropriate and timely treatment, which includes appropriate use of emergency liver transplantation. The main causes vary across the world. In the UK, it is predominantly caused by paracetamol toxicity; however, since the purchasing restrictions law there has been a 43% reduction in deaths (Hawton et al. 2013). In other countries it is most commonly hepatitis A, B, and E. Table 11.4 shows the more in-depth causes of ALF. Acute liver failure (ALF) can be classified into three subcategories based on the timing of encephalopathy development after the onset of jaundice, as outlined by the King's classification in 1993. Hyperacute liver failure refers to cases where hepatic encephalopathy arises within 7 days, typically caused by paracetamol toxicity in individuals without pre-existing liver disease. Acute liver failure occurs when encephalopathy manifests between 8 and 28 days after jaundice onset and can have various aetiologies such as viral hepatitis, drug-induced liver injury, or autoimmune hepatitis. Subacute liver failure is a rarer form, associated with encephalopathy developing between 5 and 26 weeks after jaundice onset and linked to conditions like Budd-Chiari syndrome, Wilson disease, or autoimmune hepatitis. The King's classification is significant for prognostication and guiding healthcare providers in referring patients to specialized liver management centres, with subacute liver failure generally carrying a poorer prognosis compared to acute liver failure.

CLINICAL FEATURES

Clinical features of ALF are determined by the cause and rate of severity to the liver. The range of presentation can be that of mild non-specific symptoms (nausea, vomiting, and abdominal pain) to combative, confusion, and decreased consciousness. It is therefore paramount to undertake a comprehensive

TABLE 11.4   Identifies the main causes of ALF.

Drugs and toxins	Paracetamol, Amanita phalloides, Isoniazid, Halothane, monoamine oxidase inhibitors, phenytoin, Ecstasy	**Metabolic**	Wilson disease, Reye's syndrome, Alpha-1-antitrypsin deficiency, haemachromatosis
Infection	Virus: Hepatitis A, Hepatitis B, hepatitis E, Herpes simplex virus, Epstein–Barr virus	**Autoimmune**	Autoimmune hepatitis, primary binary cirrhosis, primary sclerosis cholangitis, sarcoidosis.
Cardiovascular	Shock, heat stroke, Budd-Chiari syndrome	**Miscellaneous**	Acute fatty liver of pregnancy, lymphoma
Unknown	Approximately 15–20% of ALF cases cannot be found to have a specific cause		

history to delineate the cause. However, obtaining a detailed and accurate medical history from patients with ALF can be very challenging, if not impossible, due to the presence of an altered mental status. The practitioner is usually forced to rely on family and friends to obtain information about recent symptoms, medication use, risk factors and any significant past medical problems.

Hepatic encephalopathy is caused by hepatic insufficiency associated with ALF. It is a neuropsychiatric syndrome for which symptoms, manifested on a continuum, are deterioration in mental status, with psychomotor dysfunction, impaired memory, increased reaction time, sensory abnormalities, poor concentration, disorientation, and coma. It is caused by the accumulation of neurotoxins. The Conn score, also known as the West Haven Criteria, is a 5-point scale (0 to 4) for grading the severity of HE based upon neurocognitive function (e.g., consciousness, intellectual function, and behaviour).

Coagulopathy is an essential component of ALF syndrome and reflects the central role of liver function in haemostasis. However, the exact mechanism remains to be fully elucidated. Current evidence suggests that the coagulopathy is derived from a complex and delicate interplay between decreased synthesis of procoagulant factors and anticoagulant factors, impaired fibrinolytic systems, defective platelets, and thrombocytopenia (Santiago et al. 2009).

ALF is characterised by the development of hepatic encephalopathy and coagulopathy within 24 weeks of the onset of acute liver disease. Diagnosis should be heavily supported through biochemistry and coagulation tests (see Table 11.5).

Cardiovascular changes in ALF are similar in nature to sepsis; hypotension, tachycardia, and low systemic vascular resistance.

TABLE 11.5 Laboratory testing in acute liver failure.

Purpose	Test	Comment
Severity of ALF	• Prothrombin time/INR • Bilirubin • Albumin • Lactate • Phosphate	Prothrombin time/INR is the most useful test, however, loses prognostic value temporarily when plasma is given to prevent bleeding.
Cause of ALF	Viral serologies Autoimmune serologies Paracetamol level Ceruloplasmin Serum copper Pregnancy test	Determining the cause of ALF accurately as the prognosis depends on the cause of the ALF. The cause may only respond to specific therapy also.
Complications of ALF	Creatinine BUN Haemoglobin/ haematocrit White cell count with differential Blood cultures Urine culture Glucose Electrolytes Ammonia	The tests are used to determine whether anaemia, infection, renal failure, or other problems have been complicated by ALF. Ammonia levels also help assess the risk of cerebral oedema.

Oliguric renal failure occurs in >30% of ALF, and this is also an indicator of poor prognosis; however, paracetamol overdose renal failure is the exception.

Initial Management

Patients with coagulopathy and hepatic encephalopathy should be treated in the ICU setting. The initial management should be conducted with a systematic A-I approach. Treatment is broadly supportive until either the patient improves or needs transfer to liver specialist unit. ALF patients have high risk of complications including sepsis, haemodynamic instability, renal failure, and sepsis. Table 11.6 highlights specific treatment for the less common presenting causes of ALF.

Intubation

Intubation is recommended in patients with a grade III/IV encephalopathy for airway protection and control of carbon dioxide levels. Ventilation should be aimed with lung protection strategies and to maintain normocapnia.

Fluid Resuscitation

Fluid resuscitation is an important aspect of initial management and should be done cautiously. Excess fluid should be avoided due to potential increased associated inter cranial pressures which could lead to herniation and death. Hypotonic solutions are proving more favourable in recent trials. It is also important to have strict electrolyte control, including sodium, phosphate, potassium, and magnesium, and to correct them aggressively. Haemodynamic changes can mimic sepsis; increased portal pressure, splanchnic sequestration of blood, decreased central venous return, high cardiac output, and decreased

TABLE 11.6   Treatment for the less common presenting causes of ALF.

Herpes Simplex hepatitis	• Aciclovir: 10 mg/kg 8 hourly	**Acute Hepatitis B**	• Entecavir: 0.5 mg oral/NG once daily Or • Enofovir disoproxil: 300 mg oral/NG once daily
Acute fatty liver of pregnancy	• Refer to obstetrics • Potential expedient delivery of foetus.	**Budd-Chiari syndrome**	• Anticoagulation therapy • Transjugular intrahepatic portosystemic shunt
Amanita phalloides	• Activated charcoal: 25–100 g as a single dose, repeat every 4–6 hours, if required • Benzylpenicillin 2.4–4.8 g/a day into four divided doses	**Wilsons disease**	• Plasmapheresis, continuous veno-venous haemofiltration, albumin dialysis, or plasma exchange.
Autoimmune hepatitis	• Methylprednisolone 60 mg IV once daily.		

systemic vascular resistance. Vasopressors are recommended to maintain a MAP >60 mmHg to ensure an acceptable cerebral perfusion. Invasive monitoring is therefore essential.

Neurological

Sedation and analgesics with short half-life are preferred due to assessment of neurological status and hepatic encephalopathy e.g. Propofol and Fentanyl. Efforts should be made to minimise elevations of intracranial pressure by raising the patients head to 30°, maintain head and neck alignment, clustering care, reducing surrounding stimuli and maintaining normothermia.

Nutrition and Glycemic Control

ALF is associated with severe catabolism, metabolic consequences and therefore hypoglycemia. Glucose levels should be monitored 1–2 hours a day and corrected with IV glucose as applicable. Continuous glucose infusions increase the risk of hyponatreamia, so they should be given concurrently with sodium chloride 0.9% and potassium chloride 40 mmol/l.

Hyperammonemia can increase the risk of cerebral oedema, so nutrition can be delayed for 24–48 hours. EN via a nasogastric tube can then be commenced being mindful of ammonia levels after. A PPI should be prescribed for gut protection and lactulose to assist the removal of ammonia through the faeces.

Coagulopathy

Do not give blood products unless active bleeding is evident. If bleeding occurs discuss with the haematologist. Fibrin degradation or D-Dimers levels should be taken to exclude disseminated intravascular coagulation (DIC). Typically, FFP will be given with active bleeding and an INR >1.5 or INR >7 and platelets will be given if platelets <20×10/l and/or bleeding or invasive procedure required. Phytomenadione 10 mg once daily should be given for three days, however be mindful this is not to correct the coagulopathy but to ensure patient is replete.

N-Acetylcysteine (NAC)

N-Acetylcysteine (NAC) significantly improves survival rates, decreases complications of ALF, and decreases the overall length of hospital stay. It is used in both paracetamol toxicity and non-paracetamol toxicity (with evidence of hepatic encephalopathy). NAC is "a thiol-containing agent that scavenges free oxygen radicals and replenishes cellular, mitochondrial, and cytosolic glutathione stores by serving a source of a glutathione surrogate that combines directly with reactive metabolites or serves as a source of sulphate, thus preventing hepatic damage" (Halliwell and Gutteridge 1999). NAC should be delivered by the MHRA approved Scottish and Newcastle Acetylcysteine Protocol (SNAP) protocol (as per Toxbase) in the emergency department, and on transfer to ICU as per local policy/advise from liver specialist units. Acetylcysteine therapy should continue until end points, such as improvement of hepatic function by clinical and laboratory parameters have been achieved.

Haemodiafiltration

Haemodiafiltration should be commenced if potassium >6 mmol/l, HCO_3^- <15 mmol/l or Creatinine >400 mm/l.

Rather than wait until the strict criteria is met for transplantation, patients with severe ALF should be discussed with the local liver transplant centre at the earliest available opportunity. This should occur if:

- Prothrombin time >20 seconds or INR >2
- pH <7.3 or H+ >50 nmol/l
- Hypoglycaemia
- Conscious level impaired
- Creatinine >200 mm/l

Upper Gastro-intestinal Bleeding

Upper Gastro-intestinal bleeding (UGIB) is a common occurrence in AECC, approximately 75% of all acute GI bleeding cases are estimated to occur in up to 150 per 100 000 people a year with a mortality rate up to 15% (Kamboj et al. 2019). Any blood loss above the ligament of Treitz is classified as an UGIB. It can present as haematemesis, haematochezia, or melaena. The predominant causes of UGIB are due to PUD which can be associated with NSAIDs, *Helicobacter pylori,* and stress mucosal disease. Table 11.7 shows other causes and their prevalence in occurrence.

During history–taking, important information to gather are comorbidities, a detailed review of current medication, and a social history regarding alcohol consumption. Medications to be mindful of are NSAIDs, anti-platelet drugs, aspirin, or anticoagulants.

Clinical presentation is well-characterised with haematemesis, melaena, or haematochezia. Although haematochezia is typically seen in lower gastrointestinal bleeds, it can also be seen with profuse UGIB. Other typical presentations reflect a medical emergency with syncope and haemodynamic instability.

There are two main scoring systems used in UGIB; the Rockall score and the Glasgow Blatchford score. The Rockall risk scoring system is used to predict re-bleeding and mortality rates based on age, the presence of shock, medical comorbidity, and endoscopic findings. The Glasgow Blatchford score is based on simple clinical observations, haemoglobin, and blood urea concentrations and does not require endoscopy results. There have been studies into which is more favourable, but the conclusion is that a combination of both is the optimal approach for guidance in emergency treatment.

TABLE 11.7   Causes of upper gastro-intestinal bleeding and occurrence frequency.

Cause	Occurrence frequency (%)
Peptic ulcer disease	40–50
Duodenal ulcer	30
Erosive esophagitis	11
Duodenitis	10
Varices	5–30 (respective of chronic liver disease)
Mallory-Weiss tear	5–15
Vascular malformations	5

Initial Management

In a medical emergency, an A–E assessment and treatment plan should be performed. If anything should change through the assessment, then restart the assessment as UGIB is highly unpredictable and can deteriorate swiftly.

AIRWAY AND BREATHING

Elective intubation should be performed in severe haematemesis or if the patient is unable to protect their own airway. If the patient can protect their airway, then supplemental oxygen (unless contraindicated) should be given to maintain oxygen saturation levels of 94–98% (BTS 2017).

Circulation

Two large bore cannula (>18 g) or a CVC should be inserted to facilitate haemodynamic instability. Intravenous fluids should be given (crystalloid) to maintain a MAP >60 mmHg. If repeated boluses increase the risk of fluid overload, the patient should be reassessed each time. Persistent hypotension will require vasopressor support. All critically unwell patients should have an arterial line inserted for continuous haemodynamic and ABG monitoring. Hypotension does not occur until there has been a significant blood loss of approximately 2000 ml. Blood transfusion should occur to maintain an Hb >70 (or in higher risk patients >90) with every fourth unit of FFP. Platelets should be offered to patients who are actively bleeding with a platelet count of <50 × 109/l. Patients with pre-existing liver disease may have low platelets due to portal hypertension and splenomegaly. FFP should be given to patients who are actively bleeding and have a prothrombin time or activated partial thromboplastin time greater than 1.5 times normal. If a patient's fibrinogen level remains less than 1.5 g/l despite fresh frozen plasma use, offer cryoprecipitate as well. The haematologist on-call should be made aware of severe UGIB patients for decisions. If severe ongoing haematemesis is evident, then the major haemorrhage protocol should be activated ensuring FBC, clotting, U&E, LFT, and Ca^{2+} are taken and delivered to the laboratory after each massive haemorrhage pack is transfused. This is to reassess the patient and decide whether further products are required, or Blood Bank can stand down.

Disability

Regular monitoring of the patient's consciousness should be assessed as it may be reduced secondary to hypotension or hepatic encephalopathy (Glasgow Coma Score [GCS] is favourable). It is imperative the patient remains Nil By Mouth (NBM) until clinically indicated they have improved. Early referral to gastroenterology/endoscopist for further management and guidance is important. This could include OGD, IR, or CT angiogram. Upper GI endoscopy is required to locate the source of bleeding and stop the mechanism (through injecting adrenaline or clipping). If bleeding continues or the source cannot be identified, then a Sengstaken-Blakemore tube can be inserted.

Proton-pump Inhibitors

Proton pump inhibitors (PPI) are used to treat patients with non-variceal UGIB after OGD. A prescription of 80 mg Omeprazole IV bolus should then be followed by a continuous infusion of 8 mg/h. IV omeprazole for 72 hours.

Fields of Practice – Mental Health

Mental health impacts highly in the predisposing risk factors, care, and treatment of patients with gastrointestinal and hepatobiliary conditions and disorders. People with schizophrenia and bipolar disorder have a higher prevalence of hepatic illness compared to the general population (Menon et al. 2022), as there is an increased risk linked with other medical comorbidities and unhealthy lifestyle factors (alcohol and substance misuse). People with depressive disorders also have a high prevalence of chronic liver disease due to lifestyle and prescribed medication. Sertraline is associated with liver disease and serotonin norepinephrine reuptake inhibitors can induce liver injuries. Tricyclic antidepressants in patients with chronic liver disease have poor clearance which can increase anticholinergic side effects, seizures, sedation, orthostatic hypotension, and arrhythmogenic effects. Conversely, patients who have been diagnosed with gastrointestinal or hepatobiliary disorders have a high prevalence of depression.

It is paramount that psycho-pharmacy must be individualised being mindful of the underlying medical condition and the long-term effects they may have.

Take Home Points

- Advanced practitioners must utilise effective history-taking and physical examination skills to ensure the prompt diagnosis or differential diagnosis to minimise potential complications and deterioration.
- There are diverse presentations and the implications on wider groups such as the LGBTQIA+ community, paediatrics, and the BAME community should be considered. All patients should be approached and cared for in a holistic, timely manner with an A–E approach.
- Patients who have mental health issues or learning disabilities have higher incidents of GI/HPB problems.
- Early and appropriate referral to the relevant teams and tertiary centres has potential for better outcomes, either for guidance of management or for transfer of care.

REFERENCES

British Society of Paediatric Gastroenterology Hepatology and Nutrition & Royal College of Paediatrics and Child Health. (2017). *Quality Standards for Paediatric Gastroenterology, Hepatology and Nutrition* [online]. Available from: https://www.rcpch.ac.uk/sites/default/files/2018-03/standards_for_paediatric_gastroenterology_hepatology_and_nutrition.pdf [accessed 21 June 2023].

Curtis, J.S., Kennedy, S.E., Barrett, A. et al. (2021). Upper gastrointestinal disorders in adult patients with intellectual and developmental disabilities. *Cureus* 13 (6): e15384.

Gleadle, J. (2012). *History and Clinical Examination at a Glance*. Wiley-Blackwell.

Halliwell, B. and Gutteridge, J.M. (1999). *Free Radicals in Biology and Medicine*, 840–842. Oxford: Oxford University Press.

Hawton, K., Bergen, H., Simkin, S. et al. (2013). Long term effect of reduced pack sizes of paracetamol on poisoning deaths and liver transplant activity in England and Wales: interrupted time series analyses. *BMJ* 346: 1–9.

Health Education England. (2017). *Multi-professional Framework for Advanced Clinical Practice in England* [online]. Available from: `https://www.hee.nhs.uk/sites/default/files/documents/multi-professionalframeworkforadvancedclinicalpracticeinengland.pdf` [accessed 21 June 2023].

Health Education England (HEE). (2022). *Advanced Clinical Practice in Acute Medicine Curriculum Framework – Credentials* [online]. Available from: `https://advanced-practice.hee.nhs.uk/our-work/credentials` [accessed 20 June 2023].

Kamboj, A.K., Hoversten, P., and Leggett, C.L. (2019). Upper gastrointestinal bleeding: etiologies and management. *Mayo Clinic Proceedings* 94 (4): 697–703.

Kiriyama, S., Gabata, T., Takada, T. et al. (2010). New diagnostic criteria of acute pancreatitis. *Journal of Hepatobiliary and Pancreatic Science* 17: 24–36.

Langrish, C. (2007). *Acute Pancreatitis – A Clinical Overview (Anaesthesia Tutorial of the Week 73)*. Available from: `https://www.e-safe-anaesthesia.org/e_library/11/Acute_Pancreatitis_TOTW_073_2007.pdf` [accessed 6 July 2023].

Menon, V., Ransing, R., and Praharaj, S.K. (2022). Management of psychiatric disorders in patients with hepatic and gastrointestinal diseases. *Indian Journal of Psychiatry* 64 (2): 379–393.

NICE. (2020). *Pancreatitis: NICE Guideline* [NG104] [online]. Available from: `https://www.nice.org.uk/guidance/ng104/chapter/Context` [accessed 22 June 2023].

Santiago, J., Munoz, R., Todd Stravitz, A., and Gabriel, R. (2009). Coagulopathy of acute liver failure. *Clinics in Liver Disease* 13 (1): 95–107.

The Faculty of Intensive Care Medicine. (2018). *Curriculum for Training for Advanced Critical Care Practitioners – Syllabus. V1.1* [online]. Available from: `www.ficm.ac.uk/media/6896` [accessed 20 June 2023].

The Royal College of Emergency Medicine. (2022). *Emergency Medicine Advanced Clinical Practitioner Curriculum 2022 (Adult)* [online]. Available from: `https://rcem.ac.uk/wp-content/uploads/2022/09/ACP_Curriculum_Adult_Final_060922.pdf` [accessed 20 June 2023].

Thoeni, R. (2012). The revised Atlanta classification of acute pancreatitis: its importance for the radiologist and its effect on treatment. *Radiology* 262 (3).

Tintinalli, J.E., Ma, O.J., Yealy, D.M. et al. (ed.) (2020). *Tintinalli's Emergency Medicine: A Comprehensive Study Guide*. McGraw Hill.

Wang, S.S., Lin, X.Z., Tsai, Y.T. et al. (1988). Clinical significance of ultrasonography, computed tomography, and biochemical tests in the rapid diagnosis of gallstone-related pancreatitis: a prospective study. *Pancreas* 3 (2): 153–158.

Yadav, D., Agarwal, N., and Pitchumoni, C.S. (2002). A critical evaluation of laboratory tests in acute pancreatitis. *The American Journal of Gastroenterology* 97 (6): 1309–1318.

FURTHER READING

Kalra, A., Yetiskul, E., Wehrle, C.J. et al. (2022). *Physiology, Liver* [online]. In: StatPearls [Internet]. Treasure Island (FL): StatPearls Publishing 2022 Jan-. Available from: `https://www.ncbi.nlm.nih.gov/books/NBK535438/` [Updated 8 May 2022].

CHAPTER 12

Haematological and Oncological Presentations

Barry Hill

Aim

The aim of this chapter is to provide the reader with knowledge about some of the key haematological and oncological presentations that may be encountered in acute, emergency, and critical care (AECC) environments.

Haematology is the study of the physiology of blood and the diseases associated with it, and oncology is the study of all types of cancer. To advance practice, this chapter aides the reader in recognising the risk factors for Oncological and Haematological emergencies and supports their ability to diagnose and treat these presentations in the environments of acute, emergency, and critical care.

LEARNING OUTCOMES

After reading this chapter the reader will:

1. Gain a better understanding of acute haematological and oncological, emergency and critical care presentations.
2. Be able to identify haematological and oncological emergencies and interventional treatments.
3. Better appreciate systemic anti-cancer treatments and their side effects, including long-term late presentation.
4. Gain better understanding of the different treatment intentions and implications this will have on decision-making and ceiling of care.

The Advanced Practitioner in Acute, Emergency and Critical Care, First Edition. Edited by Sadie Diamond-Fox, Barry Hill, Sonya Stone, Caroline McCrea, Natalie Gardner, and Angela Roberts.
© 2024 John Wiley & Sons Ltd. Published 2024 by John Wiley & Sons Ltd.

SELF-ASSESSMENT QUESTIONS

1. What are haematological and oncological emergencies?
2. Explain some of the adjuvant, neo-adjuvant, and palliative treatments available.
3. What investigations are considered essential when assessing patients who present to acute care services with haematological and oncological presentations?
4. Discuss the key considerations that inform a diagnosis and differential of which aides a clinical assessment?

INTRODUCTION

In this chapter, a selection of acute, emergency, and critical haematological and oncological disorders will be presented to the reader. Haematology is the study of the physiology of blood and the diseases associated with it, and oncology is the study of all types of cancer. Haematology Oncology Advanced Practitioners specialise in treating, screening, and preventing disorders of the blood such as anaemia, sickle cell disease, bleeding disorders, haemophilia as well as different types of cancer, including leukaemia and lymphoma.

The Advanced Practitioner must consider the four pillars of advanced practice when providing acute care to patients with haematological and oncological disorders, and work within their scope of practice underpinned by their regulatory body. All Advanced Practitioners must establish and utilise kindness and compassion within their care and ensure inclusivity and a holistic approach. People with haematological and oncological conditions require a dignified approach to their care, as many of these conditions are not generally understood, and stereotyping and stigma still exist around many illnesses. Consequently, Advanced Practitioners must ensure that they are competent and knowledgeable within the haematological and oncological specialities, if they are expected to lead and manage care for patients with such disorders. This will safeguard a factual and evidence-based approach to advocate and empower their patient.

Multi-professional Framework (MPF) for Advanced Clinical Practice Guidance for Professional Development (HEE 2017)

This chapter maps to the following statements within the MPF:

1. Clinical Practice:	1.1	1.2	1.3	1.4	1.5	1.6	1.7	1.8	1.9
2. Leadership and Management:	2.1	2.7	2.8						
3. Education:	3.2								
4. Research:	3.7								

Accreditation Considerations

This chapter maps to the following statements within the following national accreditation documents:

Curriculum for Training for Advanced Critical Care Practitioners Syllabus V1.1
(The Faculty of Intensive Care Medicine 2018)

2.5	4.1	4.3	

Advanced Critical Care Outreach Competencies
(The Intensive Care Society, Critical Care Networks – National Nurse Leads and The National Outreach Forum 2022)

A1	A5	B1	C1	C3	

Emergency Medicine Advanced Clinical Practitioner Curriculum 2022 – Adult
(The Royal College of Emergency Medicine 2022)

HCP–3	HC1–9	

Advanced Clinical Practice in Acute Medicine Curriculum Framework
(Health Education England 2022)

- Presentations and Conditions of Acute Medicine by System/Specialty: Oncology and Haematology

HAEMATOLOGIC EMERGENCIES

The management of haematologic emergencies is directed towards immediate stabilisation of the acutely ill patient to prevent morbidity and mortality related to severe anaemia, infection, bleeding, and thrombosis. Patients at risk for infection and sepsis, such as neutropenic or asplenic patients, require prompt attention; quality metrics focus on time to initiation of antibiotic therapy for these patients. Simultaneously, significant haematologic findings of unknown aetiology require thorough evaluation, especially where necessary therapies may obscure the underlying diagnosis or impede later diagnostic testing. Haematologic emergencies arise in people who have been previously well, who have known blood disorders, or who have systemic disease. Initial measures of support, diagnosis, and treatment are based on general principles that often do not require a definitive diagnosis to initiate management. Some initial key factors that Advanced Practitioners should consider include:

- Haemoglobin levels may be normal in acute blood loss.
- The decision to transfuse red blood cells (pRBCs) should be based on aetiology, severity, and chronicity of the anaemia as well as on clinical symptoms and end-organ perfusion rather than haemoglobin values.
- Patients with sickle cell disease require prompt evaluation for complications including stroke, acute chest syndrome, splenic sequestration, infection, vaso-occlusive episodes, and priapism.

- Prompt evaluation and treatment of neutropenic patients is essential to decrease morbidity and mortality associated with infection. Appropriate cultures should be obtained but should not delay empiric antibiotic treatment. Disposition should be based on the underlying aetiology of the neutropenia and clinical presentation.
- Increasingly, the management of immune thrombocytopenia (ITP) is guided by bleeding symptoms rather than platelet count.
- Platelet disorders and von Willebrand disease (vWD) typically result in mucosal-type bleeding, whereas haemophilia causes haemarthrosis and deep muscle bleeds. Drugs that interfere with platelet function (e.g. aspirin, non-steroidal anti-inflammatory agents) should be avoided in patients with haemostatic defects.

ACUTE PULMONARY EMBOLISM

Acute Pulmonary Embolism (APE) is characterised by numerous clinical manifestations which are the result of a complex interplay between different organs; the symptoms are therefore various and part of a complex clinical picture. Pulmonary embolism (PE) is a potentially lethal condition; it should be seen as a medical emergency. Most patients who die because of PE will do so within the first few hours of the event. This condition may present with very few clinical signs and/or symptoms, this means it can be easily missed. A PE is a blockage in the pulmonary artery, which is the blood vessel that carries blood from the heart to the lungs. This blockage, usually a blood clot, is potentially life-threatening as it can prevent the blood from reaching the lungs. A small proportion of cases are due to the embolisation of air, fat or talc in drugs of intravenous drug abusers and a small piece of tumour (cancer) that has broken off from a larger tumour in the body. Small clots may cause no symptoms at all and medium ones cause sudden breathlessness. Sometimes, if a clot is big enough to block lung circulation, it can cause collapse or even sudden death. Smaller wandering clots can break off a clot in the leg over several days. This causes increasingly troublesome symptoms. The lungs can start to bleed temporarily, which causes sharp pains when the patient breathes. The patient can also cough up blood. Because the severity of the disease is extremely varied and all the symptoms are common in other conditions, diagnosis can be difficult. Various tests may be used to help confirm the diagnosis. These may include one or more of the following: ultrasound of the leg, blood test for D-dimer and isotope scan, and CT pulmonary angiogram (CTPA) scan.

CLINICAL INVESTIGATION – ACUTE PULMONARY EMBOLISM

Pain can be related to local disturbances in pulmonary circulation, pleural involvement, or impairment of coronary circulation. Central PE may produce typical angina also due to RV ischaemia, while pleuritic chest pain can be the consequence of pleural irritation due to pulmonary infarction secondary to small distal pulmonary artery (PA) embolisation. Dyspnoea has a multi-factorial origin, resulting from bronchospasm or vasospasm, disturbances in pulmonary circulation, immobility or diminished respiratory excursion of the diaphragm, atelectasis and/or pulmonary infarction, anoxia, or impairment of cardiac function. In patients with pre-existing heart failure or pulmonary disease, deteriorating dyspnoea may be the only symptom indicative of PE. Anoxia is manifested clinically by cyanosis. Hyperbilirubinemia may occur when hepatic congestion co-exists. Dyspnoea, chest pain, and cough are the most frequent symptoms of PE, while fever, tachycardia, abnormal pulmonary signs, and peripheral vascular collapse are the most common physical findings. Cyanosis, haemoptysis, syncope, and the various manifestations of acute cor pulmonale are less commonly observed. Incidental pulmonary embolisms (IPEs) are common in cancer patients. Examining the characteristics and outcomes of IPEs in cancer patients can help to ensure proper management, promoting better outcomes. The incidence of venous thromboembolism (VTE), including PEs, in cancer patients is usually underestimated. In addition to the usual symptomatic presentation, PE can be found incidentally during routine imaging studies, including staging computed tomography (CT) scans of the chest or abdomen.

Pharmacology – Anticoagulation

Anticoagulation is often referred to as thinning of the blood within clinical environments. However, anticoagulation does not actually thin the blood. It alters certain chemicals in the blood to stop clots forming so easily. It doesn't dissolve the clot either, which is another common misconception. Anticoagulation prevents a PE from getting larger and prevents any new clots from forming. The body's own healing mechanisms can then get to work to break up the clot. Anticoagulation treatment is usually started immediately (as soon as a PE is suspected) to prevent the clot worsening, while waiting for test results. The main anticoagulants used to treat PEs are low-molecular-weight heparin (LMWH) and warfarin. Low-molecular-weight heparin is given as an injection. Regular injections of this medication are usually used as the initial treatment for a PE because they start working immediately. Warfarin comes in tablet form, which is usually taken soon after the initial treatment with LMWH. Warfarin takes longer to start working than heparin injections, but as it is more convenient to take it is usually recommended for a longer period after the patient has stopped having these injections. Treatment with warfarin will usually be recommended for at least three months, although some patients need to take it for longer than this. Occasionally, patients may need to take warfarin for the rest of their life.

BRAIN METASTASES

Brain metastases are a common complication of cancer and the most common type of brain tumour. Anywhere from 10% to 26% of patients who die from their cancer will develop brain metastases. While few cancers that metastasise to the brain can be cured using conventional therapies, long-term survival and palliation are possible with minimal adverse effects to patients. Increasingly, neuro-cognition and quality of life are being recognised as important endpoints for patients as survival continues to increase. Primary cancers such as lung, breast, and melanoma are most likely to metastasise to the brain. Small-cell lung cancer has a high propensity to spread to the brain such that prophylactic treatment (cranial irradiation) is considered the standard of care. Other malignancies such as prostate and head and neck cancers rarely result in brain metastases. It can be difficult to predict which patients will develop brain metastases other than by using tumour type and subtype. The differential diagnoses of cerebral metastases include abscess, demyelination, parasitic infestation, and primary tumour – glioma/ependymoma (Amsbaugh and Kim 2022).

CLINICAL INVESTIGATION – BRAIN METASTASES

A neurological exam must be completed (see Neurological Examination in Chapter 9). Difficulty in one or more areas may provide clues about the part of the brain that could be affected by a brain tumour. Imaging tests such as Magnetic Resonance Imaging (MRI) is commonly used to help diagnose brain metastases. A dye may be injected through a vein during MRI. Several specialised MRI scan components including functional MRI, perfusion MRI, and magnetic resonance spectroscopy support a diagnosis of brain tumour and plan treatment. Other imaging tests may include CT and positron emission tomography (PET). For example, if the primary tumour causing the brain metastases is unknown, the patient is likely to require a chest CT scan to look for lung cancer. Collecting and testing a sample of abnormal tissue (biopsy) should be performed as part of an operation to remove a brain tumour, or it can be performed using a needle. The biopsy sample is then viewed under a microscope to determine if it is cancerous (malignant) or non-cancerous (benign), and whether the cells are metastatic cancer or from a primary tumour. This information is critical to establish a diagnosis and a prognosis and to guide treatment.

TUMOUR LYSIS SYNDROME

Tumour lysis syndrome (TLS) is an oncological emergency characterised by metabolic and electrolyte abnormalities that can occur after the initiation of any cancer treatment but can also occur spontaneously. TLS is a condition that occurs when many cancer cells die within a short period, releasing their contents into the blood. When cancer cells break down quickly in the body, levels of uric acid, potassium, and phosphorus rise faster than the kidneys can remove them. This causes TLS. Excess phosphorus can absorb calcium, leading to low levels of calcium in the blood. Changes in blood levels of uric acid, potassium, phosphorus, and calcium can affect the functioning of several organs, especially the kidneys, the heart, brain, muscles, and gastrointestinal tract.

RED FLAGS – TUMOUR LYSIS SYNDROME

These include nausea with or without vomiting; lack of appetite and fatigue; dark urine, reduced urine output, or flank pain. Numbness, seizures, or hallucinations.

Muscle cramps and spasms. Heart palpitations. The metabolic derangements associated with TLS are hyperkalaemia, hypocalcaemia, hyperphosphataemia, and hyperuricaemia.

TLS is diagnosed based on blood tests, along with signs and symptoms. Its onset may be subtle, with only a few abnormal laboratory values, but it can also present with frank kidney and organ failure.

Examination – Tumour Lysis Syndrome

TLS is most associated with highly proliferative, bulky, chemosensitive haematological malignancies, particularly high-grade non-Hodgkin's lymphoma (e.g. Burkitt's lymphoma) and acute lymphoblastic leukaemia (ALL). However, reports of TLS associated with other types of malignancies (including

(continued)

(continued)

solid tumours – see Tables 12.1 and 12.2) are increasing. Key diagnostic factors include haematological malignancy, pre-existing renal impairment, syncope/chest pain/dyspnoea, and seizures. Other diagnostic factors include nausea and vomiting, anorexia, diarrhoea, and muscle weakness (BMJ 2020). TLS can be classified as laboratory TLS (defined as the presence of two or more of the following metabolic abnormalities: hyperuricaemia, hyperphosphataemia, hyperkalaemia, or hypocalcaemia),

TABLE 12.1   Examples of molecular markers used in cancer diagnosis and prognosis.

Cancer	Genetic market	Principal application
Chronic myeloid leukaemia	Philadelphia chromosome t(9;22) (q34;q11) [BCR/ABL]	Primary diagnosis, detection of residual disease after treatment
Non-Hodgkin's lymphoma Follicular Burkitt's	t(14;18)(q32;q21) [BCL2/IGH] t(S;14)(q24;q32)	Primary diagnosis, detection of residual disease after treatment As above
Neuroblastoma	MYCN amplification	Prognosis
Breast cancer	HER2-neu/ERB2 amplification	Prognosis
Familial cancers		
Breast	BRCA1, BRCA2	Diagnosis of hereditary predisposition
Colon	APC, MSH2, MLH1	As above
Wilms' tumour	TP53 mutation	As above
Retinoblastoma	RB mutation	As above

Tumours may be classified not only by their biological behaviour but also traditionally by their tissue of origin. Most tumours retain sufficient characteristics of the normal differentiated cell to allow recognition of the type of tissue from which they were derived, which is the basis for the classification of tumours by tissue type.
Source: Peate (2019) / with permission of Elsevier.

TABLE 12.2   Classification by tissue type and malignant tumours.

Tissue of origin	Malignant tumour
Epithelial	**'Carcinoma'**
Squamous: surface epithelium, cell lining covering body cavities, organs and tracts	Squamous cell carcinoma, e.g. lung, skin, stomach
Glandular: glands or ducts in the epithelium	Adenocarcinoma, e.g. breast, lung, colon
Transitional cells: bladder lining	Transitional cell carcinoma, e.g. bladder
Basal cells: skin layer	Basal cell carcinoma (BCC), 'rodent ulcer'
Liver	Hepatocellular carcinoma
Biliary tree	Cholangiocarcinoma

TABLE 12.2   (Continued)

Tissue of origin	Malignant tumour
Placenta	Choriocarcinoma
Testicular epithelium	Seminoma, teratoma, embryonal carcinoma
Endothelial cells	Angiosarcoma
Mesothelial: covering the surface of serous membranes	Mesothelioma, e.g. pleura, peritoneum
Connective tissue	**'Sarcoma'**
Bone	Osteosarcoma
Cartilage	Chondrosarcoma
Fatty tissue	Liposarcoma
Fibrous tissue	Fibrosarcoma
Lymphoid tissue	Lymphomas
Bone marrow	Leukaemias, e.g. ALL, CML
Muscle	**'Myosarcoma'**
Smooth muscle	Leiomyosarcoma
Striated muscle	Rhabdomyosarcoma
Cardiac muscle	Cardiac sarcomas
Neural	
Meninges	Meningeal sarcoma
Glia	Glioblastoma multiforme
Neurones	Neuroblastoma, medulloblastoma

Source: Peate (2019) / with permission of Elsevier.

or clinical TLS (defined as laboratory TLS with one or more of the following clinical manifestations: acute kidney injury [i.e. increased serum creatinine], cardiac arrhythmia, seizure, or sudden death). Early identification of patients at risk of TLS and initiating appropriate preventive management is effective in most patients. Vigorous hydration in combination with hypouricaemic agents constitutes the cornerstone of both prevention and treatment.

LEUKAEMIA

Leukaemia is a cancer that starts in the blood-forming cells of the bone marrow. When one of these cells changes and becomes a leukaemia cell, it no longer matures the way it should. Often, it divides to make new cells faster than normal. Leukaemia cells also don't die when they should. They build up in the bone marrow and crowd out normal cells. At some point, leukaemia cells leave the bone marrow and spill into the bloodstream, often causing the number of white blood cells (WBCs) in the blood to increase. Once in the blood, leukaemia cells can spread to other organs, where they can keep other cells in the body from working properly. Leukaemia is different from other types of cancer that start in organs like the lungs, colon, or breast and then spread to the bone marrow. Cancers that start in another part of the body and then spread to the bone marrow are not leukaemia. Hence, it is imperative to undertake a full physical examination of patients presenting with cancer symptoms, including examinations of lumps and bumps (see Figure 12.1).

There are several different types of leukaemia (see Figure 12.2).

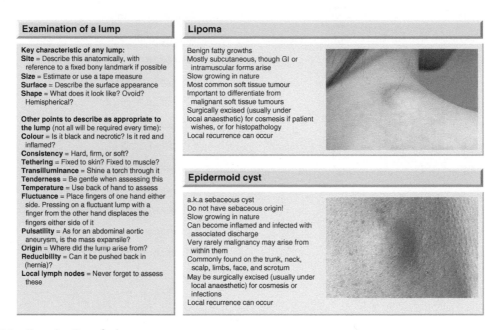

Examination of a lump

Key characteristic of any lump:
Site = Describe this anatomically, with reference to a fixed bony landmark if possible
Size = Estimate or use a tape measure
Surface = Describe the surface appearance
Shape = What does it look like? Ovoid? Hemispherical?

Other points to describe as appropriate to the lump (not all will be required every time):
Colour = Is it black and necrotic? Is it red and inflamed?
Consistency = Hard, firm, or soft?
Tethering = Fixed to skin? Fixed to muscle?
Transilluminance = Shine a torch through it
Tenderness = Be gentle when assessing this
Temperature = Use back of hand to assess
Fluctuance = Place fingers of one hand either side. Pressing on a fluctuant lump with a finger from the other hand displaces the fingers either side of it
Pulsatility = As for an abdominal aortic aneurysm, is the mass expansile?
Origin = Where did the lump arise from?
Reducibility = Can it be pushed back in (hernia)?
Local lymph nodes = Never forget to assess these

Lipoma

Benign fatty growths
Mostly subcutaneous, though GI or intramuscular forms arise
Slow growing in nature
Most common soft tissue tumour
Important to differentiate from malignant soft tissue tumours
Surgically excised (usually under local anaesthetic) for cosmesis if patient wishes, or for histopathology
Local recurrence can occur

Epidermoid cyst

a.k.a sebaceous cyst
Do not have sebaceous origin!
Slow growing in nature
Can become inflamed and infected with associated discharge
Very rarely malignancy may arise from within them
Commonly found on the trunk, neck, scalp, limbs, face, and scrotum
May be surgically excised (usually under local anaesthetic) for cosmesis or infections
Local recurrence can occur

FIGURE 12.1   Examination of a lump.

Acute Lymphocytic Leukaemia (ALL) in Adults

Acute lymphocytic (or lymphoblastic) leukaemia is sometimes called ALL. It starts in the bone marrow where blood cells are made. It is more common in children than in adults.

Acute Myeloid Leukaemia (AML) in Adults

Acute myeloid leukaemia is also called acute myelocytic leukaemia, acute myelogenous leukaemia, acute granulocytic leukaemia, acute non-lymphocytic leukaemia, or sometimes just AML. It is most common in older people.

Chronic Lymphocytic Leukaemia (CLL)

Chronic lymphocytic leukaemia (CLL) is a type of cancer that starts from white blood cells (called lymphocytes) in the bone marrow. CLL mainly affects older adults, and accounts for about one-third of all leukaemias.

Chronic Myeloid Leukaemia (CML)

Chronic myeloid leukaemia (CML), also known as chronic myelogenous leukaemia, is a type of cancer that starts in the blood-forming cells of the bone marrow and invades the blood. Only about 10% of leukaemias are CML.

Chronic Myelomonocytic Leukaemia (CMML)

Chronic myelomonocytic leukaemia (CMML) is a type of cancer that starts in blood-forming cells of the bone marrow and invades the blood. It affects mainly older adults.

Leukaemia in Children

Leukaemia is the most common cancer in children and teens, accounting for almost 1 out of 3 cancers. Most childhood leukaemias are ALL. Most of the remaining cases are AML. Chronic leukaemias are rare in children.

FIGURE 12.2   Types of leukaemia (American Cancer Society 2023). *Source*: https://www.cancer.org/cancer/leukemia.html/ last accessed February 27, 2023.

NEUTROPENIC SEPSIS

Neutropenic sepsis is a potentially life-threatening complication of neutropenia (low neutrophil count). It is defined as a temperature of greater than 38°C (or hypothermia less than 36°C), or any symptoms and/or signs of sepsis, in a person with an absolute neutrophil count of 0.5×10^9/l or lower (NICE 2020a). Sepsis is a syndrome defined as life-threatening organ dysfunction due to a dysregulated host response to infection. Febrile neutropenia is the most common complication of anticancer treatment and describes the presence of fever in a person with neutropenia. NICE (2020b) advises the following examination when suspecting neutropenic sepsis. Some of the risk factors include haematological malignancy, large tumour burden, chemosensitive tumours, and recent chemotherapy.

RED FLAGS – NEUTROPENIC SEPSIS

Generalised constitutional symptoms are common (lethargy, rigors, confusion). Patients can go from being well to being in life-threatening septic shock in just a few hours. Neutropenia markedly alters the host's immune response and makes infection more difficult to detect. Ask about respiratory, urinary, oropharyngeal, and lower GI symptoms. Enquire about recent instrumentation/dental work. Does the patient have a Hickman Line? Ask about recent line use and whether there is pain around the line. Patients with febrile neutropenia MUST receive antibiotics even if there are no localising signs of infection. During assessment inspect for red flags of shock e.g. tachypnoea, tachycardia, hypotension, altered mental state, fever, and complete a detailed examination for any localising signs of infection.

Examination – Assessment for Neutropenic Sepsis

- General appearance, level of consciousness, and cognition.
  - Consider using the Glasgow Coma Scale (GCS) or AVPU ('alert, voice, pain, unresponsive') scale, to assess level of consciousness.
- Temperature.
  - Be aware that people with neutropenic sepsis may not present with fever and may present with hypothermia.
- Heart rate, respiratory rate, and signs of respiratory distress, and blood pressure.
- Capillary refill time and oxygen saturation (abnormal results may indicate poor peripheral perfusion).
- Mottled or ashen skin; pallor or cyanosis of the skin, lips, or tongue; cold peripheries.
- Any rash.
  - A non-blanching rash which may suggest meningococcal disease.
  - Be aware that viral exanthems in people who are immunosuppressed may present atypically.
- Weak high-pitched or continuous cry (in children under five years of age).
- Any breach of skin integrity (for example, cuts, burns, or skin infections) or other skin signs suggesting infection or mucositis.

(continued)

(*continued*)

    o Dry mucous membranes or other signs of dehydration.

    o The possible underlying source of infection.

        ■ Be aware that people who are immunosuppressed and/or have neutropenia often lack an obvious source of infection.

ANTIVIRAL IMMUNODEFICIENCY

Patients with haematology and oncology disorders are susceptible to many different bacterial, fungal, and viral infections. Viral titre assay offers multiple methods to measure the amount of virus in the sample, such as Real-Time (RT) PCR, Western Blot, ELISA, and flow cytometry. These methods utilise the amount of viral DNA, RNA, or proteins to quantify the virus. However, these methods do not measure the actual biological activities of the virus. To investigate the infectivity of the virus, *in vitro* assays are required to assess the neutralising ability of antibody candidates as well as the effectiveness of antiviral small molecule drugs. An infectious viral titre assay is conducted to determine the strength of a virus against the host cells. Viral infectivity is characterised as the number of virus particles capable to invade a host cell. This is determined by using susceptible cells to the specific virus by measuring the viral infectivity. Among the viral pathogens, cytomegalovirus (CMV), Epstein–Barr virus (EBV), and adenovirus cause the greatest morbidity and mortality and have been the most common infectious causes of death, particularly in patients following the grafting of allogeneic marrow. This great susceptibility to viral infections is due to the immunodeficiency in cellular and humoral immune responses lasting for months to years. Contributing factors are high-dose chemo/radiotherapy, graft-versus-host disease (GVHD) prophylaxis/treatment, GVHD itself, the degree of HLA disparity between donor and recipient and the underlying disease. Defects of T cell helper and cytotoxic functions contribute to the great incidence of viral infections.

PLATELET DISORDERS

Thrombocytopenia means a reduction in the platelet count below the normal lower limit, which is usually defined as $150 \times 10^9/l$. This can have a variety of causes, including a reduction in platelet production, a reduction in platelet survival, and dilution of platelet numbers resulting from the transfusion of platelet-poor blood. The risk of bleeding is not based on the platelet count alone; age, comorbidity, the need for anticoagulation, risk of trauma, and any need for surgery should also be considered when managing people with thrombocytopenia. Platelet function abnormalities (thrombocytopathy) include a range of inherited and acquired defects of platelet function. Thrombocytopathy may cause a thrombotic or a bleeding tendency, or may be part of a wider disorder such as myelodysplasia. A low platelet count may be due to a variety of different causes, for example: the initial manifestation of infections such as HIV and Hepatitis C virus, or it may reflect the activity of life-threatening disorders such as the thrombotic microangiopathies.

A thorough history and examination are essential, with consideration of any history or indication of a possible underlying cause, and any history of abnormal bleeding. When a low platelet count is discovered incidentally, the full blood count (FBC) must be repeated, and a blood smear performed. Initial laboratory test should include FBC with differential and a blood film, prothrombin time, activated partial thromboplastin time (aPTT), renal function and thyroid function tests (TFTs). Bone marrow examination should be considered for patients over 60 years of age (mainly to exclude dysplasia) and in those with systemic symptoms or signs suggestive of haematological cancer. Specific assays of inherited platelet dysfunction include:

- Light transmission aggregometry: evaluates the aggregation or clumping of platelets in response to aggregating stimuli.
- Flow cytometry: should be used in the investigation or confirmation of Glanzman thrombocytopenia (GT), Bernard–Soulier syndrome (BSS), and Scott syndrome, and may also be used to investigate abnormalities in the collagen and thrombin receptors.
- Measurement of total and released nucleotides provides an important additional diagnostic tool usually in conjunction with aggregometry for determining whether there is any specific deficiency in dense granule numbers or their content (e.g. storage pool disease), or specific defect(s) in degranulation (e.g. release defects).
- Platelet alpha granule proteins and beta-thromboglobulin can be measured by ELISA, radioimmunoassay, or Western blotting and may be helpful for the diagnosis of Quebec platelet disorder.
- Electron microscopy is very useful for defining ultrastructural abnormalities associated with a variety of platelet defects.
- Molecular genetic diagnosis of heritable platelet disorders may offer valuable confirmation of diagnosis in affected individuals, in family members where phenotypic testing of platelets is impractical and for antenatal diagnosis.
- Bone marrow examination is not usually required except in those with an atypical course, or a large spleen, or if splenectomy is contemplated.
- Testing for drug-dependent platelet antibodies – this is not widely available but may be useful in severe disease where the diagnosis is in doubt.

DISSEMINATED INTRAVASCULAR COAGULATION

Disseminated intravascular coagulation (DIC) is a widespread inappropriate intravascular deposition of fibrin with consumption of coagulation factors and platelets that occur because of disorders which release pro-coagulant material into the circulation or cause widespread endothelial damage or platelet aggregation. Consequently, it is suggested that DIC is a thrombo-haemorrhagic disorder characterised by primary thrombotic and secondary haemorrhagic diathesis, causing multi-organ failure. The main clinical presentation is bleeding, but in approximately 5–10% of the population it is manifested with microthrombotic lesions, such as gangrenous limbs. In most patients in hospital, excessive bleeding may be seen after venepuncture, or around cannula sites, sutures, wound drains, and wounds. Because of the high probability of bleeding, Advanced Practitioners must be cautious of non-visible bleeding. Generalised bleeding in the gastrointestinal tract, mouth, throat, lung, urinary tract, and vaginal bleeding may become severe. Additional signs and symptoms include infections, malignancy, vascular abnormalities, hypersensitivity reactions, and obstetric complications. Less frequently, thrombi may cause acute kidney injury and ischaemia, and can sometimes cause gangrene. The diagnosis of DIC is not made from a single laboratory value. It will be made based on the collection of a variety of data, beginning with a characteristic patient history and physical examination, investigations for prolonged clotting times, deranged fibrinogen levels (fibrin degradation and D-dimer) and a declining platelet count.

Pathogenesis is believed to be a key event underlying DIC and comes from the increased activity of tissue factor. Damaged tissue will inevitably be released into the circulating volume from damaged cells or tumours, or because of increased cell release secondary to normal inflammatory processes (such as proinflammatory cytokine release by monocytes and endothelial cells). It is usual that blood is taken and sent to pathology for clotting-focused testing when:

- Patients present as being pale and complaining of fatigue.
- Patients present with abnormal bleeding, such as prolonged bleeding or with an inability to stop bleeding.
- When organ function is impaired, in multi-organ failure.
- When liver failure is suspected.

In cases such as these, it would be pertinent to explore partial thromboplastin time (PTT) and activated PTT. PTT is a test that measures the overall speed at which blood clots, by means of two consecutive series of biochemical reactions known as the intrinsic and common coagulation pathways.

Examination – Diagnosis and Management of DIC

- The diagnosis of DIC should encompass both clinical and laboratory information. The International Society for Thrombosis and Haemostasis (ISTH) DIC scoring system provides objective measurement of DIC. Where DIC is present the scoring system correlates with key clinical observations and outcomes. It is important to repeat the tests to monitor the dynamically changing scenario based on laboratory results and clinical observations.

- The cornerstone of the treatment of DIC is treatment of the underlying condition. Transfusion of platelets or plasma (components) in patients with DIC should not primarily be based on laboratory results and should, in general, be reserved for patients who present with bleeding. In patients with DIC and bleeding or at high risk of bleeding (e.g. postoperative patients or patients due to undergo an invasive procedure) and a platelet count of $<50 \times 10^9/l$ transfusion of platelets should be considered.

- In non-bleeding patients with DIC, prophylactic platelet transfusion is not given unless it is perceived that there is a high risk of bleeding. In bleeding patients with DIC and prolonged prothrombin time (PT) and aPTT, administration of fresh frozen plasma (FFP) may be useful. It should not be instituted based on laboratory tests alone but should be considered in those with active bleeding and in those requiring an invasive procedure. There is no evidence that infusion of plasma stimulates the ongoing activation of coagulation.

- If transfusion of FFP is not possible in patients with bleeding because of fluid overload, consider using factor concentrates such as prothrombin complex concentrate, recognising that these will only partially correct the defect because they contain only selected factors, whereas in DIC there is a global deficiency of coagulation factors. Severe hypofibrinogenaemia ($<1 g/l$) that persists despite FFP replacement may be treated with fibrinogen concentrate or cryoprecipitate.

- In cases of DIC where thrombosis predominates, such as arterial or VTE, severe purpura fulminans associated with acral ischaemia or vascular skin infarction, therapeutic doses of heparin should be considered. In these patients where there is perceived to be a co-existing high risk of bleeding, there may be benefits in using continuous infusion unfractionated heparin (UFH) due to its short half-life and reversibility. Weight adjusted doses (e.g. 10 l/kg/h) may be used without the intention of prolonging the aPTT ratio to 1Æ5–2Æ5 times the control. Monitoring the aPTT in these cases may be complicated and clinical observation for signs of bleeding is important.

- In critically ill, non-bleeding patients with DIC, prophylaxis for VTE with prophylactic doses of heparin or LMWH is recommended. Consider treating patients with severe sepsis and DIC with recombinant human activated protein C (continuous infusion, 24 lg/kg/h for four days). Patients at high risk of bleeding should not be given recombinant human activated protein C. Current manufacturers guidance advises against using this product in patients with platelet counts of $<30 \times 10^9/l$.

- In the event of invasive procedures, administration of recombinant human activated protein C should be discontinued shortly before the intervention (elimination half-life of 20 minutes) and may be resumed a few hours later, depending on the clinical situation. In the absence of further prospective evidence from randomised controlled trials confirming a beneficial effect of antithrombin concentrate on clinically relevant endpoints in patients with DIC and not receiving heparin, administration of antithrombin cannot be recommended. In general, patients with DIC should not be treated with antifibrinolytic agents. Patients with DIC that is characterised by a primary hyperfibrinolytic state and who present with severe bleeding could be treated with lysine analogues, such as tranexamic acid (e.g. 1 g every eight hours).

Guidelines for the diagnosis and management of DIC (British Society of Haematology, 2012).

IMMUNOTHERAPY AND CHEMOTHERAPY

Immunotherapy and chemotherapy are common cancer treatments. Both use drugs to stop the cancer from growing, but they achieve this in different ways. Immunotherapy enhances the immune system so it can target cancer cells. Chemotherapy directly acts on cancer cells, preventing them from replicating.

IMMUNOTHERAPY

There are different types of immunotherapies and are sometimes referred to as targeted therapies. Checkpoint inhibitors affect a type of WBC called a lymphocyte. Lymphocytes are an important part of the immune system. When they are active, lymphocytes can attack another cell such as a cancer cell. But if they receive a certain signal from the other cell, they switch off (become inactive) and do not attack it.

CHECKPOINT INHIBITORS

Checkpoint inhibitors block the signals that switch off lymphocytes. They do this by attaching to either the cancer cell or the lymphocyte. This means the lymphocyte stays active and can attack the cancer cell. Immune system modulators are immunotherapy drugs. They help the immune system attack and destroy cancer cells. They are given as tablets. Types of immune system modulator include: lenalidomide, pomalidomide, and thalidomide. Other immune system modulators include artificial versions of proteins called interferon and interleukin. These proteins are normally made naturally in the body. They help control how the immune system works. Interferon and interleukin are given by injection. They are not used very often, as newer drugs have become available.

BACILLUS CALMETTE-GUERIN

Another type of immune system modulator is BCG used for blood cancer. BCG is a type of bacteria which can cause tuberculosis (TB). It can be weakened, so that it is not harmful, and used as a treatment for bladder cancer. It is given directly into the bladder to stimulate the immune system to attack cancer cells. This is called intravesical immunotherapy.

VIRUS THERAPY TO TREAT CANCER

Virus therapy uses a virus that has been made or changed in a laboratory. The virus finds and infects the cancer cells. This treatment also trains the immune system to find and attack cancer cells. A virus therapy called T-VEC is sometimes used to treat melanoma that has come back in the same area.

MONOCLONAL ANTIBODIES

All cells have receptors on their surface. Receptors help cells send or receive signals. Monoclonal antibodies are made so they can only connect to one type of receptor. Most monoclonal antibodies target receptors that are mainly found on cancer cells. Some target receptors that are found on other cells in the body. By connecting to the cell's receptor, monoclonal antibody immunotherapies can help the body's immune system by: blocking signals that stop WBCs attacking cancer cells (also called a checkpoint inhibitor); and connecting to cancer cells to help the immune system find and attack them.

CANCER VACCINES

Vaccines train the immune system to find and attack certain types of abnormal cells. They are commonly used to protect us from infections such as the flu, mumps, or measles.

ADOPTIVE CELL TRANSFER AND CAR-T THERAPY

Adoptive cell transfer and T-cell therapy use a person's own WBCs to find and destroy cancer cells. WBCs usually fight infection. Some WBCs are collected from the body. Biomedical scientists then either: choose the cells that are naturally best at recognising cancer cells; and/or change cells to make them better at recognising cancer cells. More of these cells are then grown in the laboratory. They are given back into the bloodstream to find and attack cancer cells. There are different types of adoptive cell transfer. For example, T-cell therapy or CAR T-cell therapy uses WBCs called T cells. CAR-T is a highly complex and innovative new treatment. CAR-T is a type of immunotherapy which involves collecting and using the patients' own immune cells to treat their condition. NHS England (2023) note that the NHS is providing CAR-T therapies for children and young people with B cell ALL, and identify that NICE also recommended CAR-T therapy for adults with diffuse large B-cell lymphoma (DLBCL) and primary mediastinal B-cell lymphoma in England. The treatment involves several steps over several weeks. First the patient's blood is taken and is sent off to the manufacturer's laboratory. Here the patient's blood is modified to fight the cancer cells. The CAR-T blood is then transported back to the hospital and the patient is administered with the CAR-T to treat their condition. Currently, NICE has approved CAR-T use in the NHS, where all other treatment options have been unsuccessful for relapsed or refractory B-cell ALL in people up to the age of 25 years. A second one has been approved for relapsed or refractory DLBCL after two or more systemic therapies. CAR-T – chimeric antigen receptor T-cell-therapy is specifically developed for each individual patient and involves reprogramming the patient's own immune system cells which are then used to target their cancer. It is a highly complex and potentially risky treatment, but it has been shown in trials to cure some patients, even those with quite advanced cancers and where other available treatments have failed.

SIDE EFFECTS OF IMMUNOTHERAPY

Immunotherapy causes the immune system to become more active. That means it is better at finding and attacking cancer cells. But immunotherapy can also cause unwanted effects. These are very different to the side effects of other cancer treatments, such as chemotherapy or radiotherapy. For example, checkpoint inhibitors can make the immune system overly active. This causes inflammation in the body. The most common parts of the body they affect are the: skin – causing a rash, itching, or changes in skin colour; glands in the body that make hormones – causing problems such as sweating, weight changes, feeling more hungry or thirsty, passing more urine (peeing), loss of sex drive, feeling tired (fatigue) or headaches; bowels – causing diarrhoea or tummy pain; joints – causing pain and swelling. More rarely, these drugs cause problems in other major organs. Sometimes this type of side effect can start weeks or months after completion of treatment. It can also appear more than a year after treatment ends. Some people have very few side effects, but the side effects of checkpoint inhibitors can be serious.

CHEMOTHERAPY

Chemotherapy uses anti-cancer (cytotoxic) drugs to destroy cancer cells. Cytotoxic means toxic to cells. Most chemotherapy drugs are carried in the blood. This means they can reach cancer cells anywhere in the body. Chemotherapy is sometimes called systemic anti-cancer therapy (SACT). Cytotoxic chemotherapy drugs disrupt the way cancer cells grow and divide. But they also affect some of the healthy cells in the body. These healthy cells can usually recover from damage caused by chemotherapy. But cancer cells cannot recover, and they eventually die. Because chemotherapy drugs can affect some of the healthy cells in the body, this can cause side effects. Most side effects will go away after treatment finishes. Clinicians often treat cancer with two or more chemotherapy drugs. Sometimes they also combine chemotherapy drugs with other medicines, such as steroids, immunotherapy, or targeted cancer drugs. The drug combinations they use often have a name that is made up of the first letters of the drug names. Some combination chemotherapy names utilise acronyms; for example, MIC: M = mitomycin, I = ifosfamide, C = cisplatin. Another being, CHOP: C = cyclophosphamide, H = doxorubicin,

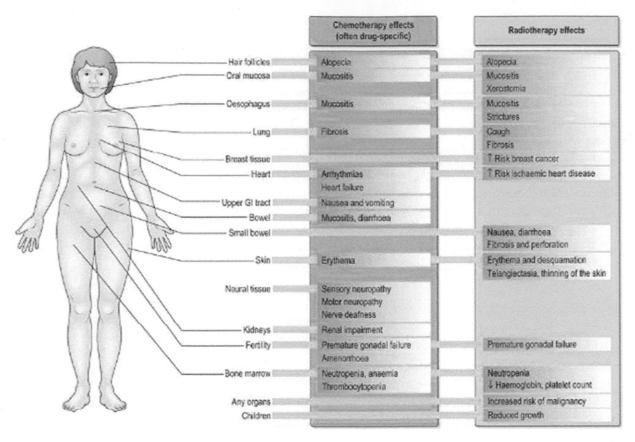

FIGURE 12.3   Side effects of chemotherapy and radiotherapy (acute/pink, and late/blue). *Source*: Peate (2019) / with permission of Elsevier.

O = vincristine (Oncovin), P = prednisolone, a steroid (Cancer Research UK 2020). Side effects of chemotherapy include the following symptoms: a temperature of 38°C/100°F or higher, shivering episodes, flu-like symptoms, gum or nose bleeds or unusual bleeding (if bleeding doesn't stop after 10 minutes of pressure), mouth ulcers that prevent effective eating or drinking, vomiting (that continues in spite of taking anti-sickness medication), diarrhoea (four or more bowel movements more than usual or diarrhoea at night), difficulty with breathing, and signs of infection (The Royal Marsden 2023). Other side effects can be seen in Figure 12.3.

Case Study – Systemic Anti-cancer Therapy

- Sarah presented to the SACT unit with deranged bloods – initially only hyperphosphataemia. She was generally unwell with high tumour burden (HTB) status. Blood profiles were checked by the Registered Nurses on the SACT day unit and were repeated after 48 hours. A physical examination by the Advanced Practitioner identified several red flags, including diarrhoea and vomiting, nausea and lethargy, loss of appetite and weakness. The second set of bloods revealed hyperkalaemia, hyperphosphataemia, hypocalcaemia, hyperuricaemia. What is the differential diagnosis, and what would initial management be?

RADIATION THERAPY

Radiation therapy (also called radiotherapy) is a cancer treatment that uses high doses of radiation to kill cancer cells and shrink tumours. At high doses, radiation therapy kills cancer cells or slows their growth by damaging their DNA. Cancer cells whose DNA is damaged beyond repair stop dividing or die. When the damaged cells die, they are broken down and removed by the body. Radiation therapy does not kill cancer cells immediately. It takes days or weeks of treatment before DNA is damaged enough for cancer cells to die. Then, cancer cells keep dying for weeks or months after radiation therapy ends. There are two main types of radiation therapy, external beam and internal. The type of radiation therapy that you may have depends on many factors, including: the type of cancer, the size of the tumour, the tumour's location in the body, how close the tumour is to normal tissues that are sensitive to radiation, the patient's general health and medical history, whether they will have other types of cancer treatment, and other factors, such as age and other medical conditions (National Cancer Institute [NCI] 2019).

HAEMOSTASIS

Haemostasis is a complex process. It involves a dynamic interaction between platelets, plasma, and coagulation factors to control active bleeding. When injury occurs to tissue, the surrounding blood vessels will narrow (a process also called vasoconstriction), encouraging platelets to thicken, form a plug, and protect the area.

Diagnostic Approach

The goal of initial examination is to differentiate bleeding caused by injured or diseased blood vessels from that caused by a systemic haemostatic disorder. A combination of clinical signs, history, and screening tests (platelet count, bleeding time, coagulation panel) will help make this distinction. Blood vessel disorders are primarily diagnosed by inspection, either visually or using ancillary diagnostics (i.e. endoscopy, radiography, ultrasonography, or biopsy). Clinical signs of bleeding from damaged vessels depend on the size of the injured vessel. Large vessel disorders are characterised by haemorrhage from a single anatomic site, often with blood loss anaemia. Small vessel disorders (vasculopathies) rarely cause anaemia. Vasculopathies typically cause multisystemic signs including cutaneous ecchymoses, uveitis, glomerulonephritis, and pulmonary or peripheral oedema.

SYSTEMIC BLEEDING DISORDERS

Systemic bleeding disorders are classified as defects of either primary haemostasis (platelet plug formation) or secondary haemostasis (fibrin clot formation). Primary haemostatic disorders are caused by failure of platelet plug formation due to quantitative or qualitative platelet disorders, or due to von Willebrand factor deficiency. Clinical signs of primary haemostatic disorders include petechiae, mucosal haemorrhage, prolonged bleeding at sites of injury. Specific primary haemostatic disorders and diagnostic tests, for example: thrombocytopenia: platelet count, platelet estimate from blood smear, platelet dysfunction: *in vivo* bleeding time, platelet aggregation, drug history, and metabolic profile. Secondary haemostatic disorders are caused by failure of fibrin clot formation due to deficiency of one or more coagulation factors.

BLOOD DYSCRASIAS

Blood dyscrasia is an abnormal or pathological condition of the blood cells. RBCs, WBCs, and platelets are created in bone marrow. Due to the accelerated rate of production of cells and limited ability to store cells in the marrow, these blood cells are particularly vulnerable to pathological changes. Primary blood disorders present when there are any blood cell problems. Secondary disorders occur from bleeding and are, therefore, a result of something other than 'the blood cell' itself.

ANAEMIA

Blood supports all the activities and functions of all of the organs and tissues in the body, providing nutrients, oxygen, and hormones, as well as defending the body against infections and getting rid of waste products. The blood cells each have different functions, which sustain life when they work together. Blood cells are produced in the bone marrow. Haematopoiesis ensures that we have the right type of mature functioning blood cells, at the right time and in the right number. When cells are immature and non-functioning, we develop diseases and chronic conditions that can seriously impact on quality of life. Anaemia is a term used to describe a deficiency of the RBCs (erythrocytes) or the Hb that attaches itself to RBCs. Signs and symptoms of anaemia include shortness of breath, palpitations, fatigue and lethargy, anorexia, sensitivity to the cold, ankle oedema, headache, and sore mouth and gums.

When examining a patient with suspected anaemia, a careful history is required. The patient who is anaemic may often have a pallor or a yellow tinge, depending on the type of anaemia they have. The diagnosis is based on a general history, which should include any chronic illness the person may have, and medication being taken. A full blood count will reflect the degree of anaemia and further analysis of the blood will uncover the type of anaemia the patient has. Further investigations may be undertaken to find the cause of any chronic blood loss if indicated. These would include:

- Urine testing for the presence of blood (haematuria)
- Faecal occult blood
- Endoscopy
- Colonoscopy
- Investigations of the bone marrow.

Making the diagnosis in anaemia is very important and assumptions should not be made about the cause. Signs and symptoms are considered carefully, blood profile is analysed, and treatment is dependent on the type of anaemia. In addition, the patient should be asked detailed questions. These questions should be applied within the clinical content and stability for the patient's presentation. Questions may include:

- Their diet: do they eat iron-rich foods?
- Their medication: do any of the drugs taken cause bleeding into the gastrointestinal tract; for example, non-steroidal anti-inflammatory drugs (e.g. ibuprofen)?
- Pregnancy and menstrual cycle.
- Any pertinent family history, not only for anaemia but also for jaundice, cholelithiasis, splenectomy, bleeding disorders, and abnormal Hb.
- Any chronic diseases or history of weight loss, sickness, and/or diarrhoea.

Iron deficiency (ID) anaemia is most often caused by long-term blood loss. Patients may describe problems with heavy menstrual periods, indigestion, or change in bowel habit. Ferritin is a protein in the body that stores iron. Blood tests may be taken to measure the ferritin in the bloodstream to help confirm ID anaemia. ID anaemia can be the presenting factor for some disorders, such as gastric ulceration, gynaecological problems, and underlying cancers. Once all of the investigations have taken place to identify chronic blood loss and treat the underlying cause if there is one, iron supplements are prescribed and the patient is given dietary advice. This will include increasing green leafy vegetables, pulses and beans, eggs, meat, and fish, to name but a few. Blood monitoring is required and a regular review of the full blood count is recommended, depending on the severity of the anaemia.

HAEMOLYTIC ANAEMIAS

Haemolytic anaemia is a term used to describe many different anaemias that all have a common characteristic: they have an abnormality that destructs red cells. This disorder leads to the reduced lifespan of RBCs, not an underproduction of them. The patient often presents with symptoms of anaemia due to haemolysis, and further investigation gives rise to diagnosis of haemolytic anaemia, which requires specialist management.

THALASSAEMIA

This describes a group of inherited disorders that affects the production of Hb. Depending on the severity of the condition, there is little Hb produced, resulting in a profound symptomatic anaemia. It is a genetic disease, often diagnosed soon after birth, with differing degrees of severity depending on the type. Patients will have severe anaemia and an overload of iron in their haematological system. Patients with thalassaemia should be reviewed by specialist haematology services, take any medications as prescribed, maintain a healthy diet, try to be as healthy as possible, not consume alcohol, and be cautious around activities that cause injury, bruising, or increase oxygen consumption. Blood transfusions may be required and bone marrow transplant in severe cases.

SICKLE CELL ANAEMIA

Sickle cell disease and sickle cell anaemia are terms used to describe a group of disorders that are hereditary and largely affect African, Caribbean, Middle Eastern, and Asian people. The RBCs are misshapen, and the lifespan of the RBCs is shorter. Patients may have sickle cell crises, which is very painful and requires hospitalisation, pain relief, and hydration. In addition, patients may have anaemia and the associated symptoms, and be more predisposed to developing infections. Figure 12.4 offers a visual depiction of acute and chronic clinical complications associated with Sickle Cell Disease. Treatment, like in thalassaemia, is for the lifespan of the patient; blood transfusions, pain relief, and antibiotics for infection help manage the disease. The complexity of anaemia is clear; when anaemia is discussed in practice it is often considered as a chronic condition. Some types of anaemia are common, particularly ID anaemia; in fact, this is one of the commonest presenting factors in primary and secondary care. It is important, however, to recognise that some of the rarer anaemias are, if not life-limiting, very debilitating. In addition, anaemia can herald the start of a chronic disease that itself is very difficult to live with. Offering care to people experiencing anaemia can be a challenge. One of the key challenges is to ensure that care is delivered in such a way that recognises the impact the symptoms of anaemia can have on quality of life, and to support the patient and their family.

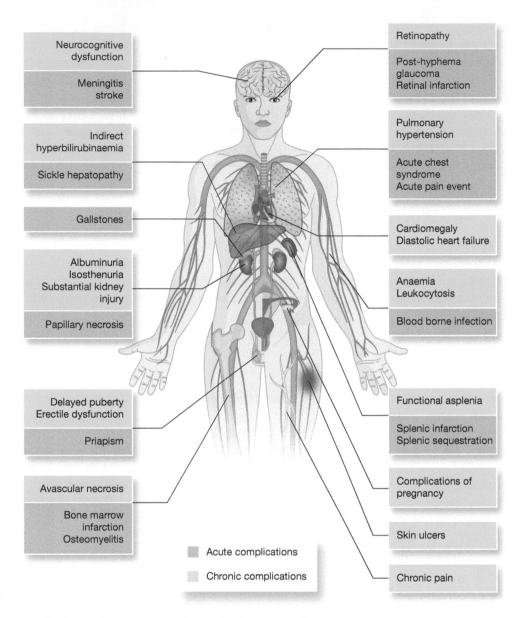

FIGURE 12.4   Sickle cell disease: acute and chronic clinical complications.

HUMAN IMMUNODEFICIENCY VIRUS

Human immunodeficiency virus (HIV) is a virus that attacks the body's immune system, specifically the WBCs called CD4 cells. HIV destroys these CD4 cells, weakening a person's immunity against opportunistic infections, such as tuberculosis and fungal infections, severe bacterial infections, and some cancers (WHO 2023). HIV belongs to the *Lentivirus* group of retroviral family. These are cytopathic and have a long latent period and a chronic course. Two distinct variants of HIV have been identified: HIV-1 and HIV-2. Retroviruses contain the enzyme reverse transcriptase that allows viral RNA to be transcribed into

DNA, which is then incorporated into the host cell genome. The virus preferentially infects T-helper lymphocytes (CD4+ T cells) and progressively destroys them, leading to increased susceptibility to opportunistic infections. Retroviruses contain the enzyme reverse transcriptase that allows viral RNA to be transcribed into DNA, which is then incorporated into the host cell genome. The virus preferentially infects T-helper lymphocytes (CD4+ T cells) and progressively destroys them, leading to increased susceptibility to opportunistic infections. Sepsis and respiratory failure (particularly if associated with pneumocystis pneumonia [PCP]) are associated with poorer survival in HIV-infected patients requiring ICU admission. The need for mechanical ventilation and the disease severity as assessed by the Acute Physiology and Chronic Health Evaluation II (APACHE II) is associated with increased hospital mortality. Low serum albumin and a history of weight loss are further predictors of a higher mortality.

GRANULOCYTOPENIA

This term is used to indicate an abnormal reduction in the numbers of circulating granulocytes. This is commonly called neutropenia, as up to 75% of granulocytes are neutrophils. In cases that involve splenomegaly (enlarged spleen), a number of these cells get trapped and are unable to circulate through veins and arteries around the body. The consequence of neutropenia is that the body will be susceptible to infections that, if unrecognised or left untreated, may result in sepsis and could lead to death.

Take Home Points
- This chapter is unable to address all haematological and oncological presentations; however, it has provided a sample and examples of valuable theoretical knowledge that will support Advanced Practitioners in their AECC roles.
- Haematological and oncological presentations are complex and multifaceted, particularly during acute presentations.
- The role of the Advanced Practitioner in AECC is to establish effective assessment and treatment interventions to stabilise acute presentations and alleviate acute symptoms.

REFERENCES

American Cancer Society. (2023). *Leukemia*. Available from: https://www.cancer.org/cancer/leukemia.html [accessed 27 February 2023]

Amsbaugh, M.J., Kim, C.S. (2022) *Brain Metastasis* [online]. Available from: https://www.ncbi.nlm.nih.gov/books/NBK470246 [accessed 21 June 2023].

BMJ. (2020). *Tumour Lysis Syndrome* [online]. Available from: https://bestpractice.bmj.com/topics/en-gb/936 [accessed 21 June 2023].

British Society of Haematology (BSH). (2012). *Diagnosis and Management of Disseminated Intravascular Coagulation* [online]. Available from: https://b-s-h.org.uk/guidelines/guidelines/diagnosis-and-management-of-disseminated-intravascular-coagulation-1 [accessed 21 June 2023].

Cancer Research UK. (2020). *Chemotherapy* [online]. Available from: https://www.cancerresearchuk.org/about-cancer/treatment/chemotherapy/what-chemotherapy-is [accessed 21 June 2023].

Health Education England (HEE). (2022). *Advanced Clinical Practice in Acute Medicine Curriculum Framework – Credentials* [online]. Available from: https://advanced-practice.hee.nhs.uk/our-work/credentials [accessed 20 June 2023].

Health Education England. (2017). *Multi-professional Framework for Advanced Clinical Practice in England* [online]. Available from: https://www.hee.nhs.uk/sites/default/files/documents/multi-professionalframeworkforadvancedclinicalpracticeinengland.pdf [accessed 21 June 2023].

NCI. (2019). *Radiation Therapy to Treat Cancer* [online]. Available from: https://www.cancer.gov/about-cancer/treatment/types/radiation-therapy [accessed 21 June 2023].

NHS England. (2023). *CAR-T Therapy* [online]. Available from: https://www.england.nhs.uk/cancer/cdf/car-t-therapy [accessed 21 June 2023].

NICE. (2020a). *Neutropenic Sepsis* [online]. Available from: https://cks.nice.org.uk/topics/neutropenic-sepsis [accessed 21 June 2023].

NICE. (2020b). *Neutropenic Sepsis: Assessing a Person with Suspected Neutropenic Sepsis* [online]. Available from: https://cks.nice.org.uk/topics/neutropenic-sepsis/diagnosis/assessment [accessed 21 June 2023].

Peate, I. (2019). *Alexander's Nursing Practice: Hospital and Home*, 5e. Elsevier (E-Book).

The Faculty of Intensive Care Medicine. (2018). *Curriculum for Training for Advanced Critical Care Practitioners – Syllabus. V1.1* [online]. Available from: www.ficm.ac.uk/media/6896 [accessed 20 June 2023].

The Intensive Care Society, Critical Care Networks – *National Nurse Leads and The National Outreach Forum*. (2022). *Advanced Critical Care Outreach Competencies* [online]. Available from: https://ics.ac.uk/asset/43B8C11B-4512-41D0-B97768FABA2C30B2 [accessed 20 June 2023].

The Royal College of Emergency Medicine. (2022). *Emergency Medicine Advanced Clinical Practitioner Curriculum 2022 (Adult)* [online]. Available from: https://rcem.ac.uk/wp-content/uploads/2022/09/ACP_Curriculum_Adult_Final_060922.pdf [accessed 20 June 2023].

The Royal Marsden. (2023). *Chemotherapy: Effects and Side Effects* [online]. Available from: https://www.royalmarsden.nhs.uk/your-care/treatments/chemotherapy/chemotherapy-effects-and-side-effects [accessed 21 June 2023].

WHO. (2023). *HIV* [online]. Available from https://www.who.int/health-topics/hiv-aids#tab=tab_1 [accessed 21 June 2023].

FURTHER READING

British Society for Haematology (BSH). *Haematology Guidelines* [onlline]. Available from: https://b-s-h.org.uk/guidelines/guidelines [accessed 21 June 2023].

NICE. (2016). *Haematological Cancers: Improving Outcomes* [online]. Available from: www.nice.org.uk/guidance/ng47/resources/haematological-cancers-improving-outcomes-pdf-1837457868229 [accessed 21 June 2023].

CHAPTER 13

Rheumatological and Immunological Presentations

Caroline McCrea, Barry Hill, Sonya Stone, and Sadie Diamond-Fox

> **Aim**
> The aim of this chapter is to provide the reader with knowledge about some of the key rheumatological and immunological presentations that may be encountered in acute, emergency, and critical care (AECC) environments.

LEARNING OUTCOMES

After reading this chapter the reader will:

1. Be more aware of common and uncommon rheumatological/immunological conditions, and their clinical presentations and complications.
2. Gain enhanced knowledge about rheumatological and autoimmune diseases.
3. Better understand specific investigations that can be used in the diagnosis of rheumatological/immunological conditions.
4. Consider different examinations to support clinical decision-making and differential diagnosis.

SELF-ASSESSMENT QUESTIONS

1. Choose a rheumatological and immunological disorder that you see frequently in your practice and write down a definition of the disorder.
2. Think about a Subjective, Objective, Assessment and Plan (SOAP) approach to your assessment, referring to the history-taking chapter, what subjective and objective assessment would you take, and how would you plan the care of a symptomatic patient.

The Advanced Practitioner in Acute, Emergency and Critical Care, First Edition. Edited by Sadie Diamond-Fox, Barry Hill, Sonya Stone, Caroline McCrea, Natalie Gardner, and Angela Roberts.

3. As an autoimmune disease, consider type 1 diabetes mellitus (T1DM) and its pathophysiology. Can you explain the altered pathophysiology of T1DM. Can you explain how these manifests into signs and symptoms?

INTRODUCTION

In this chapter, a selection of acute, emergency, and critical rheumatological and immunological disorders will be presented to the reader. Rheumatology covers the diagnosis, care, and treatment of a wide range of conditions, which affect the joints and surrounding tissues. This includes arthritis, connective tissue and autoimmune diseases, all long-term conditions that can severely impair mobility and movement, if left untreated. Immunology is the study of the immune system or immunity, a range of defences developed by humans, for example, to protect against infection by surrounding microorganisms i.e. viruses, bacteria, fungi, and other parasites, and pathologies.

Multi-professional Framework (MPF) for Advanced Clinical Practice Guidance for Professional Development (HEE 2017)

This chapter maps to the following statements within the MPF:

1. Clinical Practice:	1.2	1.6	1.7

Accreditation Considerations

This chapter maps to the following statements within the following national accreditation documents:

Curriculum for Training for Advanced Critical Care Practitioners Syllabus V1.1
(The Faculty of Intensive Care Medicine 2018)

2.1	4.3	

Advanced Critical Care Outreach Competencies
(The Intensive Care Society, Critical Care Networks – National Nurse Leads and The National Outreach Forum 2022)

A1	A5	B1	C1	C3	

Emergency Medicine Advanced Clinical Practitioner Curriculum 2022 – Adult
(The Royal College of Emergency Medicine 2022)

MuC6	

RHEUMATOLOGICAL EMERGENCIES

Rheumatological conditions can sometimes present as emergencies. These can occur due to the disease process or may be iatrogenic. Some of the important articular emergencies are septic arthritis, acute polyarthritis, and atlanto-axial dislocation. Classical polyarteritis nodosa may present with massive gastro-intestinal bleeding, intestinal perforation, or acute pancreatitis. Adult respiratory distress syndrome, bilateral pneumonitis, and diffuse alveolar haemorrhage due to systemic lupus erythematosus or systemic necrotising vasculitis and ventilatory failure due to polymyositis are some of the respiratory emergencies. Scleroderma is well known to cause renal crisis, which can be fatal if not diagnosed and managed promptly. Microscopic polyangiitis and Wegener's granulomatosis may cause rapidly progressive renal failure. Cerebrovascular accident, cortical vein thrombosis, seizures, and acute psychosis are important neurological complications of rheumatic disease. Cardiac emergencies include tamponade, acute myocarditis, and acute myocardial infarction. Vision can be threatened in Behcet's disease, temporal arteritis and seronegative spondylarthritis. Catastrophic antiphospholipid syndrome is a devastating emergency. The management of these emergencies includes critical care, immunosuppression when indicated, and withdrawal of the offending drug. Anticoagulants must be used in the management of antiphospholipid syndrome. A good understanding of these conditions is of paramount importance for proper management. A variety of conditions, presentations and associated complications, and recommended treatments and supportive measures can be seen in Table 13.1 (Gutiérrez-González 2015).

TABLE 13.1   Classification of rheumatologic emergencies.

Condition	Presentations and associated complications	Potential treatments/ supportive measures
Catastrophic antiphospholipid syndrome (cAPS)	<ul><li>Rapidly evolving, severe form of antiphospholipid syndrome</li><li>Leads to multi-organ failure:<ul><li>Renal – 78%</li><li>Pulmonary – 66%</li><li>Central nervous system (CNS) – 56%</li></ul></li><li>Causes vessel occlusion or occlusive impact on organs, systems, and/or tissues</li><li>Associated with syphilis and related non-venereal treponematoses</li><li>Presents with thrombocytopenia and pancytopenia, may also have positive antiglobulin test</li></ul>	<ul><li>Anticoagulation</li><li>Glucocorticoid therapy</li><li>Plasmapheresis</li></ul>

(Continued)

TABLE 13.1   (Continued)

Condition	Presentations and associated complications	Potential treatments/ supportive measures

Pulmonary-renal syndrome/Goodpasture's syndrome/Anti-glomerular basement membrane disease	• Rapidly progressing glomerulonephritis (RPGN) and diffuse alveolar bleeding (DAB)
	• May be due to one of three immune causes:
	  • Type 1: Antibody mediated – anti-glomerular basal membrane antibodies (anti-GBM) positive (12.5–17.5% cases)
	  • Type 2: Immune complex mediated – associated with systemic lupus erythematous (SLE)
	  • Type 3: Pauci-immune – anti-neutrophil cytoplasmic antibody (ANCA) positive (56–77.5% cases)
		Glucocorticoids
		Immunological agents – Rituximab
		Mechanical ventilation
		Haemodialysis

Central nervous system (CNS) vasculitis	• Inflammation of blood vessels resulting in tissue damage from ischaemia • Subsequent activation of the inflammatory cascade that leads to blood vessel occlusion and necrosis • Antigen–antibody complex that triggers an inflammatory cascade mostly mediated by cytokines Th1 (Salvarani et al. 2008)	

Anti-Ro syndrome (neonatal lupus)	• Transplacental passage of the maternal anti-SSA/Ro and anti-SSB/La to the foetus
	• Typical clinical manifestations (Tincani et al. 2006):
	  ➢ Transient eruption
	  ➢ Congenital heart block
	  ➢ Hepatobiliary dysfunction
	  ➢ Haematological and neurological dysfunction
	  ➢ Pulmonary abnormalities
	• In utero mortality is 23%, while at 1 year of age is 54%
		Determine if anti-Ro and anti-LA antibodies are present
		Management of baby in neonatal ICU ± permanent pacemaker

Macrophage activation syndrome (MAS)	• Mortality close to 70% often undiagnosed (30% post-mortem)
	• Acute presentation of liver failure, consumption coagulopathy and encephalopathy
	• Clinical presentation:
	  ➢ Extended fever >39°C (for at least 7 days)
	  ➢ Internal bleeding—melena
	  ➢ CNS alterations
	  ➢ Jaundice and lymphadenopathies
		Supportive therapy:
		• Plasmapheresis
		• Antibiotics if infection caused activation
		First-line therapy IV/PO Cyclosporine 3–5 mg/kg per day

TABLE 13.1   (Continued)

Condition	Presentations and associated complications	Potential treatments/ supportive measures
Scleroderma renal crisis	Characterised by: • The acute onset of renal failure. • The abrupt onset of moderate to marked hypertension (although some patients remain normotensive). • A urine sediment that is usually normal or reveals only mild proteinuria with few cells or casts	Initiation of angiotensin-converting inhibitor (ACE) ± calcium channel blocker
Septic arthritis	• Inflammatory process in specific joint with rapid joint destruction • Possible systemic sepsis	Source control à joint washout + appropriate antimicrobials

Atlanto-axial subluxation	• Most common symptom is pain either neck or headache
	• Neurological manifestations
	  ➢ Lack of co-ordination
	  ➢ Unusual gait
	  ➢ Upper motor neurone signs
	  ➢ Paraplegia/hemiplegia
		Urgent radiological diagnosis Surgical intervention may be required

Source: Adapted from Gutiérrez-González (2015).

IMMUNOLOGIC EMERGENCIES

The immune system is a complex defence mechanism designed to protect human beings from infection and other invasion from outside sources. It usually works perfectly, but at times it can over respond, causing disease and even assault on the tissues of the body that it is designed to protect. Emergency providers will face immunologic emergencies that range from mild allergic reactions to life-threatening anaphylaxis. Immunosuppressive drugs, used in a variety of situations, including in transplant recipients, can place patients at risk for infection and other disease processes. To note, children and young people can also present to an emergency department with their first episode of an immunologic disorder, such as Kawasaki disease or juvenile rheumatoid arthritis.

Table 13.2 presents disorders of adaptive immunity and provides examples and clinical presentations.

AUTOIMMUNE DISORDERS

These are a collection of diseases that can either be organ specific; antibodies and T cells react in a specific tissue, or systemic conditions; reactivity against antigens spread throughout tissues (Wang et al. 2015) (see Figure 13.1). Currently there are several different classifications to help in the diagnosis of autoimmune diseases, which ultimately incorporates serology, clinical features, and histopathology. Autoimmune disease happens when the body's natural defence system cannot tell the difference between the body's own cells and foreign cells, causing the body to mistakenly attack normal cells. There are more

TABLE 13.2   Classification of immunological conditions.

Classification and examples	Clinical presentation
Disorders of adaptive immunity	
T-cell (cellular) immunodeficiency	
• IFN-γ/IL-12	Atypical mycobacterial and salmonella infections
• AIRE mutations	Mucocutaneous candidiasis (thrush) and autoimmune endocrinopathy
B-cell (antibody-mediated) immunodeficiency	
• Selective IgA deficiency	Recurrent sinopulmonary infections with encapsulated bacteria
• Specific antibody deficiency	Autoimmune disease and increased risk of malignancy in CVID
• IgG subclass deficiency	Recurrent upper respiratory tract infections
CID (combined immunodeficiency)	
• Wiskott-Aldrich syndrome	Thrombocytopenia with bleeding and bruising; eczema; recurrent bacterial and viral infections; autoimmune disease
• Ataxia telangiectasia	Chronic sinopulmonary disease; cerebellar ataxia (difficulty with control of movement); small, dilated blood vessels of the eyes and skin; malignancy
• DiGeorge syndrome	Hypoparathyroidism; seizures; cardiac abnormalities; abnormal facies; infection
• Hyper IgE syndrome	Chronic dermatitis; recurrent, severe lung infections; skin infections; bone fragility; failure to shed primary teeth
SCID (severe combined immunodeficiency)	
• JAK3 deficiency	Severe, recurrent opportunistic infections; failure to thrive; diarrhoea; rash
T⁻, B⁻	
• Adenosine deaminase (ADA) deficiency	Lack virtually all immune protection against bacteria, virus, and fungi. Prone to repeated and persistent infections often life-threatening.
• RAG 1/2 deficiency	Associated with life-threatening infections (bacterial/viral/fungal) early on in infancy
Disorders of innate immunity	
Phagocyte defects	
• Chronic granulomatous disease	Severe infection; abscesses with granuloma formation
• Leukocyte adhesion deficiency	Recurrent, severe bacterial infections; poor wound healing; delayed separation of the umbilical cord
Complement defects	
• Deficiency in early complement pathway components (C1q, C1r, C2, C4)	SLE–like syndrome, rheumatoid disease, multiple autoimmune diseases, infections
• Deficiency in late complement pathway components (C5, C6, C7, C8, C9)	Neisserial infections, SLE-like syndrome
• C3 and regulatory components	Recurrent infections with encapsulated bacteria

TABLE 13.2   (Continued)

Classification and examples	Clinical presentation
Disorders of immune dysregulation	
Hemophagocytic lymphohistiocytosis (**HLH**)	Fever, splenomegaly, cytopenia, rash
Autoimmune lymphoproliferative syndrome (**ALPS**)	Splenomegaly, adenopathy
Immunodysregulation polyendocrinopathy (**IPEX**)	Autoimmune enteritis, early onset diabetes, thyroiditis, haemolytic anaemia, thrombocytopenia, eczema
Autoimmune polyendocrinopathy-candidiasis-ectodermal dystrophy (**APECED**)	Autoimmunity affecting parathyroid, adrenal, other endocrine organs; candidiasis; dental enamel hypoplasia

Source: Adapted from Notarangelo (2010), Al-Herz et al. (2014), Bonilla et al. (2015), Picard et al. (2015).

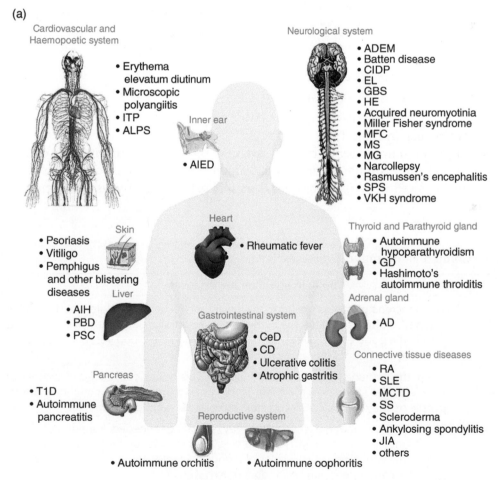

FIGURE 13.1   (a), (b) Representative organ-specific and systemic autoimmune diseases. *Source*: Wang et al. (2015) / John Wiley & Sons.

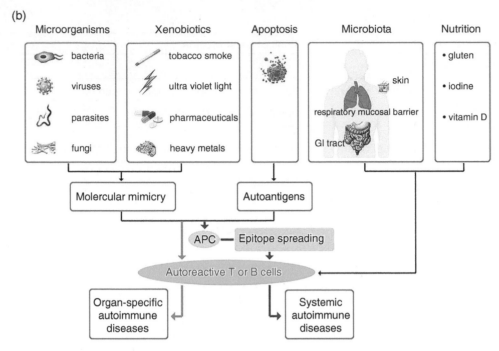

FIGURE 13.1   (Continued)

than 80 types of autoimmune diseases that affect a wide range of body parts. The most common autoimmune diseases can be seen in Table 13.3.

Symptoms of autoimmune disease may be severe in some people and mild in others. Common autoimmune diseases share similar symptoms. Common symptoms of autoimmune disease include fatigue, joint pain and swelling, skin problems, abdominal pain or digestive issues, recurring fever, and swollen glands.

TABLE 13.3   Common autoimmune diseases.

Common autoimmune diseases	
Type 1 Diabetes Mellitus	The pancreas produces the hormone insulin, which helps regulate blood sugar levels. In type 1 diabetes mellitus, the immune system attacks and destroys insulin-producing cells in the pancreas. Hyperglycaemia will damage the blood vessels and organs, including the heart, kidneys, eyes, and nerves.
Rheumatoid arthritis (RA)	In RA, the immune system attacks the joints. This attack causes redness, warmth, soreness, and stiffness in the joints. Unlike osteoarthritis, which commonly affects people as they get older, RA can start as early 30 years old or sooner.
Psoriasis/psoriatic arthritis	Skin cells grow and then shed when they're no longer needed. Psoriasis causes skin cells to multiply too quickly. The extra cells build up and form inflamed, red patches, commonly with silver-white scales of plaque on lighter-toned skin. On darker skin, psoriasis can appear purplish or dark brown with grey scales. Up to 30% of people with psoriasis also develop swelling, stiffness, and pain in their joints. This form of the disease is called psoriatic arthritis.

TABLE 13.3   (Continued)

Multiple sclerosis (MS)	Multiple sclerosis (MS) damages the myelin sheath, the protective coating surrounding nerve cells in the central nervous system. Damage to the myelin sheath slows the transmission speed of messages between the brain and spinal cord to and from the rest of the body. This damage can lead to numbness, weakness, balance issues, and trouble walking. The disease comes in several forms that progress at different rates. About 50% of people with MS need help walking within 15 years after the disease starts.
Systemic lupus erythematosus (SLE)	Although doctors in the 1800s first described lupus as a skin disease because of the rash it commonly produces, the systemic form, which is most common, affects many organs, including the joints, kidneys, brain, and heart. Joint pain, fatigue, and rashes are among the most common symptoms.
Inflammatory bowel disease	Inflammatory bowel disease (IBD) describes conditions that cause inflammation in the lining of the intestinal wall. Each type of IBD affects a different part of the GI tract. Crohn's disease can inflame any part of the GI tract, from the mouth to the anus. Ulcerative colitis affects only the lining of the large intestine (colon) and rectum.
Addison's disease	Addison's disease affects the adrenal glands, which produce the hormones cortisol and aldosterone as well as androgen hormones. Too little cortisol can affect how the body uses and stores carbohydrates and sugar (glucose). Deficiency of aldosterone will lead to sodium loss and excess potassium in the bloodstream. Symptoms include weakness, fatigue, weight loss, and hypoglycaemia.
Graves' disease	Graves' disease attacks the thyroid gland in the neck, causing it to produce too much of its hormones. Thyroid hormones control the body's energy usage, known as metabolism. Having too much of these hormones increases metabolism, causing symptoms like nervousness, a fast heartbeat, heat intolerance, and weight loss. One potential symptom of this disease is bulging eyes, called exophthalmos. It can occur as a part of Graves' ophthalmopathy, which occurs in around 30% of those with Graves' disease.
Sjögren's syndrome	This condition attacks the glands that provide lubrication to the eyes and mouth. The hallmark symptoms of Sjögren's syndrome are dry eyes and dry mouth, but it may also affect the joints or skin.
Hashimoto's thyroiditis	In Hashimoto's thyroiditis, thyroid hormone production slows to a deficiency. Symptoms include weight gain, sensitivity to cold, fatigue, hair loss, and swelling of the thyroid (goitre).
Myasthenia gravis	Myasthenia gravis affects nerve impulses that help the brain control the muscles. When the communication from nerves to muscles is impaired, signals cannot direct the muscles to contract. The most common symptom is muscle weakness, which worsens with activity and improves with rest. Muscles that control eye movements, eyelid opening, swallowing, and facial movements are often involved.
Autoimmune vasculitis	Autoimmune vasculitis happens when the immune system attacks blood vessels. The inflammation that results narrows the arteries and veins, allowing less blood to flow through them.
Pernicious anaemia	This condition causes a deficiency of a protein made by stomach lining cells, which is an intrinsic factor needed for the small intestine to absorb Vitamin B12 from food. Without enough of this vitamin, one will develop anaemia, and the body's ability for proper DNA synthesis will be altered. Pernicious anaemia is more common in older adults. According to a 2012 study, it affects 0.1% of people in general but nearly 2% of people over age 60.
Celiac disease	People with celiac disease cannot eat foods containing gluten, a protein found in wheat, rye, and other grain products. When gluten is in the small intestine, the immune system attacks this part of the gastrointestinal tract and causes inflammation. Celiac disease affects about 1% of people in the United States. Many people have reported gluten sensitivity, which is not an autoimmune disease but can have similar symptoms such as diarrhoea and abdominal pain.

Autoimmune conditions can have a variety of diagnostic and clinical classifications, but they are not always particularly specific or sensitive.

CLINICAL INVESTIGATIONS: ANTI-NEUTROPHIL CYTOPLASMIC ANTIBODIES (ANCA)

Anti-neutrophil cytoplasmic antibodies (ANCA) are autoantibodies that target a type of human white blood cell called neutrophils, which are important in health for fighting infection partly through the release of toxic substances that destroy bacteria. Representative organ-specific and systemic autoimmune diseases are usually considered in three subtypes; granulomatosis with polyangiitis (GPA), microscopic polyangiitis (MPA), and eosinophilic GPA (EGPA) (see Figure 13.2). When testing patients, ANCA can be used in two formats: indirect immunofluorescence assay (IFF) or immunoassay such as enzyme-linked immunosorbent assay (ELISA). These formats are important as not all patients with systemic vasculitis are ANCA IFF positive, so this test alone may not be sensitive enough. This is why clinicians need to have insight into the sensitivity and specificity of these tests. Patients should only be screened if the clinician has high suspicion of a vasculitic picture, as the test can produce a false positive result (Phatak et al. 2017; Elena 2013). ANCA has a sensitivity of 75.2% and a pooled specificity of 98.4% to diagnose ANCA-associated vasculitis (AAV) (Guchelaar et al. 2021).

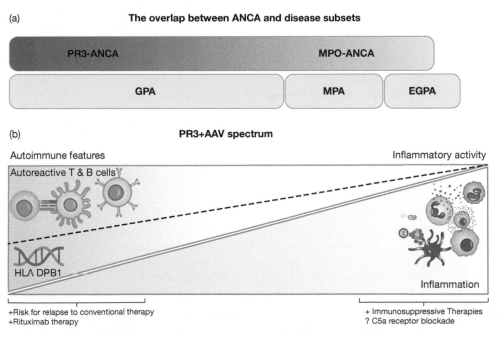

FIGURE 13.2   ANCA-associated Vasculitis disease subsets and immune features. *Source*: Sharma et al. (2020) / John Wiley & Sons.

CLINICAL INVESTIGATIONS IMMUNOLOGICAL CONDITIONS: LABORATORY TESTS

It is extremely difficult to diagnose potential autoimmune diseases solely on laboratory tests. However, they can be used to aid diagnosis with the understanding that a combination of tests will be required. Laboratory investigations can help determine disease severity and potentially prognosis, but the clinician must be aware that the test might not be disease-specific. Inflammatory conditions will cause abnormalities in routine blood results.

Inflammatory Markers

These markers are not diagnostic of inflammation, but can help in the diagnosis of autoimmune diseases, infections, and malignancies.

Erythrocyte Sedimentation Rate (ESR)

It is the measure of the quantity of red blood cells that develop over time. There are a multitude of factors that can influence an increase in ESR, one of which is inflammation. Clinicians need to be aware of factors that can affect or influence ESR:

★ Age
★ Gender
★ Haemoglobin concentration
★ Red blood cell morphology

ESR is not considered a diagnostic test but can be used to monitor disease activity, such as with rheumatoid arthritis (RA) (Lahita and Weinstein 2007; Klippel et al. 2008).

C-Reactive Protein (CRP)

C-Reactive Protein is an innate immune protein that is used to activate the complement system. It is a better indicator of inflammation than ESR as the concentration changes more quickly, thus considered more sensitive.

Ferritin

It is a protein that stores iron, and elevated levels can indicate acute sepsis, inflammation, or malignancy. Clinicians should be aware of the implications of raised ferritin levels as it can be indicative of specific diseases (Breda et al. 2009; Koulaouzidis et al. 2009):

★ Adult Stills disease
★ Juvenile idiopathic arthritis
★ Haemophagocytic lymphohistiocytosis
★ Haemochromatosis

Examination Scenarios – Rheumatological Examination

Head and neck

Alopecia
Red/sore/dry eyes
Nasal crusting/epistaxis
Oral ulcers
Dry mouth
Hearing loss

Joint disease

Pain and early morning
  stiffness
Duration, distribution of
  synovitis
Disability

Rash

Psoriasis, SLE,
  dermatomyositis
Erythema nodosum
Circinate balanitis
Keratoderma
  blennorrhagica
Vasculitis
Livedo reticularis

Nails

Psoriatic nail changes
Vasculitis
Dermatomyositis

Genitourinary

Previous STD
Vaginal dryness

Vascular

Raynaud's phenomenon
DVT/CVT recurrent
  miscarriage

Cardiac

Pericarditis

Respiratory

Pleuritis
Fibrosis, effusions
Pulmonary embolus
Pulmonary hypertension

Gastrointestinal

Diarrhoea
Jaundice

Neurological

Mononeuritis mutiplex
Compression
  neuropathy
Myelopathy
Peripheral neuropathy

Haematopoietic

Anaemia
Lymphadenopathy
Splenomegaly

The purpose of joint examination is the detection of joint swelling, differentiation between inflammatory and degenerative joint disease, and the assessment of disease activity in an individual patient. Joint swelling in inflammation (synovitis) is boggy in nature. The joint is often warm, with overlying erythema, and there is often pain at the extremes of movement. Swelling due to degenerative disease is bony hard. Different inflammatory diseases have predilections for different sites. Rheumatoid arthritis, for example, favours the metacarpophalangeal (MCP) and proximal interphalangeal (PIP) joints in the hand, with relative sparing of the distal interphalangeal (DIP) joints. However, osteoarthritis in the hand focuses on the first carpometacarpal (CMC) joint, the PIP joints (forming Bouchard's nodes) and the DIP joints (forming Heberden's nodes). Many rheumatological conditions are systemic diseases. Potential extra-articular manifestations of disease must be sought in clinical examination. The gait, arms, legs, spine (GALS) screen and detailed examination of the arm, leg, and spine has already been described. For RA patients, the focus is not only the description of the classic bony deformity but also the detection of active synovitis (swollen and tender joints).

Diagnosis and Referral of Inflammatory Arthritis

Inflammatory arthritis is a collective term for a group of conditions, including RA and spondyloarthritis (SpA), that cause inflammation of the tissues around affected joints. Inflammatory arthritis has a range of genetic and environmental risk factors. RA onset peaks between 40 and 60 years of age, and is more common in women, people who smoke, and people who are obese. Axial SpA usually begins between 20 and 30 years of age, is equally common in men and women, and can be more severe in people who smoke. NICE (2023) recommends that adults with suspected axial SpA should be referred to a rheumatologist, indicating the need for a specific referral pathway from primary to secondary care for inflammatory back pain. The All-Party Parliamentary Groups (APPG) for axial SpA report shows that only 21% of clinical commissioning groups (CCGs) have a specific pathway in place. Some CCGs indicated that they had alternative arrangements, such as referral to musculoskeletal triage services; however, this could increase time to diagnosis. It is also important that commissioners have programmes to raise awareness of the signs and symptoms of axial SpA in primary care, as recommended by NICE. However, of the 44% (85/191) of CCGs that responded, only 34% (29/85) had these programmes in place.

Fields of Practice – Paediatrics

There are many conditions that can be treated by paediatric rheumatology clinicians working in advanced practice; however they are often disorders of inflammation or auto-immunity. Common rheumatic conditions in children include:

- Juvenile arthritis
- Juvenile dermatomyositis
- Paediatric vasculitis, such as Kawasaki disease
- Lupus
- Auto-inflammatory syndromes
- Localised and systemic scleroderma
- Juvenile rheumatoid arthritis
- Joint hypermobility
- Osteomyelitis

Fields of Practice – Mental Health

Lwin et al. (2020) identifies that depression is two times more common in RA patients than in the general population, and intriguingly a bi-directional relationship with RA has been shown in cross-sectional studies. Chronic inflammation impairs the physiological responses to stress, including effective coping behaviours, resulting in depression, which leads to a worse long-term outcome in RA. In RA patients, the pain score is not always solely related to inflammatory arthritis and immunological disease activity.

RED FLAGS – PATHOLOGICAL CONSIDERATIONS

Ocular involvement is a common manifestation of inflammatory rheumatic diseases, often requiring a multidisciplinary collaboration between rheumatologists and ophthalmologists.

Case Study – Cutaneous Small-vessel Vasculitis (CSVV)

Presenting complaint: A 54-year-old male presented with pyrexia >39, palpable purpura on lower limbs, and arthritis of knees and ankles.

History of presenting complaint: Five-day history of fever with associated joint pain, no recent travel or risky sexual behaviours

Examination: Pyrexia 38.8, normotensive and respiratory function normal
Bilateral palpable purpura on lower extremities and abdomen (see picture below)
Significant swelling of the knees extending to suprapatellar pouch
GCS E4V5M6 = 15/15

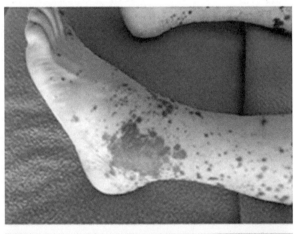

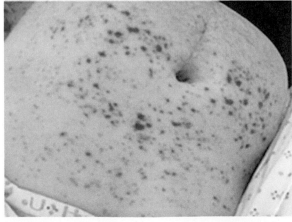

Biochemical investigations: C-Reactive protein (CRP) 109 U/l (Normal <5 U/l)
Alanine aminotransferase 680 U/l (Normal 5–50 U/l)
Alkaline phosphatase 123 IU/l (Normal 40–130 U/l)
All other biochemical tests were within normal range

Serology investigations: Infective cause was ruled out
Hepatitis A, B, C viruses, HIV-1 and 2 were negative
Anti-cytomegalovirus and Epstein-Barr virus immunoglobulins (Ig) (IgG but no IgM) were found

Other investigations: Transthoracic ECHO showed no evidence of vegetations
CXR clear
Liver ultrasound showed normal gallbladder appearance and hepatopetal blood flow

Histological investigation: Histological section of a purpuric lesion showing evidence of leukocyto-clastic vasculitis with fibrinoid necrosis of small blood vessels in the upper dermis.

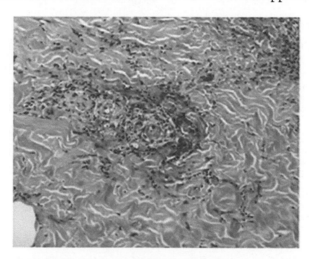

Differential diagnosis: Likely viral in origin given skin purpura and cytolytic hepatitis. Further virology screening sent for emergent viruses; Hepatitis E virus was reactive.
Rash spontaneously disappeared within two weeks; laboratory results normalised within four weeks

Learning points: 45–55% of CSVV cases are idiopathic
15–20% maybe caused by; autoimmune conditions, hypersensitivity drug reactions, lymphoprolifera-tive disorders or malignancies, and infections

In the above case, patient was not taking any medications thus ruling out hypersensitivity vasculitis. Other than raised CRP other inflammatory markers were normal making infective cause less likely.

Case Study – Hemophagocytic Lymphohistiocytosis (HLH)

Presenting complaint: A 42-year-old Nepalese male presented with fever, rigors, and myalgia.

History of presenting complaint: A five-day history of fever, rigors, and myalgia. No past medical history and took no medications. Non-smoker and minimal alcohol intake and reports no illicit drug use. Lives in the UK for the past 12 years, and most recently returned to Nepal four months ago. Of note, during his stay in Nepal, he met a family member with Tuberculosis (TB).

On Examination

Pyrexic with temperature 38.8°C, Blood pressure 92/52 mmHg, Heart rate 120/min (sinus tachycardia), and a respiratory rate of 24/min with saturations of 95% on room air.

Cardiovascular and respiratory examination unremarkable.

Abdominal examination revealed mild splenomegaly with no palpable lymphadenopathy.

Initial investigation	Value	Reference range
Haemoglobin	77 g/l	12.5–15 g/l
White cell count	15.2×10^9/l	$4.0–11.0 \times 10^9$
Platelet count	147×10^9/l	$150–400 \times 10^9$
Bilirubin	25 mmol/l	3–17 mmol/l
Alanine aminotransferase (ALT)	48 IU/l	10–40 IU/l
Alkaline phosphatase (ALP)	372 IU/l	44–147 IU/l
Albumin	37 g/l	30–50 g/l
Ferritin	168–962 ng/ml	13–300 ng/ml
Triglycerides	3.84 mmol/l	<1.7 mmol/l
Renal function normal		

Investigations

- chest X-ray – clear
- urine dipstick – negative
- blood cultures – negative
- CT scan of his chest, abdomen, and pelvis revealed mediastinal lymphadenopathy and splenomegaly
- mediastinal lymph node fine-needle aspirate (FNA)-negative for lymphoma and TB
- Peripheral blood TB ELISPOT was negative

Management and Outcome

- Due to cardiovascular instability the patient was referred to the intensive care unit for inotropic support
- Had multiple courses of antimicrobials with no improvement

- Note to have five out of eight second line criteria for the diagnosis of HLH (fevers, splenomegaly, a progressive pancytopenia, raised ferritin, and raised fasting triglyceride levels)
- Bone marrow biopsy confirmed diagnosis, with 1 in 200 cells demonstrating haemophagocytosis
- Underlying pathoaetiology unclear-->screened for both congenital and acquired causes which all came back negative
- Due to unclear cause, patient was started on treatment according to the Histiocyte Society HLH-2004 guideline
- Failed first line HLH treatment that included; etoposide, ciclosporin, full course of dexamethasone, and empirical treatment for TB
- After multiple readmissions and a variety of different treatments, the patient eventually required work-up for a haematopoietic stem-cell transplantation
- This included a repeat peripheral blood TB ELISPOT that was now reactive

Learning Points

- Patients are generally diagnosed with HLH if they meet at least five of the eight criteria listed below:
  1. Fever $\geq 38.5\,°C$
  2. Splenomegaly
  3. Cytopenias (affecting at least two of the below):
     Haemoglobin $<90\,g/l$ (in infants <4 weeks: haemoglobin $<100\,g/l$)
     Platelet count $<100 \times 10^9/l$
     Neutrophil count $<1.0 \times 10^9/l$
  4. Hypertriglyceridaemia (fasting, $>3.0\,mmol/l$) and/or hypofibrinogenaemia ($<1.5\,g/l$)
  5. Haemophagocytosis in bone marrow, spleen, lymph nodes, liver, or other tissue
  6. Low or absent Natural Killer (NK) cell activity
  7. Ferritin $>500\,\mu g/l$
  8. Elevated soluble CD25 (soluble interleukin 2 receptor):
  9. $>2400\,\mu g/ml$ or elevated based on the laboratory-defined normal range

  Criteria commonly used to aid in the diagnosis of haemophagocytic lymphohistiocytosis (HLH)

- Care should be taken in the early phase of the disease process as not all patients will exhibit all five criteria.
- There is a misconception that the above are 'gold standard' in the diagnosis of HLH, which is not strictly the case.
- Mistakenly thought that the absence of haemophagocytosis means no presence of HLH.
- The presence of haemophagocytosis has poor specificity (Goel et al. 2012; Gupta et al. 2008; Ho et al. 2014; Lao et al. 2016).

INVESTIGATION

A diagnostic platform for autoimmune diseases can be seen below.

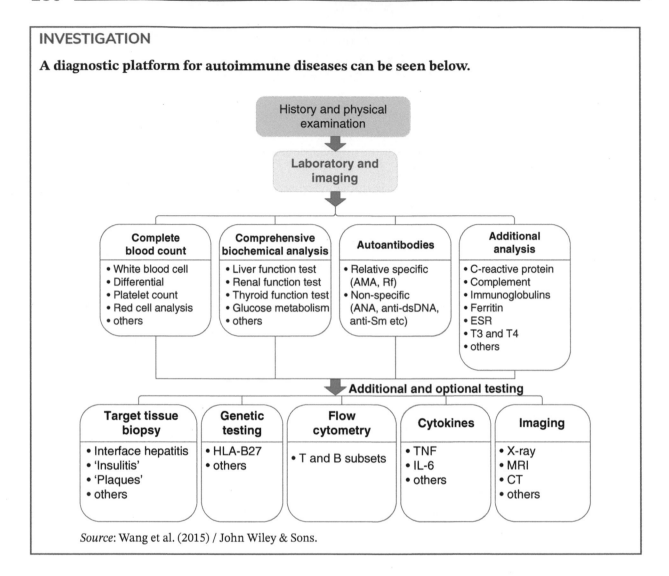

Source: Wang et al. (2015) / John Wiley & Sons.

Take Home Points
- Rheumatological and immunological presentations are complex and require through subjective and objective assessment by the advanced practitioner.
- Rheumatic disease refers to arthritis and conditions that affect the joints, tendons, muscle, ligaments, bones, and muscles. Therefore, differential diagnosis can be challenging.
- Immune system disorders cause abnormally low activity or over activity of the immune system. Advanced Practitioners must look out for signs of overactivity, whereby the body attacks and damages its own tissues (autoimmune diseases).
- Immune deficiency diseases decrease the body's ability to fight invaders, causing vulnerability to infections.

REFERENCES

Al-Herz, W., Bousfiha, A., Casanova, J.L. et al. (2014). Primary immunodeficiency diseases: an update on the classification from the international union of immunological societies expert committee for primary immunodeficiency. *Frontiers in Immunology* 5: 162.

Bonilla, F.A., Khan, D.A., Ballas, Z.K. et al. (2015). Joint task force on practice parameters, representing the American Academy of Allergy, Asthma & Immunology; the American College of Allergy, Asthma & Immunology; and the Joint Council of Allergy, Asthma & Immunology. Practice parameter for the diagnosis and management of primary immunodeficiency. *The Journal of Allergy and Clinical Immunology* 136 (5): 1186–1205.

Breda, L., Nozzi, M., de Sanctis, S., and Chiarelli, F. (2009). Laboratory tests in the diagnosis and follow-up of pediatric rheumatic diseases: an update. *Seminars in Arthritis and Rheumatism*.

Elena, C. (2013). L28. Relevance of detection techniques for ANCA testing. *Presse Médicale* 42: 582–584.

Goel, S., Polski, J.M., and Imran, H. (2012). Sensitivity and specificity of bone marrow hemophagocytosis in hemophagocytic lymphohistiocytosis. *Annals of Clinical and Laboratory Science* 42: 21–25.

Guchelaar, N.A.D., Waling, M.M., Adhin, A.A. et al. (2021). The value of anti-neutrophil cytoplasmic antibodies (ANCA) testing for the diagnosis of ANCA-associated vasculitis, a systematic review and meta-analysis. *Autoimmunity Reviews* 20 (1): 102716. https://doi.org/10.1016/j.autrev.2020.102716. Epub 2020 Nov 13. PMID: 33197574.

Gupta, A., Weitzman, S., and Abdelhaleem, M. (2008). The role of hemophagocytosis in bone marrow aspirates in the diagnosis of hemophagocytic lymphohistiocytosis. *Pediatric Blood & Cancer* 50: 192–194.

Gutiérrez-González, L.A. (2015). Rheumatologic emergencies. *Clinical Rheumatology* 34 (12): 2011–2019. https://doi.org/10.1007/s10067-015-2994-y. Epub 2015 Jun 24. PMID: 26099604; PMCID: PMC7101757.

Health Education England (HEE). (2022). *Advanced Clinical Practice in Acute Medicine Curriculum Framework – Credentials* [online]. Available from: https://advanced-practice.hee.nhs.uk/our-work/credentials [accessed 20 June 2023].

Health Education England. (2017). *Multi-professional Framework for Advanced Clinical Practice in England* [online]. Available from: https://www.hee.nhs.uk/sites/default/files/documents/multi-professionalframeworkforadvancedclinicalpracticeinengland.pdf [accessed 21 June 2023].

Ho, C., Yao, X., Tian, L. et al. (2014). Marrow assessment for hemophagocytic lymphohistiocytosis demonstrates poor correlation with disease probability. *American Journal of Clinical Pathology* 141: 62–71.

Klippel, J.H., Stone, J.H., Crofford, L.J., and White., P.H. (2008). *Primer on rheumatic diseases. Thirteenth. Chapter 2*, 15–20. Springer.

Koulaouzidis, A., Cottier, R., Bhat, S. et al. (2009). A ferritin level >50 μg/L is frequently consistent with iron deficiency. *European Journal of Internal Medicine* 20: 168–170.

Lahita, R.G. and Weinstein, A. (2007). *Educational review manual in rheumatology*, 4e. Chapter 1, 1–42. New York, NY: Castle Connolly Graduate Medical Publishing, Ltd.

Lao, K., Sharma, N., Gajra, A., and Vajpayee, N. (2016). Hemophagocytic lymphohistiocytosis and bone marrow hemophagocytosis: a 5-year institutional experience at a tertiary care hospital. *Southern Medical Journal* 109: 655–660.

Lwin, M.N., Serhal, L., Holroyd, C., and Edwards, C.J. (2020). Rheumatoid arthritis: the impact of mental health on disease: a narrative review. *Rheumatology and Therapy* 7 (3): 457–471. https://doi.org/10.1007/s40744-020-00217-4.

NICE. (2023). *Diagnosis and Referral of Inflammatory Arthritis* [online]. Available from: www.nice.org.uk/about/what-we-do/into-practice/measuring-the-use-of-nice-guidance/impact-of-our-guidance/nice-impact-arthritis/diagnosis-and-referral-of-inflammatory-arthritis [accessed 21 June 2023].

Notarangelo, L.D. (2010). Primary immunodeficiencies. *The Journal of Allergy and Clinical Immunology* 125 (2 Suppl 2): S182–S194.

Phatak, S.A., Aggarwal, V., Agarwal, A., and Lawrence, R.M. (2017). Antineutrophil cytoplasmic antibody (ANCA) testing: audit from a clinical immunology laboratory. *International Journal of Rheumatic Diseases* 20: 774–778.

Picard, C., Al-Herz, W., Bousfiha, A. et al. (2015). Primary immunodeficiency diseases: an update on the classification from the International Union of Immunological Societies Expert Committee for Primary Immunodeficiency 2015. *Journal of Clinical Immunology* 35 (8): 696–726.

Salvarani, C., Brown, R.D. Jr., Calamia, K.T. et al. (2008). Primary CNS vasculitis with spinal cord involvement. *Neurology* 70 (24 Pt 2): 2394–2400. https://doi.org/10.1212/01.wnl.0000314687.69681.24.

Sharma, R.K., Lovstrom, B., Gunnarsson, I., and Malmstrom, V. (2020). Proteinase 3 autoreactivity in anti-neutrophil cytoplasmic antibody-associated vasculitis—immunological versus clinical features. *Scandinavian Journal of Immunology* 92 (5): 1–9.

The Faculty of Intensive Care Medicine. (2018). *Curriculum for Training for Advanced Critical Care Practitioners – Syllabus. V1.1* [online]. Available from: www.ficm.ac.uk/media/6896 [accessed 20 June 2023].

The Intensive Care Society, Critical Care Networks – *National Nurse Leads and The National Outreach Forum*. (2022). *Advanced Critical Care Outreach Competencies* [online]. Available from: https://ics.ac.uk/asset/43B8C11B-4512-41D0-B97768FABA2C30B2 [accessed 20 June 2023].

The Royal College of Emergency Medicine. (2022). *Emergency Medicine Advanced Clinical Practitioner Curriculum 2022 (Adult)* [online]. Available from: https://rcem.ac.uk/wp-content/uploads/2022/09/ACP_Curriculum_Adult_Final_060922.pdf [accessed 20 June 2023].

Tincani, A., Rebaioli, C.B., Taglietti, M., and Shoenfeld, Y. (2006). Heart involvement in systemic lupus erythematosus, antiphospholipid syndrome and neonatal lupus. *Rheumatology* 45: 8–13.

Wang, L., Wang, F.S., and Gershwin, M.E. (2015). Human autoimmune diseases: a comprehensive update. *Journal of Internal Medicine* 278 (4): 369–395.

FURTHER READING

NICE. (2020). *Rheumatoid Arthritis in Adults: Management* [online]. Available from: www.nice.org.uk/guidance/ng100 [accessed 21 June 2023].

NICE. (2023). *Immune System Condition* [online]. Available from: www.nice.org.uk/guidance/conditions-and-diseases/blood-and-immune-system-conditions [accessed 21 June 2023].

BNF. (2023). *Immune Response* [online]. Available from: https://bnf.nice.org.uk/treatment-summaries/immune-response [accessed 21 June 2023].

CHAPTER 14

Mental Health Presentations

Clare Allabyrne

Aim

The aim of this chapter is to review the fundamental principles of working with clients with mental health issues, and more specifically, to explore mental health presentations in acute, emergency, and critical care. This should then help to elevate and advance skills particularly around assessment for these clients in line with Health Education England's (HEE) Multi-professional Advanced Clinical Practice Framework (HEE 2017). This will further enable practitioners to work confidently and effectively with these clients.

LEARNING OUTCOMES

After reading this chapter the reader will:

1. Understand the importance of their own mental health.
2. Be aware of the parity of esteem agenda, including consideration of diagnostic overshadowing and therapeutic communication.
3. Understand how to undertake a mental state examination as part of a holistic, biopsychosocial assessment.
4. Appreciate the importance of assessment including the suicidality and psychosis.
5. Understand Post-Traumatic Stress Disorder (PTSD) and Post-Intensive Care Syndrome (PICS) for patients and their families.

The Advanced Practitioner in Acute, Emergency and Critical Care, First Edition. Edited by Sadie Diamond-Fox, Barry Hill, Sonya Stone, Caroline McCrea, Natalie Gardner, and Angela Roberts.
© 2024 John Wiley & Sons Ltd. Published 2024 by John Wiley & Sons Ltd.

SELF-ASSESSMENT QUESTIONS

1. Name the different groups of antidepressants available? How do they differ from each other?
2. What is the benefit of recognising diagnostic overshadowing within mental health?
3. Can you describe the different assessment/screening tools available to you?
4. List the differentials that you would have for a 32-year-old female presenting with acute confusion.

INTRODUCTION

This chapter can only introduce the salient points for these clients very briefly and it is hoped it will offer a foundation for further and continued thinking about how they are worked with in your service(s). Before looking at specifics, it is important to understand some underlying principles when working with mental health. Mental health issues occur on a spectrum, and they affect all of us. Understanding your own mental health and your attitudes and beliefs around mental illness/disorders, is a vital component of working with those who are known to have or present with mental health issues. We all get anxious, stressed, sad, or low at times. It is the degree to which these issues impact your life that determines whether professional or other support is needed.

In working with clients with mental health issues, it is important to have a high degree of self-awareness, particularly around the impact their mental health has on you and the interaction this has with your own mental health. It is not within the scope of this chapter to go into detail as to how you can do this, but simply connecting to how you are feeling day to day. It is recognised that awareness of changes to your mental health (often, but not always, in reaction to external events) and the use of supervision in the workplace around the impact of the work is a good place to start. Working with this often disenfranchised and stigmatised group of clients' needs to come from a place of respect for them and their experiences, acknowledging the intrinsic value of their individual worth as people.

Multi-professional Framework (MPF) for Advanced Clinical Practice Guidance for Professional Development (HEE 2017)

This chapter maps to the following statements within the MPF:

1. Clinical Practice:	1.4	1.5	1.6	1.7	1.10
2. Leadership and Management:	2.1	2.10			
3. Education:	3.1				

Accreditation Considerations

This chapter maps to the following statements within the following national accreditation documents:

Curriculum for Training for Advanced Critical Care Practitioners Syllabus V1.1
(The Faculty of Intensive Care Medicine 2018)

3.2	3.13	3.15	3.16	3.17	3.21	3.22

Advanced Critical Care Outreach Competencies
(The Intensive Care Society, Critical Care Networks – National Nurse Leads and The National Outreach Forum 2022)

A1	B1

Emergency Medicine Advanced Clinical Practitioner Curriculum 2022 – Adult
(The Royal College of Emergency Medicine 2022)

MHP1	MHP2	MHP4	MHP5	MHC2	MHC8

Advanced Clinical Practice in Acute Medicine Curriculum Framework
(Health Education England 2022)

Presentations and Conditions of Acute Medicine by System/Specialty: Psychiatry & Geriatric medicine

PARITY OF ESTEEM

Understanding the individual worth of each client, means it is also important to understand the parity of esteem agenda in relation to working with clients who present with mental health issues. This is either as a singular presentation, as psychological sequelae of physical health issues, or as a comorbidity. Parity of esteem in relation to mental health was enshrined in law in the Health and Social Care Act 2012 (Baker and Gheera 2020). It describes the imperative to give equal value to both mental and physical health and originated from the mortality gap that had been identified, in which people with mental illnesses were dying 15–20 years before the general population (Centre for Mental Health 2013). There were and still are many reasons for this mortality gap, that include both discrimination and stigma, unconscious bias, and inadequate funding (RCN 2019). The improvement required to achieve parity of esteem is a big undertaking and there is much work going on to achieve this. Awareness and acknowledgement of these issues are fundamental, and further reading is recommended.

Diagnostic Overshadowing and Unconscious Bias

"The Interpretation of new information depends on what you believed beforehand."

(Sox et al. 2013)

These are vital issues to be aware of in relation to working with patients who present with mental health issues. Diagnostic overshadowing is a term that originally came from the field of Learning Disabilities. Diagnostic overshadowing has been described as the tendency to attribute all behavioural, emotional, and social issues to a certain diagnosis and other issues are not considered. It can also occur when symptoms of physical illness are attributed to the service user's mental illness. As a result, people get inadequate diagnosis or treatment of their overall condition (Jones et al. 2008). This has been a significant contributor to the previously mentioned mortality gap.

As unconscious bias can contribute to diagnostic overshadowing, it is therefore important to have some awareness of this phenomenon. Lang (2019) describes two types of bias: conscious bias, or explicit bias, which is intentional – you are aware of your attitudes and the behaviours that result from them. You may wish to revisit these in yourself. Unconscious bias, or implicit cognitive bias represents the set of biases that are unintentional; you are not aware of your attitudes and the behaviours that result from them (Lang 2019). Unconscious bias functions below the level of consciousness and is evolutionary in nature. When speed was more important than accuracy, it led to information processing shortcuts. They are associated with, amongst other things, stereotypes, social influence, and emotional and moral motivation. It requires work and self-awareness to identify them in yourself, and in others, as they can also be institutional and societal. There are numerous identified unconscious biases and I recommend you become more familiar with them, as this will allow you to identify the bias(es) that you or your colleagues/service may be most prone to. Examples of unconscious bias are ascertainment bias, whereby we see what we expect to see, like a self-fulfilling prophecy and confirmation bias, whereby we look for information that confirms what we suspect/think and disregard information that does not fit this picture. Both types of unconscious biases can be directly linked to diagnostic overshadowing.

Therapeutic Communication

Working with this client group requires an expert communicator with high-level interpersonal skills. We have already touched on self-awareness and will touch briefly here on therapeutic communication. It can be difficult to define therapeutic communication precisely; van Servellen (1997) defines therapeutic communication in this way: "interpersonal exchange, using verbal and non-verbal messages, that culminates in someone being helped to overcome stress, anxiety, fear, or other emotional experiences that cause distress" (van Servellen 1997). This could describe any client in our service(s); therefore, therapeutic communication should underpin all our communication in healthcare settings.

Epstein et al. (2000) have suggested that all therapeutic communication is based on a therapeutic relationship with the client, which is determined by your therapeutic use of self. Therapeutic use of self is the ability to use your personality consciously and in full awareness to establish a relationship with your client. Therapeutic communication always has a context. Things to be aware of in yourself and if possible, your client, are your/their values, attitudes, and beliefs; culture and spirituality; gender, social status, age, and developmental level (Epstein et al. 2000). These all determine how you both will interact and react to each other. Some techniques for therapeutic communication include open ended questioning, active listening techniques, non-verbal and verbal cues to continue the conversation, and summarising (Sharma and Gupta 2022).

MENTAL HEALTH AND ETHNICITY

MIND (2021) has identified several noteworthy facts in relation to mental health and ethnicity. Black men are more likely to have experienced a psychotic disorder in the last year compared with white men. Additionally, black people are four times more likely to be detained under the Mental Health Act than white people; older south Asian women are an at-risk group for suicide; refugees and asylum seekers are more likely to experience mental health problems than the general population, including higher rates of depression, anxiety, and PTSD. People of Indian, Pakistani, and African-Caribbean origin show higher levels of mental wellbeing than other ethnic groups. Suicidal thoughts and self-harm are less common in Asian people than Caucasian people. Mental ill-health is lower among Chinese people than in Caucasian people. The caveat to this is there may be under-reportage from some communities, perhaps in relation to stigma and different cultural perceptions of mental illness.

INVESTIGATION

There are a multitude of screening tools that can be used in the assessment of mental health issues and as a pointer to further services including specialist services, if required. The two most used screening tools, which you may be familiar with are the Generalised Anxiety Disorder 7 (GAD 7) and the Patient Health Questionnaire 9 (PHQ 9). The first screens for symptoms of anxiety and the second for depression. Depression is said to be the predominant mental health issue worldwide, followed by anxiety (Vos et al. 2013). If you or your service choose to use screening tools, you must ensure there is a clinical governance structure around them, including prescribed actions in relation to any score.

HOLISTIC ASSESSMENT IN MENTAL HEALTH

While the focus is on holistic assessment in mental health, it is important that all assessments are holistic, as a person's internal and external systems will have an impact on their health presentation(s). Therefore, the use of a biopsychosocial framework in health as a basis for assessment is a good place to start. For the purposes of this chapter, the biopsychosocial framework in the assessment of mental health will be focused on.

The biopsychosocial framework offers a basis for understanding the impact of an illness presentation, whether acute or chronic, on a person's life and how that may be expressed in the biological, psychological, and social domains. This allows for a more in-depth understanding and synthesis of the information gathered to inform the formulation of the person's difficulties and leads directly to a more targeted, specific management plan. This use of the biopsychosocial model in mental health has more recently been supported in the proposed Research Domain Criteria (RDoC) by the National Institute of Mental Health (NIMH) as part of a framework for research into mental health, which brings both physical and mental health together, rather than looking at them separately, which has previously been identified as an issue (Bolton and Gillett 2019). It may also still be an issue today and you are encouraged to think about how you/your service works holistically with both, regardless of what the presentation is.

To undertake holistic assessments in mental health within a biopsychosocial framework, it necessary to consider the following:

- Interpersonal skills and therapeutic communication
- The purpose of the assessment and any limitations of the service

Before undertaking a mental health assessment, some useful questions to think about are (Garlick and Rhodes 2011):

WHY?

This is usually based on information from the referrer and/or carers or other agencies. Consider: does the person know they have been referred? Why have they been referred to now? Triggers? What is the level of risk? Do they have a communication issue?

WHAT?

What is the aim of the assessment? Is it an emergency? Are you assessing whether the person can be treated at your service or for treatment elsewhere?

WHERE?

Where will the assessment take place? Your service, home, online? Risk in relation to environment should be considered here.

WHO?

Who should undertake the assessment? Should it be a joint assessment? Should parents/carers be there? Do you need an interpreter?

WHEN?

This is based on local definitions of timelines for emergencies: is this an emergency; is it urgent; is it routine?

(Garlick and Rhodes 2011)

Other matters to consider in a mental health assessment include:

➢ Whether your service has a local protocol for conducting a mental health assessment
➢ The reason for referral, including the person being referred/referrer/carer's perception of why they have been referred as appropriate, particularly in relation to how much you involve a carer
➢ Individual information including personal history, spiritual beliefs, and cultural practices
➢ Mental and Physical Health history, past and current, including medication
➢ Substance use
➢ Current Social Circumstances
➢ Synthesis and formulation

All mental health assessments must include a Mental State Examination (MSE). This is conducted as part of the overall assessment and has specific things to pay attention to.

Ten Point Guide to Mental State Examination

Examples of what to look for in each category from Hufton et al. (2022):

Appearance: posture, gait, dress, self-care, physical health
Behaviour: Facial expression, eye contact
Speech: Rate and flow, volume
Mood: How does the patient describe how they are feeling?
Affect: Patients' expression, what you observe?
Thoughts: What does the patient talk about? Any abnormalities?
Perception: Consider the presence of hallucinations
Cognition: An awareness of self and environment, do they know what day it is?
Insight: Do they recognise and understand their experiences? What is their understanding of the problem?
Clinical Judgement and risk assessment: Summarise your findings including an assessment of risk.
(Hufton et al. 2022)

Risk Assessment Mental Health

Risk assessment is an essential and intrinsic component of any mental health assessment.
There are three primary risks to consider in a mental health assessment:

- Risk to self (Self-harm, suicidality, neglect, substance use)
- Risk to others (violence)
- Risk from others (safeguarding). This is the risk that gets overlooked the most in a mental health presentation. It needs to be remembered that these are vulnerable adults, and safeguarding must always be considered.

Fields of Practice – Paediatrics

Brief Tips for Assessing Children and Young People (CYP) Presenting with Mental Health Issues

It is not within the scope of this chapter to go into detail here, but a young person should always be assessed in the context of their wider systems (family, school, etc.). Genograms are a particularly useful way of obtaining a history and identifying patterns. A genogram is a diagram outlining the history of the behaviour patterns (e.g. divorce or suicide) of a family over several generations (Merriam Webster 2022). They are a useful tool to engage the family with their story and to highlight both mental and physical health issues generationally.

PHARMACOLOGICAL PRINCIPLES IN MENTAL HEALTH

The same universal principles that apply for all patients should also be followed in relation to pharmacology and prescribing for patient's presenting with mental health issues. National, regional, and local guidelines should be adhered to in relation to first line prescribing of medications for psychiatric disorders.

Most psychiatric disorders use both psychosocial and pharmacological interventions. In relation, specifically, to mental health patients who use medication to help manage their illness, concordance may be an issue, especially for those whose symptoms are severe. Not taking a prescribed medication can lead to a worsening of the illness, further interventions, and admission to hospital. The input and expertise of a pharmacist is said to be a good practice when prescribing and monitoring a medication for severe mental health conditions (RPS 2022).

There are four primary types of medication for mental health problems (MIND 2022)

- Hypnotics and anxiolytics – These medications can be prescribed for severe anxiety or insomnia (difficulty getting to sleep or staying asleep).
- Antidepressants – usually for moderate to severe depression. Some are also licensed to treat anxiety, phobias, bulimia, and some physical conditions including managing severe pain.
- Antipsychotics – to reduce the symptoms of schizophrenia, schizoaffective disorder, psychosis, and sometimes severe anxiety or bipolar disorder, as well as the psychotic symptoms of a personality disorder. Some are also licensed to treat physical problems, such as persistent hiccups, problems with balance and nausea, agitation and psychotic experiences in dementia. This is only recommended if there is a risk to self or others, or in severe distress.
- Lithium and other mood stabilisers – They are licensed to be used as part of the treatment for: bipolar disorder, mania and hypomania, recurrent, severe depression, and schizoaffective disorder. Lithium, anticonvulsants, and antipsychotics are the three main types of medication which are used as mood stabilisers.

LITHIUM TOXICITY

Lithium has a very narrow therapeutic index and can be highly toxic when levels in the body fall outside that index. Therefore, lithium levels are usually measured one week after starting treatment, one week after every dose change, and weekly until levels are stable, at which point they should be measured every three months (Taylor et al. 2012; NICE 2020). All patients admitted to hospital should have their last lithium level reviewed or a new level sent.

Lithium toxicity can present with a variety of symptoms including diarrhoea, vomiting, anorexia, muscle weakness, lethargy, dizziness, ataxia, lack of coordination, tinnitus, blurred vision, coarse tremor of the extremities and lower jaw, muscle hyper-irritability, choreoathetoid movements, dysarthria, and drowsiness. Patients with severe lithium toxicity can also present with hyperreflexia and hyperextension of limbs, syncope, toxic psychosis, seizures, polyuria, renal failure, electrolyte imbalance, dehydration, circulatory failure, coma, and occasionally death (NICE 2022a).

Lithium toxicity needs rapid assessment and the risk for toxicity is higher for patients who have a pre-existing diagnosis of hypertension, diabetes, congestive heart failure, chronic renal disease, schizophrenia, or Addison's disease. If lithium toxicity is suspected, an urgent lithium level should be carried out immediately and specialist advice sought. Lithium toxicity has no specific antidote, in secondary care the treatment is supportive and lithium levels are normally rechecked every 6–12 hours. On occasion, osmotic or forced alkaline diuresis may be required (Taylor et al. 2012; Joint Formulary Committee 2019).

RED FLAGS – EMERGENCY

Current actions endangering self or others
Overdose/suicide attempt/violent aggression
Possession of a weapon

RED FLAGS – VERY HIGH RISK

Acute suicidal ideation or risk of harm to others with clear plan or means
Ongoing history of self-harm or aggression with intent
Very high-risk behaviour associated with perceptual or thought disturbance, delirium, dementia, or impaired impulse control

---

RED FLAGS – HIGH RISK

Suicidal ideation with no plan or ongoing history of suicidal ideas with possible intent
Rapidly increasing symptoms of psychosis and/or severe mood disorder
High-risk behaviour associated with perceptual or thought disturbance, delirium, dementia, or impaired impulse control
Overt/unprovoked aggression in care home or hospital ward setting
Wandering at night (community)
Vulnerable isolation or abuse

RED FLAGS – MODERATE RISK

Significant patient/carer distress associated with severe mental illness (but not suicidal)
Absent insight/early symptoms of psychosis
Resistive aggression/obstructed care delivery
Wandering (hospital) or during the day (community)
Isolation/failing carer or known situation requiring priority intervention or assessment.

THINKING ABOUT ACUTE CARE

Perception of Illness

Disease itself is pathological, and the way an individual perceives physical or emotional discomfort is not easily measured. The perception of illness might be influenced by cultural beliefs, psychological needs, or something else that may have little to do with the identified illness. An understanding of a person's illness perception is necessary both in diagnosis and in treatment.

Perception is subjective, so having a structure and language to describe their perception can be helpful to the patient. Gregory (2022) describes a way of carrying this out by focusing on four key areas:

Identity: What does the patient believe is true about the disease, what do they think the symptoms are?
Cause: What does the patient believe started it?
Timeline: The initial illness appearance. What is the trajectory? How long will it take? What will be the conclusion, is it acute or chronic?
Consequences: What does having this illness mean? Will it have a negative effect on their life?
(Gregory 2022)

Threats to health and how an individual responds to them are fundamental processes for survival and maintenance of everyday functioning. The Common-Sense Model of Illness Regulation also provides a framework to understand how threats to health are detected, processed, and managed (Hagger and Orbell 2022) and could provide a more detailed way of exploring these issues (see Figure 14.1).

Chronic Illness and Depression

People can experience symptoms of depression after being diagnosed with a medical illness. These symptoms may or may not decrease as the condition is treated, or they adjust to the impact the condition has on their life. Certain medications used to treat various illness can also trigger depression, so it is worth being mindful of this when treating your patients and/or prescribing.

Some of the risk factors for depression include a personal or family history of depression and/or a family member(s) who have died by suicide. For the purposes of this chapter, the risk factors for depression to be particularly mindful of are directly related to having another illness. For example, conditions such as Parkinson's disease and stroke cause changes in the brain. In some cases, these changes may have a direct role in depression. Illness-related anxiety and stress can also trigger symptoms of depression.

As well as the above, the same factors that increase the risk of depression in otherwise healthy people will also raise the risk in people with physical health issues/illnesses, particularly if those illnesses are chronic. Depression is common among people who have chronic illnesses such as: Alzheimer's disease,

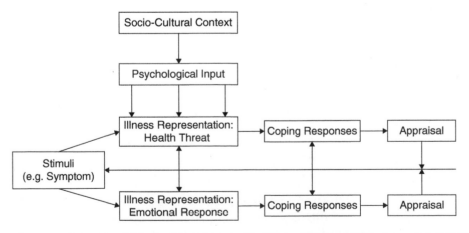

FIGURE 14.1   The common-sense model of self-regulation of health and illness (Richardson et al. (2016)).
Source: Adapted from Diefenbach and Leventhal (1996).

Autoimmune diseases, including systemic lupus erythematosus, rheumatoid arthritis, and psoriasis; Cancer, Coronary heart disease, Diabetes, Epilepsy, HIV/AIDS, Hypothyroidism, Multiple sclerosis, Parkinson's disease, Stroke (National Institute of Mental Health [NIMH] 2021).

Research suggests that people who have depression and another medical illness tend to have more severe symptoms of both illnesses (NIMH 2021). A collaborative, holistic, individualised approach to care that includes both mental and physical health care can improve a person's heath overall. Treating both conditions together can help people better manage both their depression and their chronic disease.

Case Study

Harry is a 54-year-old White Irish male.

He lives with his wife and two sons (23 and 25) and is a lorry driver, so spends long periods of time away from home and on the road.

There is a history of Type 1 diabetes in his family (father). His mother has suffered from depression and anxiety.

Harry was diagnosed with Type 1 diabetes six months ago, and is on a multiple daily injection basal-bolus insulin regimen.

Harry presents to you with the following symptoms:

Not wanting to do anything, he is beginning to miss work.

Feeling tired and sleeping a lot.

Overeating.

Irritable with his family.

- What are the differential diagnoses?
- What are the risks?
- What would your management plan be?

THINKING ABOUT EMERGENCY CARE

The Royal College of Emergency Medicine (RCEM) has produced a toolkit to improve care for those who present with mental health issues to the emergency department (ED). It is hoped and strongly recommended that this is available for all EDs and is used as a reference point for caring for these patients. Below is a list of auditable standards for individual patients from this toolkit.

1. Patients should have mental health triage by ED nurses on arrival to briefly gauge their risk of self-harm, suicide, and risk of leaving the department before assessment or treatment is complete. This is used to determine what level of observation the patient requires while in the ED.

2. Patients at medium or high risk of self-harm or suicide should be searched for objects or medication that may be used to self-harm.

3. Patients at medium or high risk of suicide or of leaving before assessment and treatment are complete should be observed closely while in the ED. There should be documented evidence of either continuous observation or intermittent checks (recommended every 15 minutes), whichever is most appropriate.

4. If a patient states that they want to leave or decline treatment, then there should be documentation of the assessment of that patient's capacity to make that decision at that time, based on a face-to-face conversation and not rely on records from previous attendances.

5. When an ED doctor reviews a patient presenting with self-harm or a primary mental health problem, they should conduct a brief risk assessment of suicide and further self-harm.

6. Previous psychiatric history should be documented in the patient's ED clinical record. This should include previous self-harm or suicide attempts, previous admissions and current treatment.

7. An MSE should be recorded in the patient's ED clinical record.

8. From the time of referral, a member of the mental health team should see the patient face-to-face and offer appropriate assistance to both patient and referrer within one hour. Full assessment may be delayed if the patient is not yet fit for assessment.

9. People who have attended the ED for help with self-harm should receive a comprehensive biopsychosocial assessment with appropriate safety or care planning at every attendance, unless a joint ED/Psychiatric written management plan states that this is not necessary or unhelpful.

10. Details of any referral or follow-up arrangements should be documented in the patient's ED notes.

Patients Presenting with Psychotic Symptoms in the ED

A person presenting with psychotic symptoms will have their own unique set of symptoms and experiences. However, there are three main symptoms associated with a psychotic episode: confused and disturbed thoughts, hallucinations, and delusions.

There are many conditions known to trigger psychosis, the most well-known being schizophrenia and bipolar disorder, as well as alcohol or substance use. However, it is important to remember in differential diagnoses that stress, anxiety, depression, and sleeplessness can also cause psychosis. There are also several physical health conditions, such as HIV and AIDS, Malaria, Syphilis, Alzheimer's Disease, Parkinson's Disease, Hypoglycaemia, Systemic Lupus Erythematosus, and Brain Tumour, that have an increased risk of causing psychosis (NHS 2019).

Case Scenario

Josie is a 17-year-old Black British female. She presents to the ED with acute pain and tenderness in her right shoulder, arm, and wrist. There is no apparent injury.

She lives at home with his mother, father, and younger sister (12).

She has no past medical history.

She does not drink alcohol, but does some 'weed', two to three 'spliffs' daily and often uses it to manage her pain.

Her hobbies are skateboarding and weight training.

She has presented before with similar complaints and injuries. These have been treated and she has been discharged with no follow up.

When you ask about the pain this time, she says it is because the government have planted an electronic device in her shoulder, so they can monitor and control her. It hurts particularly when they are activating it and that's when she comes to the ED. Lately, the implanted device has been sending her messages telling her to find people who do not have an implant and make them ready to receive one.

1. What are your differentials?
2. What clinical investigations will you do?
3. What will you ask next?
4. What are the risks?
5. How will you manage them? Now? In the longer term?
6. Will you notify her parents?
7. What are the specific issues you might need to be aware of?

Patients Presenting with Self-harm and Suicidality in EDs

For the purposes of this chapter, the National Institute of Clinical Excellence (NICE) (2022b) definition of self-harm and the National Institute of Mental Health (NIMH) (2022) definitions for suicide-related behaviour and thinking will be focused on.

NICE (2022b) defines self-harm as intentional self-poisoning or injury, irrespective of the apparent purpose. While many people who engage in self-harming behaviour do not wish to die, it is a risk factor for suicide as there is an increased risk of attempting or completing suicide, either deliberately or accidentally.

The National Institute of Mental Health (2022) defines suicide as death caused by self-directed injurious behaviour with intent to die as a result of the behaviour. A suicide attempt is a non-fatal, self-directed, potentially injurious behaviour with intent to die as a result of the behaviour. A suicide attempt might not result in injury. Suicidal ideation refers to thinking about, considering, or planning suicide (National Institute for Mental Health 2022).

The NICE guideline (NG225 2022) makes many recommendations for good practice in working with people of all ages who self-harm and it is recommended this is referred to in service(s) when planning care pathways/protocols, etc. for working with this client group.

In relation to risk assessment, it very clearly states that risk assessment tools should **NOT** be used to predict future self-harm or suicide attempts, they should **NOT** be used to decide who should or should not be offered treatment or discharged. This also precludes the use of any global risk stratification, such as low, medium, or high for the same purposes.

It is well known that the same people can present to EDs on multiple occasions following an episode of self-harm. It is important to remember to treat the person with dignity and compassion and to treat each individual episode as a singular presentation, within the context of their overall presentation, dependent on the previous history if known; to remember diagnostic overshadowing and potential cognitive bias(es); and to be mindful of the use of any punitive measures.

NICE (2022b) suggests that following a patient presenting with an episode of self-harm, the triage or initial assessor needs to assess the following:

- the severity of the injury and how urgently physical treatment is needed
- the person's emotional and mental state, and level of distress
- whether there is immediate concern about the person's safety
- whether there are any safeguarding concerns
- the person's willingness to accept medical treatment and mental healthcare

- the appropriate nursing observation level
- if they are a repeat attendee, whether the person has a care plan

It is then necessary to offer referral to age-appropriate liaison psychiatry services, or for children and young people, crisis response service (or an equivalent specialist mental health service or a suitably skilled mental health professional) as soon as possible after arrival, for a psychosocial assessment and support and assistance alongside physical healthcare (NICE 2022b).

Red Flags for Suicide

A sense of hopelessness, a feeling of entrapment, well-formed plans, perception of no social support, distressing psychotic phenomena, significant pain/physical chronic illness.

Learning Event

Lucy's Story

"I have had a severe mental illness for over 20 years, involving a nine-year inpatient stay and several shorter inpatient stays since then. I have often gone to emergency departments when I'm in crisis and have required surgery for my self-harm injuries. My experiences in emergency departments have often made my physical and mental health worse. Being acutely psychotic and in pain is hard enough, but the environment of 'safe rooms' in emergency departments often makes this harder. I'm left to sleep on the floor – sometimes for days on end – while waiting for a mental health bed. Often, I do not have access to proper food, aside from sandwiches (which I cannot eat as I need a gluten-free diet). My antidepressant medication is stopped suddenly; it's taken away from me when I arrive, and the emergency department do not stock it. This leads to horrendous withdrawal symptoms including nausea, vomiting, tremors, anxiety – and a wors-ening of my psychotic state" (CQC 2020).

Could this happen in your department? How do we learn from patient experiences?

PSYCHOLOGICAL WELLBEING IN THE CRITICAL CARE ENVIRONMENT

A stay in a critical care environment can be traumatic. It forces patients to confront their own mortality and can be quite emotive.

The main mental health presentations that are encountered in critical care are depression, PTSD, and PICS. A depression has previously been discussed, the focus will now be on PTSD, and then more specifically PICS.

POST-TRAUMATIC STRESS DISORDER

"Endless days and nights filled with strange broken sleep. A sea of fragmented menacing faces and shadows swimming through erratic beeps and bells." (Wake and Kitchiner 2013, p. 1). This is from a patient describing their experience of being in the Intensive Care Unit (ICU). These disturbing memories affected her psychological recovery and led to the development of PTSD.

There appears to be a paucity of data around the occurrence of this phenomenon and there are varying statistics about how many patients develop PTSD following a stay in ICU from 1 in 10, to 1 in 5, or around 25% (Wake and Kitchiner 2013; PTSD UK 2022; Burki 2019).

The strongest risk factor for developing PTSD after being in ICU appears to be a pre-existing diagnosis of anxiety and not necessarily the condition that necessitated the stay in ICU (Burki 2019). According to Calsavara et al. (2021), there is also a strong correlation between sepsis and psychiatric sequelae, including PTSD.

While you will not see the symptoms of PTSD necessarily manifest in the ICU, what is helpful during the ICU stay is to be mindful that any patient can develop PTSD, to be aware of the risk factors above in particular, and to consider the psychological support that is offered both during admission and especially after discharge.

POST-INTENSIVE CARE SYNDROME

Surviving the illness/incident that brought a patient to ICU is not always the end of the story. Some of those survivors will go to develop cognitive, psychological/psychiatric, and/or physical disabilities, which have been grouped together into a syndrome, PICS (see Figure 14.2). For the purposes of this chapter, the primary focus will be on the cognitive and mental health presentation of this syndrome.

The definition of PICS in this context is new and worsening symptoms in cognitive and mental health that arise in the critical care setting and persist after discharge (Rawal et al. 2017).

ICU is also known to have a psychological impact on families and carers of the patient, and this is described separately in Post-intensive Care Syndrome-Family (PICS-F). Rawal et al. (2017) describe it as the acute and chronic effects on the family psychologically during admission, discharge, and sometimes death of their loved one.

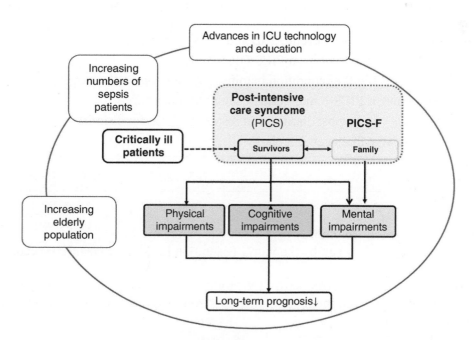

FIGURE 14.2 Conceptual framework for post-intensive care syndrome. *Source*: Inoue et al. (2019) / John Wiley & Sons.

Again, as with PTSD, it is useful to think about/assess patients on admission for any predisposing factors such as their ability to adapt to stress in the past, medication history, current mental and clinical status, and environmental and family factors (Rawal et al. 2017).

The management of PICS starts on admission requiring a multidisciplinary approach for best outcomes. The ABCDE bundle has been used with good preventive rates for PICS (Kress 2013; Morandi et al. 2011; Pandharipande et al. 2010). This consists of:

Awakening (using light or minimal sedation)
Breathing (spontaneous breathing trials)
Coordination of care and communication among various disciplines
Delirium monitoring, assessment, and management
Early ambulation in the ICU.

Amongst other additional measures, there are two others mentioned in Rawal et al. (2017) that are pertinent. The first is diary keeping either by the family, the health care professional, or both. This can be used to support both the patient and family, and there is evidence that it can decrease symptoms of PTSD (Garrouste-Orgeas et al. 2014; Jones et al. 2010). The second is further supported by evidence, and is the creation or continuation of post-ICU clinics that provide support and follow up counselling to the patient and their family (Mehlhorn et al. 2014).

Case Scenario

Nawar, an 80-year-old Asian male has been admitted to your ICU with severe symptoms of COVID-19 leading to pneumonia and acute respiratory distress syndrome requiring ventilation.

He is a widower with five children. He lives with his eldest daughter Sabira (58).

Nawar had been suffering from anxiety prior to his admission and been prescribed Citalopram.

1. What steps will you take to prevent PTSD and PICS for Nawar?
2. What steps will you take to prevent PICS-F for Sabira?
3. How will you know if either condition manifests in Nawar post discharge?
4. How will you know if PICS-F manifests in Sabira post discharge?
5. What is your duty of care post discharge in respect to these conditions?
6. What is the discharge management plan?

Learning Event

To take part in World Mental Health Day.

World Mental Health Day is run by the World Federation for Mental Health. It occurs with a different theme, each October.

Mental Health UK are partnering with ITN Productions Industry News to produce 'Play Your Part', a digital news-style programme highlighting how everyone has a role to play, when it comes to the future of mental health.

Mental Health UK states:

"The programme will raise awareness around the cost-of-living crisis and the effect this has on mental health, highlight the positive stories surrounding the recovery phase of the pandemic and showcase the changing conversations around mental health in the workplace. Showing how prevention is key, the programme will also explore the importance of educating the digital first generation at an early age, provide information to empower individuals to understand and manage their own mental health and will highlight the role of the NHS and local community initiatives."

Please consider how you and/or service can take part in this and future World Mental Health Days/Weeks.

Take Home Points
- Working with people who are mentally unwell requires a high degree of self-awareness, enhanced and advanced communication skills, as well as an understanding of the conditions, risks, and how they present.
- A multidisciplinary team approach is called for when individuals are mentally unwell.
- Good quality care for this group hinges upon a commitment to therapeutic communication, holism, person-centred care, as well as an appreciation of the value of all individuals.

REFERENCES

Baker, C and Gheera, M. (2020). *Mental Health: Achieving 'Parity of Esteem'. House of Commons Library. UK Parliament* [online]. Availbale from: parliament.uk [accessed 9 June 2022].

Bolton, D. and Gillett, G. (2019). *The Biopsychosocial Model of Health and Disease: New Philosophical and Scientific Developments* [online]. Cham (CH): Palgrave Pivot. Chapter 4, Biopsychosocial Conditions of Health and Disease. Available from: https://www.ncbi.nlm.nih.gov/books/NBK552028/ doi: 10.1007/978-3-030-11899-0_4 [29 Mar 2019].

Burki, T.K. (2019). Post-traumatic stress in the intensive care unit. *Spotlight* 7 (10): 843–844. https://doi.org/10.1016/S2213-2600(19)30203-6.

Calsavara, A.J., Costa, P.A., Nobre, V., and Teixeira, A.L. (2021). Prevalence and risk factors for post-traumatic stress, anxiety, and depression in sepsis survivors after ICU discharge. *Brazilian Journal of Psychiatry [online]* 43 (3): 269–276. https://doi.org/10.1590/1516-4446-2020-0986. PMID: 33053073; PMCID: PMC8136386. Available from: https://www.scielo.br/j/rbp/a/HHLCcD8XzVpkQLjWDCnWqWq/?lang=en [accessed 22 June 2023].

Care Quality Commission. (2020). *Assessment of Mental Health Services in Acute Trusts Programme. How Are People's Mental Health Needs Met in Acute Hospitals, and How Can this Be Improved?* [online]. Available from: http://Microsoft Word - 20201014_AMSAT_FINAL FOR WEB (cqc.org.uk) [accessed 22 June 2023].

Centre for Mental Health. (2013). *Briefing Note: Parity of Esteem.* [online]. Availble from: https://www.centreformentalhealth.org.uk/sites/default/files/2018-09/parity.pdf [accessed 17 August 2022].

Diefenbach, M.A. and Leventhal, H. (1996). The common-sense model of illness representation: theoretical and practical consideration. *Journal of Social Distress and Homelessness* 5 (1): 11–38.

Epstein, R.M., Borrell, F., and Caterina, M. (2000). Communication and mental health in primary care. In: *New Oxford Textbook of Psychiatry* (ed. M.G. Gelder, J.J. López-Ibor, and N.C. Andreasen), 2000. Oxford University Press.

Garlick, D. and Rhodes, L. (2011). *Holistic Adult Mental Health Assessment Tool.* Pavilion Publishing & Media Limited.

Garrouste-Orgeas, M., Périer, A., Mouricou, P., Grégoire, C., Bruel, C., Brochon, S., Harris, F. et al. (2014). *Writing in and Reading ICU Diaries: Qualitative Study of Families' Experience in the ICU* [online]. 9(10):e110146. ed. Available from: PLoS ONE. [PMC free article] [PubMed] [Google Scholar] [accessed 22 June 2023].

Gregory, C. (2022). What Is Illness Perception? (with pictures) [online]. Available from: wise-geek.com [accessed 8 September 2022].

Hagger, M.S. and Orbell, S. (2022). The common sense model of illness self-regulation: a conceptual review and proposed extended model. *Health Psychology Review* 16 (3): 347–377. https://doi.org/10.1080/17437199.2021.1878050.

Health Education England. (2017). *Multi-professional Framework for Advanced Clinical Practice in England* [online]. Available from: https://www.hee.nhs.uk/sites/default/files/documents/multi-professionalframeworkforadvancedclinicalpracticeinengland.pdf [accessed 22 June 2023].

Health Education England (HEE). (2022). *Advanced Clinical Practice in Acute Medicine Curriculum Framework – Credentials* [online]. Available from: https://advanced-practice.hee.nhs.uk/our-work/credentials [accessed 20 June 2023].

Hufton, F., Petch, J., Rege, S. (2022). *Ten Point Guide to Mental State Examination (MSE) in Psychiatry* [online]. Available from: psychscenehub.com [accessed 13 July 2022].

Inoue, S., Hatakeyama, J., Kondo, Y. et al. (2019). Post-intensive care syndrome: its pathophysiology, prevention, and future directions. *Acute Medicine and Surgery* 6 (3): 233–246.

Joint Formulary Committee. (2019). *British National Formulary* [online]. BMJ Group and Pharmaceutical Press. Available from: https://bnf.nice.org.uk [accessed 27 September 2022].

Jones, S., Howard, L., and Thornicroft, G. (2008). Diagnostic overshadowing: worse physical health care for people with mental illness. *Acta Psychiatric Scandinavica* 118: 169–171.

Jones, C., Bäckman, C., Capuzzo, M. et al. (2010). Intensive care diaries reduce new onset posttraumatic stress disorder following critical illness: a randomised, controlled trial. *Critical Care* 2010;14: R168. [PMC free article] [PubMed] [Google Scholar].

Kress, J.P. (2013). Sedation and mobility: changing the paradigm. *Critical Care Clinics* (2013);29: 67–75.

Lang, R. (2019). *What Is the Difference Between Conscious and Unconscious Bias?: FAQs* [online]. Available from: https://engageinlearning.com/faq/compliance/unconscious-bias/what-is-the-difference-between-conscious-and-unconscious-bias [accessed 1 August 2022].

Mehlhorn, J., Freytag, A., Schmidt, K. et al. (2014). Rehabilitation interventions for post-intensive care syndrome: a systematic review. *Critical Care Medicine* 42: 1263–1271.

Merriam Webster (2022). *Genogram.* Merriam-Webster.com Dictionary, Merriam-Webster https://www.merriam-webster.com/dictionary/genogram. Accessed 25 Aug. 2022.

MIND. (2021). *Black, Asian and Minority Ethnic (BAME) Communities* [online]. Available from: www.mental-health.org.uk/explore-mental-health/a-z-topics/black-asian-and-minority-ethnic-bame-communities [accessed 31 August 2022].

MIND. (2022). *A to Z of Psychiatric Drugs – MIND* [online]. Available from: https://www.mind.org.uk/information-support/drugs-and-treatments/medication/drug-names-a-z/ [accessed 22 June 2023].

Morandi, A., Brummel, N.E., and Ely, E.W. (2011). Sedation, delirium and mechanical ventilation: the 'ABCDE' approach. *Current Opinion in Critical Care* 2011;17: 43–49.

National Health Service. (2019). *Mental Health Conditions: Psychosis* [online]. Available from: https://www.nhs.uk/mental-health/conditions/psychosis/causes [accessed 13 September 2022].

National Institute for Health and Care Excellence (NICE). (2020). *Bipolar Disorder: Assessment and Management (NICE Guideline)* [online]. Available from: https://www.nice.org.uk/guidance/cg185 [accessed 22 June 2023].

National Institute of Mental Health. (2021). *Chronic Illness and Mental Health: Recognizing and Treating Depression* [online]. Available from: https://www.nimh.nih.gov/health/publications/chronic-illness-mental-health [accessed 22 June 2023].

National Institute of Mental Health. (2022). NIMH: Suicide [online]. Available from: nih.gov [accessed 15 September 2022].

NICE. (2022a). *Bipolar Disorder: Lithium* [online]. Available from: https://cks.nice.org.uk/topics/bipolar-disorder/prescribing-information/lithium [accessed 27 September 2022].

NICE. (2022b). *Self-harm: Assessment, Management and Preventing Recurrence* [online]. Available from: https://www.nice.org.uk/guidance/ng225 [accessed 22 June 2023].

Pandharipande, P., Banerjee, A., McGrane, S., and Ely, E.W. (2010). Liberation and animation for ventilated ICU patients: the ABCDE bundle for the back-end of critical care. *Critical Care* 14: 157.

PTSD UK. (2022). *PTSD from Being in an Intensive Care Unit* [online]. Available from: https://www.ptsduk.org/ptsd-from-being-in-an-intensive-care-unit/#:~:text=How%20common%20is%20PTSD%20among,persist%20for%20longer%20than%20this [accessed 21 September 2022].

Rawal, G., Yadav, S., and Kumar, R. (2017). Post-intensive care syndrome: an overview. *Journal of Translational Internal Medicine* 5: 90–92.

Richardson, E.M., Schuz, N., Sanderson, K. et al. (2016). Illness representations, coping, and illness outcomes in people with cancer: a systemic review and meta-analysis. *Journal of the Psychological, Social and Behavioural Dimensions of Cancer* 26 (6): 724–737.

Royal College of Nursing (2019). *Parity of esteem – delivering physical health equality for those with serious mental health needs*. Royal College of Nursing.

Royal Pharmaceutical Society. (2022). *The Role of Pharmacy in Mental Health and Wellbeing* [online]. Available from: rpharms.com [accessed 30 August 2022].

van Servellen, G. (1997). *Communication Skills for the Health Care Professional: Concepts and Techniques*. Gaithersburg, MD: Aspen.

Sharma, N. and Gupta, V. (2022). Therapeutic communication. In: *StatPearls* [online]. Treasure Island (FL): StatPearls Publishing Jan. Available from: https://www.ncbi.nlm.nih.gov/books/NBK567775 [accessed 11 August 2022].

Sox, H.C., Higgins, M.C., and Owens, D.K. (2013). *Medical Decision Making*, 2e. Oxford: Wiley-Blackwell.

Taylor, D., Paton, C., and Kapure, S. (2012). *The Maudsley Prescribing Guidelines*, 11e. London: Informa Healthcare.

The Faculty of Intensive Care Medicine. (2018). *Curriculum for Training for Advanced Critical Care Practitioners – Syllabus. V1.1* [online]. Available from: www.ficm.ac.uk/media/6896 [accessed 20 June 2023].

The Intensive Care Society, Critical Care Networks – *National Nurse Leads and The National Outreach Forum*. (2022). *Advanced Critical Care Outreach Competencies* [online]. Available from: https://ics.ac.uk/asset/43B8C11B-4512-41D0-B97768FABA2C30B2 [accessed 20 June 2023].

The Royal College of Emergency Medicine. (2022). *Emergency Medicine Advanced Clinical Practitioner Curriculum 2022 (Adult)* [online]. Available from: https://rcem.ac.uk/wp-content/uploads/2022/09/ACP_Curriculum_Adult_Final_060922.pdf [accessed 20 June 2023].

Vos, T., Barber, R.M., Bell, B. et al. (2013). Global, regional, and national incidence, prevalence, and years lived with disability for 301 acute and chronic diseases and injuries in 188 countries, 1990–2013: a systematic analysis for the Global Burden of Disease study. *The Lancet* 386 (9995): 743–800.

Wake, S. and Kitchiner, D. (2013). Post-traumatic stress disorder after intensive care. *BMJ* (2013);346: f3232. https://doi.org/10.1136/bmj.f3232.

UNIT 4

DIAGNOSIS AND MANAGEMENT IN ACUTE, EMERGENCY, AND CRITICAL CARE

CHAPTER 15

Radiology

Joe Wood, Stephanie Shea, and Tracey Maxfield

Aim

This chapter aims to provide the advanced practitioner with the knowledge to underpin safe selection of radiological investigations. It will cover the risks and benefits of the common modalities and integrate clinical context into the diagnostic decision-making process using a problem-based approach.

LEARNING OUTCOMES

After reading this chapter the reader will:

1. Be familiar with legislation and safety practices surrounding radiological investigations.
2. Understand the strengths and weaknesses of common imaging modalities including x-ray, computed tomography, and magnetic resonance imaging.
3. Recognise which clinical questions can be answered by each imaging modality and how the subsequent report impacts management plan.
4. Be able to apply clinical reasoning and context to select appropriate and proportionate radiological investigations for a variety of clinical presentations.

SELF-ASSESSMENT QUESTIONS

1. Which type of x-ray results in most radiation for the patient – knee, chest, or abdomen?
2. Which modality is most sensitive for the detection of pleural effusions – CXR or ultrasound?

The Advanced Practitioner in Acute, Emergency and Critical Care, First Edition. Edited by Sadie Diamond-Fox, Barry Hill, Sonya Stone, Caroline McCrea, Natalie Gardner, and Angela Roberts.
© 2024 John Wiley & Sons Ltd. Published 2024 by John Wiley & Sons Ltd.

3. When might an MRI be deemed an urgent or emergency investigation?
4. Radiation in pregnancy – what might be your approach to explaining risk versus benefit to the patient?
5. A colleague advises you to request a chest x-ray to assess for possible rib fractures. Is this an appropriate request?

Multi-professional Framework (MPF) for Advanced Clinical Practice in England (HEE 2017)

1.1	1.2	1.3	1.6	1.8	1.4	1.5	1.8
2.3	2.4						

Accreditation Considerations

This chapter maps to the following statements within the following national accreditation documents:

Curriculum for Training for Advanced Critical Care Practitioners Syllabus V1.1
(The Faculty of Intensive Care Medicine 2018)

2.3

Advanced Critical Care Outreach Competencies
(The Intensive Care Society, Critical Care Networks – National Nurse Leads and The National Outreach Forum 2022)

A4

Emergency Medicine Advanced Clinical Practitioner Curriculum 2022 – Adult
(The Royal College of Emergency Medicine 2022)

SLO1	SLO3	SLO4

Advanced Clinical Practice in Acute Medicine Curriculum Framework
(Health Education England 2022)

- Specialty Clinical CiPs: 2

INTRODUCTION

Radiology is a branch of clinical practice that uses imaging technology to diagnose and treat disease. Radiology may be divided into two different areas, including diagnostic radiology and interventional radiology.

There are several Ionising Radiation (Medical Exposure) Regulations (IR[ME]R) Considerations to be made.

IONISING RADIATION (MEDICAL EXPOSURE) REGULATIONS (IR[ME]R) CONSIDERATIONS

The ionising radiation (medical exposure) regulations aim to protect patients by ensuring radiation is used safely. They outline the responsibilities of radiation protection and basic safety standards for the employer, referrer, practitioner, and operator including:

- Minimising unintended, excessive, or incorrect medical exposure
- Justifying each exposure to ensure the benefits outweigh the risks
- Optimising diagnostic doses to ensure they are 'as low as reasonably practicable' for their intended use.

As a non-medical referrer, ensure that you comply with national and local competencies and remain up to date on the advanced practice register held by your employer. Table 15.1 compares the radiation dose for commonly ordered investigations. Dose, urgency, pre-test probability, and diagnostic yield should all contribute to your decision-making when choosing the most appropriate imaging modality (see Table 15.2).

TABLE 15.1   Radiation doses for commonly ordered investigations in acute care.

Examination	Typical dose (mSV)	Equivalent period of natural background radiation for context
XR limbs or joints	<0.01	<1.5 days
XR teeth (bitewing)	<0.01	<1.5 days
XR PA chest	0.014	3 days
XR neck (cervical spine)	0.08	2 weeks
XR hip	0.3	7 weeks
XR thoracic spine, abdomen, pelvis	0.7	4 months
XR lumbar spine	1.3	7 months
CT head scan	1.4	1 year
CT thorax	6.6	3.6 years
CT abdomen or pelvis	10	4.5 years

Source: Adapted from https://www.gov.uk/government/publications/ionising-radiation-dose-comparisons/ionising-radiation-dose-comparisons.

TABLE 15.2   Pros and cons of key imaging modalities.

	+	−
CT	Quick, detailed, available 24/7 3d reconstruction, excellent anatomical definition	Radiation Soft tissue definition less than MRI
MRI	No radiation Multiple anatomic planes Most detailed assessment of soft tissues Better assessment of brainstem (avoids artefacts of CT)	Prolonged study times May not be available out of hours Bony differentiation worse than CT Implanted devices must be MRI safe Long-term effects on foetus are not known so ideally should delay in pregnancy.
US	Good for soft tissue and vascular assessments	Formal ultrasound may not be available out of hours May have less utility in trauma setting where subcutaneous emphysema impacts image acquisition.

The strengths and weaknesses of each key modality need to be considered in conjunction with the patient's history (see Table 15.2). The patient's condition and presentation will determine the direction and type of investigation required. Table 15.3 highlights some of the specialist imagery that can be done for patients with cardiological conditions, whilst Table 15.4 describes tests that focus on musculoskeletal presentations.

GYNAECOLOGY

Abdominal pain is a common acute presentation. In women, diagnosing the cause is challenging as gynaecological conditions have non-specific symptoms and can be mistaken for other intra-abdominal pathology. Despite these difficulties, rapid radiological imaging is vital due to the significant risk of bleeding/infection and to preserve fertility (Impey and Child 2016). Identifying the correct modality depends on the category of acute gynaecological pathology, which can be divided into three main categories (see Table 15.5).

Ultrasound is the primary modality (abdominal or transvaginal) utilised when caring for the stable patient. Access to this out of hours is often restricted and inadequate views cannot rule out pathology. This needs to be considered when revising your clinical question. Computerised tomography (CT) scans in the emergency setting for non-pregnant patients, can identify signs of hemoperitoneum, large pelvic lesions, and exclude non-gynaecological causes (Roche et al. 2012). The dual-CT setting reduces radiation exposure, particularly key for younger patients (Marin et al. 2014). For ongoing gynaecological management, MRI is used to confirm the presence of endometriosis and the extent of the disease.

UROLOGY

Acute urinary retention is a recognised urological emergency. It is easily managed using a readily available ultrasound bladder scan device, which is non-invasive and requires minimal training. Renal ultrasound may reveal associated hydronephrosis or possible obstructive cause (Hughes and Cruickshank 2011).

TABLE 15.3 Imaging investigations for cardiac presentations.

	Description	Indication	Benefits/rationale
Echocardiogram	Dynamic images of the moving heart using transoesophageal or transthoracic ultrasound.	• Aortic dissection • Aortic/mitral valve regurgitation • Determining systolic and/or diastolic ventricular impairment • Pericardial effusion • Valvular disease • Endocarditis: valvular vegetation (>2 mm), aortic root abscess • Hypertrophic cardiomyopathy	• Assessment of anatomy • Heart failure cause, to assist in management. • Plan intervention • Non-invasive • Can be performed at bedside if patient is unwell
Angiography	Imaging of cardiac anatomy and blood flow using contrast agent under fluoroscopic control.	• Coronary artery disease: diagnostic/therapeutic. • STEMI • Valvular disease. • Cardiomyopathy; congenital heart disease; biopsy • Pericardial disease	• For interventional procedures such as angioplasty, valvuloplasty, biopsy, septal defect correction • Electrophysiology studies • Radiofrequency ablation • Determine types and origins of arrhythmia; monitor response to pharmacological intervention
Cardiac CT	Coronary angiography without catheterisation	• Less invasive than angiography • Coronary calcium score calculation • Accurate assessment of coronary artery disease with >50% stenosis • Aortic dissection: shows flap and true and false lumen • Assessment of chronic chest pain.	• Low-dose radiation • Accessible, relatively quick
Cardiac MRI	Radiation free imaging Detailed cardiac structure and functionality Best for diseases affecting myocardium	• Previous MI • Cardiac myopathy • Check if pacemaker in situ and discuss with Radiology prior to requesting	• Contrast agent used to assess ischemia • Can detect subtle pathological changes in anatomy

TABLE 15.4   Imaging investigations for musculoskeletal presentations.

	Presentation	Indication	Considerations
Plain film (X-ray)	Minor injury to axial or appendicular skeleton Secondary survey targeting injuries after polytrauma imaging Detection of subcutaneous/ingested foreign bodies (dependent on radiopacity) Non-accidental injury (all patient groups)	Post intervention imaging such as reduction of fractures and dislocations. Detection of joint effusions and instability prior to more detailed imaging To inform more detailed imaging requests if clinically appropriate	Any neurovascular injury of the extremity must be assessed and managed prior to XR imaging Ensure analgesia optimisation to ensure patient comfort and subsequent best images possible
CT	Major trauma Acute onset symptoms of suspected MSK origin Skeletal disease progression	Haemodynamic instability secondary to trauma Suspected intra-abdominal fluid detected on focused ultrasound scan If initial plain films detect significant trauma	Access required to CT scanning within 60 minutes of trauma and reporting within 60 minutes of the scan Availability of interventional radiologist within 60 minutes of referral
MRI	Cauda equina syndrome Spinal cord compression Myeloproliferative disorders Spondylodiscitis Suspected occult fracture.	Acute neurological emergencies requiring urgent diagnosis and treatment Malignancy, intervertebral disc prolapse and trauma Acute or chronic symptoms of known disease Assist future management and referrals	Discussion with senior clinician and on-call radiologist to arrange urgent MRI if indicated Early referral to specialist tertiary centre after comprehensive initial assessment

TABLE 15.5   Gynaecological pathologies.

Non-pregnant	Pregnant women	Post-partum
Ovarian cyst (haemorrhagic or functional) Rupture of ovarian tumours Luteal body bleeding Ovarian/Adnexal torsion Pelvic inflammatory disease Tubo-ovarian abscesses Coital laceration Retained tampons/foreign bodies	Miscarriage (threatened or missed) Ectopic pregnancy Ischaemia of myoma Torsion of enlarged adnexa Abruption	Ovarian vein thrombosis Post-partum Haemorrhage Uterine infection

Source: Adapted from Doumouchtsis and Arulkumaran (2016).

TABLE 15.6 Imaging investigations for urological presentations.

Clinical presentation	Differential diagnosis	Imaging modalities
Scrotal pain and swelling	Testicular torsion Epididymitis Strangulated inguinal hernia Orchitis Hydrocele	Doppler ultrasound Scrotal US
Flank pain ± infection	Renal colic Pyelonephritis	CT KUB Intravenous urography (IVU) (if CT unavailable) USS/Doppler (pregnancy or renal disease)
Haematuria (microscopic or macroscopic)	Renal colic Renal disease Urinary tract infection Renal or bladder cancer Benign prostatic hyperplasia	CT KUB Renal tract US Cystography
Trauma	Ruptured urethra Renal laceration Intra or extraperitoneal bladder rupture	CT cystography

Source: Adapted from Wyatt et al. (2012).

To avoid misdiagnosis of urological emergencies, a detailed history of symptoms and examination is crucial to identify the precise radiological investigation (see Table 15.6). Further, imaging requires highly skilled users and advanced methods.

VASCULAR

Deep Vein Thrombosis (DVT)

Ultrasound is the first-line investigation for suspected Deep Vein Thrombosis (DVT) with a sensitivity and specificity of approximately 95% (Mettler 2018). Department protocols vary, but generally vessels are visualised from the iliacs proximally to the deep calf veins distally, including the femoral and popliteal vessels in between. Occasionally, ultrasound may also be ordered to risk stratify those with confirmed pulmonary embolism (PE) and guide intervention.

Acute Limb Ischaemia

CT angiogram uses IV contrast agent to evaluate the vascular system. It is useful to map vasculature to assess severity of stenosis or vessel occlusion and plan intervention – angioplasty/stenting, etc. (Jongkind et al. 2022). Drawbacks include radiation and the risk of contrast-induced nephropathy.

Magnetic resonance angiography (MRA) avoids these but cannot be used in those with certain implanted devices, such as cochlear implants and pacemakers. Digital subtraction angiography is considered gold standard but is invasive and hence often not first-line (Olinic et al. 2019).

Aortic Pathologies

Suspicious findings on chest x-ray include a prominent aorta in the left paratracheal region, notching of inferior aspect of ribs and a widened mediastinum. Detailed evaluation can be achieved by contrast-enhanced CT (Bhave et al. 2018). Transoesophageal echocardiography may also be utilised where available. If abdominal aortic aneurysm is suspected, ultrasound offers an effective bedside screening tool (Fraleigh and Duff 2022). In symptomatic patients or those suggestive of leak or rupture, urgent surgical opinion should be sought.

RESPIRATORY

CXR

Chest x-rays will be performed on almost all patients presenting with acute shortness of breath (SOB). It is important to have a structured approach to interpretation (see Table 15.7) as distribution of chest x-ray findings will help guide likely diagnosis and inform necessity of alternate imaging modalities (see Table 15.8).

Red Flag: Where history, examination, and observation point towards tension pneumothorax (loss of air entry on affected side, deviated trachea, tachycardia, hypotension), treatment should not be delayed for imaging confirmation.

LUNG ULTRASOUND

Lung ultrasound is particularly useful in identifying pleural fluid and identifying the position of the diaphragm to ensure safe thoracocentesis when indicated (Demi et al. 2023). It is also helpful in evaluation of consolidation and pulmonary oedema (covered in Chapter 7).

TABLE 15.7   Structured approach to x-ray interpretation.

D	Details	Date, time, name, type of film (AP versus PA)
R	RIPE	Rotation, inspiration, picture (are all areas of interest included), exposure
S	Soft tissues	Ribs, sternum, clavicles, breast shadows, calcifications, surgical emphysema
A	Airway	Trachea, mediastinal width, aortic knuckle
B	Breathing	Lung field outlines, symmetry, pleura
C	Circulation	Heart size, shape, and borders
D	Diaphragm	Shape, contour, relative heights, costophrenic angles
E	Extras	Tubes, lines, pacemakers

TABLE 15.8   Findings and investigations in common respiratory pathologies.

Potential diagnosis	CXR findings	Other imaging/investigations
Pulmonary oedema	Bilateral, widespread opacities, upper lobe diversion, Kerley B lines, cardiomegaly, or signs of cardiac devices/surgery if cardiogenic.	Echocardiography Fluid assessment Lung ultrasound: B line distribution BNP
Pleural effusion	Blunting of costophrenic angle, meniscus sign	Lung ultrasound (most sensitive)
Right lower lobe pneumonia	Opacity obscuring right hemidiaphragm	Lung ultrasound
Right middle lobe pneumonia	Opacity obscuring right heart border	Lung ultrasound
Left upper lobe consolidation	Opacity obscuring left heart border	Lung ultrasound
Pneumothorax/ bullae	Loss of lung markings	CT if non-resolving with initial intervention
Left lower lobe consolidation	Opacity obscuring left hemidiaphragm	Lung ultrasound
Lobar collapse	Loss of volume with mediastinal shift Silhouette signs	Consider bronchoscopy CT if non-resolving (e.g. is the cause of collapse and obstructing mass)
Possible aortic pathology	Widened mediastinum >8 cm at level of aortic arch	CT in right clinical context
Pneumomediastinum	Lucency along aortic arch/cardiac border	CT

APPROACH TO PULMONARY EMBOLISM

Chest x-rays are neither sensitive nor specific for PE but may help to exclude differential diagnoses (Moore et al. 2018). History, physical exam, and use of pre-test probability are key when considering how to investigate PE. Scores such as Wells and Geneva can guide investigation and subsequent management (Duffett et al. 2020). In the stable patient, where nuclear medicine scans are available, ventilation/perfusion (V/Q) scans can be performed to assess the flow of blood and air within the lungs. This involves inhalation of specialised gas and IV injection of a labelled solution. Images are then produced for ventilation and perfusion stages, respectively. If this demonstrates a perfusion defect without a corresponding ventilation defect, this is concerning for PE (Bajc et al. 2009). In pregnancy V/Q may be the modality of choice owing to reduced ionising radiation to breast tissue when compared to CT (Tester et al. 2020). Although evidence is conflicting, interobserver reliability has been questioned, and it is generally accepted that both sensitivity and specificity of this modality is reduced in co-existing lung disease such as COPD (Chowdhury 2017). Thus, Computed Tomography pulmonary angiography (CTPA) is often preferred in the acute setting and carries a sensitivity of over 83% (Hepburn-Brown et al. 2019) Classic CT features of PE include filling defect in the pulmonary arterial tree, enlarged pulmonary trunk and right heart (features of right heart strain), wedge lung infarction, and hypoperfusion of lung in the distribution of the occluded vessel.

SEVERE/ATYPICAL OR UNRESOLVING SYMPTOMS

Urgent plain CT of the chest alone is rarely warranted outside of the trauma setting. If, however, initial chest x-ray shows features of concern (mass, total collapse, bullae, tethered lung, upper lobe pathologies), or presentation is atypical or unresolving, CT may be valuable to further characterise pathology (Whiting et al. 2015).

Case Study – Acute Shortness of Breath

- History: three-day history of worsening SOB, right-sided chest pain and productive green sputum.
- Medical History: hypertension, no other formal diagnoses, 20 pack year history.
- Examination: crepitations throughout right lung on auscultation, dullness to percussion right base, left lung clear, no peripheral stigmata of lung disease, no swelling of the limbs, sharp chest pain reproducible on deep inspiration and localised laterally on chest wall.
- Investigations: raised inflammatory markers, D-dimer of 200, troponin of 6, ECG sinus tachycardia.
- Choice of imaging: Chest x-ray ordered initially, which showed right basal opacification without loss of volume, tracheal or mediastinal shift. Lung ultrasound subsequently ruled out significant pleural fluid.
- Diagnosis and rationale: chest pain unlikely to be cardiac in nature given negative troponin, lack of ECG changes and described character, location, and reproducibility, therefore most likely source is pleural. Patient medical history, negative D-dimer and lack of any peripheral signs of DVT make PE very unlikely in this instance and thus CTPA is not warranted. Chest x-ray shows right basal pathology with differential being pneumonia or effusion. Although very large effusions may be easy to identify on x-ray, lung ultrasound is more sensitive at identifying smaller volumes. Here no fluid was identified and thus the likely diagnosis is a right-sided pneumonia.

NEUROLOGY

Acute Reduction in Consciousness

Where there is suspicion of raised intracranial pressure or an intracranial event, CT is preferred in the acute phase due to the speed of image acquisition and widespread out-of-hours availability. However, MRI is superior to CT for detecting haemorrhage in subacute and chronic phases and parenchymal shearing injuries (Mettler 2018). Diffusion weighted MRI may be useful when differentiating acute from chronic infarcts. In evaluation of brain tumours, MRI with gadolinium is the investigation of choice. Table 15.9 details first-line investigations for suspected neurological presentations.

STROKE/TRANSIENT ISCHAEMIC ATTACK

Non-contrast CT head is the initial investigation of choice for haemorrhagic stroke with a sensitivity of 98% within 24 hours of symptoms (Chan 2013) although early ischaemic strokes may be difficult to visualise. MRI can easily detect acute ischaemic strokes but is rarely used in the emergency setting as

TABLE 15.9   Imaging investigations for neurological pathologies.

Suspected pathology/presentation	Imaging modality
Acute stroke	Non-contrast CT (or MRI if available)
Acute haemorrhage	Non-contrast CT
Major head trauma	CT initially/MRI later if stable
Acute severe headache	Non-contrast CT
Seizure	CT acutely/MRI with and without contrast later especially if cause not found
Venous sinus thrombus	CT with contrast
Unexplained confusion	CT without contrast/MRI if sustained
Meningitis/encephalitis	Consider CT with contrast
Carotid/vertebral dissection/aneurysm	CT angiogram
Tumour or metastases	MRI ± contrast
Intracranial infection	MRI

CT can adequately rule out haemorrhage (a contraindication for anticoagulation for ischaemic stroke management) (Mendelson and Prabhakaran 2021). CT venograms may visualise venous sinus thrombosis (Ghoneim et al. 2020). In cases of transient ischaemic attack (TIA), carotid Dopplers may help risk stratify further events (Rudkin et al. 2018) and guide surgical intervention (endarterectomy). Where timing of symptoms is unclear, a CT perfusion scan may help determine if there is any reversible damage (salvageable brain tissue) (Demeestere et al. 2020).

HEAD INJURY/TRAUMA

Facial and cervical spine x-rays lack sensitivity and are difficult to interpret with multiple pitfalls and thus there should be a low threshold for CT evaluation (Joseph et al. 2014). Linear fractures are represented by a lucent line; depressed fractures are often seen as dense white areas (due to overlapped bone fragments). Where fractures are depressed, CT is indicated. Basilar skull fractures may lead to tears in dura mater with cerebrospinal fluid (CSF) leak and again require further imaging. Where head injury is substantial or associated with reduced consciousness non-contrast CT of the head and neck will likely be the first-line investigations to rule out significant intracranial pathology and assess bone cortex abnormalities (Rincon et al. 2016). Initial evaluation of the brain in the emergency setting is to detect mass effect or blood (see Table 15.10).

Red Flag: If CT head scan is normal within six hours of symptom onset but subarachnoid haemorrhage is still suspected, consider consented lumbar puncture for exclusion (Kameda-Smith et al. 2021).

CONFUSION/ENCEPHALITIS

Approach to acute confusion or personality change can be extremely nuanced. While CT and MRI can highlight pathologies which may cause this presentation, often other investigations such as blood tests and lumbar punctures alongside appropriate antimicrobial or antiviral therapy are often instigated prior

TABLE 15.10 CT findings in neurological pathologies.

Pathology	CT findings
Haemorrhage	High density (bright) if acute (approx. 1–7 days), reducing density over few days to weeks, hypodense after 1 month (chronic)
EDH	Lentiform (bi-convex lens shape), rarely crosses sutures, often associated with temporal skull fracture
SDH	Crescentic, usually crosses sutures, does not cross midline
SAH	Blood in CSF spaces/ventricles, CT angiogram often follows plain CT
ICH	Intra-axial/parenchymal blood
Infarct	Low density in vascular territory – cytotoxic oedema affects both grey and white mater
Tumour	Usually enhancing focal parenchymal lesion, vasogenic oedema
Mass effect	Gyral expansion, crowding of foramen magnum, effacement of ventricles and or CSF spaces

Source: Adapted from Holmes and Misra (2017).

TABLE 15.11 National Institute of Health and Care Excellence (NICE) Guidance (2014) on imaging in head injuries.

CT within 1 hour	CT within 8 hours
GCS <13 on initial assessment OR GCS <15 2 hours after injury	Age >65
Suspected open or depressed skull fracture	History of bleeding or clotting disorders
Signs of basal skull fracture (haemotympanum, Battle's sign, panda eyes, CSF leak from ears or nose)	Dangerous mechanism of injury (fall from >1 m or 5 stairs, ejected from motor vehicle, pedestrian, or cyclist versus motor vehicle)
Post-traumatic seizure	>30 minutes retrograde amnesia
Focal neurological deficit	
Repeated vomiting	

to such imaging. If a central cause of confusion is suspected, CT head is often the first-line investigation. Outside of the acute phase, MRI may be useful in determining ongoing inflammation or hypoxic brain injuries (Hijazi et al. 2018) (see Table 15.11).

CASE STUDY – COLLAPSE AND REDUCED GCS

- Presentation – 58-year-old found collapsed by Wife, breathing but not rousable, bruising to left temple.
- Medical History – atrial fibrillation on warfarin, diabetic, epilepsy, normally GCS 15, and fully independent.
- Examination – pupils equal and reactive to light, GCS 10/15, normal reflexes, slight increase in flexor tone, no facial asymmetry, no clonus.

- Investigations – blood sugars 7, INR 2.1, troponin normal, other bloods normal, ECG sinus 65 bpm, urinary tox-screen negative, blood gas shows raised lactate of 5.
- Imaging choice – CT head performed due to evidence of head injury and additional risk factor of anticoagulation and raised INR, this showed no acute intracranial pathology. Patient then had a self-terminating seizure of 30 seconds. Repeat CT was not warranted but patient was loaded on IV anti-epileptics and supported with supplemental oxygen and cardiac monitoring. GCS slowly improved to 14/15 with some residual confusion. Repeat blood gas showed a normalised lactate.
- Diagnosis – in this case the patient was likely post-ictal from epileptic related seizures; however, alternate causes needed to be addressed. Given risk factors and evidence of head injury, CT head was a proportionate first-line investigation to rule out immediately life-threatening pathologies. If the patient continued to seize, escalation of medical management would be appropriate, and potential intubation if in status epilepticus. If ongoing reduced GCS and seizures, MRI could be considered to investigate cause alongside investigations such as EEG.

GASTROINTESTINAL

Abdominal pain may be secondary to a vast array of pathologies and first-line imaging differs accordingly (see Table 15.12). Abdominal x-ray may be useful in suggesting bowel obstruction or toxic megacolon, but CT is often the preferred modality – allowing accurate assessment of soft tissues (Cartwright and Knudson 2015). Erect CXR is useful in detecting free air within the abdomen to suggest perforation. Ultrasound of the abdomen may also be extremely useful (and is preferred in suspected cholecystitis and biliary colic) but is often not available out of hours (Abdolrazaghnejad et al. 2019). Use of point of care abdominal ultrasound for abdominal aortic aneurysms is now widespread in the emergency setting. Contrast-enhanced CT is the mainstay of acute abdominal imaging. In cases of abdominal trauma with haemodynamic instability, immediate surgical input should be considered prior to imaging.

TABLE 15.12   Imaging investigations in abdominal presentations.

Suspected pathology	Modality
Appendicitis	US/CT
Aneurysm	CT
Pancreatitis	US (gallstones)/CT if not improving
Bowel obstruction	CT (AXR if stable)
Bowel perforation	Erect CXR, CT
Cholecystitis	US
Renal calculi	CT KUB
Ectopic pregnancy	US

Source: Adapted from Cartwright and Knudson (2015).

CASE STUDY – ABDOMINAL PAIN

- 40-year-old female, 1/52 history of abdominal pain related to eating meals.
- Past history: high cholesterol, HTN, BMI 37, type 2 diabetes.
- Abdominal exam – right upper quadrant pain, tender at Murphy's point.
- Investigations – CRP 130, WCC 14, ALP 300 ALT 35, amylase normal, cardiovascularly stable.
- Imaging choice – abdominal ultrasound revealed an inflamed gallbladder with multiple gallstones, with dilated common bile duct suggestive of obstruction, no other abnormality was identified.
- Diagnosis and further imaging – acute cholecystitis and choledocholithiasis requiring follow-up with therapeutic endoscopic retrograde cholangiopancreatography (ERCP). General surgical opinion or percutaneous drainage via interventional radiology may also be considered.
- Points to consider – if diagnosis was not apparent from ultrasound OR if the same patient presented with haemodynamic compromise, then emergent CT would be preferred. ERCP in itself has many risks and may lead to worsening clinical picture with development of pancreatitis amongst others.

Case Study

- Presenting Complaint – 87-year-old man who sustained a fall while walking. He is complaining of right hip pain and unable to weight-bear.
- Past Medical History – Type 2 diabetic on metformin and PRN co-codamol for osteoarthritis pain. Lives independently and mobilises with a stick.
- Examination – Tender over right greater trochanter on palpation. Unable to weight-bear or straight leg raise on the right side. No obvious shortening/rotation. Pedal pulse present.
- Imaging Choice – X-ray of pelvis and right hip with lateral/AP views. Severe osteoarthritis of the hip joint and presence of an old inferior pubic Rami fracture. No disruption to Shenton's line and no obvious sign of a fracture on close inspection.
- Diagnosis – After sufficient pain relief, you re-examine to find the clinical signs of a neck or femur fracture remain but no sign on the x-ray. In the presence of ongoing pain and clinical uncertainty, the views are insufficient to rule out a possible occult fracture. In line with NICE guidelines, a CT scan is ordered and discussed with the orthopaedic team.
- Learning Points:
  - Interpretation of x-rays in older adults becomes more challenging with age. It is user dependant and complicated by the presence of osteoarthritis (Kessler and Dean 2017).
  - Non-displaced hip fractures may not be visible on an initial x-ray and the risk of complications requires a timely intervention. Adopt a safe radiological approach by maintaining a high index of suspicion and low threshold for advanced imaging (NICE 2017).
  - Important to focus on the findings of the physical examination and to use radiological modalities as an adjunct to answer your clinical question.

Case Study

- Presenting Complaint – 64-year-old female presents to the emergency department with a 7-day history of left-sided abdominal pain and constipation. In the last 48 hours she has developed acute vomiting, with severe abdominal pain and distension.
- Past Medical History – She is prescribed omeprazole for gastric reflux and lives independently. She has a history of extensive abdominal surgery including laparotomy for a perforated appendix, hysterectomy, and x2 hernia repairs.
- Examination – Initial observations show signs of sepsis and bloods indicate raised inflammatory markers. Her abdomen is rigid/tender globally, and bowel sounds are absent.
- Imaging Choice – She is clinically unwell requiring fluid resuscitation and sepsis treatment. An erect chest and abdominal x-ray at the bedside are appropriate, especially if CT imaging is not readily available. This will provide an initial clinical impression alongside ongoing observation for signs of large or small bowel obstruction (Day and Fordyce 2020). Plain x-rays have limitations however – subtle signs can be missed dependant on the proficiency of the interpreter. In a critically unwell patient with a surgical abdomen, CT would be the 'gold standard' (Royal College of Surgeons 2017). CT provides further detail to confirm the diagnosis and identify the underlying cause. Consider how the chosen modality will support IR(ME)R principles and answer your clinical question.
- Diagnosis and Rationale – History of abdominal pain, constipation, and extensive surgical operations has led to the likely presence of adhesions causing a bowel obstruction. She is clinical unwell, with signs of sepsis and at high risk of perforation. CT would provide further detail and aid a surgical intervention. However, in some cases, CT may not be sensitive to identifying more unusual diagnoses such as mesenteric ischaemia. Early discussions with the radiologist will establish the most appropriate first-line scan for prompt diagnosis and avoid unnecessary exposure (Fitzpatrick et al. 2020). Remember to treat the patient, not the scan.

PHARMACOLOGY

Contrast Reactions

Most CT IV contrasts are iodinated and primarily excreted by the kidneys. For MRI, gadolinium is the most common; this crosses the placenta and is again primarily excreted by the kidneys. They can be nephrotoxic and induce acute tubular necrosis, and, in the case of gadolinium, nephrogenic systemic fibrosis (especially in those already dialysis dependent). Contrast induced nephropathy is defined as acute renal impairment within three days of contrast without another cause. Risk factors are pre-existing renal disease, diabetes, myeloma, other allergies/atopy, and nephrotoxic medications (Shams and Mayrovitz 2021). Although published evidence is conflicting, contrast-induced nephropathy in those with eGFR less than 30 is generally considered high risk (Rudnick et al. 2020); hence, risk must be carefully weighed against clinical benefit for each patient. Consider PO/IV hydration, withholding nephrotoxics and monitoring renal function post scan in the at-risk patient. Discuss options with the duty radiologist to see if your clinical question can be answered without contrast or with an alternate modality. In cases of severe pre-existing renal impairment, consider a discussion with critical care to establish if haemodialysis would be considered if necessary.

Other reactions range from mild (metallic taste in the mouth, flushing, nausea, urticaria) to severe (wheeze, laryngospasm, anaphylaxis). These may be immediate or delayed. Asthmatics and those with renal impairment are at higher risk of reaction. Consider pre-emptive prescription of antihistamine or steroids and follow local policies if reaction is confirmed.

NUCLEAR MEDICINE

Radiopharmaceuticals essentially make patients radioactive for a short period of time and thus hospital staff and patients must be advised of how to manage this risk. Isolation is advised, if practical, as well as avoiding prolonged exposure or contact with children and pregnant women. The British Nuclear Medicine Society offer further guidance.

SEDATION

Compliance with positioning for image acquisition is often challenging, especially in an acutely confused patient. This can mean patients are exposed to radiation, with the resulting images being non-diagnostic due to poor image quality or movement artefacts. When there are concerns about patient tolerance or compliance, alternative imaging modalities need to be considered. If these will not answer your question and the decision/scan cannot be reasonably delayed to address pain, confusion, etc., then sedation or anxiolytics can be considered. This should be discussed with a senior clinician and anaesthetist as subsequent airway support may be required.

DRUG HISTORY

A thorough drug history can help risk stratify patients and guide imaging choice. Anticoagulation is of particular importance in the case of head injuries.

LEARNING EVENTS

Unexpected Pathology

You are caring for a 28-year-old male who was involved in a road traffic collision while riding his electric scooter. He was not wearing a helmet and sustained a head injury. Witnesses reported a loss of consciousness, and he is amnesic to events. He is complaining of a persistent headache and had recurrent episodes of vomiting, so a CT head scan is requested under NICE guidance. You receive a call from the on-call radiologist who reports no acute traumatic pathology. However, there is an incidental finding of a space occupying lesion with mass effect and indicative of a primary malignancy. They recommend a neuro-surgical opinion.

Consider the following:

1. What would be your next steps?
2. How would you approach this conversation?

Access to extensive advanced imaging modalities provides us with rapid detection of acute pathology. However, in a small number of cases, it may identify an unexpected or incidental finding which is unrelated to the presenting complaint (Royal College of Radiologists 2018). Breaking bad news can be challenging, especially with limited information and when the imaging may not provide a conclusive result as it was for a different purpose. For example, it may identify the presence of malignancy but not provide any further detail. However, it is the clinician's responsibility to communicate these results to the patient in a timely and sensitive manner, ensuring an open and honest conversation of the findings and your understanding including any limitations. This can be difficult to do, so you may require senior support. It is key to provide a clear follow up plan and appropriate safety net advice.

DELAYED REPORTING

You are managing a caseload of patients on a busy assessment unit. A 19-year-old male presents with sudden onset of left-sided pleuritic chest pain and mild SOB. He reports the pain is worse on deep inspiration and occurred after carrying heavy boxes. On initial examination he appears comfortable and SpO2 97% on air. On auscultation you hear decreased breath sounds at the left base. You request a chest x-ray and ask the nursing staff to inform you once this has been done. The unit becomes busy, and a few hours have passed. You reassess the patient who looks very unwell, acutely SOB and SpO2 88% on air. When you review the x-ray, it shows a left sided pneumothorax.

Consider the following:

1. What are your initial steps?
2. What are the learning points?
3. How would you approach the conversation?

The use of X-rays in the acute setting often relies on interpretation at the point of care and the user being adequately trained to identify significant abnormalities (RCEM 2020). The clinician requesting the investigations is responsible for interpretation of the images. Failure to review in a timely manner and identify the abnormality can result in delayed diagnosis and treatment. This is important to consider when managing your caseload and maintaining your clinical accountability. Patient safety is paramount, underpinned by the principles of IR(ME)R and duty of candour. There are certain imaging considerations that need to be taken into account with different patient populations. Table 15.13 highlights some of those areas, focusing on; pathological, psychological, and sociocultural issues that might arise.

TABLE 15.13 Imaging considerations in special populations.

Patient population	Imaging considerations	RED FLAG = pathological considerations	AMBER FLAG = psychological considerations	GREEN FLAG = social/cultural issues.
Paediatrics	• Avoid unnecessary ionising radiation exposure • Thorough history-taking and physical assessment • Observe patient outside of examination room • Use of play specialists • Can the patient follow instructions to ensure optimal imaging? • Collateral history from parents or carers	Awareness of non-accidental injury in all groups of patients when timeline and pattern appear inconsistent		
Child-bearing age	• Patients between the ages of 12 and 55. • Discretion when asking first day of last menstrual period • If patient's dates outside of 28-day rule, consider pregnancy testing • Explain risk/benefit prior to referral	Pregnant patient; delay imaging until second trimester if possible		
Mental health Learning disability Cognitive impairment temporary or permanent	• Liaise with parents, carers, key workers to establish baseline and assist with management/choosing best approach. • Ensured appropriate consent in place • Mental health support team involvement • Check medical notes for hospital passports/identification of special requirements • Does the patient have a current section 2 or 3 order in place? • Consider deprivation of liberty safeguards (DOLS) if the patient is at risk of causing significant harm to themselves	Optimise pain relief prior to imaging referral	Consider anxiety – is patient able to comply with examination requirements? Claustrophobia with CT & MRI?	Seek advice from Radiology: Extra time/quiet environment/support for patient at the time of radiation exposure

TABLE 15.13   (Continued)

Patient population	Imaging considerations	RED FLAG = pathological considerations	AMBER FLAG = psychological considerations	GREEN FLAG = social/cultural issues.
Older people	• Higher pain threshold • Low threshold for advanced imaging in older adults (silver trauma guidance)	Minimal trauma can cause severe injuries Classic signs/red flags often not present e.g. raised ICP in subdural haemorrhage If patient fails to mobilise following fall and initial imaging normal, consider occult fracture and more detailed imaging		
Ethnicity	• Cultural competency required throughout. • Consider the patient's ethnic origin/gender/genealogy/epidemiology in diagnostic differentials		Undressing for examination may cause anxiety	Language barrier. Engage services of professional interpreter where possible Ensure any considerations required by radiology are included e.g. patient preference for gender-specific operator

Take Home Points

- Use history, physical examination, and bloods to establish a likely diagnosis and pre-test probability to establish the clinical question you want answered.
- Understand the clinical application of the radiology modalities available to you. Establish which modalities can effectively rule in or out your differential diagnoses.
- Seek advice from the radiology department with regards to most appropriate imaging modality to request if you are unsure.
- Select the modality which best balances diagnostic yield and radiation exposure. Always rationalise your choices.
- Ensure patients are well-informed – what should they expect, what are the risks?
- Treat the patient based on clinical assessment, do not delay treatment while awaiting imaging.
- If there is clinical suspicion of a diagnosis, but inconclusive imaging results, escalate to a senior and consider further detailed imaging.

REFERENCES

Abdolrazaghnejad, A., Rajabpour-Sanati, A., Rastegari-Najafabadi, H. et al. (2019). The role of ultrasonography in patients referring to the emergency department with acute abdominal pain. *Advanced Journal of Emergency Medicine* 3 (4): e43. https://doi.org/10.22114/ajem.v0i0.152.

Bajc, M., Neilly, J.B., Miniati, M. et al. (2009). EANM guidelines for ventilation/perfusion scintigraphy. *European Journal of Nuclear Medicine and Molecular Imaging* 36 (8): 1356–1370.

Bhave, N.M., Nienaber, C.A., Clough, R.E., and Eagle, K.A. (2018). Multimodality imaging of thoracic aortic diseases in adults. *JACC: Cardiovascular Imaging* 11 (6): 902–919.

Cartwright, S.L. and Knudson, M.P. (2015). Diagnostic imaging of acute abdominal pain in adults. *American Family Physician* 91 (7): 452–459.

Chan, O. (2013). *ABC of Emergency Radiology*, 3e. London: Wiley-Blackwell.

Chowdhury, R. (2017). *Radiology at a Glance*, 2e. Chichester, UK: Wiley.

Day, R. and Fordyce, J. (2020). 7.2 Approach to abdominal pain – Section 7 Digestive emergencies. In: *Textbook of Emergency Medicine*, 5e (ed. P. Cameron, M. Little, B. Mitra, and C. Deasy). Elsevier.

Demeestere, J., Wouters, A., Christensen, S. et al. (2020). Review of perfusion imaging in acute ischemic stroke: from time to tissue. *Stroke* 51 (3): 1017–1024.

Demi, L., Wolfram, F., Klersy, C. et al. (2023). New international guidelines and consensus on the use of lung ultrasound. *Journal of Ultrasound in Medicine: Official Journal of the American Institute of Ultrasound in Medicine* 42 (2): 309–344. https://doi.org/10.1002/jum.16088.

Doumouchtsis, S.K. and Arulkumaran, S. (ed.) (2016). *Emergencies in Obstetrics and Gynaecology*, 2e. Oxford, UK: Oxford University Press.

Duffett, L., Castellucci, L.A., and Forgie, M.A. (2020). Pulmonary embolism: update on management and controversies. *BMJ (Clinical Research Ed.) 370*: m2177. https://doi.org/10.1136/bmj.m2177.

Fitzpatrick, L.A., Rivers-Bowerman, M.D., Thipphavong, S. et al. (2020). Pearls, pitfalls, and conditions that mimic mesenteric ischemia at CT. *Radiographics* 40 (2): 545–561.

Fraleigh, C.D. and Duff, E. (2022). Point-of-care ultrasound: an emerging clinical tool to enhance physical assessment. *The Nurse Practitioner* 47 (8): 14.

Ghoneim, A., Straiton, J., Pollard, C. et al. (2020). Imaging of cerebral venous thrombosis. *Clinical Radiology* 75 (4): 254–264.

Health Education England (HEE). (2017). *Multi-professional Framework for Advanced Clinical Practice in England* [online]. Available from: https://www.hee.nhs.uk/sites/default/files/documents/multi-professionalframeworkforadvancedclinicalpracticeinengland.pdf [accessed 20 June 2023].

Health Education England (HEE). (2022). *Advanced Clinical Practice in Acute Medicine Curriculum Framework – Credentials* [online]. Available from: https://advanced-practice.hee.nhs.uk/our-work/credentials [accessed 20 June 2023].

Hepburn-Brown, M., Darvall, J., and Hammerschlag, G. (2019). Acute pulmonary embolism: a concise review of diagnosis and management. *Internal Medicine Journal* 49 (1): 15–27.

Hijazi, Z., Lange, P., Watson, R., and Maier, A.B. (2018). The use of cerebral imaging for investigating delirium aetiology. *European Journal of Internal Medicine* 52: 35–39.

Holmes, E.J. and Misra, R.R. (2017). *Interpretation of Emergency Head CT: A Practical Handbook*. Cambridge University Press.

Hughes, T. and Cruickshank, J. (2011). *Adult Emergency Medicine at a Glance*. Hoboken, NJ: Wiley-Blackwell.

Impey, L. and Child, T. (2016). *Obstetrics & Gynaecology*, 5e. Wiley-Blackwell.

Jongkind, V., Earnshaw, J.J., Bastos Gonçalves, F. et al. (2022). Editor's Choice - Update of the European Society for Vascular Surgery (ESVS) 2020 Clinical Practice Guidelines on the Management of Acute Limb Ischaemia in Light of the COVID-19 Pandemic, Based on a Scoping Review of the Literature. *European Journal of Vascular and Endovascular Surgery: The Official Journal of the European Society for Vascular Surgery* 63 (1): 80–89. https://doi.org/10.1016/j.ejvs.2021.08.028.

Joseph, A.P., Harris, R., and Dimmick, S. (2014). 3.8 Radiology in major trauma. In: *Textbook of Adult Emergency Medicine E-Book*, 117.

Kameda-Smith, M., Aref, M., Jung, Y. et al. (2021). Determining the diagnostic utility of lumbar punctures in computed tomography negative suspected subarachnoid hemorrhage: a systematic review and meta-analysis. *World Neurosurgery* 148: e27–e34.

Kessler, R. and Dean, A.J. (2017). Chapter 11 – Plain radiography in the elderly. In: *Clinical Emergency Radiology*, 2e (ed. C. Fox). Cambridge, UK: Cambridge University Press.

Marin, D., Boll, D.T., Mileto, A., and Nelson, R.C. (2014). State of the art: dual-energy CT of the abdomen. *Radiology* 271 (2): 327–342.

Mendelson, S.J. and Prabhakaran, S. (2021). Diagnosis and management of transient ischemic attack and acute ischemic stroke: a review. *JAMA* 325 (11): 1088–1098.

Mettler, F. (2018). *Essentials of Radiology*, 4e. London: Elsevier.

Moore, A.J., Wachsmann, J., Chamarthy, M.R. et al. (2018). Imaging of acute pulmonary embolism: an update. *Cardiovascular Diagnosis and Therapy* 8 (3): 225.

National Institute for Health and Care Excellence. (2014). *Head Injury: Assessment and Early Management (NICE Guidelines No. 176)* [online]. Available from: www.nice.org.uk/guidance/cg176 [accessed 22 June 2023].

National Institute for Health and Care Excellence. (2017). *The Management of Hip Fractures in Adults, 2011. Updated 2017. ([NICE Guidelines No. 124].)* [online]. Available from: www.nice.org.uk/guidance/cg124 [accessed 22 June 2023].

Olinic, D.M., Stanek, A., Tătaru, D.A. et al. (2019). Acute limb ischemia: an update on diagnosis and management. *Journal of Clinical Medicine* 8 (8): 1215.

Rincon, S., Gupta, R., and Ptak, T. (2016). Imaging of head trauma. *Handbook of Clinical Neurology* 135: 447–477.

Roche, O., Chavan, N., Aquilina, J., and Rockall, A. (2012). Radiological appearances of gynaecological emergencies. *Insights Into Imaging* 3 (3): 265–275.

Royal College of Emergency Medicine. (2020). *RCEM Guidance on Management of Investigation Results in the Emergency Department* [online]. Available from: RCEM_BPC_InvestigationResults_200520.pdf [accessed 22 June 2023].

Royal College of Surgeons. (2017). *Emergency General Surgery (Acute Abdominal Pain) – Commissioning Guide 2014. Updated 2017* [online]. Available from: http://rcseng.ac.uk [accessed 22 June 2023].

Rudkin, S., Cerejo, R., Tayal, A., and Goldberg, M.F. (2018). Imaging of acute ischemic stroke. *Emergency Radiology* 25 (6): 659–672.

Rudnick, M.R., Leonberg-Yoo, A.K., Litt, H.I. et al. (2020). The controversy of contrast-induced nephropathy with intravenous contrast: what is the risk? *American Journal of Kidney Diseases* 75 (1): 105–113.

Shams, E. and Mayrovitz, H.N. (2021). Contrast-induced nephropathy: a review of mechanisms and risks. *Cureus* 13 (5): e14842.

Tester, J., Hammerschlag, G., Irving, L. et al. (2020). Investigation and diagnostic imaging of suspected pulmonary embolism during pregnancy and the puerperium: a review of the literature. *Journal of Medical Imaging and Radiation Oncology* 64 (4): 505–515.

The Faculty of Intensive Care Medicine. (2018). *Curriculum for Training for Advanced Critical Care Practitioners – Syllabus. V1.1* [online]. Available from: `www.ficm.ac.uk/media/6896` [accessed 20 June 2023].

The Intensive Care Society, Critical Care Networks – *National Nurse Leads and The National Outreach Forum.* (2022). *Advanced Critical Care Outreach Competencies* [online]. Available from: `https://ics.ac.uk/asset/43B8C11B-4512-41D0-B97768FABA2C30B2` [accessed 20 June 2023].

The Royal College of Emergency Medicine. (2022). *Emergency Medicine Advanced Clinical Practitioner Curriculum 2022 (Adult)* [online]. Available from: `https://rcem.ac.uk/wp-content/uploads/2022/09/ACP_Curriculum_Adult_Final_060922.pdf` [accessed 20 June 2023].

The Royal College of Radiologist (2018). *Standards for Interpretation and Reporting of Imaging Investigations*, 2e. London: The Royal College of Radiologists.

Whiting, P., Singatullina, N., and Rosser, J.H. (2015). Computed tomography of the chest: I Basic principles. *BJA Education* 15 (6): 299–304.

Wyatt, J.P., Illingworth, R.N., Graham, C.A. et al. (2012). *Oxford Handbook of Emergency Medicine*, 4e. Oxford: Oxford University Press.

FURTHER READING

Herring, W. (2019). *Learning Radiology: Recognising the Basics*, 4e. London: Elsevier.

Mettler, F. (2018). *Essentials of Radiology*, 4e. London: Elsevier.

CHAPTER 16

Principles of Point of Care Ultrasound

Hannah Conway

Aim

The aim of this chapter is to explore the clinical application of Point-of-Care Ultrasound (PoCUS) within acute, emergency, and critical care (AECC). We will cover the key modalities utilised within these clinical areas and will categorise per body system:

- Heart
- Lung
- Vascular
- Abdomen

For each modality a diagnostic reasoning framework will be provided, which combines the sonographic data with clinical history and presentation. The goal of this is to enable the Advanced Clinical Practitioner (ACP) to improve their clinical decision-making skills, by taking advantage of this valuable diagnostic tool.

LEARNING OUTCOMES

After reading this chapter the reader will:

1. Understand the basics of ultrasound physics and image generation.
2. List the clinical applications of ultrasound within AECC.

The Advanced Practitioner in Acute, Emergency and Critical Care, First Edition. Edited by Sadie Diamond-Fox, Barry Hill, Sonya Stone, Caroline McCrea, Natalie Gardner, and Angela Roberts.
© 2024 John Wiley & Sons Ltd. Published 2024 by John Wiley & Sons Ltd.

3. Recognise the sonographic features of common red flag pathology.
4. Apply the sonographic reasoning method to aid clinical decision–making.
5. Understand the importance of the five pillars of PoCUS practice.

SELF-ASSESSMENT QUESTIONS

1. How is an ultrasound image generated?
2. What ultrasound modality do you or would you find most helpful to aid in your clinical decision-making?
3. What are the benefits of ultrasound over other imaging modalities?
4. What are the five pillars of PoCUS? And how could you as an ACP improve ultrasound governance within your clinical specialty?

Multi-professional Framework (MPF) for Advanced Clinical Practice Guidance for Professional Development (HEE 2017)

This chapter maps to the following statements within the MPF:

1. Clinical:	1.2	1.4	1.6	1.8	1.9

Accreditation Considerations

This chapter maps to the following statements within the following national accreditation documents:

Curriculum for Training for Advanced Critical Care Practitioners Syllabus V1.1
(The Faculty of Intensive Care Medicine 2018):

2.2	3.2	3.5	4.2	4.3	4.5	4.12	4.14

Advanced Critical Care Outreach Competencies
(The Intensive Care Society, Critical Care Networks – National Nurse Leads and The National Outreach Forum 2022):

A4	

Emergency Medicine Advanced Clinical Practitioner Curriculum 2022 – Adult
(The Royal College of Emergency Medicine 2022):

SLO 6	

Advanced Clinical Practice in Acute Medicine Curriculum Framework
(Health Education England 2022):

- Appendix 1 - Agreed Practical Procedures

INTRODUCTION

The acute specialties share some common themes. Patients are acutely unwell, requiring time-critical management within a highly stressed environment. As such, rapid and accurate diagnosis is required to ensure patients are treated safely and effectively.

NHS England (2017) published a set of proposed standards to support acute care services in providing access to high-quality care for patients admitted acutely. One clinical standard pertains to seven-day access to urgent diagnostic imaging, inclusive of ultrasound. As a result of these standards, widening access to bedside ultrasound training and accreditation has been prioritised within AECC. Multiple approved accreditation pathways are now in existence, some of which are now integrated into specialty curriculum (BSE 2022; FAMUS 2022).

Ultrasound is a minimally invasive, non-ionising tool which provides the user with a 'window' into the patient's body, through which pathology can be detected. One of the key benefits of this tool, is its portability. This allows the responsible clinician to perform diagnostic investigations at the bedside, where clinical decisions can be made, and goal-directed management can be commenced without delay (Carroll et al. 2023). In comparison to gold standard imaging modalities, ultrasound is found to be comparable and, in some cases, superior in the detection of many acute pathologies (Bierig and Jones 2009).

When considering how to clinically apply ultrasound findings, a structured approach is essential. Penny and Zachariason (2015) propose a method which combines critical thinking with diagnostic reasoning skills; the Sonographic Reasoning Method (SRM) (see Figure 16.1).

SRM links the key elements of diagnostic reasoning and places importance on application of clinical context when performing and interpreting ultrasound examinations. The available data gathered during step 1 of the SRM, will enable the clinician to establish a pre-test probability of disease likelihood, prior to undertaking diagnostic imaging (Duggan et al. 2020). Equally as important, is the awareness of

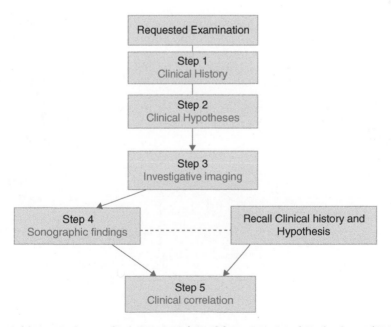

FIGURE 16.1   Sonographic reasoning method. *Source*: Adapted from Penny and Zachariason (2015).

the diagnostic limitations of PoCUS, with this always influencing the decision to perform additional or alternative imaging. Limitations of each ultrasound modality will be discussed in greater detail as we progress through the chapter.

HOW IS ULTRASOUND GENERATED?

Before exploring the clinical application of PoCUS within AECC, it is first important to gain a basic understanding of how ultrasound is generated. This will enable clinicians to appreciate how placing an ultrasound probe over a three-dimensional (3D) organ can produce the two-dimensional (2D) image, we see on the ultrasound monitor.

An ultrasound probe is a transducer, which is designed both to 'send' and 'receive' sound waves (see Figure 16.2). Built within the footprint of the probe, is a layer of piezo electric (PZE) crystals that when exposed to an electrical current, begin to oscillate. It is through this oscillation, that a sound wave is produced (Otto 2016). The sound wave is emitted from the probe into the patient's body, where it will encounter tissues, fluids, air, bone, and the interfaces between these various mediums (Abu-Zidan et al. 2011) (see Figure 16.3). A proportion of the sound waves will reflect off these various interfaces, back towards the probe. The remaining waves will either fade (or attenuate), change direction or scatter if the interface happens to be irregular (Au and Zwank 2020). Once received by the probe, the PZE crystals once again begin to oscillate, converting mechanical energy back to an electrical current.

Through this process, the ultrasound machine is able to 'build' a sonographic picture of the structure of interest. Two key pieces of information are extrapolated: distance to interface and amplitude of reflected wave. Distance is determined by the time taken between sending and receiving a reflected sound wave (Otto 2016). The amplitude of the reflected wave is represented as a dot, enabling creation of a grey scale image. The stronger the amplitude, the brighter the dot. A single dot on its own would not

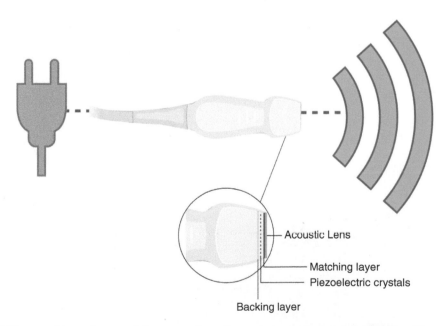

FIGURE 16.2   Ultrasound transducer and the generation of sound waves. *Source*: Adapted from Biorender.com (2022).

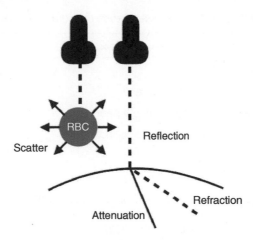

FIGURE 16.3   Ultrasound and its interaction with tissue. *Source*: Conway (2022b) / John Wiley & Sons.

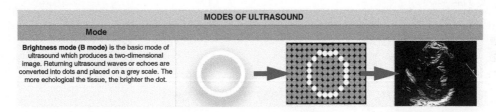

FIGURE 16.4   Production of a 2D image using B Mode technology. *Source*: Conway (2022b) / John Wiley & Sons.

provide us with any helpful information. But when we consider this process is happening in real time, a moving 2D representation of the 3D structure starts to form on our monitor (see Figure 16.4).

HEART ULTRASOUND

Introduction

Ultrasound of the heart, also known as echocardiography, has become a widely accepted diagnostic tool within AECC. Clinicians not only use echocardiography to detect cardiac pathology, but routinely use to serially assess the impact of various goal-directed strategies This may include fluid resuscitation (or de-resuscitation), inotrope titration, guiding thrombolysis management (Longobardo et al. 2018).

Clinical Application

Echocardiography within AECC is usually confined to a focussed dataset, using a clinical question-based approach (see Table 16.1). It is a powerful tool in rapidly detecting red flag pathology in patients with haemodynamic compromise or shock (Lancellotti et al. 2014).

The heart is visualised via three 'acoustic windows' on the chest wall. Through these windows the probe is positioned at agreed points to obtain specific tomographic views of the heart. In a focussed data-set, we can obtain five views of the heart and vasculature (see Figure 16.5).

TABLE 16.1 Focussed heart clinical questions.

Clinical question-based approach
Is the heart dilated?
Are the ventricles impaired?
Is there any evidence of low preload?
Is there a pericardial or pleural collection?
Is there valvulopathy?
Are there increased right-sided pressures
Is there low stroke volume or cardiac output?

Source: Adapted from FUSIC (2022).

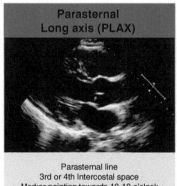

Parasternal Long axis (PLAX)

Parasternal line
3rd or 4th Intercostal space
Marker pointing towards 10–10 o'clock

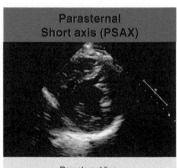

Parasternal Short axis (PSAX)

Parasternal line
3rd or 4th Intercostal space
Marker pointing towards 1–2 o'clock

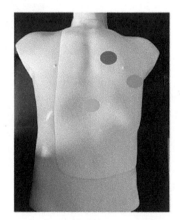

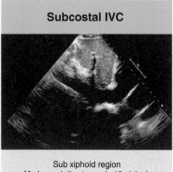

Subcostal IVC

Sub xiphoid region
Marker pointing towards 12 o'clock

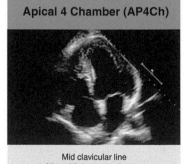

Apical 4 Chamber (AP4Ch)

Mid clavicular line
4th or 5th Intercostal space
Marker pointing towards 3 o'clock

Subcostal 4 Chamber (SC4Ch)

Sub xiphoid region
Marker pointing towards 3 o'clock

FIGURE 16.5 Basic ultrasound views of the heart. *Source*: Conway (2022a) / John Wiley & Sons.

RED FLAG PATHOLOGY

Cardiogenic Shock

Cardiogenic shock (CS) is characterised by severe ventricular dysfunction, leading to low cardiac output, poor end organ perfusion resulting in tissue hypoxia and death (Diepen et al. 2017). The leading cause of CS is acute myocardial infarction (AMI), which carries a high mortality (McMurray et al. 2012). Performing an echocardiogram should not delay cardiac catheterisation in event of a suspected AMI; however, it is an invaluable tool in assessing the degree of ventricular dysfunction and presence of any associated pathology (Sia et al. 2008).

Often when we describe CS, we are referring to the left ventricle (LV); however, it can affect the right ventricle (RV) or even both ventricles. Several mechanical complications associated with AMI include:

- **Ventricular wall rupture** occurs as a result of tear in the poorly perfused myocardium. It can occur early (<72 hours) or late (>96 hours) and is usually accompanied by a pericardial collection (Sia et al. 2008).
- **Ventricular dysfunction or failure** is common in AMI as a result of ischaemic myocardium. It can affect the myocardium regionally or globally, and echocardiography can aid in the determination of this (Otto 2016).
- **Valve regurgitation** may occur as a result of rupture of sub-valvular apparatus (primary) or chamber dilatation and altered geometry of the ventricle (secondary regurgitation) (Izquierdo-Gomez et al. 2018).

Obstructive Shock

Two examples of obstructive shock seen within AECC are cardiac tamponade and pulmonary embolism (PE). While different pathologies, they are linked by the same mechanism, which is obstruction to blood flow through the cardiopulmonary circulation (McLean 2016). Both pathologies can lead rapidly to cardiac arrest and death, however, thankfully are highly reversible if detected and treated immediately (Durila 2018).

Focused echocardiographic signs of cardiac tamponade include, a visible pericardial collection, right atrial 'systolic' collapse, right ventricular 'diastolic' collapse, and a dilated, plethoric inferior vena cava (IVC) (see Figure 16.6). Additional signs do exist but fall into a more advanced dataset. Right ventricular diastolic collapse is a highly specific sign, although less sensitive than the presence of right atrial systolic collapse (Alerhand and Carter 2019; Trivedi and Kokkirala 2022). It is important to note that cardiac tamponade remains a clinical diagnosis, and therefore if clinically suspected, treatment should not be delayed in place of organising an echocardiogram (Dragoi et al. 2022). Figure 16.7 shows the importance of clinical correlation and history taking with the sonographic findings.

Common echocardiographic signs of PE include dilated and impaired RV, paradoxical septal wall motion and plethoric IVC (caused by the increased right-sided pressures) (see Figure 16.8). Due to failure of the RV, the LV cardiac output is significantly reduced and therefore appears empty and hyperdynamic (Anderson and Buckland 2019). This phenomenon is referred to as ventricular interdependence, when one ventricle's loading conditions, alter the other (Naeije and Badagliacca 2017).

One highly specific sign that has been historically associated with PE is the McConnell's sign (see Figure 16.9). This characteristic regional wall motion abnormality comprises of RV free wall akinesis and

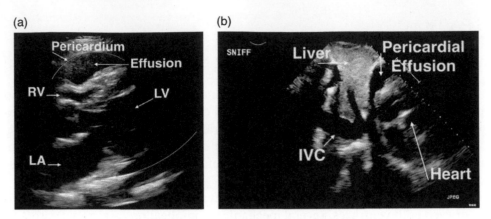

FIGURE 16.6 (a) Parasternal view demonstrating pericardial effusion collapsing RV during diastole. (b) subcostal view demonstrating dilated, plethoric inferior vena cava (IVC). *Source*: Shyy et al. (2017) / John Wiley & Sons.

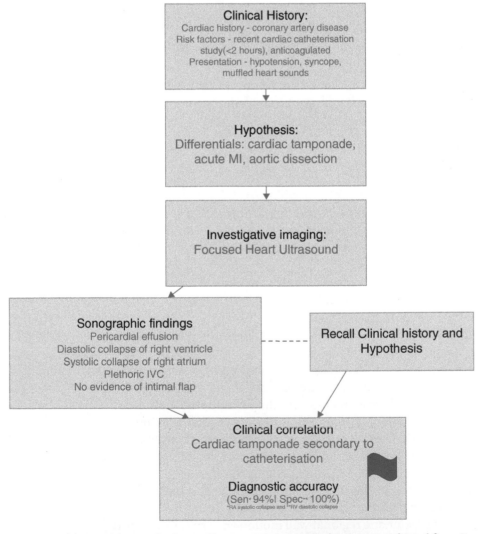

FIGURE 16.7 Sonographic reasoning method – cardiac presentation exemplar. *Source*: Adapted from Penny and Zachariason (2015) using diagnostic accuracy data from Trivedi and Kokkirala (2022).

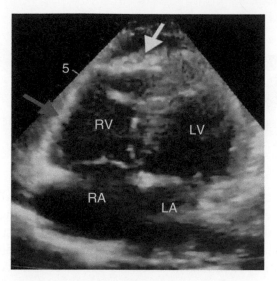

FIGURE 16.8   Parasternal short axis view demonstrating dilated RV, paradoxical interventricular wall motion and resultant small, empty LV. *Source*: Zaalouk et al. (2021) / John Wiley & Sons.

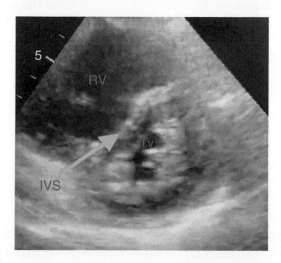

FIGURE 16.9   Apical four chamber view demonstrating dilated RV and McConnell's sign. Red arrow = akinetic RV free wall, yellow arrow = apical sparing. *Source*: Zaalouk et al. (2021) / John Wiley & Sons.

apical sparing (López-Candales et al. 2010). This pattern is thought to be more representative of tethering of the RV apex to a hyperdynamic LV, than a true sparing of RV apical function. While all these signs can aid in the diagnosis and risk stratification of PE, it is important to note that unless a clot is seen in transit within the right heart, a diagnosis of PE cannot be confirmed using ultrasound alone (Konstantinides et al. 2019). Furthermore, presence of a normal RV on ultrasound, does not exclude PE.

DISTRIBUTIVE (OR VASOPLEGIC) SHOCK AND HYPOVOLEMIC SHOCK

Clinicians find it extremely challenging to differentiate between distributive and hypovolemic shock using ultrasound alone. The sonographic findings of both pathophysiological states are almost identical, therefore clinical correlation is fundamental (Lafon et al. 2020).

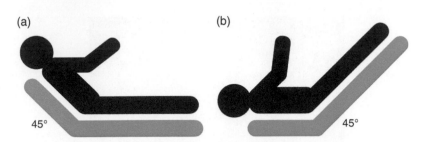

FIGURE 16.10   (a) Patient in the semi-recumbent position. (b) Patient in the passive leg raise (PLR) position.

In hypovolemia, the ventricles will appear hyperdynamic with small internal areas, creating a characteristic 'kissing ventricle' whereby the walls collapse during end systolic (McLean 2016). The size and respiratory variation of the IVC has been used for decades as a fluid status tool, however there are several studies that question its predictive value, due to multiple confounding factors that affect its reliability, including increased intra-abdominal, intrathoracic pressures, and RV function (Millington 2019).

In distributive shock, for example sepsis, the classic 'early' sonographic presentation will mimic hypovolemia. However, unlike truly hypovolemic patients, septic patients will demonstrate a limited response to fluid resuscitation in terms of increasing ventricular areas and improving blood pressure (Via et al. 2011). Therefore, when using ultrasound in these cases, focus must be shifted towards assessing fluid responsiveness to help differentiate between these two states. One simple, yet effective, technique to test fluid responsiveness is the passive leg raise (PLR) test (see Figure 16.10). An alternative is to administer a mini fluid challenge (i.e. 100 ml) (McLean 2016). Studies have demonstrated both techniques to be effective at predicting fluid responsiveness (Maizel et al. 2007; Muller et al. 2011).

LUNG ULTRASOUND

Introduction

Lung ultrasound (LUS) is an established tool in AECC and has been quoted by many to be the modern-day stethoscope, whereby the user can see, rather than just listen (Gillman and Kirkpatrick 2012). It has been proven to have higher diagnostic accuracy compared to clinical physical examination and chest radiography (CXR) combined (Lichtenstein et al. 2004). Furthermore, it has been found to be comparable to computed tomography (CT) in diagnosing many respiratory diseases (Bandi et al. 2008; Wang et al. 2021; Zieleskiewicz et al. 2020), thus making lung ultrasound a safe alternative to traditional modalities.

Unlike other ultrasound modalities, whereby a recognisable organ is seen, interpretation of LUS is based mainly on presence of lung artefact. Lung artefact is generated by the interfaces that exist between tissue, fluid air, and bone (Saraogi 2015). Certain disease processes create characteristic patterns, which clinicians can use to detect pathology (Lichtenstein 2014).

Clinical Application

Like in ultrasound of the heart, a clinical question-based approach (see Table 16.2) is used to aide in the rapid detection of red flag pathology using a systematic approach. Often the trigger for performing an LUS examination is hypoxia or signs of respiratory distress (Mojoli et al. 2019).

TABLE 16.2   Focussed lung clinical questions.

Clinical question-based approach
Are there any signs of pneumothorax?
Is there any evidence of interstitial syndrome?
Is there any evidence of consolidation or atelectasis?
Is there a pleural collection?

Source: Adapted from FUSIC (2022).

To examine the chest with ultrasound, two probes are recommended, dependent on anatomical location of the scan. For anterior lung scanning, a linear probe is recommended to facilitate high-resolution imaging for superficial structures such as pleura. And for examination of lung bases, a low frequency curvilinear probe is recommended. This will provide both a wider and deeper field of view, which makes it ideal for assessing consolidations and effusions (Miller 2015).

The most recognised and established protocol used by clinicians in AECC, is the Basic Lung Ultrasound Examination (or BLUE) protocol (Lichtenstein and Mezière 2011). By placing one's hands on the patient's chest, as shown in (see Figure 16.11), three points can be identified per lung.

1. The upper BLUE point – Anterior zone
2. The lower BLUE point – Antero-lateral zone
3. 'PLAPS' points – Postero-lateral zone

In a landmark study, LUS has been found to have an overall diagnostic accuracy of 90.5% for the most common causes of respiratory failure: pneumonia, pulmonary oedema, COPD, asthma, PE, and pneumothorax (Lichtenstein and Mezière 2008). A decision tree was formulated (see Figure 16.11) to aid clinicians in differentiation of these respiratory pathologies, by assessing specific lung patterns or profiles.

RED FLAG PATHOLOGY

Pneumothorax

Lung ultrasound is more accurate in ruling in/out, the diagnosis of pneumothorax than on CXR (Volpicelli et al. 2012). In the healthy lung, the visceral and parietal pleura layers will be in apposition and will slide during respiration. Absence of lung sliding does not on its own indicate pneumothorax but warrants a high index of suspicion until proven otherwise. It is recommended that 'four signs' in total should be assessed within a particular sequence to aid diagnosis (Volpicelli 2011) (see Figure 16.12).

Consolidation

Consolidation on LUS have various appearances dependant on severity and location (Miller 2015). Anterior or peripheral consolidations appear as a hypoechoic region beneath the pleura. The interface between abnormal lung and normal aerated lung creates an irregular line, termed the shred sign (see Figure 16.13). More significant postero-basal consolidation appears as homogenous tissue; termed

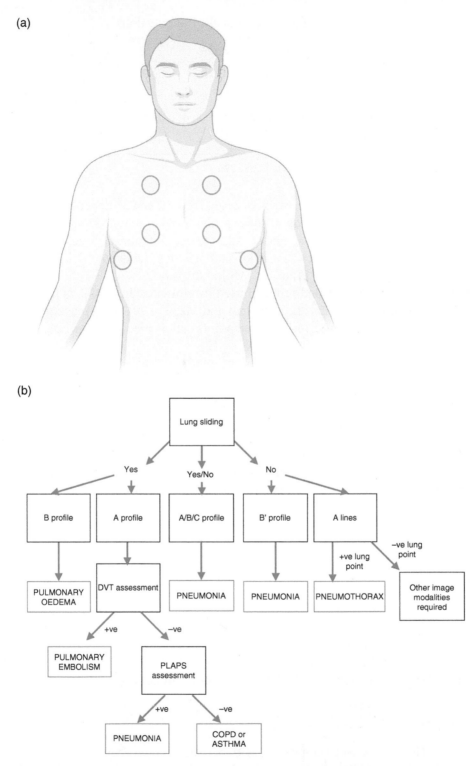

FIGURE 16.11   (a) BLUE points. *Source*: Adapted from Biorender.com (2022). (b) BLUE protocol decision tree. *Source*: Lichtenstein and Mezière (2008) / with permission of Elsevier.

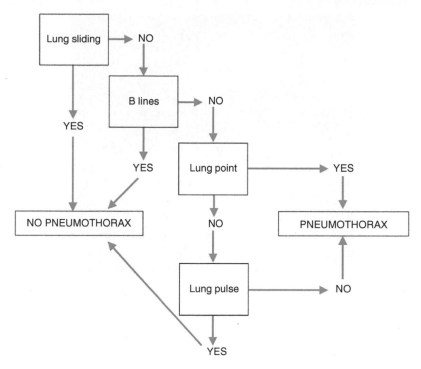

FIGURE 16.12   Flowchart on diagnosis of pneumothorax. *Source*: Volpicelli (2011) / Springer Nature.

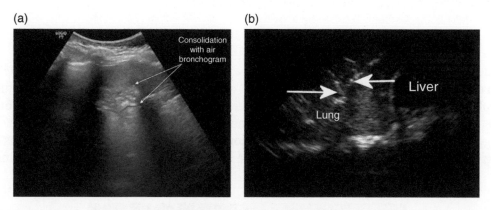

FIGURE 16.13   (a) Anterior lung zone with small area of subpleural consolidation and shred sign = red line. *Source*: Adapted from Biorender.com (2022). (b) Postero-lateral lung zone demonstrating tissue-like sign, also referred to lung hepatisation. *Source*: Adapted from Blaivas (2012).

tissue-like sign (see Figure 16.13). If severe enough, the lung may take on the sonographic appearance of the liver, hence the name – hepatised lung (Durant and Nagdev 2010).

Interstitial Syndrome

A specific lung artefact, coined the B line artefact, is created from the contiguity between alveolar air and septal thickening, as seen in pulmonary fibrosis, pneumonitis, and/or pulmonary oedema (see Figure 16.14). This artefact is characterised by vertical hyperechoic lines, arising from the pleural

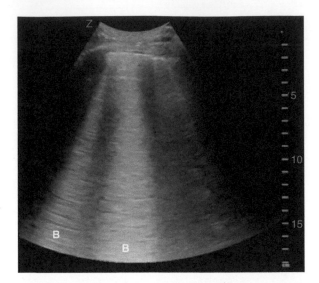

FIGURE 16.14　Anterior lung zone demonstrating B-lines (B) in a patient with pulmonary oedema. *Source*: Adapted from Russell et al. (2020).

line, descending to the bottom of the image without fading (Dietrich et al. 2016). True B lines erase all underlying lung artefact and move in concert with lung sliding. In normal lungs, up to two B lines between one rib space is considered normal; however, if there are more than two B lines present between rib spaces, this signifies interstitial pathology (Miller 2015).

Effusion

Pleural effusions can be easily missed or mistaken for collapse or consolidations on CXR. LUS is highly sensitive in detection of even small effusions (<20 ml) and is 100% sensitive in detection of effusions over 100 ml in volume (Soni et al. 2015). LUS can help determine the nature of the pleural collection based on appearance. Transudative collections often appear anechoic or black, whereas exudative collections are more echogenic with or without loculations or fibrinous strands (Soni et al. 2022). Clinicians can determine the size and volume of effusions using LUS (see Figure 16.15), which will aid in deciding whether

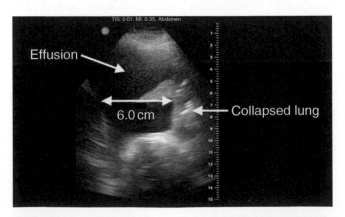

FIGURE 16.15　Posterolateral lung zone demonstrating a large simple pleural effusion and collapsed lung. Using the Balik formula, this effusion is estimated to be 1200 ml (20 × 60 mm). *Source*: Adapted from Cid et al. (2020).

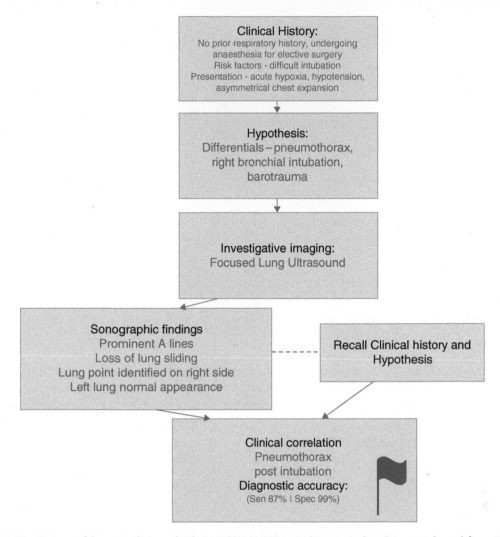

FIGURE 16.16 Sonographic reasoning method – respiratory presentation exemplar. *Source*: Adapted from Penny and Zachariason (2015) using diagnostic accuracy data from Ebrahimi et al. (2014).

drainage is necessary. Thereafter, LUS can guide percutaneous placement of a chest drain, which has several reported advantages over traditional landmark techniques (Taylor et al. 2018; Wong et al. 2016).

Figure 16.16 shows the importance of clinical history and its implications on sonographic findings.

VASCULAR ULTRASOUND

Introduction

Many clinicians are already well versed in the use of ultrasound to guide vascular access. Within AECC, this modality of ultrasound plays two main roles:

1. Ultrasound guided placement of intravenous catheters
2. Assessment of lower limb deep vein thrombosis (DVT)

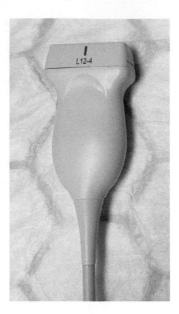

FIGURE 16.17   High frequency, linear probe.

A high frequency, linear probe is used for vascular applications, which has a thin rectangular footprint (see Figure 16.17). As explained earlier within the chapter, a high frequency probe makes this a perfect tool for assessing superficial, in high resolution. However, caution must be taken when scanning patients with significant tissue oedema or obesity, as the quality of imaging may be limited by attenuation at increased depths of scanning (Uppot 2018).

Clinical Application

Vascular Access

Central venous access is commonly required in acutely unwell patients. Rationale for placement includes haemodynamic monitoring, blood, fluid and drug administration, haemodialysis, and total parenteral nutrition. Historically, these catheters were placed using a 'landmark' technique, however this has been associated with failure rates as high as 35% (NICE 2002).

The National Institute of Health and Clinical Excellence (NICE 2002) recommends the use ultrasound guidance (USG) for placement of central venous catheters, following appraisal of 20 randomised trials. Key themes that emerged from this guidance include:

- USG is significantly better than landmark approach in the placement of internal jugular venous catheters in adults and infants. Additionally, there is no difference in time taken between approaches.
- USG is associated with fewer complications and fewer failure rates in the placement of subclavian venous catheters in adults.

More recently the European Society of Anaesthesiology (ESA) taskforce produced clinical guidance on placement of 'all' forms of vascular access, including peripheral venous access. While evidence base is weak to support use of USG for peripheral access routinely, what is recommended is to use USG for patients with moderate to difficult venous access. USG will enable clinicians to evaluate the vessel prior to attempting cannulation in an attempt to maximise chances of success and reduce risk of complications (Lamperti et al. 2020).

The vessel of interest can be visualised via two approaches. 'Transverse', whereby the ultrasound beam is perpendicular to the long axis of the vessel, and 'Longitudinal', whereby the ultrasound beam is in line with the long axis vessel (see Figure 16.18). Realtime assessment of the needle is key. In the transverse view, the needle is visualised in cross section, therefore the actual tip of the needle can easily be mistaken for a cross section of the shaft. To avoid this, the probe can be angulated or preferably switched to using the longitudinal approach. The longitudinal view provides the user with a visual of the entire needle, shaft and tip. It also allows the user to follow the trajectory of the needle to avoid puncturing the posterior wall. This technique is more challenging than the transverse approach, therefore a more skilled user is required (Chapman et al. 2006).

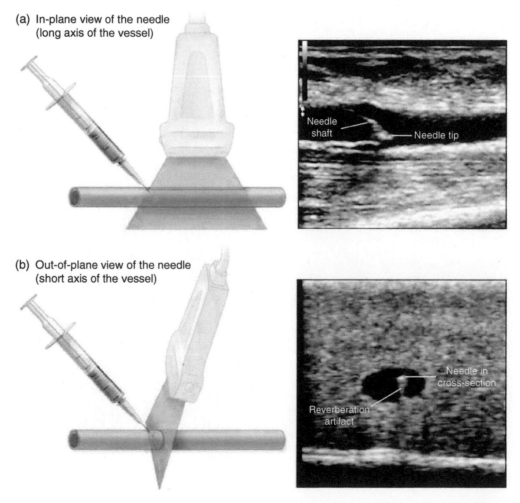

FIGURE 16.18   (a) Transverse view, needle out of plane. (b) Longitudinal view, needle in plane. *Source*: AIUM (2019) / John Wiley & Sons.

DEEP VEIN THROMBOSIS (DVT) ASSESSMENT

Critically ill patients are at higher risk for developing DVT, which is associated with an increased in-hospital mortality (Malato et al. 2015). There are multiple risk factors that increase the risk in this patient population. This includes immobility, indwelling catheters, renal failure, and premorbid state e.g. obesity. It has been reported that DVT occurs in up to 10% of patients, despite the routine use of thromboprophylaxis (Cook et al. 2005).

Therefore, DVT assessment using focussed ultrasound is an invaluable tool for clinicians practising within critical care. The recommended approach is a two-point-compression ultrasound (CUS) of the lower limb (see Figure 16.19). In trained hands, and alongside D-dimer testing, CUS has been found to be a safe and efficient to more comprehensive modalities (Gibson et al. 2009). Once again, a clinical based question approach is used (see Table 16.3).

To perform the assessment, first the patient should be positioned supine, with the hip externally rotated and a slight flexion of the knee. The probe should be placed at two points on the lower leg, the sapheno-femoral junction (SFV) and the popliteal vein (PV).

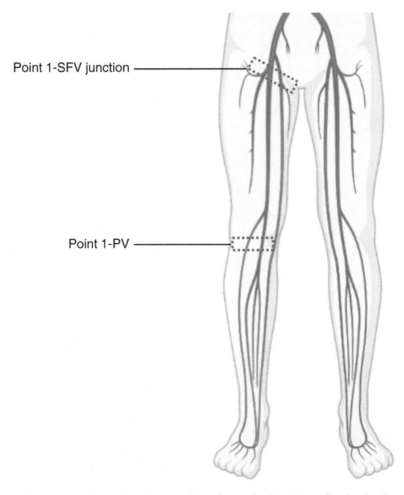

Point 1-SFV junction

Point 1-PV

FIGURE 16.19   Two-point compression points. SFV, saphenofemoral vein, PV, popliteal vein. *Source*: Adapted from Biorender.com (2022).

TABLE 16.3   Focussed DVT clinical Questions.

Clinical question-based approach
Is the vessel patent and compressible?
Is there any evidence occlusive or non-occlusive thrombus?
Is there any evidence of venous flow with calf compression?
Is there any evidence of phasic flow with respiration?

Source: Adapted from FUSIC (2022).

(a)   (b)

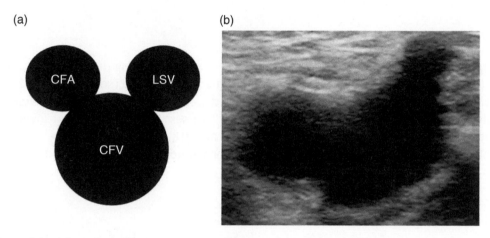

FIGURE 16.20   (a) Mickey Mouse sign. CFA, common femoral artery. LSV, long saphenous vein. CFV, common femoral vein. (b) sonographic Mickey Mouse sign.

Point 1

The first point of assessment is the saphenofemoral junction. This can be located by applying the probe transversely at the inguinal ligament. From here the probe should be moved caudally until three vessels are seen: the common femoral artery, the common femoral vein, and the saphenous vein. The combined appearance of these vessels, sonographically, is often referred to as the 'Mickey Mouse' sign (see Figure 16.20), owing to the shape (Almasarei and Knipe 2017).

Point 2

The second point of assessment is the popliteal vein. This can be located by applying the probe transversely within the popliteal fossa, posterior to the knee. This is easiest to perform with the knee flexed, either in the supine or sitting position. Once the popliteal vein is identified, it should be followed until it is positioned lateral to the artery.

At both points, the veins should be visually patent, fully compressible (wall to wall) and demonstrate no filling defect on colour Doppler assessment. There is a third point that can be added to assess the common femoral vein, however a recent meta-analysis by Lee et al. (2019) demonstrated no statistically significant difference in diagnostic accuracy, between two-point and three-point compression.

RED FLAG PATHOLOGY

Direct Thrombus Visualisation and Compressibility

Ruling out a DVT based on absence of a visual thrombus must not be used as a sole diagnostic criterion. Acute thrombi appear dark (hypoechoic) on ultrasound (see Figure 16.21); this makes it difficult to differentiate from the appearance of blood, which appears black. Chronic thrombi are brighter (hyperechoic), therefore easier to detect. It is therefore deemed a secondary diagnostic criterion. Failure to compress the vein is the primary diagnostic criteria for DVT of the lower extremities, associated with a high sensitivity and specificity (Karande et al. 2016).

Partial Filling Defect

Colour Doppler should be applied to assess for a partial or complete filing defect; a calf squeeze can be useful here to augment flow to this area and reveal the true filling pattern (see Figure 16.22).

Despite the associated high diagnostic accuracy of two-point CUS, it is still recommended that a formal duplex scan is organised with a one-week period to assess full vasculature of lower extremities. This however should not delay treatment (Needleman et al. 2018).

Figure 16.23 shows the importance of clinical history, sonographic findings and their correlation with the diagnosis.

ABDOMINAL ULTRASOUND

Introduction

Focused abdominal ultrasound is not as established as the other ultrasound modalities within AECC. However, one clinical area it is synonymous with is the trauma setting, which necessitates rapid diagnosis of intra-abdominal pathology to determine whether emergency intervention (i.e. laparotomy) is

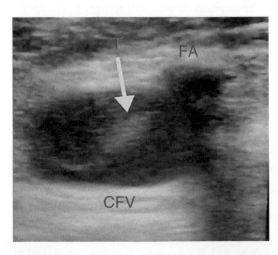

FIGURE 16.21   Non-compressible common femoral vein (CFV) secondary to early thrombus (T). FA = femoral artery. *Source*: Adapted from Zaalouk et al. (2021).

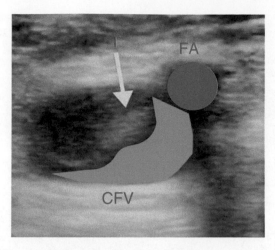

FIGURE 16.22 Partial filling defect (blue) identified on colour flow doppler. Red, arterial flow CFV, common femoral vein, FA, femoral artery, T, thrombus. *Source*: Image credit: Adapted from Zaalouk et al. (2021).

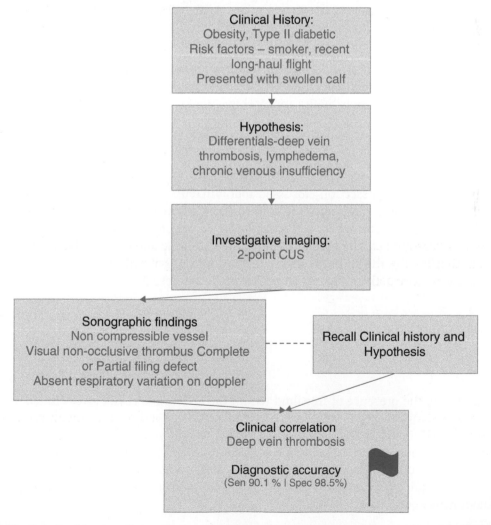

FIGURE 16.23 Sonographic reasoning method – vascular presentation exemplar. *Source*: Adapted from Penny and Zachariason (2015) using diagnostic accuracy data from Bhatt et al. (2020).

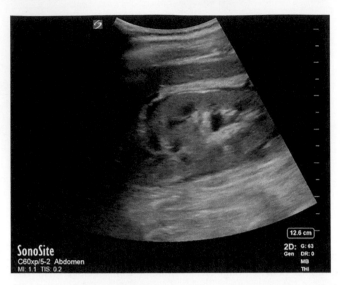

FIGURE 16.24   Transverse view of right kidney displaying moderate hydronephrosis. Anechoic spaces within the kidney signify the presence of fluid in the renal collecting system. *Source*: Adapted from Alberter and Sauer (2022).

required (Boutros et al. 2016). The FAST scan (Focused Abdominal Sonography in Trauma) was developed in the late 1900s (Bloom and Gibbons 2022) and is used routinely by emergency clinicians to rapidly identify hemoperitoneum, with sensitivities approaching 100% (Pearl and Todd 1996).

Clinical Application

In addition to FAST, which is focused on identifying signs of gross intra-abdominal pathology (i.e. bleeding, aortic aneurysm, or dissection), focussed abdominal ultrasound can be utilised to aid decision-making in relation to acute kidney injury (Boniface and Calabrese 2013). This is particularly useful in the critical care environment, where a large majority of patients will be catheterised. In anuric or oliguric patients, ultrasound can be used to assess bladder volume and correct placement and function of the catheter. Additionally, the kidneys can be inspected for signs of hydronephrosis (see Figure 16.24), which may signify an obstructive uropathy (Boniface and Calabrese 2013).

RED FLAG PATHOLOGY

Free Fluid

In the trauma setting, the presence of free fluid within the abdominal cavity gives clinicians two pieces of information (see Figure 16.25). Firstly, there is evidence of hemoperitoneum, and thus indirectly there may be organ injury (Kameda and Taniguchi 2016). In non-trauma settings, there is still a role for abdominal ultrasound when there is clinical suspicion of intra-abdominal pathology. Examples of this include the suspected ruptured ectopic pregnancy (Moore et al. 2007) or in advanced liver disease, to assess the degree of ascites and guide paracentesis (Blaivas 2005). See Table 16.4 for focused clinical questions that can aid in diagnosing abdominal pathology.

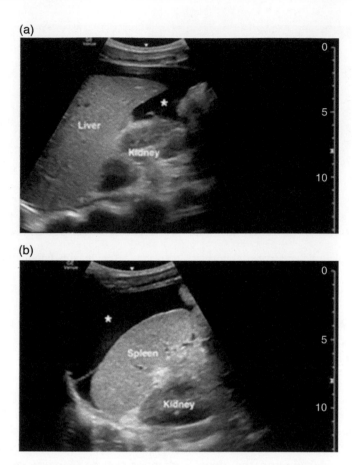

FIGURE 16.25   (a) Intra-abdominal free fluid (asterisk) adjacent to the caudal liver edge in the right upper quadrant view and (b) in the subdiaphragmatic space, in the left upper quadrant view. Fluid appears anechoic sonographically. *Source*: Adapted from Harris et al. (2022).

TABLE 16.4   Focussed abdomen clinical questions.

Clinical question-based approach
Is there any free fluid in the abdomen?
Is the aorta dilated, are there any signs of intimal flap?
Are there any signs of hydronephrosis?
Is the bladder empty or full, is the foley catheter visible?
Is the stomach full?

Source: Based on Intensive Care Society FUSIC and Society of Acute Medicine FAMUS protocol (FAMUS 2022; FUSIC 2022).

Dilated Aorta

A dilated section of the abdominal aorta, measuring over 3 cm in maximal diameter, is referred to as an abdominal aortic aneurysm or AAA. AAA is associated with a high morbidity and mortality and is more common in males, and patients over the age of 65 (Vorp 2007). Focused ultrasound of the abdominal

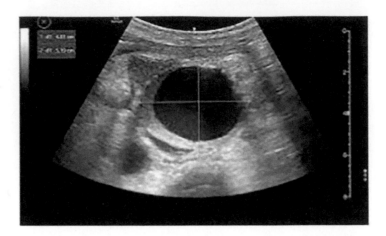

FIGURE 16.26   Abdominal aortic aneurysm. Abnormal dimensions >3 cm maximal diameter. *Source*: Adapted from Rhudy et al. (2022).

aorta has a high sensitivity 93% and specificity 97%for diagnosis of AAA, which makes it an ideal screening tool (Smallwood and Dachsel 2018). Clinicians can assess the maximal aortic dimensions, as seen in Figure 16.26, as well as inspect for evidence of rupture (Rhudy et al. 2022).

Aortic Dissection

Aortic dissection has been estimated to be the aetiology of cardiac arrest in 7% of out-of-hospital cardiac arrests (Carroll et al. 2020). Mortality increases 1–2% per hour, as such focussed abdominal ultrasound plays an important role in reducing the 'door to diagnosis' time (Možina et al. 2012). Sonographic findings associated with dissection include identifiable intimal flap (see Figure 16.27), aortic dilation,

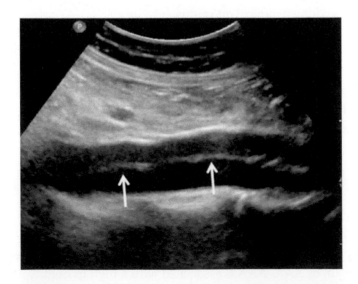

FIGURE 16.27   Abdominal aortic dissection. Intimal flap indicated by arrows. *Source*: Adapted from Wang et al. (2020).

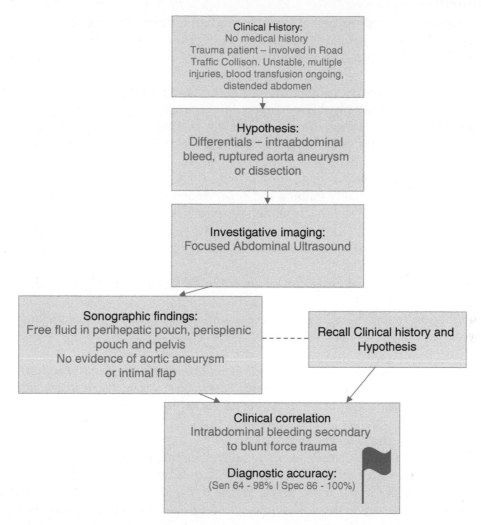

FIGURE 16.28   Sonographic reasoning method – trauma presentation exemplar. *Source*: Adapted from Penny and Zachariason (2015) using diagnostic accuracy data from Kameda and Taniguchi (2016).

calcification, and peri-aortic/pericardial collection. If a flap is identified within the abdominal exam, a focussed ultrasound scan of the heart is indicated to assess the extent and classification of dissection (i.e. A or B), which will influence the surgical plan (Earl-Royal et al. 2019).

Clinical correlation with sonographic findings are key, particularly in cases where trauma is involved (see Figure 16.28).

DISCUSSION

Point-of-care ultrasound is a versatile and effective tool used routinely within the AECC settings. There are many advantages to this form of imaging, perhaps the most important being the associated diagnostic accuracies in identification of many red flag pathologies.

There are however, several recognised limitations when utilising ultrasound in the acutely unwell patients (Smallwood and Dachsel 2018). All of which can influence image quality and thus, reliability of the findings. Key limitations can be categorised into 'patient and operator factors' (Abu-Zidan 2012).

Patient factors: Often unwell patients are unable to move into the recommended scanning positions. This limits the clinician's ability to apply the ultrasound probe effectively and optimise the view of the structure of interest. Some patients are mechanically ventilated or are undergoing advanced monitoring, which can obscure views of vital organs. Finally, there is a growing population of obese patients, who, due to increased body habitus, are challenging to scan due to the increased depth of imaging (Uppot 2018).

Operator factors: Good, quality training and supervision is key to safeguard high-quality practice (BMUS 2022). Despite established accreditation programmes, there is still work that needs to be done within local clinical areas, to improve ultrasound governance. The reported diagnostic accuracies will be heavily influenced if the operator is not adequately trained or is inexperienced.

Cormack et al. (2019) suggests using 'five pillars of PoCUS' to safeguard highest standards of clinical quality and safety (see Table 16.5).

Beyond training and supervision, there are several important initiatives that clinicians should prioritise to improve ultrasound governance within clinical areas (BMUS 2022):

Identification of a dedicated PoCUS lead. An appropriately qualified clinician, usually to an advanced level, should take overarching responsibility of governance, to ensure all staff who perform PoCUS have undergone high-quality training and accreditation. This individual should maintain good links with both cardiology and radiology departments, so that cases which fall outside the scope of PoCUS datasets, can be escalated appropriately.

Reporting and archiving. Outside of sonography departments, there is usually a lack of robust archiving systems and often scans are reported at the bedside, without a report being generated or images being stored for future review. This is not the best practice and as such, a simple report (ideally electronic), appropriate to the level of practice of the operator, should be filled out and included in the medical records. Imaging systems, such as PACS can be used to upload all PoCUS studies, to accompany this electronic report.

Regular case reviews. Organising a forum in which clinicians, from all specialties can gather to review cases, usually monthly, is an example of best practice. Challenging cases, or cases where PoCUS made a significant difference to patient management can be presented. These forums are incredibly helpful in creating a community of practice.

TABLE 16.5   Five pillars of point-of-care ultrasound.

Five pillars of PoCUS				
Governance	Infrastructure	Administration	Education	Quality
Medical executive	Equipment	Workflow	Structure	Clinical audit
Director/Lead	Networks	Reporting	Training	Case review
Steering group	Archiving	Patient records	Credentialling	Feedback
Teaching faculty	Infection control	Logbooks	Skills maintenance	Compliance

Source: Based on Cormack et al. (2019).

Take Home Points

- Point of care ultrasound is an invaluable tool that, when used by an appropriately trained professional, can aid diagnosis of a multitude of conditions.
- Ultrasound has been found to be comparative and, in some cases, superior to other imaging modalities in the diagnosis of common acute pathologies.
- In the UK, there are several training programmes available to healthcare professionals that wish to utilise ultrasound as a diagnostic modality within their scope of practice.
- Deciding which accreditation is most suitable for the individual practitioner depends on three fundamental factors:
    1. Practical exposure to a range of pathology
    2. Support from an accredited mentor
    3. Minimum requirement for your area of practice

REFERENCES

Abu-Zidan, F.M. (2012). Point-of-care ultrasound in critically ill patients: where do we stand? *Journal of Emergencies, Trauma, and Shock* 5 (1): 70–71.

Abu-Zidan, F.M., Hefny, A.F., and Corr, P. (2011). Clinical ultrasound physics. *Journal of Emergencies, Trauma, and Shock* 4 (4): 501–503.

AIUM (2019). AIUM practice parameter for the use of ultrasound to guide vascular access procedures. *Journal of Ultrasound in Medicine* 38 (3): E4–E18.

Alberter, A. and Sauer, J. (2022). Hydronephrosis and free fluid identified by point-of-care ultrasound leads to diagnosis. *Journal of the American College of Emergency Physicians Open* 3 (5): e12824.

Alerhand, S. and Carter, J.M. (2019). What echocardiographic findings suggest a pericardial effusion is causing tamponade? *The American Journal of Emergency Medicine* 37 (2): 321–326.

Almasarei, H. and Knipe, H. (2017). *Mickey Mouse Sign (Ultrasound)* [online]. Available from: radiopedia. org2022 [accessed 12 January 2023].

Anderson, R. and Buckland, J. (2019). *Pulmonary Embolism in Echo* [online]. Available from: https://www. cardioserv.net/pulmonary-embolism-echo/ [accessed 26 June 2023].

Au, A. and Zwank, M. (2020). *Ultrasound PHYSICS and Technical Facts for the Beginner* [online]. Available from: https://www.acep.org/sonoguide/basic/ultrasound-physics-and-technical-facts-for-the-beginner [accessed 26 June 2023].

Bandi, V., Lunn, W., Ernst, A. et al. (2008). Ultrasound vs. CT in detecting chest wall invasion by tumour: a prospective study. *Chest* 133 (4): 881–886.

Bhatt, M., Braun, C., Patel, P. et al. (2020). Diagnosis of deep vein thrombosis of the lower extremity: a systematic review and meta-analysis of test accuracy. *Blood Advances* 4 (7): 1250–1264.

Bierig, S.M. and Jones, A. (2009). Accuracy and cost comparison of ultrasound versus alternative imaging modalities, including CT, MR, PET, and angiography. *Journal of Diagnostic Medical Sonography* 25 (3): 138–144.

Biorender.com. (2022). Original figures (not created using BioRender templates).

Blaivas, M. (2005). Emergency diagnostic paracentesis to determine intraperitoneal fluid identity discovered on bedside ultrasound of unstable patients. *The Journal of Emergency Medicine* 29 (4): 461–465.

Blaivas, M. (2012). Lung ultrasound in evaluation of pneumonia. *Journal of Ultrasound in Medicine* 31 (6): 823–826.

Bloom, B. and Gibbons, R. (2022). *Focused Assessment with Sonography for Trauma* [online]: StatPearls. Available from: `https://www.ncbi.nlm.nih.gov/books/NBK470479/2022` [accessed 12 January 2023].

Boniface, K.S. and Calabrese, K.Y. (2013). Intensive care ultrasound: IV. Abdominal ultrasound in critical care. *Annals of the American Thoracic Society* 10 (6): 713–724.

Boutros, S.M., Nassef, M.A., and Abdel-Ghany, A.F. (2016). Blunt abdominal trauma: the role of focused abdominal sonography in assessment of organ injury and reducing the need for CT. *Alexandria Journal of Medicine* 52 (1): 35–41.

British Medical Ultrasound Society (BMUS). (2022). *Guidlines for Professional Ultrasound Practice* [online]. Available from: `https://www.bmus.org/media/resources/files/SoR_and_BMUS_guidelines_2022_7th_Ed.docx_FrypvRQ.pdf` [accessed 12 January 2023].

British Society of Echocardiography (BSE). (2022). *Level 1 Accreditation (L1)* [online]. Available from: `https://www.bsecho.org/Public/Accreditation/Personal-accred/L1-accred.aspx2021` [accessed 12 January 2023].

Carroll, B.J., Schermerhorn, M.L., and Manning, W.J. (2020). Imaging for acute aortic syndromes. *Heart* 106 (3): 182.

Carroll, D., Bell, D. and Bandura, P. 2023 *Point-of-care Ultrasound (Curriculum)* [online]. Available from: `https://radiopaedia.org/articles/62779` [accessed 26 June 2023].

Chapman, G.A., Johnson, D., and Bodenham, A.R. (2006). Visualisation of needle position using ultrasonography. *Anaesthesia* 61 (2): 148–158.

Cid, X., Wang, A., Heiberg, J. et al. (2020). Point-of-care lung ultrasound in the assessment of patients with COVID-19: a tutorial. *Australasian Journal of Ultrasound in Medicine* 23 (4): 271–281.

Conway, H. (2022a). Focused echocardiography. In: *Advanced Clinical Practice: at a glance* (ed. S. Diamond-Fox, B. Hill, and I. Peate). Wiley.

Conway, H. (2022b). Fundamental ultrasound skills. In: *Advanced Clinical Practice: at a glance* (ed. S. Diamond-Fox, B. Hill, and I. Peate). Wiley.

Cook, D., Douketis, J., Crowther, M.A. et al. (2005). The diagnosis of deep venous thrombosis and pulmonary embolism in medical-surgical intensive care unit patients. *Journal of Critical Care* 20 (4): 314–319.

Cormack, C.J., Wald, A.M., Coombs, P.R. et al. (2019). Time to establish pillars in point-of-care ultrasound. *Australasian Journal of Ultrasound in Medicine* 22 (1): 12–14.

Diepen, S., Katz, J.N., Albert, N.M. et al. (2017). Contemporary management of cardiogenic shock: a scientific statement from the American Heart Association. *Circulation* 136 (16): e232–e268.

Dietrich, C.F., Mathis, G., Blaivas, M. et al. (2016). Lung B-line artefacts and their use. *Journal of Thoracic Disease* 8 (6): 1356–1365.

Dragoi, L., Teijeiro-Paradis, R., and Douflé, G. (2022). When is tamponade not an echocardiographic diagnosis. . . or is it ever? *Echocardiography* 39 (7): 880–885.

Duggan, N.M., Selame, L.A., and Shokoohi, H. (2020). Why pretest probability matters when we do point-of-care ultrasound. *Journal of the American College of Emergency Physicians Open* 1 (6): 1778.

Durant, A. and Nagdev, A. (2010). Ultrasound detection of lung hepatization. *The Western Journal of Emergency Medicine* 11 (4): 322–323.

Durila, M. (2018). Reversible causes of cardiac arrest 4H's and 4T's; can be easily diagnosed and remembered following general ABC rule, Motol University Hospital approach. *Resuscitation* 126: e7.

Earl-Royal, E., Nguyen, P.D., Alvarez, A., and Gharahbaghian, L. (2019). Detection of type B aortic dissection in the Emergency Department with Point-of-Care Ultrasound. *Clinical Practice and Cases in Emergency Medicine* 3 (3): 202–207.

Ebrahimi, A., Yousefifard, M., Mohammad Kazemi, H. et al. (2014). Diagnostic accuracy of chest ultrasonography versus chest radiography for identification of pneumothorax: a systematic review and meta-analysis. *Tanaffos* 13 (4): 29–40.

Gibson, N.S., Schellong, S.M., Kheir, D.Y. et al. (2009). Safety and sensitivity of two ultrasound strategies in patients with clinically suspected deep venous thrombosis: a prospective management study. *Journal of Thrombosis and Haemostasis* 7 (12): 2035–2041.

Gillman, L.M. and Kirkpatrick, A.W. (2012). Portable bedside ultrasound: the visual stethoscope of the twenty-first century. *Scandinavian Journal of Trauma, Resuscitation and Emergency Medicine* 20: 18.

Harris, J., Vassallo, S., Finan, C.D., and Kalivoda, E.J. (2022). Point-of-care ultrasound evaluation of blunt abdominal trauma. *Journal of the American College of Emergency Physicians Open* 3 (4): e12786.

Health Education England (HEE). (2022). *Advanced Clinical Practice in Acute Medicine Curriculum Framework – Credentials* [online]. Available from: https://advanced-practice.hee.nhs.uk/our-work/credentials [accessed 20 June 2023].

Health Education England (HEE). (2017). *Multi-professional Framework for Advanced Clinical Practice in England* [online]. Available from: https://www.hee.nhs.uk/sites/default/files/documents/multi-professionalframeworkforadvancedclinicalpracticeinengland.pdf [accessed 20 June 2023].

Intensive Care Society. (2022). *Focused Ultrasound in Intensive Care (FUSIC)* [online]. Available from: www.ics.ac.uk/Society/Learning/FUSIC_Accreditation2021 [accessed 12 January 2023].

Izquierdo-Gomez, M., Mari-Lopez, B., and Lacalzada-Almeida, J. (2018). Ischaemic mitral valve regurgitation. *e-Journal of Cardiology Practice* 16 (12).

Kameda, T. and Taniguchi, N. (2016). Overview of point-of-care abdominal ultrasound in emergency and critical care. *Journal of Intensive Care* 4 (1): 53.

Karande, G.Y., Hedgire, S.S., Sanchez, Y. et al. (2016). Advanced imaging in acute and chronic deep vein thrombosis. *Cardiovascular Diagnosis and Therapy* 6 (6): 493–507.

Konstantinides, S.V., Meyer, G., Becattini, C. et al. (2019). 2019 ESC guidelines for the diagnosis and management of acute pulmonary embolism developed in collaboration with the European Respiratory Society (ERS). *The task force for the diagnosis and management of acute pulmonary embolism of the European Society of Cardiology (ESC)* 54 (3): 1901647.

Lafon, T., Appert, A., Hadj, M. et al. (2020). Comparative early hemodynamic profiles in patients presenting to the emergency department with septic and nonseptic acute circulatory failure using focused echocardiography. *Shock* 53 (6): 695–700.

Lamperti, M., Biasucci, D.G., Disma, N. et al. (2020). European Society of Anaesthesiology guidelines on perioperative use of ultrasound-guided for vascular access (PERSEUS vascular access). *European Journal of Anaesthesiology | EJA* 37 (5): 344–376.

Lancellotti, P., Price, S., Edvardsen, T. et al. (2014). The use of echocardiography in acute cardiovascular care: Recommendations of the European Association of Cardiovascular Imaging and the Acute Cardiovascular Care Association. *European Heart Journal Cardiovascular Imaging* 16 (2): 119–146.

Lee, J.H., Lee, S.H., and Yun, S.J. (2019). Comparison of 2-point and 3-point point-of-care ultrasound techniques for deep vein thrombosis at the emergency department: a meta-analysis. *Medicine (Baltimore)* 98 (22): e15791.

Lichtenstein, D.A. (2014). Lung ultrasound in the critically ill. *Annals of Intensive Care* 4 (1): 1.

Lichtenstein, D.A. and Mezière, G.A. (2008). Relevance of lung ultrasound in the diagnosis of acute respiratory failure: the BLUE protocol. *Chest* 134 (1): 117–125.

Lichtenstein, D.A. and Mezière, G.A. (2011). The BLUE-points: three standardized points used in the BLUE-protocol for ultrasound assessment of the lung in acute respiratory failure. *Critical Ultrasound Journal* 3 (2): 109–110.

Lichtenstein, D., Goldstein, I., Mourgeon, E. et al. (2004). Comparative diagnostic performances of auscultation, chest radiography, and lung ultrasonography in acute respiratory distress syndrome. *Anesthesiology* 100 (1): 9–15.

Longobardo, L., Zito, C., Carerj, S. et al. (2018). Role of echocardiography in the intensive care unit: overview of the most common clinical scenarios. *Journal of Patient Centered Research Reviews* 5 (3): 239–243.

López-Candales, A., Edelman, K., and Candales, M.D. (2010). Right ventricular apical contractility in acute pulmonary embolism: the McConnell sign revisited. *Echocardiography* 27 (6): 614–620.

Maizel, J., Airapetian, N., Lorne, E. et al. (2007). Diagnosis of central hypovolemia by using passive leg raising. *Intensive Care Medicine* 33 (7): 1133–1138.

Malato, A., Dentali, F., Siragusa, S. et al. (2015). The impact of deep vein thrombosis in critically ill patients: a meta-analysis of major clinical outcomes. *Blood Transfusion* 13 (4): 559–568.

McLean, A.S. (2016). Echocardiography in shock management. *Critical Care* 20 (1): 275.

McMurray, J.J., Adamopoulos, S., Anker, S.D. et al. (2012). ESC Guidelines for the diagnosis and treatment of acute and chronic heart failure 2012: The task force for the diagnosis and treatment of acute and chronic heart failure 2012 of the European Society of Cardiology. Developed in collaboration with the Heart Failure Association (HFA) of the ESC. *European Heart Journal* 33 (14): 1787–1847.

Miller, A. (2015). Practical approach to lung ultrasound. *BJA Education* 16 (2): 39–45.

Millington, S.J. (2019). Ultrasound assessment of the inferior vena cava for fluid responsiveness: easy, fun, but unlikely to be helpful. *Canadian Journal of Anesthesia/Journal canadien d'anesthésie* 66 (6): 633–638.

Mojoli, F., Bouhemad, B., Mongodi, S., and Lichtenstein, D. (2019). Lung ultrasound for critically ill patients. *American Journal of Respiratory and Critical Care Medicine* 199 (6): 701–714.

Moore, C., Todd, W.M., O'Brien, E., and Lin, H. (2007). Free fluid in Morison's pouch on bedside ultrasound predicts need for operative intervention in suspected ectopic pregnancy. *Academic Emergency Medicine* 14 (8): 755–758.

Možina, H., Jug, B., and Podbregar, M. (2012). Point-of-care ultrasound in patients with aortic dissection – two year experience at Ljubljana Emergency Medical Unit. *Critical Ultrasound Journal* 4 (1): A14.

Muller, L., Toumi, M., Bousquet, P.J. et al. (2011). An increase in aortic blood flow after an infusion of 100 ml colloid over 1 minute can predict fluid responsiveness: the mini-fluid challenge study. *Anesthesiology* 115 (3): 541–547.

Naeije, R. and Badagliacca, R. (2017). The overloaded right heart and ventricular interdependence. *Cardiovascular Research* 113 (12): 1474–1485.

National Institute for Health and Care Excellence (NICE). (2002). *Guidance on the Use of Ultrasound Locating Devices for Placing Central Venous Catheters* [online]. Available from: www.nice.org.uk/guidance/ta49 [accessed 26 June 2023].

Needleman, L., Cronan, J.J., Lilly, M.P. et al. (2018). Ultrasound for lower extremity deep venous thrombosis. *Circulation* 137 (14): 1505–1515.

Otto, C. (2016). *Textbook of clinical echocardiography*, 6e. Elsevier.

Pearl, W.S. and Todd, K.H. (1996). Ultrasonography for the initial evaluation of blunt abdominal trauma: a review of prospective trials. *Annals of Emergency Medicine* 27 (3): 353–361.

Penny, S.M. and Zachariason, A. (2015). The sonographic reasoning method. *Journal of Diagnostic Medical Sonography* 31 (2): 122–129.

Rhudy, A.K., Patel, S., Houser, A. et al. (2022). Point-of-care ultrasound for identification of ruptured infrarenal abdominal aortic aneurysm. *Echocardiography* 39 (6): 841–843.

Russell, F.M., Ferre, R., Ehrman, R.R. et al. (2020). What are the minimum requirements to establish proficiency in lung ultrasound training for quantifying B-lines? *ESC Heart Failure* 7 (5): 2941–2947.

Saraogi, A. (2015). Lung ultrasound: present and future. *Lung India* 32 (3): 250–257.

Seven Day Services Clinical Standards (2017). *Diagnostics*, 4–5. NHS England.

Shyy, W., Knight, R.S., Kornblith, A., and Teismann, N.A. (2017). Point-of-care diagnosis of cardiac tamponade identified by the flow velocity paradoxus. *Journal of Ultrasound in Medicine* 36 (11): 2197–2201.

Sia, Y.T., O'Meara, E., and Ducharme, A. (2008). Role of echocardiography in acute myocardial infarction. *Current Heart Failure Reports* 5 (4): 189–196.

Smallwood, N. and Dachsel, M. (2018). Point-of-care ultrasound (POCUS): unnecessary gadgetry or evidence-based medicine? *Clinical Medicine (London, England)* 18 (3): 219–224.

Society for Acute Medicine. (2022). *Focused Acute Medicine Ultrasound (FAMUS)* [online]. Available from: www.acutemedicine.org.uk/famus [accessed 26 June 2023].

Soni, N.J., Franco, R., Velez, M.I. et al. (2015). Ultrasound in the diagnosis and management of pleural effusions. *Journal of Hospital Medicine* 10 (12): 811–816.

Soni, N.J., Dreyfuss, Z.S., Ali, S. et al. (2022). Pleural fluid echogenicity measured by ultrasound image pixel density to differentiate transudative versus exudative pleural effusions. *Annals of the American Thoracic Society* 19 (5): 857–860.

Taylor, L.A., Vitto, M.J., Joyce, M. et al. (2018). Ultrasound-guided thoracostomy site identification in healthy volunteers. *Critical Ultrasound Journal* 10 (1): 1–5.

The Faculty of Intensive Care Medicine. (2018). *Curriculum for Training for Advanced Critical Care Practitioners – Syllabus. V1.1* [online]. Available from: www.ficm.ac.uk/media/6896 [accessed 20 June 2023].

The Intensive Care Society, Critical Care Networks – *National Nurse Leads and The National Outreach Forum.* (2022). *Advanced Critical Care Outreach Competencies* [online]. Available from: https://ics.ac.uk/asset/43B8C11B-4512-41D0-B97768FABA2C30B2 [accessed 20 June 2023].

The Royal College of Emergency Medicine. (2022). *Emergency Medicine Advanced Clinical Practitioner Curriculum 2022 (Adult)* [online]. Available from: https://rcem.ac.uk/wp-content/uploads/2022/09/ACP_Curriculum_Adult_Final_060922.pdf [accessed 20 June 2023].

Trivedi, V. and Kokkirala, A. (2022). *Cardiac tamponade. Ferri's Clinical Advisor*, 316–318. Elsevier.

Uppot, R.N. (2018). Technical challenges of imaging & image-guided interventions in obese patients. *The British Journal of Radiology* 91 (1089): 20170931.

Via, G., Price, S., and Storti, E. (2011). Echocardiography in the sepsis syndromes. *Critical Ultrasound Journal* 3 (2): 71–85.

Volpicelli, G. (2011). Sonographic diagnosis of pneumothorax. *Intensive Care Medicine* 37 (2): 224–232.

Volpicelli, G., Elbarbary, M., Blaivas, M. et al. (2012). International evidence-based recommendations for point-of-care lung ultrasound. *Intensive Care Medicine* 38 (4): 577–591.

Vorp, D.A. (2007). Biomechanics of abdominal aortic aneurysm. *Journal of Biomechanics* 40 (9): 1887–1902.

Wang, J., Yao, C., Wu, Y., and Lai, B. (2020). Asymptomatic long-segmental type A aortic dissection diagnosed by transthoracic echocardiography: a case report and literature review. *Journal of Clinical Ultrasound* 48 (9): 574–578.

Wang, M., Luo, X., Wang, L. et al. (2021). A comparison of lung ultrasound and computed tomography in the diagnosis of patients with COVID-19 : a systematic review and meta-analysis. *Diagnostics (Basel)* 11 (8).

Wong, A., Kingwill, A., and Barker, G. (2016). Chest drains: is the triangle of safety really safe? An ultrasonographic study of enshrined practice to improve patient outcome and safety. *Intensive Care Medicine Experimental* 4 (Suppl 1): A376–A376.

Zaalouk, T.M., Bitar, Z.I., Maadarani, O.S., and Ragab Elshabasy, R.D. (2021). Modified BLUE protocol ultrasonography can diagnose thrombotic complications of COVID-19 with normal lung ultrasound. *Clinical Case Reports* 9 (5): e04075.

Zieleskiewicz, L., Markarian, T., Lopez, A. et al. (2020). Comparative study of lung ultrasound and chest computed tomography scan in the assessment of severity of confirmed COVID-19 pneumonia. *Intensive Care Medicine* 46 (9): 1707–1713.

CHAPTER 17

Laboratory Tests

Sarah Henry and Natalie Gardner

Aim

The aim of this chapter is to help you develop and apply understanding of common laboratory tests, the significance of their results with which to inform your diagnostic decision-making.

LEARNING OUTCOMES

After reading this chapter the reader will be able to:

1. List and describe common laboratory tests.
2. Discuss how to interpret results of laboratory tests.
3. Explain the pathophysiology of individual tests.
4. Understand the key investigations required to aid in the diagnosis of common conditions.

SELF-ASSESSMENT QUESTIONS

1. What key lab tests would you order in a patient with suspected DKA?
2. Which tests form part of a standard biochemistry profile?
3. What colour bottle would you send if you wanted to run coagulation studies?
4. What conditions could form part of your differential diagnosis from results of low WBCs in a 21-year old male patient.

The Advanced Practitioner in Acute, Emergency and Critical Care, First Edition. Edited by Sadie Diamond-Fox, Barry Hill, Sonya Stone, Caroline McCrea, Natalie Gardner, and Angela Roberts.

INTRODUCTION

Patient's do not present with a diagnosis but instead provide the clinician with signs and symptoms. It is only through a combination of a comprehensive history, a physical examination, and the utilisation of appropriate diagnostic testing that a diagnosis can be reached and a treatment plan implemented. In this chapter, we will discuss common laboratory tests requested in acute, emergency and critical care (AECC) settings. As an Advanced Clinical Practitioner (ACP), it is crucial to be competent in the interpretation of laboratory investigations. This interpretation coupled with the patient's clinical history will allow for the formulation of both diagnosis and a subsequent treatment and management plan. In the AECC setting, this interpretation and diagnostic decision-making often occurs under operational pressure and so it is imperative that the clinician responsible for requesting the laboratory investigations has a sound knowledge of the pathophysiology of each test to underpin the clinical reasoning behind performing a specific test. With each laboratory test performed, there are both risks and benefits for the patient, and so it is imperative that consideration is given to how the test results will alter patient management. However, in many cases laboratory tests are performed in line with local and national guidelines, pathways, and polices. It must be remembered that the laboratory tests discussed in this chapter are not exhaustive and each patient should be assessed and managed on an individual basis.

Within the constraints of this chapter, it is unrealistic to attempt to comprehensively study every laboratory test available. Instead, common laboratory tests will be discussed and symptoms examined according to the following systems:

1. Cardiovascular
2. Endocrinology
3. Gastroenterology
4. Haematology
5. Renal
6. Respiratory

As a clinician, developing an understanding of which laboratory investigations to perform employing a structured approach to their interpretation will provide a robust toolkit from which to help identify and support the diagnosis formed. It must be remembered that the reference, or normal, range of laboratory investigations can vary according to the following factors:

- Age
- Sex
- Sample collection time
- Pre-existing health conditions
- Pregnancy

In addition, each clinician should ensure that they are working within their own level of competency and within the boundaries of their current role. Due to the nature of working at an Advanced level of Practice it must be remembered that this may fall outside the traditional scope of practice of the Clinician's base-profession.

Multi-professional Framework (MPF) for Advanced Clinical Practice Guidance for Professional Development (HEE 2017)

This chapter maps to the following statements within the MPF:

1. Clinical:	1.1	1.2	1.4	1.6

Accreditation Considerations

This chapter maps to the following statements within the following national accreditation documents:

Curriculum for Training for Advanced Critical Care Practitioners Syllabus V1.1
(The Faculty of Intensive Care Medicine 2018)

2.2	2.2	2.2	2.2	2.2
3.1	3.1	3.1	3.1	3.1
3.2	3.2	3.2	3.2	3.2
4.2	4.2	4.2	4.2	4.2

Advanced Critical Care Outreach Competencies
(The Intensive Care Society, Critical Care Networks – National Nurse Leads and The National Outreach Forum 2022)

A1	C2

Emergency Medicine Advanced Clinical Practitioner Curriculum 2022 – Adult
(The Royal College of Emergency Medicine 2022)

SLO3

Advanced Clinical Practice in Acute Medicine Curriculum Framework
(Health Education England 2022)

- Generic Clinical CiPs: 1, 2, 3
- Specialty Clinical CiPs: 3

BLOOD COLLECTION

Blood should be collected from a vein where there is no intravenous infusion running, using an appropriately sized needle in order to prevent both damage to cells and damage to veins which could lead to erroneous results.

Blood is collected in colour coded bottles. The colour indicates the chemical contained within the bottle. These chemicals are present for the following purposes:

- Prevent clotting
- Accelerate clotting
- Preserve the structure of blood cells
- Preserve the concentration of some constituent of the sample

The order of draw of samples is important to prevent cross-contamination and false-positive results due to additives from the venous blood collection tubes.

Bloods should be drawn in the following order:

- Blood Cultures: aerobic followed by anaerobic
- Coagulation testing
- Tests drawn in tubes without additives
- Tests drawn in tubes with additives

See Table 17.1 for details of each blood collection tube, the additive, and the associated use in testing.

In the instance that a sample needs to be mixed with the tube additive, this should be done by inversion of the tube and not shaking so as to prevent cellular breakdown.

TABLE 17.1   Common blood collection tubes.

Venous blood collection tube colour	Additive	Uses
Light blue	Citrate	Coagulation studies, INR, D-dimer, Fibrinogen
Red	Silica particles	Biochemistry tests requiring a serum, which acts as a clot activator. Hormone testing, drug levels, toxicology, bacterial and viral serology, antibodies.
Gold	Clot activator	Speeds up blood clotting and separation of serum. Use for routine biochemistry tests requiring blood serum, B12, Ferritin, Folate.
Purple	EDTA	Anticoagulant and preserves the structure of blood cells. FBC and other haematological tests, HbA1c, electrophoresis.
Pink	Cross match	Blood group Cross matching
Grey	Fluoride oxalate	Blood glucose, ethanol, Lactate

In the AECC setting, it is helpful to consider laboratory investigations in the following categories:

- Haematology
- Biochemistry

The most common laboratory investigations performed are listed in the tables below along with possible causes for their abnormal results.

Haematology

In haematology, the main investigations sit within the full blood count (FBC). This looks at the cellular components of the blood, and evaluation of the values associated with these will help form your differential diagnosis. Within a standard FBC, it can be helpful to divide the results into three main sections; red cells, white cells, and platelets. Tables 17.2–17.4 look at these components and values in detail, and what the values correspond to.

Haematinics are another important part of haematology laboratory investigations, as they consist of the nutrients required for haematopoiesis in the bone marrow, and without which cytopenias can develop. Table 17.5 summarises haematinics.

Biochemistry

In biochemistry, the main investigations discussed here are split into urea and electrolytes (U&Es) and liver function tests (LFTs). Other biochemistry tests are discussed later in this chapter.

U&ES

U&Es are a marker of both kidney function and levels of electrolytes, and are primarily used for looking at renal disease, dehydration, and cardiac risk. Table 17.6 summarises the normal U+E range values and the common causes for being outside of these values.

LIVER FUNCTION TESTS

Within the AECC population, we can use LFTs to help determine the source of any damage to the liver, and to help us distinguish between two main patterns of injury; a hepatocellular pattern, and a cholestatic pattern. A hepatocellular pattern will show as predominantly elevated aminotransferases, and a cholestatic pattern will be predominantly elevated alkaline phosphatase (ALP), gamma glutamyl transferase (GGT), and bilirubin. Table 17.7 presents a detailed analysis of LFTs.

ARTERIAL BLOOD GASES (ABGS)

Arterial Blood Gases (ABGs) sit under biochemistry as part of point-of-care testing. Within the AECC populations, this can be an invaluable tool for getting immediate feedback regarding key physiology within your patient, that you can then take action on. Table 17.8 summarises ABGs.

OTHER KEY BIOCHEMISTRY INVESTIGATIONS

There are many biochemistry investigations that are very pertinent to the AECC populations, but do not sit under an overall heading. These are reviewed in Table 17.9.

TABLE 17.2 Full blood count: red cells.

Full blood count		
Red cells		
RBC Made in bone marrow	♂ 4.6–5.7 ♀ 4.0–5.2 × 1012/l	Raised
Hb Oxygen carrying ability	♂130–180 ♀ 115–165 g/l	Excess production of RBC 90% genetic, Hypoxia (altitude sickness/COPD) Disease usually renal or liver. Can be elevated in cerebellar dysfunction. Reduced plasma volume from fluid loss or dehydration. Low Anaemia – check Hb and MCV to aid classification. Acute versus chronic. Normocytic anaemia: Reduced production of RBC secondary to bone marrow dysfunction e.g. aplastic anaemia. Diet deficiency/absorption problem/loss of cells from bleeding, haemolysis or chronic inflammation. Haemoglobinopathy e.g. sickle cell. Chronic disease e.g. Liver/GI/Renal
MCV Mean Cell Volume	80–100%	Raised Macrocytic anaemia – occurs with Vitamin B12/folate deficiency. Can occur secondary to Liver disease, Hypothyroid, Medications, SLE. Low Microcytic anaemia – occurs with chronic disease or iron deficiency. Check ferritin when low MCV identified.
MCH Mean corpuscular haemoglobin	27–32 Picograms/cell	Mean cell haemoglobin mass. This should mirror MCV. It is important to remember smaller cells have lower Hb.
MCHC Mean cell haemoglobin concentration	320–370 g/l	Raised Hereditary Spherocytosis B12/folic acid deficiency Low Microcytic anaemia Iron deficiency
Haematocrit Ratio of volume of red blood cells to the total volume of blood	♂ 42–52 ♀ 35–47	Raised Bleeding OR Haemodilution

TABLE 17.3   Full blood count: white cells.

Full Blood Count		
White Cells		
WBC Protect from infection	3.6–11 x 10⁹/l	<u>Raised</u> (Leucocytosis) Infection Systemic illness Secondary to allergy or inflammation Can be raised with certain cancers even if no obvious infection e.g. leukaemia <u>Low</u> (Leukopenia) Some Medications e.g. SACT Autoimmune disease Secondary to virus Severe bacterial infection Bone marrow failure Liver disease Excess alcohol Blasts are types of immature white blood cells. They usually constitute <1% of white cells. They can be raised in bone marrow overdrive. This indicates possible leukaemia.
Neutrophils Fight infection and heal injuries	2–7.5 x 10⁹/l (50–70%)	<u>Raised</u> (Neutrophilia) Bacterial/viral infection Steroids Exercise Necrosis Vasculitis Malignancy Myeloid leukaemia <u>Low</u> (Neutropenia) SACT Rheumatoid arthritis Medications e.g. azothiaprene, carbimazole, NSAIDs Epstein Barr Virus Late sign of overwhelming bacterial infection Patients of Afro-Caribbean heritage

(Continued)

TABLE 17.3   (Continued)

Full Blood Count		
Lymphocytes Memory cells	1.5–3.5 x 10⁹/l (25–35%)	Two main types: B cells which produce antibodies that attack bacteria, viruses, toxins, and T cells, which destroy the body's cells which have become malignant or have been attacked by viruses. Raised (Lymphocytosis) Secondary to virus Stress following an acute illness/episode e.g. MI or seizure Epstein Barr Virus Lymphocytic Leukaemia Low (Lymphopenia) HIV Secondary to steroids RA SLE Sarcoidosis Immunocompromised Lymphoma Secondary to medications
Monocytes Ingest and remove dead cells, boost immune response	0.2–0.8 x 10⁹/l (4–6%)	Raised Chronic Infection TB Syphilis Crohn's Disease Ulcerative colitis Malignancy
Eosinophils Disease fighting cell	0.04–0.4 x 10⁹/l (1–3%)	Raised Secondary to parasites Secondary to allergies Asthma Neoplasm
Basophils Protect from pathogens	0.01–0.1 x 10⁹/l	Raised Secondary to parasites Hypersensitivity

Coagulation

Coagulation screens allow us to assess the synthetic function of the liver, as well as assess and monitor any suspected or diagnosed coagulopathies. Many patients in the AECC populations will be on prescribed anticoagulants, and coagulation screen can be used to monitor their coagulation status during an inpatient stay. The key components of a coagulation screen are reviewed in Table 17.10.

TABLE 17.4   Full blood count: platelets.

Full blood count		
Platelets		
Platelets	150–440 x 10^9/l	Raised (Thrombocytosis)
Crucial for clotting		Chronic Infection
		Malignancy
		Bone marrow over production
		Medications
		Chronic bleeding
		Low (Thrombocytopenia)
		Sepsis
		Secondary to virus
		HIV
		Rheumatoid Arthritis
		SLE
		Bleeding
		Transfusion
		DIC
		Leukaemia
		Alcohol
		Medications
		HELLP
		Bone Marrow Dysfunction
		Portal hypertension.
		When clumping in tube occurs, this should be discussed with the haematology laboratory.

TABLE 17.5   Haematinics.

Haematinics	
Serum ferritin	Low iron/low serum ferritin
Serum iron	
Vitamin B12 (Cobalamin)	Iron deficiency can lead to microcytic anaemia
Serum folate	
	Low vitamin B12/low serum folate
Required by bone marrow to make red blood cells in haematopoiesis	Secondary to malabsorption
	Poor diet
	Secondary to infection

TABLE 17.6 U&Es

U&Es		
Sodium (Na)	135–145 mmol/l	Check patient's volume status
		Normal Na with fluid overload = euvolemic hyponatraemia and is secondary to SIADH, renal problems, hypothyroid
		Raised Na with hypovolaemia causes include:
		IV fluids High salt intake
		Low Na with hypovolemia causes include:
		Gastric loss Sweating Burns Adrenal insufficiency Diuresis
		Low NA with hypervolemia causes include:
		Heart failure Liver failure Nephrotic syndrome
Potassium (K)	3.5–5.5 mmol/l	<u>Raised</u> If raised >7 check ECG
		Increased oral Intake Secondary to blood transfusion Renal failure Potassium sparing diuretics Secondary to medications: ACE inhibitors NSAIDs, Beta blockers Rhabdomyolysis Acidosis Diabetes Addison's disease
		<u>Low</u>
		Secondary to gastric loss Poor oral intake
Urea	2.0–6.5 mmol/l	<u>Raised</u> Non-renal causes include:
		High protein intake Breakdown of protein secondary to steroids/starvation/burns GI bleed Dehydration

TABLE 17.6   (Continued)

		U&Es
		Renal causes include:
		Dehydration Reduced GFR Obstruction Kidney disease
		CHECK IS THERE AN AKI?
		Low Liver failure Pregnancy Low protein diet
Creatinine	55–120 mmol/l	Raised
		Usually originating from renal cause (AKI or CKD). Check GFR
		Urea/serum creatinine ratio can help distinguish between pre-renal and renal cause of raised creatinine. If Urea is raised and creatinine stays stable indicates pre-renal AKI – see further reading.
		NB. Look at trend in creatinine value. If not available treat as acute change.
Chloride	98–108 mmol/l	Raised
		Excess IV sodium chloride Metabolic acidosis Secondary to medications Low
		Poor oral intake Bodily loss e.g. Diahorrea and vomiting Secondary to medications e.g. bicarbonates, laxatives, diuretics, steroids
		NB. When low there is a risk of alkalosis.
Magnesium (Mg) 50–60% found in bone	0.75–0.95 mmol/l	Mg stabilises membranes, and is regulated by the kidneys
		Raised Severe renal disease Low Reduced oral intake Poor absorption Increased excretion
		Low K can lead to low potassium and low Calcium in severe cases. Ensure check these

TABLE 17.7 LFTs.

LFTs		
Bilirubin	Total 0–21 Unconjugated <10 Conjugated <17 umol/l	<u>Raised</u> (Total) Total haemolysis secondary to: Sepsis Medications e.g. anabolic steroids, Antibiotics, Antimalarials, Vitamin C and A, Codeine, NSAIDs Pregnancy (HELLP) Transfusion reaction <u>Raised</u> (Unconjugated – Hepatic) Liver cell problems e.g. hepatitis Paracetamol overdose Gilbert's syndrome (affects 10% of population) <u>Raised</u> (Conjugated – Post Hepatic) Obstruction e.g. gall stones, Pancreatic cancer, Liver obstruction
Alk Phos In Bones, Intestine, Kidneys, Liver, placenta	40–130 IU/l	<u>Raised</u> Bone disease with associated raised Calcium and Phosphate Liver damage (plus raised GGT) – usually post liver. CCF Hyperthyroid Advanced age Paget's disease
ALT Enzyme found *mainly* in liver. Also skeletal and cardiac muscle	7–40 IU/l	<u>Raised (Significant)</u> Released when damage to hepatocytes e.g. Acute hepatitis, paracetamol overdose <u>Raised (Moderate)</u> Cirrhosis Malignancy Obstructive jaundice Severe burns <u>Raised (Mild)</u> Pancreatitis MI Infectious mononucleosis Shock

TABLE 17.7   (Continued)

		LFTs
		Compare with ALP usually raised for 6–8 weeks then returns to normal unless chronic disease. Usually raised in chronic disease x10
AST In liver but also skeletal and cardiac muscle	5–40 IU/l	Raised Liver disease Systemic disease/illness
GGT Liver, pancreas, and kidney	5–80 IU/l	Raised Liver and biliary disease Alcohol Phenytoin Low Oral contraceptive pill
Total Protein	63–78 g/l	Raised Usually raised immunoglobulins indicative of infection/Myeloma Low Usually low albumin secondary to poor oral intake, Liver disease or infection
Albumin 1/2 life = 20 days	35–50 g/l	Raised Dehydration Low Poor oral intake Liver dysfunction Infection Kidney damage Malabsorption Nephrotic syndrome

Clinical Pictures

Trying to memorise lab tests and values can be challenging without context. One way to approach this and add context is to look at the results within clinical picture frames. Most conditions will have a typical clinical picture associated with it, and using these pictures can help you form and narrow your differential diagnosis. The common clinical pictures experienced within the AECC populations are summarised in Table 17.11.

TABLE 17.8   ABGs.

ABGs		
pH	7.35–7.45	Amount of H+ in blood <7.35 = acidosis >7.35 = alkalosis
PaO_2	11–14.4 KPa	Measures unbound (1%) O_2 in arterial blood Should be −10 from inspired O_2 concentration <u>Low</u> Indicates hypoxaemia possible causes: Hypoventilation Obstruction Atelectasis Chronic Respiratory disease
$PaCO_2$	4.6–6.4 KPa	<u>Raised</u> hypoventilation and acidosis acid. Shifts Oxyhaemoglobin curve to the right> That is the same if PaO_2 = lower SaO_2 the tissues will give up O_2 faster <u>Low</u> Hyperventilation and alkalosis Oxyhaemoglobin curve shifts to the left
Bicarbonate	22–28 mmol/l	Acts as a buffer Calculated from PCO_2 and pH
Base excess	−2.0 to +2.0 mmol/l	Calculated from amount of base that needs to be added/removed to achieve neutral pH <u>Raised</u> Alkalosis <u>Low</u> Metabolic acidosis
Oxyhaemoglobin	95–98%	Represents fraction of oxygenated haemoglobin in relation to total haemoglobin
Carboxyhaemoglobin	0.5–1.5%	5% smoker 10% definite exposure, 20% significant exposure, 30% life threat
Metmyoglobin	0–1.5%	Oxidised Hb which is unable to carry O2 Shifts oxyhaemoglobin curve to the left which can cause tissue hypoxia
O_2 sat	94–98%	Demonstrates the % of Hb binding sites occupied
Anion gap	10–18 mmol/l	Cations K and N – anions Cl and HCO

TABLE 17.9   Other biochemistry investigations.

		Other investigations
Amylase	0–100 IU/l	Usually found in pancreas and saliva, breaks down starch Raised Activation and blockage hence forced into plasma
Lipase	0–160 IU/l	Hydrolyses fat, secreted from pancreas rises after 48 h in acute pancreatitis, remains high for 5–7 days. Raised Pancreatitis GI obstruction Duodenal ulcer Gastroenteritis Cholecystitis
Troponin T	0–14 ng/l	>99th percentile AND symptoms or ECG changes = 90% sensitive and 95% specific to cardiac muscle at 8–12 h post symptoms Raised MI Vasospasm Post PCI/CABG CCF CKD Sepsis Hypertension Pulmonary Embolism Arrhythmias
Total calcium 99% in bone 40% plasma Ca bound to Albumin	2.2–2.65 mmol/l ionised (unbound) 1.15–1.30	Sedates nerves, causes clotting, involved in muscle contraction Raised Malignancy – bone invading or PTH mimicking Primary hyper parathyroid Acidosis Increased Albumin can give a false raised calcium therefore check corrected Ca. Total Calcium >3.5 check ECG for arrhythmia Low Tissue necrosis as draws Ca in Malignancy Hypo parathyroid Rhabdomyolysis Pancreatitis Sepsis CKD Low Albumin (false low). NB corrected calcium estimates Ca as if Albumin were normal

(Continued)

TABLE 17.11   (Continued)

Clinical pictures		
DKA pH ↓	↑ glucose ↑ ketones ↑ Na ↓ K if ++ urine ↑ K if in AKI	>11.1 >3 Glucose in urine pulls out H_2O K will decrease with insulin treatment
AKI	**Prerenal:** ↑ Na and Urea and Creatinine **Renal:** ↓ Na ↑ Ur and Creatinine ↑ K Ca ↓ and ↑ Phosphate pH ↓	Pre renal: Decreased flow and ↑ in Na and urea reabsorption, Raised urine concentration as H_2O is reabsorbed Renal: No reabsorption so Na and Urea excreted in large amounts e.g. glomerular nephritis Creatinine never reabsorbed so raised in both *Urea rise > creatinine rise* Calcium returned to bone so when phosphate increases the kidney no longer excretes hydrogen
CKD	↓ GFR (similar to % of renal function) ↑ Creatinine (after 60% of GFR is lost) Metabolic acidosis ↓ Hb ↓ bicarbonate ↑ K ↓ Ca/↑ PTH	Stage 1 – <90 Normal 2–60 – 89 Mild 3–30 – 59 Moderate – Check Hb as possible anaemia due to reduced EPO 4–15 – 29 Severe – Check Ca/P/PTH 5 – <15 End Stage Creatinine rise > urea rise
Rhabdomyolysis	↑ CK ↑ urea ↑ creatinine ↑ K ↓ Ca ↑ phosphate ↑ lactate Myoglobinuria Metabolic Acidosis	CK released from damaged muscle cells. X5 normal value indicates Rhabdomyolysis ↑ Urea and AKI K comes out of damaged cells Calcium absorbed by hypoxic tissue Phosphate increases as Ca decreases Lactate released by damaged cells causing metabolic acidosis along with sulphate, phosphate and uric acid.

TABLE 17.11   (Continued)

Clinical pictures		
Pancreatitis Cell breakdown and autolysing the pancreas Causes include: Alcohol Gall stones, Toxins Virus Scorpion Trauma Hight mortality rate is due to ARDS as lungs are next organ in line from pancreas and highly vascular so protease causes damage to vessels	Amylase >1000 Lipase ⬆ LFTs +/– ⬆ Albumin ⬇ Na, Ur and Creatinine ⬆ Ca ⬇ Mg ⬇ K ⬆ or ⬇ Glucose ⬆ PT and PPT ⬆ Platelets and Hb ⬇ Haematocrit ⬆	Pancreatic enzymes escape into plasma from broken down vessels. Lipase rises after 48 hours, both return to normal after five days even if pancreatitis not resolved. Raised lipase and protease can lead to SIRS LFTs disrupted if hepatic involvement or cause Albumin leaves plasma and enters tissues Raised Na, Urea and Creatinine indicates dehydration Ca and Mg sucked into dying pancreatic tissue and Trypsin inactivates PTH Mg can also be low due to alcohol, malnutrition, nausea/vomiting and urinary loss if in AKI/CKD K lost in vomiting and excessive aldosterone or raised in renal damage Glucose raised due to lack of insulin production from damaged pancreas PT prolonged as reduced absorption of Vitamin K from GI tract PTT and Platelets altered due to coagulopathy (Trypsin is also released which activates clotting cascade leading to micro emboli and DIC) Hb low due to bleeding as enzymes produced break down vessel walls Haematocrit elevated due to fluid shifting of fluid
Disseminated intravascular Coagulation (DIC)	Haemolysis + ⬇ platelets ⬇ platelets PT OK ⬆ APTT ⬆ D-Dimer	Over activation of coagulation, intravascular Fibrin, depletion of platelets and coat proteins causing severe haemorrhage and in some cases thrombosis. Causes: Infection Trauma particularly crush injuries CV disease Obstetric complications (HELLP) Malignancy Vasculitis Dead tissue in circulation i.e. collagen exposed

(Continued)

TABLE 17.11   (Continued)

Clinical pictures		
		Presentation: GI Bleed Dyspnoea Haematuria Oliguria AKI Intracerebral bleed Delirium Petechiae Ischaemia Gangrene
Microcytic anaemia **Iron deficiency** **Thalassemia** **Liver disease** **Haemolytic anaemia**	RBC ± ⬆ Hb ⬇ MCV ⬇ MCH ⬇ Haematocrit ⬇ Blood film shows microcytic hypochromic cells	Raised RBC can be a response to decreased O2 in tissues. Iron forms part of Haemoglobin and carries O2. If decreased less Hb made, so Mean Cell Volume is decreased as the size of cells is small Mean Cell Haemoglobin (mass of Hb in cell) is decreased or normal as haemoglobin splits to ensure normal concentration. Haematocrit is low due to smaller cells
Leukaemia	⬆ WCC ⬆ Blasts ⬇ Platelets ⬇ RBCs	Sudden rise in Neutrophils is Acute myeloid leukaemia (AML) Sudden rise in Lymphocytes = Acute Lymphocytic leukaemia (ALL) Both have chronic versions (CML, CLL) Raised Blasts = Lymphoblastic leukaemia Rise of WCC to 14 or 15 can be normal with infection, but up to 20 with no infection is probable leukaemia sepsis, lymphoma Differential diagnosis: Sepsis Lymphoma

Common Symptoms, Differential Diagnosis, and Laboratory Investigations

In order to form clinical pictures, it is important to know which tests should be considered for various presentations of reported symptoms, and how they can help form the differential diagnoses. This section highlights these within the biological system approach.

CARDIOVASCULAR

See Table 17.12.

TABLE 17.12 Cardiovascular symptom plan.

Clinical sign/ symptom	Description	Laboratory test to consider	Potential differential diagnosis
Non-pleuritic chest pain	Commonly central or left-sided. Radiates to left arm or jaw. Associated neck pain	FBC U&Es LFTs CRP Amylase Troponin	ACS Myocardial ischaemia/disease Hypoxia Anaemia Polycythaemia Coronary artery disease Drugs/Toxins Musculoskeletal Aortic pathology Oesophageal pathology Trauma Psychological cause
Palpitations	Feeling of regular or irregular fast beating of heart Heart Flutter Pounding heart	FBC CRP Troponin TFT	Abnormal pulse rate or rhythm Arrhythmia Anaemia Electrolyte abnormality Postural Orthostatic tachycardia syndrome Hypothyroidism Drugs/Toxins Endocrine/metabolic cause Psychological cause Structural abnormality
Dyspnoea	Shortness of breath at rest or on exertion Exacerbated by lying down (orthopnoea)	FBC CRP U&Es TFT ABG D-dimer Glucose	Congestive Cardiac Failure Angina Cardiac Arrhythmia Cardiac structural abnormality Abdominal Aortic Dissection Metabolic Acidosis Sepsis Decreased Oxygen Delivery Hyperthyroidism GORD Diabetic ketoacidosis Psychological Cause
Syncope	Temporary loss of consciousness usually secondary to reduced cerebral perfusion. Can be associated with exertion, chances in posture or occur randomly	FBC U&Es Calcium Magnesium Glucose	Cardiac Arrhythmia Cardiac outflow obstruction Hypovolemia Autonomic dysfunction Head injury Seizure Drugs/Toxins Hypoxia Anaemia
Oedema	Fluid retention in tissues which occurs either peripherally or centrally	FBC U&Es LFTs CRP Albumin D-dimer if suspect DVT Urinalysis	Nephrotic Syndrome Renal failure Hepatic Failure Infection VTE

GASTROENTEROLOGY

See Table 17.13.

TABLE 17.13   Gastroenterology symptom plan.

Clinical sign/ symptom	Description	Laboratory test to consider	Potential differential diagnosis
Vomiting	Projectile Non-projectile	FBC CRP	Gastroenteritis GORD
Haematemesis	Fresh red blood Coffee ground	FBC U&Es LFTs	Oesophageal Varices Rupture/Mallory-Weiss tear Gastric/duodenal ulcer
Jaundice	Skin, sclera and mucous membranes are yellow in colour	FBC U&Es LFT's	Hepatitis Liver cirrhosis Gallstones, pancreatic cancer
Dysphagia	Difficulty swallowing	FBC U&Es LFTs Calcium Magnesium	Oesophageal Cancer Psychological cause
Mouth Ulcers	Ulcers in oral mucosa	Serum Iron Serum Folate Vitamin B12	Iron deficiency anaemia Vitamin B12 Deficiency Stress
Malena	Black tar like offensive smelling stools	FBC U&Es LFTs Haematinics	UGIB
Fresh PR Bleed	Fresh red blood passed via rectum	FBC U&Es LFTs Haematinics	Haemorrhoids Lower GI malignancy Anal fissure
Systemic Symptoms	Nausea Weight Loss Fatigue Anorexla Fever Pruritis Confusion	FBC U&Es LFT Mg Ca CRP	Anorexia Nervosa Malignancy Malabsorption Infection Hepatic encephalopathy Cholestasis

HAEMATOLOGY

See Table 17.14.

TABLE 17.14   Haematological symptom plan.

Clinical sign/symptom	Description	Laboratory test to consider	Potential differential diagnosis
Evidence of compromised immune response	Recurrent infections	FBC Immunoglobulins	Compromised immunity
Decreased Exercise tolerance Recent onset increased shortness of breath at rest/on exertion Worsening angina Pedal oedema	Chest pain Shortness of breath Fatigue Lower limb swelling	RBC CRP U&Es LFT Albumin	Anaemia Pancytopenia
Skin infections Oral Sepsis Frequent oral ulcers	Ulcers in oral mucosa, discharge on tongue.	FBC CRP	Neutropenia Stress Dermatological cause
Bruising Bleeding Rashes	Unexplained and easy bruising Nosebleeds Excessive bleeding	FBC Clotting screen Immunoglobulins Vitamin K	Haemostatic disorders Multiple myeloma
Bone Pain	Common areas are hips, spin and ribs	FBC Blood Film Bone profile CRP Clotting Screen Immunoglobulins	Myeloma Hemochromatosis Sickle Cell Lymphoma Leukaemia Rheumatological disorders
Systemic Symptoms	Fatigue Fevers Night Sweats Weight Loss	FBC Blood Film Bone profile CRP U&Es LFTs Clotting Screen Immunoglobulins	Benign and malignant haematological conditions

RESPIRATORY

See Table 17.15.

TABLE 17.15   Respiratory symptom plan.

Clinical sign/ symptom	Description	Laboratory test to consider	Potential differential diagnosis
Dyspnoea	Shortness of breath at rest or on exertion	FBC CRP U&Es CRP D-dimer depending on history ABG	Pneumonia Pulmonary Embolism Deconditioning Dysfunctional Breathing
Cough	Productive or non-productive	FBC CRP U&Es Chest x-ray Sputum MSU	COPD Bronchiectasis Pulmonary Fibrosis Medication
Haemoptysis	Productive of blood when coughing	FBC CRP U&Es D-dimer Chest x-ray	Pulmonary embolism Lung cancer
Chest pain	Pleuritic chest pain (worse on inspiration)	FBC CRP U&Es D-Dimer Chest x-ray	Pleurisy Pulmonary embolism
Systemic symptoms	Fatigue Weight loss Fever	FBC CRP U&Es D-dimer Chest X-ray	Lung cancer COPD Pneumonia

RENAL

See Table 17.16.

ENDOCRINOLOGY

See Table 17.17.

TABLE 17.16 Renal symptom plan.

Clinical sign/ symptom	Description	Laboratory test to consider	Potential differential diagnosis
Dysuria	Pain or discomfort when passing urine	FBC CRP U&Es Urinalysis	UTI Sexually transmitted disease
Haematuria	Blood in urine	FBC CRP U&Es LFTs Urinalysis	UTI Trauma Bladder Malignancy Renal Malignancy
Nocturia	Waking at night to urinate	FBC CRP U&Es LFTs PSA Urinalysis	Benign prostatic hyperplasia Prostate Malignancy
Systemic Symptoms	Nausea Vomiting Weight loss Fevers Confusion Puritis	FBC CRP U&Es LFTs PSA Urinalysis	Uremic Cause Pyelonephritis AKI

TABLE 17.17 Endocrinology symptom plan.

Clinical sign/ symptom	Description	Laboratory test to consider	Potential differential diagnosis
Fatigue	Feeling tired Daytime somnolence	Early morning cortisol	Addison's Disease
Dehydration	Euvolemic Dizzy Dry mucous membranes	Early morning cortisol	Addison's Disease Hypothyroidism
Weight Loss	Muscle wasting Lose skin Decreased BMI	TFTs HbA1c Calcium U&Es	Hyperthyroid Type 1 Diabetes Pheochromocytoma Hypercalcaemia
Sweating	At rest or on exertion	TFTs Calcium U&Es	Hyperthyroidism Anxiety

(Continued)

TABLE 17.17   (Continued)

Clinical sign/ symptom	Description	Laboratory test to consider	Potential differential diagnosis
Tachycardia Palpitations	Racing heart Irregular heart	TFT	Hyperthyroidism
Weight Gain	Raised BMI	HbA1c Serum osmolality	Hypothyroid Cushing's Disease Type 2 Diabetes
Diarrhoea	Lose stools	TFT HbA1c	Hyperthyroid Hyper parathyroid Adrenal Insufficiency Diabetes
Nausea and Vomiting	Non-projectile	HbA1c Calcium PTH U&Es	DKA Hypercalcaemia Diabetes Hyper parathyroid
Constipation	Fewer than three bowel movements a week	HbA1c Calcium PTH U&Es	Hypercalcaemia Hypothyroid

FIELDS OF PRACTICE – PAEDIATRICS

It should be noted that the values of normal ranges in this chapter are based on adults. Paediatric laboratory medicine (PLM) is a sub-specialty of its own, and provides diagnostic services tailored to babies and children. Many challenges are faced in PLM, such as small sample volumes, the instruments used to acquire and transport samples, and age-specific reference intervals and critical values. To highlight this, a 10 ml adult blood collection bottle could be up to 10% of a baby's circulating blood volume. Further reading, specifically on PLM, is suggested if working with children and babies.

FIELDS OF PRACTICE – MENTAL HEALTH

Laboratory testing in patients presenting primarily with mental health concerns needs to be patient specific, based on individualised history-taking and assessments, rather than routine. A 2017 literature review (Brown et al. 2017) concluded that routine lab testing, including toxicological screening, should not be done on patients with acute psychiatric symptoms, and diagnostic evaluation should instead be directed by history-taking and physical examination.

FIELDS OF PRACTICE – LEARNING DISABILITIES

Understanding around laboratory testing in individuals with learning disabilities is an important consideration, which has been brought to light by the 2013 'Confidential Inquiry into the Deaths of People with Learning Disability' (CIPOLD) report. The report highlighted how the most common reasons for premature deaths in this patient population were problems with diagnosis and treatment, of which blood tests where emphasised. It highlighted the barriers to obtaining blood tests such as significant patient fear of contact with medical professionals, including a fear of needles. It also recognises difficulties around informed consent and knowledge of the Mental Capacity Act. Armed with this information, APs should consider approaches utilising desensitising techniques to help relieve anxiety, and build professional trusting relationships.

LEARNING EVENTS

It is essential that when considering the results of laboratory investigations performed, the clinician is able to look at the results, identify why the result is abnormal, and consider the implications that this has for the patient. The clinician should then decide what they are going to do about the abnormal result in order to be able to formulate a treatment and management plan for each patient.

Patients' symptoms should also be considered when deciding which laboratory investigations to perform. This can be guided by the above information but should also be used in collaboration with other tools to aid clinical decision-making, such as scores e.g. Wells score in VTE.

PHARMACOLOGICAL PRINCIPLES

There are a large number of medications that require routine blood tests to monitor the effects of the medication on various organ functions. An example of this in the AECC community could be demonstrated in Heparin Induced Thrombocytopenia (HIT). HIT is mainly associated with treatment with unfractionated heparin (UFH), but it can also occur with low-molecular weight heparin (LMWH). An HIT screen here acts as a negative predictive indicator for the presence of HIT. It is beyond the scope of this chapter to list all, and instead the AP should always consider the effects of any medications they prescribe as part of good prescribing practice, and consider which lab tests should be ordered and considered at the time of prescribing.

Case Study 1 – Haemolytic Anaemia

A 60-year-old female presents to same day emergency care (SDEC) via her GP with a three-week history of fatigue, dizziness, and shortness of breath. Patient looks pale. She has recently been on a skiing holiday.

Past medical history: Type 1 diabetes and has a prosthetic aortic valve.

GP has performed routine blood tests which show:

- Deranged LFTs
- U&Es – Creatinine and urea both elevated
- FBC – Reduced MCV and Hb

Clinical examination: Unremarkable other than splenomegaly and appears jaundiced in the sclera.

What other investigations would you consider?

- Family History
- Blood film: Identify abnormal red blood cell shapes
- Direct Coombs Test: Identify antibodies on RBC present in autoimmune haemolytic anaemia
- Urinalysis: positive for blood but no RBC
- Antinuclear antibodies (ANA) antibody: positive in systemic lupus erythematosus (SLE). SLE screen as associated with autoimmune haemolytic anaemia

What would your differential diagnosis be?

Anaemia due to blood loss.

Exclude by history: obvious source of bleeding and investigations.

Excluded as differential by: Bilirubin, haptoglobin, and LDH would not be elevated. Microcytic iron deficiency picture. Positive FIT test likely.

Investigations confirm a diagnosis of Autoimmune haemolytic anaemia.

What would your management plan be?

- Refer to haematologist
- Steroids with PPI cover
- Specialist advice for rituximab, intravenous immunoglobulins and other immunosuppressant medications
- Consideration of splenectomy.

Case Study 2 – Primary Hyperparathyroidism

A 47-year-old female attended SDEC via GP with an incidental finding of hypercalcemia on bloods taken by GP following gastric sleeve surgery, in Turkey. Patient reports feeling fatigued, nauseous, low in mood, and has generalised abdominal pain.

Observations: BP 126/92 HR 99 SaO2 98% RR 16 Temp. 36.2°C

On clinical examination patient has generalised abdominal pain with no guarding and a trace of bilateral pedal oedema.

What additional investigations would you perform in view of hypercalcaemia?

- U&Es
- Phosphate

- PTH
- Vitamin D
- TFTs
- LFTs
- Serum Electrophoresis
- Bence Jones Protein
- ECG (Results return as ECG sinus rhythm with sinus ectopics)
- PTH – elevated
- Phosphorous – low
- AKI 1
- Vitamin D Deficiency
- LFT's – normal range
- TFT's – normal range

What is your diagnosis?

- Primary hyperparathyroidism

What is your management plan?

- IV Fluids
- Replace Vitamin D
- Refer to endocrine for investigation of cause

Are patients' symptoms related to recent gastric sleeve or hypercalcaemia?

Impossible to tell – needs specialist investigation +/− referral for surgeon for removal of parathyroid.

Case Study 3 – Rhabdomyolysis

A 45-year-old male attended ED via ambulance following an accident at work. He is a stonemason and was trapped for two hours by some fallen stone slabs. He was assessed by the trauma team and taken for surgical repair of a fractured right femur. On primary survey patient was identified to have a right-sided flail segment and fractured right clavicle. There is no surgical intervention recommended for the fractured right clavicle.

Past medical history: Nil

Smokes five cigarettes per day and drinks five cans of lager per week.

Observations: HR 64 regular, BP 110/60, SaO_2 99% RA, RR 15, Temp. 36.2°C

Clinical examination is unremarkable other than the fractures above and widespread right-sided bruising.

Post operatively patient becomes tachycardic, HR 107, and feels nauseous. Blood tests are taken for the patient, and you are asked to interpret the results.

Hb	10.5 g/l
WBC	9.2 x 10⁹/l
Platelets	233 x 10⁹/l
Na	137 mmol/l
K	7.8 mmol/l
Urea	22.6 mmol/l
Creatinine	422 µmol/l
Bicarbonate	14 mmol/l
Glucose	4.1 mmol/l
Calcium	1.64 mmol/l
Phosphate	3.9 mmol/l
Creatinine kinase (CK)	69 000U/l

What is your interpretation of these blood results?

Hb	10.5 g/l	
WBC	9.2 x 10⁹/l	
Platelets	233 x 10⁹/l	
Na	137 mmol/l	
K	7.8 mmol/l	Raised
Urea	22.6 mmol/l	Raised
Creatinine	422 µmol/l	Raised
Bicarbonate	14 mmol/l	Low
Glucose	4.1 mmol/l	
Calcium	1.64 mmol/l	Low
Phosphate	3.9 mmol/l	Raised
Creatinine Kinase (CK)	69000U/l	Raised

Tachycardic
Hyperkalaemia
Bicarbonate low. Metabolic acidosis can affect cardiovascular system
Urea is raised likely secondary to AKI as it is too high for dehydration
Creatinine is raised which supports diagnosis of AKI
Calcium is low and phosphate is high
CK is elevated. This demonstrates rhabdomyolysis as the key diagnostic indicator is an elevated serum CK to at least five times its normal range.
Patients' urine is dark brown. What might this mean?

Another finding often seen in rhabdomyolysis is myoglobinuria. Myoglobin is an oxygen binding protein pigment found in the skeletal muscle. This can be excreted in urine following the breakdown of muscle fibres and the subsequent release of muscle contents into the circulation. This supports a diagnosis of rhabdomyolysis.

It must be remembered that a lack of myoglobinuria does not exclude a diagnosis of rhabdomyolysis.

What is the patient's diagnosis?

- AKI secondary to rhabdomyolysis

An ABG is also taken and this shows metabolic acidosis. Why?
Phosphate, sulphate, uric acid, and lactic acid are released from cells following crush injury.
What is your management?

- ABCDE Assessment
- Fluid resuscitation – large volume will be required
- Monitoring of BP, CVP, and urine output
- Management of hyperkalaemia which could be life-threatening
- Dialysis if required
- Where is the best place to carry out this management plan?
- Level 2 Care: High Dependency Unit for strict monitoring and intervention

Take Home Points

- Ensuring robust patient-centred clinical reasoning and knowledge of clinical conditions and human physiology underpins the decision to carry out each laboratory investigation performed.
- Develop a systematic method for the interpretation of laboratory investigations.
- When assimilating factors which contribute to abnormal values of the laboratory investigations performed it is essential to take into account all evidence gained from a thorough patient history and clinical examination.

REFERENCES

Brown, M.D., Byyny, R., Diercks, D.B. et al. (2017). Clinical policy: critical issues in the diagnosis and management of the adult psychiatric patient in the emergency department. *Annals of Emergency Medicine*, Elsevier 69 (4): 480–498. https://doi.org/10.1016/j.annemergmed.2017.01.036.

Health Education England. (2017). *Multi-professional Framework for Advanced Clinical Practice in England* [online]. Available from: https://www.hee.nhs.uk/sites/default/files/documents/multi-professionalframeworkforadvancedclinicalpracticeinengland.pdf [accessed 23 June 2023].

Health Education England. (2022). *Advanced Clinical Practice in Acute Medicine Curriculum Framework* [online]. Available from: https://healtheducationengland.sharepoint.com/sites/APWC/Shared%20Documents/Forms/AllItems.aspx?id=%2Fsites%2FAPWC%2FShared%20Documents%2FCreden

tials%2FCredentials%20Endorsement%20Documents%2FAdvanced%20clinical%20practice%20
in%20acute%20medicine%20curriculum%20framework%2Epdf&parent=%2Fsites%2FAPWC%2FSha
red%20Documents%2FCredentials%2FCredentials%20Endorsement%20Documents&p=true&ga=1
[accessed 23 June 2023].

The Faculty of Intensive Care Medicine. (2018). *Curriculum for Training for Advanced Critical Care Practitioners – Syllabus. V1.1* [online]. Available from: www.ficm.ac.uk/media/6896 [accessed 20 June 2023].

The Intensive Care Society, Critical Care Networks – *National Nurse Leads and The National Outreach Forum.* (2022). *Advanced Critical Care Outreach Competencies* [online]. Available from: https://ics.ac.uk/asset/43B8C11B-4512-41D0-B97768FABA2C30B2 [accessed 20 June 2023].

The Royal College of Emergency Medicine. (2022). *Emergency Medicine Advanced Clinical Practitioner Curriculum 2022 (Adult)* [online]. Available from: https://rcem.ac.uk/wp-content/uploads/2022/09/ACP_Curriculum_Adult_Final_060922.pdf [accessed 20 June 2023].

FURTHER READING

Grey, V.L., Loh, T.P., Metz, M. et al. (2017). Paediatric laboratory medicine – some reflections on the sub-specialty. *Clinical Biochemistry.* Elsevier 50 (12): 648–650. https://doi.org/10.1016/j.clinbiochem.2017.04.005.

CHAPTER 18

Pharmacology and Prescribing for the Acute, Emergency, and Critical Care Populations

Jill Bentley, David Thom, and Joseph Tooley

Aim

The aim of this chapter is to give an overview of the concepts of good prescribing practice in the acute, emergency, and critical care settings with reference to underpinning pharmacological principles.

LEARNING OUTCOMES

After reading this chapter the reader will:

1. Understand the best practice principles of prescribing and relevant legislation.
2. Understand altered pharmacology in different patient groups, such as how pharmacokinetics and pharmacodynamics of drugs may be altered in critical illness.
3. Know the underpinning principles for prescribing in 'special groups' seen in the acute, emergency, and critical care setting (e.g. renal impairment, hepatic impairment, older adults, pregnancy, extremes of body weight, patients on extracorporeal therapies).
4. Be familiar with the basic clinical principles of governance around authorisation of blood and blood products in these settings.

The Advanced Practitioner in Acute, Emergency and Critical Care, First Edition. Edited by Sadie Diamond-Fox, Barry Hill, Sonya Stone, Caroline McCrea, Natalie Gardner, and Angela Roberts.
© 2024 John Wiley & Sons Ltd. Published 2024 by John Wiley & Sons Ltd.

SELF-ASSESSMENT QUESTIONS

1. Describe the key principles of good prescribing as set out by the Royal Pharmaceutical Society Framework for prescribers.
2. Discuss the importance of assessing physiology when making prescribing decisions.
3. Discuss the pharmacokinetic changes that occur in acutely unwell patients and how this influences drug dosing.
4. List the minimum requirements for authorising, in writing, the administration of blood components.

INTRODUCTION

The Acute, Emergency, and Critical Care (AECC) populations present with complex, often unknown conditions with altered pharmacokinetics and dynamics that change frequently as the disease progresses or regresses. The legal and ethical challenges within the AECC are multifaceted and highly sensitive in nature. This chapter shares the knowledge and insight needed for this interesting yet complex group of patients.

Multi-professional Framework (MPF) for Advanced Clinical Practice Guidance for Professional Development (HEE 2017)

This chapter maps to the following statements within the MPF:

1. Clinical:	1.2	1.4	1.5	1.7	1.8
2. Leadership:	2.8				
3. Education:	3.3				
4. Research:	4.3				

Accreditation Considerations

This chapter maps to the following statements within the following national accreditation documents:

Curriculum for Training for Advanced Critical Care Practitioners Syllabus V1.1 (The Faculty of Intensive Care Medicine 2018)			
2.6	3.15	3.3	3.5

Advanced Critical Care Outreach Competencies (The Intensive Care Society, Critical Care Networks – National Nurse Leads and The National Outreach Forum 2022)
A2

Emergency Medicine Advanced Clinical Practitioner Curriculum 2022 – Adult
(The Royal College of Emergency Medicine 2022)

SLO-2

Advanced Clinical Practice in Acute Medicine Curriculum Framework
(Health Education England 2022)

- Generic Clinical CiPs: 1, 2
- Speciality Clinical CiPs: Acute Medicine: 3

GENERAL PRESCRIBING FRAMEWORKS AND GOVERNANCE CONSIDERATIONS

Prescribing frameworks detail the knowledge, skills, characteristics, qualities, and behaviours that are expected from those clinicians that meet the competencies within them, supporting the highly complex, multidimensional process of prescribing. This provides standardised levels of assurance for the public, service users, and stakeholders, and establishes commonality regardless of professional background. They aid development and push boundaries to directly improve practice.

The Royal Pharmaceutical Society (RPS) Competency Framework for all prescribers (RPS 2021) sets out to ensure safe and effective performance for those in a prescribing role, covering Independent, Supplementary prescribers, and Community Practitioners regardless of the underlying professional regulatory body (see Figure 18.1).

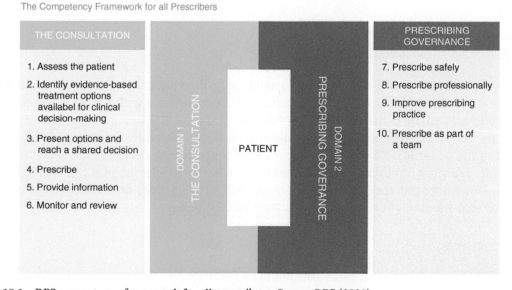

FIGURE 18.1   RPS competency framework for all prescribers. *Source*: RPS (2021).

The 10 competencies are split into two key domains. Each competency expands on the necessary skills and attributes prescribers need to demonstrate. In relation to governance, a few of the competencies have been selected for further discussion:

Competency 7: Prescribe Safely

This focuses on the prescriber's scope of practice. Recognising limits of their competence and development needs. Minimising risk, prescriber error, and patient safety through challenging practice, and the use of monitoring and reporting mechanisms.

Competency 8: Prescribe Professionally

Ensures prescribers understand their professional accountability for clinical decision-making within scope of practice. Maintaining competence through ongoing continuous professional development. Comprehension of external influences on their practice and how to mitigate these.

Competency 9: Improve Prescribing Practice

This is a key dimension that places reflection central to moving practice forward and the development of prescribers and the services they work in. Supporting peers through education, networking, and learning. Also looking at wider factors such as sustainability and environmental impact of medicines.

Competency 10: Prescribe as Part of a Team

The need for collaborative working to ensure continuity of care. Prescribers need to build and maintain relationships based on trust and mutual respect to ensure all needs of the patients are met.

LEGAL AND ETHICAL CONSIDERATIONS IN PRESCRIBING

This maps against the following RPS competencies (see Figure 18.2).

Legalities

The Medicines Act 1968 controls the production and supply of medicinal products. The remit, to protect the public from harm by stipulating that treatment must be carried out with proper skill and care by all members involved, and the patient must give consent to treatment.

Within the AECC populations assessing capacity can be complex due to a multitude of clinical reasons. Utilising the wider MDT for support, knowing what prescribing decisions are time-critical versus what can wait, can support clinical decision-making. Medical ethical principles can also aid in clinical judgements. Remember that the Mental Capacity Act (MCA) (2005) does not define what it considers as 'best interests' but stipulates factors that must always be considered.

Ethical Principles

Four key ethical principles are well-established in the application to healthcare practice. They have equal standing, and although inter-relate, stand strong also in their own right. Ethical problems arise when

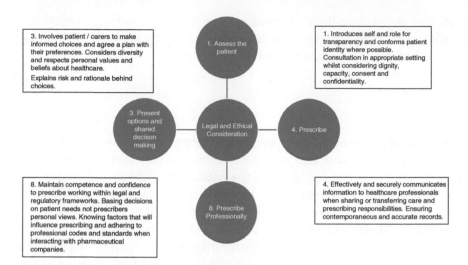

FIGURE 18.2   Prescribing competencies within legal and ethical considerations. *Source*: Original J Bentley.

there is more than one course of action but also when our patients are unable to communicate their wishes. These principles are reviewed below.

Autonomy – The individual's right to come to their own decision. Independent prescribers (IP) should practice in a way that does not coerce individuals into making choices. No decision is a wrong decision if it is informed. Capacity is key to this. The patient populations that present in the acute, emergency department and critical care settings have the potential to have fluctuating capacity or none at all. Continuous assessment and clinical judgement will be key to prescribing decisions in this area. When acting in the patient's best interest, the least restrictive action should be taken.

Beneficence – To do or maximise good. IP optimises outcomes for the patients, from ensuring non-pharmacological options are considered, to medication reviews and de-prescribing. This is a key part of prescriber's role, and links to admission avoidance and preventative strategies for long-term conditions.

Non-maleficence – To do no or minimise harm. Interrelated with beneficence; by not causing harm you are doing good. Ensure prescribing and clinical decision-making are based on best practice guidance and up-to-date credible evidence.

Justice – Ensuring there is no discrimination in terms of resources and access to healthcare, it also highlights that justice will be served if we breach non-maleficence and intentional harm through prescribing. Reflection plays a key role in Justice as we explore and deepen our understanding of own values, principles, and bias in order to prevent inferring these on the decision of others.

CLINICAL ASSESSMENT FOR PRESCRIBING

Prescribing extends beyond the act of choosing a medicine from the formulary and completing the legal requirements for its administration. Factors that may affect the choice of medicines or the dose prescribed can be affected by both quantitative measurements (blood results, patient observations) and by less quantifiable factors, such as physical assessment.

Patient acuity may necessitate timely intervention in the AECC settings, which can limit the time available for detailed assessment. Information can be gained swiftly and succinctly to safely and appropriately guide the pharmacological management of these patients.

GUIDED ASSESSMENT

Clinical reasoning and experience will aid assessment decisions in the immediate management of patients, but it is important to ensure that you do not introduce bias into the clinical reasoning. Type 1 processes will ensure rapid working diagnoses for the critically ill, but the clinician should actively work to introduce a cognitive pause and employ a type 2 cognitive process prior to prescribing. This will reduce error by confirming the clinician's initial diagnosis prior to prescribing.

During assessment, a structured approach, such as A–E, concurrently with physiological observations provides a good grounding from which to base the diagnosis or initial management. Pertinently, the initial prescribing choices may not be, in totality, to treat the underlying cause of the physiology, but in some circumstances may be to manage the physiology such that the patient is stabilised to progress on to diagnosis. An example of this is in managing cardiovascular collapse following an acute brain injury, where the patient will require immediate support and potentially intubation/ventilation in order to safely gain a diagnosis by scanning. As such, the AECC practitioner will be required to prescribe medications to manage the physiology and not necessarily the underlying issue.

IMPLICATIONS OF RESULTS

Formal laboratory results can guide prescribing choices i.e. renal function for dosing, but results can be slow to return at times. In the initial phase of resuscitation/treatment, practice may be guided by point-of-care testing, such as an arterial blood gas (ABG). Although advances in technology have increased the accuracy of point-of-care testing, the clinician should familiarise themselves with the equipment and be aware of sampling errors that may affect the results and sway the decision. This is particularly pertinent if there is a human–technology interface where there is an increased risk of error.

PHARMACOLOGY–PHYSIOLOGY INTERFACE

Patients may present with malperfusion pathologies resulting in metabolic dysfunction; this may present as acidaemia on an ABG in the initial phases of resuscitation. In normal homeostasis, the intracellular and extracellular pH of cardiac cells and the vasculature smooth muscle are in fine balance; during metabolic acidosis, both the extracellular and intracellular pH are reduced.

Cardiac muscle is affected in a multitude of ways during acidosis (see Table 18.1).

In addition, the effect of acidosis on the vasculature smooth muscle as well as vasculature endothelium is described similarly (see Table 18.2).

Clinically, this may explain a potential role for pH normalising pharmacological intervention, such as the administration of sodium bicarbonate. However, the physiological result of the administration of IV bicarbonate may result in an increased CO_2 which would require physiological compensation (increased minute volume ventilation) for which the patient may not be able to respond i.e. comatose states or tiring. The act of prescribing, in this instance, needs to consider the patient as a whole and not

TABLE 18.1   The effect of acidosis on cardiac muscle.

Effect	Explanation
Increased calcium transient amplitude	Net result of intracellular acidosis as a result of increased sarcoplasmic reticulum calcium content by desensitising the ryanodine receptor and decreased calcium release from the sarcoplasmic reticulum.
Active H^+ removal from intracellular space	H^+ is actively removed from the intra-cellular space to normalise pH. This is done by Na^+/H^+ exchange. In turn, this causes a rise in intra-cellular Na^+ concentration. This stimulates Na^+/Ca^{2+} exchange drawing in calcium from the extracellular space increasing the intracellular concentration of Ca^{2+}
Cellular hyperpolarisation	Potassium is actively removed from the intra-cellular space causing hyperpolarisation of the cell membrane
Adrenoreceptor internalisation	Reduction in the total number of adrenoreceptors available on the cell membrane
Apoptosis	Intracellular acidosis can promote apoptosis by stimulating BNIP3 activating cell death pathways

TABLE 18.2   The effect of acidosis on vasculature smooth muscle and endothelium.

Effect	Consequences
Increased calcium transient amplitude	As described in cardiac muscle, reduced effectiveness
Reduction in adrenoreceptor expression	Internalisation of adrenoreceptor reduces the active binding sites for vasoactive medications
Opening of ATP-sensitive K^+ channels	Vascular smooth muscle relaxation
Expression of inducible nitric oxide synthase	Vasodilation by overproduction of nitric oxide

just the interpretation of an ABG. By normalising the pH, there is an argument for an increased efficacy of vasoactive medications and therefore an increased dose-response curve which may prove beneficial; however, this effect in clinical reality is disputed. As such the prescriber should consider beyond the medication and intervention.

Keeping with the theme of acidosis, the concept of pKa is pertinent to AECC. Local anaesthetics and thiopentone are good examples of this. At an acidic pH lidocaine is almost completely ionised and therefore unable to cross the membrane to exert effects on sodium channels. Conversely, thiopental rapidly becomes unionised and therefore a greater proportion is free to exert its effect – as a result the dose should be reduced (see Figure 18.3 and Table 18.3).

In clinical practice, this should be considered when using thiopentone for induction in status epilepticus; the prescribing clinician should consider if an extended period of tonic-clonic seizure and hypoventilation has resulted in a metabolic and lactic acidosis. As a result, the dose required before reaching toxic levels may be reduced. An example of the opposite effect would be an infected abscess requiring incision and drainage; this will have a decreased pH due to the acidity of inflammation. This greatly reduces the

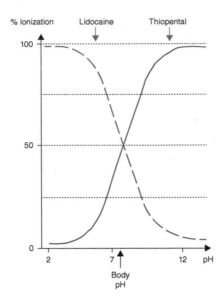

FIGURE 18.3 The effect of pH on drug ionisation.

TABLE 18.3 Worked example of use of the Henderson-Hasselbalch equation in clinical practice.

Weak acid:
pH = pKa + log [A⁻/AH]

Weak base
pH = pKa + log [B/BH⁺]

where, A-/BH⁺ are the ionised forms, AH/B are the unionised forms and pKa = the pH at which 50% drug is ionised.

Lidocaine is weakly basic with a pKa of ~7.8:
Normal tissue pH = ~7.4

7.4 = 7.8 + log [B/BH⁺]
−0.4 = log [B/BH⁺]
Ratio of conjugate acid to base [B/BH⁺] = 10⁻⁰·⁴ = 0.39
% ionised = 1 / (1 + ratio) x 100%
% ionised = 1/1.39 x 100% = 72% ionised
Therefore, only 28% drug is unionised and able to partition membranes.

In infected tissues, pH may be lower (e.g. 6.4)

6.4 = 7.8 + log [B/BH⁺]
−1.4 = log [B/BH⁺]
Ratio of conjugate acid to base [B/BH⁺] = 10⁻¹·⁴ = 0.039
% ionised = 1/1.039 x 100% = 96.2% ionised
Therefore, only 3.8% is unionised and able to partition membranes

efficacy of lidocaine, and it may be an alternative approach that should be undertaken i.e. proximal ring block rather than local infiltration.

This demonstrates the importance of the clinician performing physical examination as well as reviewing laboratory results when considering prescribing.

PHARMACOLOGICAL FACTORS

Patient Factors

AECC patients can respond differently to the same dose or drug and therefore the clinical history and examination may provide insight into how the patient might react. For example, smoking may increase the chances of patients rapidly metabolising medicines.

An example of altered metabolism, and therefore therapeutic effect, is the difference in the expression of CYP2D6 (a CYP450 subtype) enzyme responsible for the conversion of codeine into morphine for analgesia within the liver. Different groups have been shown to either have reduced expression or no expression of CYP2D6 and therefore unable to achieve analgesia with codeine.

Shock states also present unique factors to consider when prescribing. The three-compartment model for pharmacokinetics provides a basis for the relationship between shock states and altered patient responses (see Figure 18.4). Consider these scenarios: firstly, where the body is in a state of fight-or-flight, the rate constant K_{12} will be increased by the increased blood flow to skeletal muscle and reduced to the fat stores, and as such, K_{13} will be decreased. Additionally, if the clinical assessment is such that the patient is deemed intra-vascularly depleted either through haemorrhage or hypovolaemia through endovascular leakage, the volume of the first compartment is reduced, thus the concentration of any IV bolus has an increase relative to total circulating volume, and dose reduction may be a consideration (see Figure 18.5).

Clinicians should consider the individual pharmacological factors relevant to the procedure when guiding their prescribing choice. When considering analgesia or sedation, a clinician may require short-term sedation to allow for successful manipulation of a joint, however once the joint has been relocated,

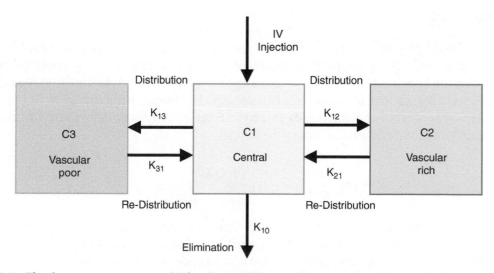

FIGURE 18.4   The three-compartment model for pharmacokinetics. *Source*: Original Thom (2022).

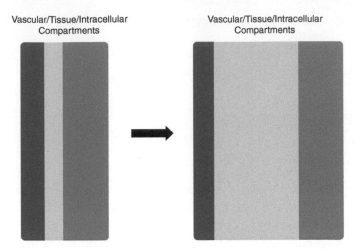

FIGURE 18.5   Increase in tissue in the intravascular space due to capillary leakage and extravasation during critical illness.

the relative pain felt by the patient will be largely diminished. The clinician should consider the safety of long-acting strong analgesics which will continue to exert their effects after the joint has been relocated and the sympathetic tone and stimulus has diminished. In this instance it may be beneficial to utilise shorter-acting agents which will provide analgesia for the procedure but are less likely to continue exerting their effects long after the stimulus has been removed. Likewise, not all sedative agents provide analgesia, and therefore, a combined approach or a choice of alternative agent may be required.

Moreover, this is also pertinent while considering a regional anaesthesia approach for a patient who has received significant volumes of strong analgesics. While managing pain is paramount, the clinician should be alert to the additional risks posed by the pharmacology already onboard, and manage these appropriately.

Environmental Factors

Consideration should be given to the environment the patient is being cared in. Consider rocuronium; in a healthy patient undergoing a short procedure in theatre, the patient may only require a low dose as the clinician has the benefit of time to allow the drug to work prior to intubation, and would not want to unduly paralyse the patient for longer than necessary. However, in the critically ill patient in the emergency department requiring emergency intubation, the priority is to gain control of the patient's airway in a timely manner, and a larger dose is beneficial.

KINETIC CHANGES IN ACUTE AND CRITICAL ILLNESS

When prescribing medications in acute and critical illness, a number of physiological changes to the normal handling, action and metabolism of drugs must be considered. Standard guidelines often do not account for them and if followed dogmatically may lead to under-dosing and treatment failure, or over-dosing and toxicity.

A full review of basic pharmacokinetics is beyond the scope of this chapter. Readers should first familiarise themselves with these general principles.

Absorption

First the prescriber must consider how to administer the drug and whether physiology will alter bioavailability (F). In early acute illness the intravenous route is preferred. Gastric emptying is often delayed, observed with rising nasogastric residual volumes and ileus may occur, particularly in critically ill post-operative patients. Vasoactive medications and stress hormones alter GI perfusion, generally shunting blood flow to more critical organs. The use of stress-ulcer prophylaxis increases gastric pH affecting absorption of weak bases, such as itraconazole. Nutrition on critical care can affect bioavailability. The DOAC rivaroxaban, for example, needs to be taken with a meal to be absorbed to therapeutic levels. Patients may be fed via nasogastric tube and feeds may interact with enteral medicines either in the feeding tube (e.g. phenytoin) or the gut (e.g. high-protein feeds and Parkinson's medications). Some medicines require protracted breaks in enteral feeding such as phenytoin which may compromise nutrition. Discuss with the pharmacist and dietitian.

It is not only enteral bioavailability which may be affected; other routes similarly can be compromised. Reduced muscle and skin perfusion can reduce absorption of subcutaneous/intramuscular injections. The IM route is also unfavourable in patients with coagulopathy due to the risk of bleeding. Transdermal absorption of medicines through patches may also be altered through reduced perfusion ($\downarrow$) or pyrexia ($\uparrow$).

Distribution

In acute illness, particularly in hyperinflammatory conditions causing distributive shock (e.g. sepsis, pancreatitis), the volume of distribution (Vd) of certain medicines can be dramatically altered (see Figure 18.5). Inflammation leads to damage to the glycocalyx on the vascular endothelium. Gap junctions between cells widen and significant vasodilation occurs (see Figure 18.6). Combined with large volumes of administered crystalloids early in the acute phase of illness, this leads to profound increase in volume of the extracellular compartment.

For hydrophilic molecules, this will significantly increase the initial Vd. It is crucial the prescriber remembers this with initial dosages for drugs like antibiotics in sepsis. The concept can be captured through the equation for loading doses:

$$\text{Loading Dose}\left(\text{LD}\right) = \frac{\text{Vd} \times \text{Cp}}{\text{F}}$$

F = bioavailability, Cp = desired plasma concentration, Vd = volume of distribution.

If volume of distribution is increased, a correspondingly larger loading dose is needed to achieve the same desired plasma concentration.

In practice, the current advice is to not adjust loading doses based on acute kidney injury. For medicines such as beta-lactam antibiotics, tranexamic acid or levetiracetam (water soluble renally cleared molecules) use normal or potentially even increased doses for the first 24–48 hours of admission then re-assess renal function and adjust dosage.

Protein binding is altered in critical illness. Many drugs are highly protein bound with only the free fraction being bio-active or available for renal/extra-corporeal clearance. Albumin is the most abundant

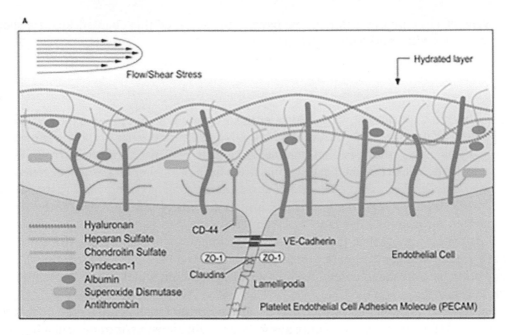

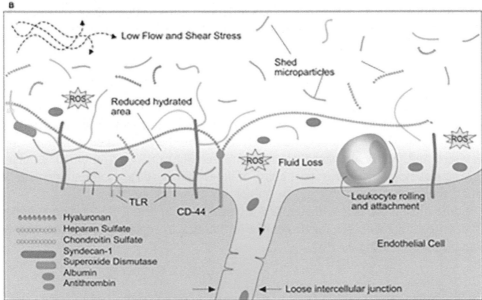

FIGURE 18.6   Barrier breakdown during sepsis. *Source*: Lupu (2020) / John Wiley & Sons / CC BY 4.0.

serum protein to which many medicines (e.g. phenytoin, warfarin, valproate) bind. Albumin falls dramatically in critical illness due to increased capillary escape, increased metabolism, and reduced synthesis. This should be accounted for when monitoring levels or adjusting maintenance doses.

Penetration of drugs to various tissue compartments is also altered. Lung and muscle penetration by Tazocin is notably erratic in sepsis, possibly due to microcirculatory impairment, and standard dosages may be insufficient. Conversely, blood-brain barrier permeability may be increased. This is advantageous in meningitis because it allows improved penetration of antibiotics. It is however disadvantageous when the CNS penetration of sedative/deleriogenic medicines is elevated, increasing vulnerability to CNS toxicity.

Metabolism

The majority of drug metabolism takes place in the liver. A few medicines are decomposed entirely in plasma either chemically (atracurium through Hoffman degradation) or via tissue enzymes (remifentanil, anidulafungin). Critical illness can alter hepatic metabolism. Shock can reduce hepatic blood flow; less drug is presented to hepatocytes per unit time to be cleared. Conversely, early in sepsis with hyperdynamic high-output state hepatic blood flow and drug metabolism may be increased. Inflammatory cytokines may also alter the levels of hepatic enzymes which may in turn affect clearance. When prescribing drugs that are highly hepatically metabolised, consider if either the effect of the drug or the plasma level can be measured to determine dose adjustment as the effect is complex and highly variable.

Elimination

Ultimately all drugs are eliminated from the body, be it as bio-transformed metabolites or as intact parent molecules. The most common route of elimination is via the kidneys, particularly water-soluble compounds, such as the beta-lactam antibiotics (e.g. penicillins). Renal function in acute illness is highly changeable; monitor renal function and consider whether it alters the clearance of the drug you prescribe. *The Renal Drug Database (RDD)* (Ashley and Dunleavy 2022) is a valuable resource for determining drug dosing in renal dysfunction which you can access through your pharmacist.

Determining renal function in acute illness is challenging, and 50% of nephrons can be lost before a rise in creatinine is detected. It can take over 48 hours after an insult for plasma creatinine to peak, and conditions such as sepsis reduce production. Additionally, following protracted courses of ventilation, substantial muscle loss occurs further impairing creatinine synthesis.

Equations such as the 'MDRD GFR equation', which estimates glomerular filtration rate based on creatinine and patient characteristics, are not validated in such patients. Where possible, 24 hour-urine creatinine collection should be undertaken. Close attention to other markers and observation of trends in levels (e.g. urea, potassium, urine output) should be used along with creatinine.

The British National Formulary (BNF) recommends use of Cockcroft and Gault to determine drug dosing over MDRD as it is more reliable in patients with extreme weights. The formula is shown below:

$$\text{Creatinine clearance}\left(\text{ml}/\min\right)=\frac{\left[140-\text{Age}\left(\text{years}\right)\right]\times\text{weight}\left(\text{kg}\right)\times\text{C}}{\text{Serum Creatinine}\left(\mu\,\text{mol/l}\right)}$$

Where, C = 1.23 (men) and 1.04 (women).

Various factors alter renal clearance in acute illness. Hypovolaemia, nephrotoxic drugs, PEEP, and rhabdomyolysis among others may all adversely affect GFR and reduce renal clearance. Conversely, vasoactive medications and early hyperdynamic states may significantly enhance renal blood flow and profoundly increase elimination (termed augmented renal clearance). Various studies have demonstrated close correlation between a GFR >130 ml/min and sub-therapeutic antibiotic levels in sepsis; a growing body of thought is that we should be using maximal if not greater than licensed doses of renally cleared antibiotics in such patients (Sime et al. 2015).

Narrow therapeutic index drugs such as gentamicin and vancomycin are almost entirely eliminated via the kidneys and are ototoxic and nephrotoxic if they are allowed to accumulate to toxic levels. Therapeutic drug monitoring according to local policy should be used to ensure therapeutic efficacy with minimal toxicity. If using a policy designed for the whole hospital, consider more frequent monitoring than advised by the guideline, given the rapidly changing nature of acutely ill patients.

PRESCRIBING FOR PATIENTS UNDERGOING CONTINUOUS RENAL REPLACEMENT THERAPY (CRRT)

AECC patients may require artificial support for severe renal dysfunction. The most common modes used are continuous veno-venous haemofiltration (CVVHF) and continuous veno-venous haemodiafiltration (CVVHDF). The modes of clearance are conceptualised in Figure 18.7.

The clearance of drugs through CRRT is complex and incompletely understood. Limited data is published by manufacturers or the BNF, and even the *Renal Drug Database* has only minimal guidance, often using references with lower flow rates and surface area filters than used in current practice. Citrate anticoagulation in some units has also contributed by allowing significantly longer filter-life-spans which minimises down-time that previously reduced delivered clearance. Advice from an ICU pharmacist should be sought when designing dosing regimens.

Drug clearance will be determined by:

- Protein binding: Only unbound drug can clear through the membrane.
- Molecular weight: Modern CCUs use high-porosity membranes, so most drugs will clear, though haemodialysis may clear larger molecules (heparins, teicoplanin) less efficiently than haemofiltration.
- Blood flow and exchange rates.
- Non-renal clearance: The percentage of the drug that is normally renally versus hepatically cleared.
- Degree of drug binding directly to membrane (significant for gentamicin, vancomycin and colistin).

A simple approach to start with is to estimate the artificial 'creatinine clearance' of the filter which may be easily approximated as the sum of the pre- and post-filter replacement rates, dialysis rate, and

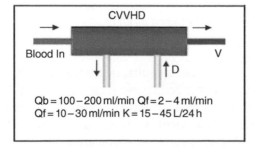
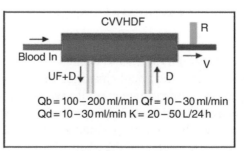

FIGURE 18.7   Differing clearance mechanisms of CVVHD and CVVHDF. *Source*: Macedo and Cerdá (2021) / John Wiley & Sons.

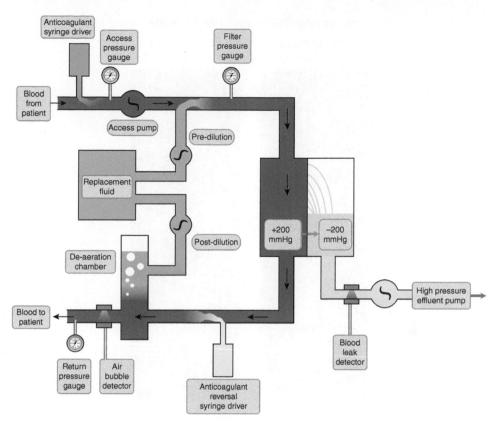

FIGURE 18.8   Conceptualised CVVHDF circuit. *Source*: https://derangedphysiology.com/main/required-reading/renal-failure-and-dialysis/Chapter%203.1.6/cvvhf-circuit-diagram last accessed February 27, 2023.

fluid removal rate divided by 60 to give a value in ml/min. Use this as a starting point to estimate filter clearance when referring to drug reference texts such as the RDD. Discuss with a pharmacist at a convenient point to refine this. Figure 18.8 conceptualises a CRRT circuit in CVVHDF mode.

PRESCRIBING IN OBESITY

Increasingly, prescribers need to consider the effect of obesity on prescribing decisions; data suggests over 11 000 hospital admissions in 2018–2019 were related to obesity. Obesity may increase likelihood of organ dysfunction leading to heart, kidney, and liver failure, all of which alter drug handling. Additionally, estimating weight-based dosing is complex. Use of actual body weight (ABW) in some drugs may lead to toxicity while use of ideal body weight (IBW) in others leads to under-dosing. Factors relevant include percentage fat-free mass and drug properties (lipophilicity versus hydrophilicity, protein binding). For water-soluble drugs IBW or adjusted body weight (AdjBW) should be used; while for lipophilic drugs ABW is preferable. The mass of lean tissue is increased in obesity along with adipose tissue, complicating the use of IBW in morbidly obese patients (use AdjBW) (see Figure 18.9 and Table 18.4).

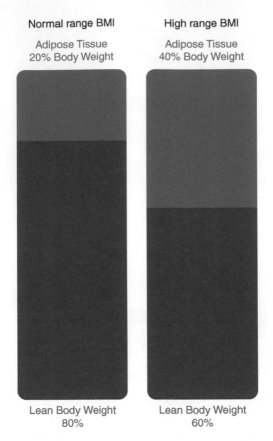

FIGURE 18.9   Ratio of adipose tissue to lean body weight in normal BMI and High BMI. *Source*: Gardner.

TABLE 18.4   Adjusting doses for extremes of weight.

Drugs which should be dosed using IBW or AdjBW*	Drugs using ABW
Acyclovir	Ambisome
Gentamicin*	Daptomycin
Ganciclovir	Fluconazole
Intravenous immunoglobulin*	Penicillins (not weight based but
Phenytoin*	consider dosing at upper end of range)
Voriconazole	

PRESCRIBING IN PREGNANCY

Prescribing in pregnancy is complex; expertise should be sought promptly. Pregnancy induces multiple changes in pharmacokinetics including altered Vd, hepatic clearance, and protein binding. Pregnancy VTE dosing of low-molecular-weight heparins, for example, uses an altered BD dose to account for enhanced clearance. Furthermore, prescribers must consider the risk of harm to the foetus including birth defects (teratogenicity). This depends on the inherent properties of the drug and its ability to cross the placenta. Small lipid-soluble drugs will cross easier than larger/more water-soluble drugs. Prescribing advice may change throughout the pregnancy-teratogens, such as trimethoprim are most dangerous in the first trimester, while NSAIDs carry the greatest risk after 30 weeks as they may close the ductus arteriosus. Consult with obstetrics/pharmacy early for advice.

PRESCRIBING IN LIVER IMPAIRMENT

Many drugs are hepatically metabolised and liver impairment is common in the acute, emergency, and critical care patient populations. Drugs can be metabolised by Phase 1 and Phase 2 reactions as shown in Figure 18.10.

The liver's ability to clear drugs is extensive, and only in very significant impairment is drug clearance affected. Phase 2 reactions tend to be better preserved than Phase 1 reactions.

Drugs may be divided into those that have a high extraction ratio and low extraction ratio. High extraction ratio drugs are highly affected by changes in liver blood flow. Low extraction ratio drugs depend only on intrinsic liver clearance, and are not significantly altered by liver blood flow. The BNF frequently cautions or contraindicates drugs in severe liver failure, but this may often be due to lack of data.

The Child-Pugh score can be used as an estimate of severity of liver dysfunction in chronic liver failure patients. Of note, in ICU do not score low albumin when calculating, as this will be low for multiple reasons. Drugs such as caspofungin have dose reductions where Child Pugh B-C is calculated. Markers of liver function in acute liver failure are not precise compared with creatinine clearance but elevated bilirubin and INR indicate poor clearance and synthetic function, respectively. If the drug in question is highly hepatically cleared (>20% eliminated), consider avoiding or dose reducing/increasing dosing interval particularly where therapeutic range is narrow and extraction ratio high.

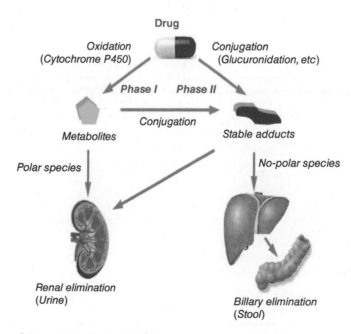

FIGURE 18.10   Phase 1 and 2 reactions. *Source*: Author.

Other considerations should include:

- Avoid nephrotoxins such as NSAIDs; risk of worsening ascites and hepatorenal syndrome
- Avoid ulcerating medicines
- Low albumin from liver failure
- Avoid unnecessary sedation in encephalopathy
- Avoid constipating drugs
- Drugs with a high bleeding risk should be avoided where possible
- Avoid hepatotoxic drugs if possible.

AUTHORISATION OF BLOOD AND BLOOD PRODUCTS

APs should consider the important legal distinction between Blood and Blood Products. All medicinal products are covered within The Medicines Act (1968) which, following an amendment in 2005, states that whole human blood and blood components are excluded from this legal definition, meaning they cannot be legally prescribed by any practitioner.

The World Health Organisation (WHO) has defined Blood Products as 'any therapeutic substance derived from human blood and plasma' (WHO 2021). These are regulated by the Medicines Act, and there are no special training requirements for IPs to prescribe these as long they are clearly defined in their scope of practice.

Blood components that are not licensed medicines are Packed Red Cells (RBC); Platelets, Cryoprecipitate, and Fresh Frozen Plasma (FFP). A framework supports 'appropriately trained, competent practitioners to make the clinical decision and provide written instructions (often referred to as authorisation) for blood component transfusion' (JPAC 2022). Table 18.5 highlight's the essential requirements for the written authorisation of blood to optimise patient safety.

TABLE 18.5   Minimum requirements for written authorisation of blood.

Minimum requirements that written authorisation of blood components must include.	
The patient's identifiers	First and last name, date of birth, unique patient id (where possible a national ID). *In emergency situations where patients cannot be immediately identified at least one unique identifier such as trauma/A&E number can be used.*
Specify the component to be given[a]	Red Blood Cells, Fresh Frozen Plasma, Platelets, Cryoprecipitate
Dose and volume required[a]	i.e. 1 pool of platelets, 1 pack of FFP, 1 unit of blood
Rate of transfusion	Remember 'maximum time' to transfuse products must include travel time from the laboratory to collect it. Blood 4 hours, Platelets 30 minutes, FFP 15 minutes
Any special requirements	i.e. irradiated component

[a] Do not use abbreviations on the written authorisation document to reduce the risk of error.

While there are no legal barriers to authorising blood, local recommendations need to be followed. Transfusion practitioners and hospital transfusion committees will have expert knowledge on your local process to follow and surrounding governance. Some NHS trusts have developed their own educational packages but the nationally recognised course remains that run by NHSBT. Developed after a 2008 collaborative project by NHSBT and SNBTS to assess the feasibility of Nurse and Midwifes authorisation of blood components, it has been adapted to cover AHP in advancing roles titled Non-Medical Authorisation of Blood Components. Training must deliver the core theoretical knowledge required for the role followed by the practice element achieved through experiential learning in the clinical area, assessed by a medical mentor. This has been successfully implemented in AHP, for example, by the training of critical care paramedics for the authorisation of blood (Smith and Doughty 2022) to use pre-hospital.

CONSENT AND TRANSFUSION

Clinicians have an ethical and legal duty to ensure shared decision-making with the patients wherever possible. Consent should be obtained prior to transfusion. Where this is not possible, clear unambiguous documentation to support the decision-making process is essential. These patients should be informed prior to discharge that transfusion has taken place during their hospital stay. The Advisory Committee on the Safety of Blood, Tissues and Organs (SaBTO) have produced guidelines on patient consent for transfusion (SaBTO 2011). Many of the AECC population will lack capacity to give informed valid consent. APs should have excellent knowledge of assessing capacity and the application of the Mental Capacity Act in the decision-making process of transfusion.

RISK FACTORS

APs should have the knowledge to consider the associated risk factors around the use of blood products. In particular, compilations such as Transfusion-associated Circulatory Overload (TACO) and Transfusion-related Acute Lung Injury (TRALI) ensure benefits outweigh the risks, and these are mitigated. Documentation supports the clinical decision-making process. Tools such as SHOT (Serious Hazards of Transfusion) and the TACO checklist can be used to support APs in this process; particularly relevant in the ED and critical care population, where massive transfusion might be required in patients who do not have capacity to consent.

SPECIALIST REQUIREMENTS

It is the responsibility of the authorising ACP to be aware of the potential need for specific requirements. CMV negative components, washed red cells, irradiated products are available at request from the blood laboratory. Scope of practice comes into play if this decision needs to be made in patients where little or no history is known. MDT working and making decisions as a team in best interests is key.

Considerations in the Clinical Decision-making Process for Transfusion

Local policy should be adhered to when authorising blood components. The British Society for Haematology guidelines and SHOT's A–E decision-making tree are evidence-based reference guides to support clinical decision-making.

Health Education England (HEE). (2017). *Multi-professional Framework for Advanced Clinical Practice in England* [online]. Available from: `https://www.hee.nhs.uk/sites/default/files/documents/multi-professionalframeworkforadvancedclinicalpracticeinengland.pdf` [accessed 20 June 2023].

JPAC. (2022). *Clinical decision-making and authorising blood component transfusion – a framework to support non-medical healthcare professionals*. Produced by the United Kingdom & Ireland Blood Transfusion Network Education Working Group.

Lupu, F., Kinasewitz, G., and Dormer, K. (2020). The role of endothelial shear stress on haemodynamics, inflammation, coagulation and glycocalyx during sepsis. *Journal of Cellular and Molecular Medicine* 24 (21): 1582–1838.

Macedo, E. and Cerdá, J. (2021). Choosing a CRRT machine and modality. *Seminars in Dialysis* 34 (6): 0894–0959.

RCEM. (2022). *Emergency Medicine Advanced Clinical Practitioner Curriculum V2.*

RPS. (2021). *A Competency Framework for all Prescribers*. Available from: `https://www.rpharms.com/resources/frameworks/prescribing-competency-framework/competency-framework` [accessed 23 June 2023].

SaBTO. (2011). *Guidelines from the Expert Committee on the Safety of Blood, Tissues and Organ's (SaBTO) on Patient Consent for Blood Transfusion.*

Sime, F.B., Udy, A.A., and Roberts, J.A. (2015). Augmented renal clearance in critically ill patients: aetiology, definition and implications for beta-lactam dose optimization. *Current Opinion in Pharmacology* 24: 1–6.

Smith, H. and Doughty, H. (2022). Training trial of critical care paramedics for non-medical authorisation of blood. *British Paramedic Journal* 6 (4): 55–59.

The Faculty of Intensive Care Medicine. (2018). *Curriculum for Training for Advanced Critical Care Practitioners – Syllabus. V1.1* [online]. Available from: www.ficm.ac.uk/media/6896 [accessed 20 June 2023].

The Intensive Care Society, Critical Care Networks – *National Nurse Leads and The National Outreach Forum*. (2022). *Advanced Critical Care Outreach Competencies* [online]. Available from: `https://ics.ac.uk/asset/43B8C11B-4512-41D0-B97768FABA2C30B2` [accessed 20 June 2023].

The Royal College of Emergency Medicine. (2022). *Emergency Medicine Advanced Clinical Practitioner Curriculum 2022 (Adult)* [online]. Available from: `https://rcem.ac.uk/wp-content/uploads/2022/09/ACP_Curriculum_Adult_Final_060922.pdf` [accessed 20 June 2023].

WHO. (2021). *Global Report on Blood Safety and Availability.*

FURTHER READING

Duconge, J. (2008). Applying organ clearance concepts in a clinical setting. *American Journal of Pharmaceutical Education* 72 (5): 121.

Erstad, B. (2004). Dosing of medications in morbidly obese patients in the intensive care unit setting. *Intensive Care Medicine* 30: 18–32.

Gregory, T. and Smith, M. (2012). Cardiovascular complications of brain injury. *Continuing Education in Anaesthesia, Critical Care and Pain* 12 (2): 67–71.

Keats, K., Powell, R., Rocker, J. et al. (2022). Evaluation of phenytoin loading doses in overweight patients using actual versus adjusted body weight. *Epilepsy & Behaviour* 134.

Kenakin, T. (2022). *Comprehensive pharmacology*. Edinburgh: Elsevier.

Kiang, T.K.L. and Ensom, M.H.H. (2016). A comprehensive review on the predictive performance of the Sheiner-Tozer and derivative equations for the correction of phenytoin concentrations. *Annals of Pharmacotherapy* 50 (4): 311–325.

Kimmoun, A. et al. (2015). Haemodynamic consequences of severe lactic acidosis in shock states: from bench to bedside. *Critical Care* 19 (1): 175.

Ritter, J. et al. (2018). *Rang and Dale's pharmacology*, 9e. Edinburgh: Elsevier.

Roberts, F. and Freshwater-Turner, D. (2007). Pharmacokinetics and anaesthesia. *Continuing Education in Anaesthesia, Critical Care and Pain* 7 (1): 25–29.

Royal College of Emergency Medicine. (2012). *Safe Sedation of Adults in the Emergency Department.*

Royal College of Emergency Medicine. (2020). *Pharmacological Agents for Procedural Sedation and Analgesia in the Emergency Department.*

Schotola, H., Toischer, K., Popov, A.F. et al. (2022). Mild metabolic acidosis impairs the beta-adrenergic response in isolated human failing myocardium. *Critical Care* 16: R153.

Thom, D.W. (2021). *The paramedic revision guide.* Chichester: Wiley Blackwell.

Thom, D. (2021). A decision theory overview and case-based discussion. *Journal of Paramedic Practice* 13 (8).

Wilcox, R.A. and Owen, H. (2000). Variable cytochrome P 450 2D6 expression and metabolism of codeine and other opioid prodrugs: implications for the Australian Anaesthetist. *Anaesthesia and Intensive Care* 28: 611–619.

CHAPTER 19

Advanced and Extended Procedures for AECC Populations

Phil Evans and Sean Buchanan

> **Aim**
> The aim of this chapter is to discuss the indications, practical considerations, risks, and benefits for common procedures that may be performed by the ACP in the acute hospital environment.

LEARNING OUTCOMES

After reading this chapter the reader will:

1. Understand the indications for common clinical procedures faced by the ACP.
2. Understand the role of governance surrounding practical procedures.
3. Be aware of the theoretical and technical process of performing common clinical procedures.
4. Be aware of the common contraindications and safety considerations for performing clinical procedures.

SELF-ASSESSMENT QUESTIONS

1. List the common pre-procedure considerations the ACP should assess before commencing a clinical procedure?
2. What are the benefits of using a lateral approach for a Lumbar Puncture?

The Advanced Practitioner in Acute, Emergency and Critical Care, First Edition. Edited by Sadie Diamond-Fox, Barry Hill, Sonya Stone, Caroline McCrea, Natalie Gardner, and Angela Roberts.
© 2024 John Wiley & Sons Ltd. Published 2024 by John Wiley & Sons Ltd.

3. What are the two main types of Local Anaesthetic? Give examples of a drug from each class.
4. List the commonly used sites for a CVC line. How to locate them?

INTRODUCTION

The ACP is well positioned to perform common clinical procedures within their scope of practice and competence. While most of the procedures may be significantly advanced of their base registration, there is increasing evidence showing that this is a safe workforce to perform such interventions.[1,2]

It should be acknowledged that while there is often a clear expectation of procedural competence according to national specialist curricula (such as RCEM), the individual ACP scope of practice lies with their employer. Governance arrangements should be clear and unambiguous, and any procedural requirements should be clearly identified in the individual job plan providing security for both patient and practitioner.

Appropriate theoretical and practical knowledge, support and experience is required to gain and maintain competence, and each practitioner should be able to clearly demonstrate their training and ongoing competence.

This chapter covers the general approach to practical procedures, governance, medication, and documentation. It discusses some of the more common procedures the ACP may face in clinical practice with associated practical tips, however, this list is not exhaustive, and the ACP should ultimately be guided by local policy and governance arrangements. Indeed, additional procedures such as suturing, reduction of fractures or dislocations, bronchoscopy and endotracheal intubation which may be performed by advanced practitioners with appropriate training and governance structures.

Multi-professional Framework (MPF) for Advanced Clinical Practice Guidance for Professional Development (HEE 2017)

This chapter maps to the following statements within the MPF:

1. Clinical:	1.1	1.2	1.7	1.11
2. Leadership:	2.11			

[1] Kocka et al. (2022). Nurse-led sedation for transfemoral transcatheter aortic valve implantation seems safe for a selected patient population. *European Heart Journal Supplements*, 24(B), pp. B23–B27.
[2] Trunz et al. (2021). National trends in lumbar puncture from 2010 to 2018: a shift reversal from the emergency department to the hospital setting for radiologists and advanced practice providers. *American Journal of Neuroradiology*, January, 42(1) pp. 206–210.

Accreditation Considerations

This chapter maps to the following statements within the following national accreditation documents:

Curriculum for Training for Advanced Critical Care Practitioners Syllabus V1.1
(The Faculty of Intensive Care Medicine 2018)

3.16	4.5	

Advanced Critical Care Outreach Competencies
(The Intensive Care Society, Critical Care Networks – National Nurse Leads and The National Outreach Forum 2022)

A1	

Emergency Medicine Advanced Clinical Practitioner Curriculum 2022 – Adult
(The Royal College of Emergency Medicine 2022)

SLO1	SLO6	

Advanced Clinical Practice in Acute Medicine Curriculum Framework
(Health Education England 2022)

General Clinical CiPs: 1, 2, 3
Speciality Clinical CiPs: 3

GOVERNANCE, NATIONAL SAFETY STANDARDS FOR INVASIVE PROCEDURES (NATSSIPS) AND LOCAL SAFETY STANDARDS FOR INVASIVE PROCEDURES (LOCSSIPS)

Procedural knowledge is a core requirement for advanced specialist training; however, their employer must also agree that there is a need for them to perform a particular clinical procedure. Any procedure requires both experience and technical skill. Therefore, there should be enough demand for the procedure to justify the governance overhead and allow the accumulation of sufficient experience by the ACPs. A clear mandate with formal governance support should be in place before any procedure is performed. This is essential to protect the patient and the practitioner in the event of an unexpected complication of the procedure.

Many employers recognise the advantages of enabling ACPs to perform key procedures. As a substantive team member, the ACP accumulates institutional knowledge as they become more experienced with the procedure, the available equipment, and the local methodology. This translates into a higher success rate, better patient satisfaction, and a more efficient service.

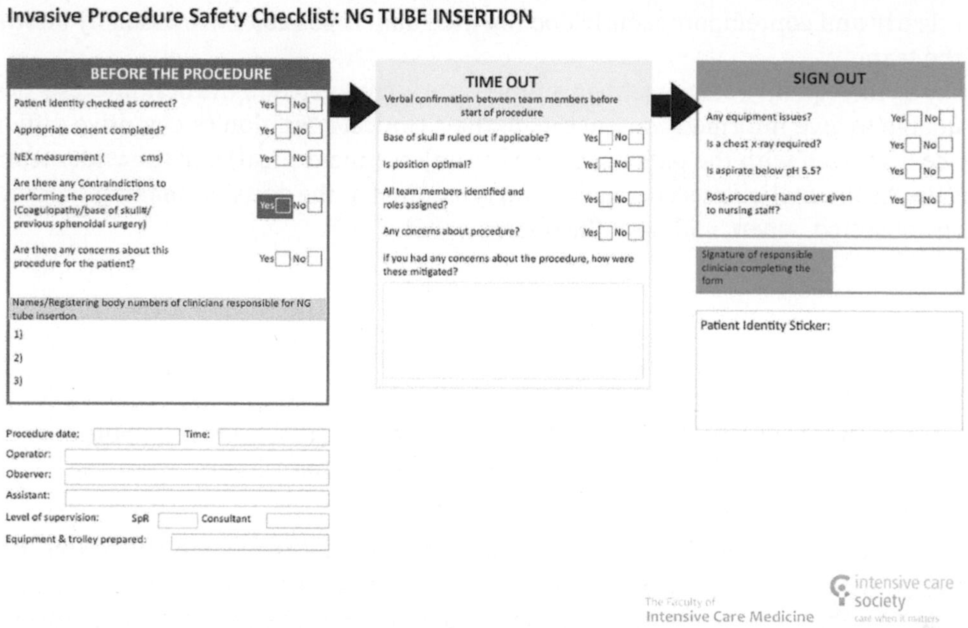

Invasive Procedure Safety Checklist: NG TUBE INSERTION

FIGURE 19.1   Example of nasogastric tube insertion LocSSIPP. *Source*: https://ficm.ac.uk/sites/ficm/files/documents/2021–10/safety_checklist_–_ng_tube_insertion_–_final_0.pdf/ last accessed 27 February 2023.

The NHS England report *National Safety Standards for Invasive Procedures (NatSSIPs)* (2015) highlighted the significance of non-technical skills in clinical procedures, and how the use of a clear framework can help reduce error. While it was developed primarily from a surgical perspective, its use was extended to include all significantly invasive procedures. It mandated the use of locally produced protocols for all significant invasive procedure based on the NatSSIP format – the Local Safety Standards for Invasive Procedures (LoCSSIP). The LoCSSIP should be developed according to a standard template and include key procedural steps, such as team briefing, consent, timings, equipment, and close out procedure (see Figure 19.1). It also acts as a record of the procedure and can be audited allowing appropriate governance.

CONSIDERATIONS FOR ALL PROCEDURES

Consent

Consent is required for all our actions in the healthcare environment to differing degrees. When the ACP is performing a clinical procedure, informed written consent is the gold standard for all elective procedures. The benefit is twofold: it ensures that there is a clear, written record of the consent process, and it also allows time to build rapport with the patient. So, the process should be viewed as part of the procedure rather than a separate task. A good rapport, in turn, is associated with patient satisfaction and allows more time for the ACP to be successful.

There are times when written consent is either impossible, such is during emergency treatment, or inappropriate, such as for routine blood tests. Verbal consent is appropriate in such circumstances but must be clearly and contemporaneously documented and, if possible, witnessed by another, named, member of the team.

There may be infrequent occasions when a procedure is completed in the best interests of the patient as they are unable to give informed consent due to their clinical condition or cognitive difficulties. This should then be discussed with the patient's advocate (unless time-critical) and the wider team to ensure it is appropriate. Again, meticulous documentation is required of the decision-making process, including who has been consulted, when, and what the outcome was.

Pre-procedure

- **Clinical review**

  It is good practice to complete a focussed history and physical examination in order to confirm that the procedure is both indicated and in the best interests of the patient.

- **Laboratory investigations**

  Before embarking on any significantly invasive procedure, it is recommended that tests of renal and liver function (metabolism of local anaesthetic/medication), as well as clotting studies are available. In some circumstances, these may be omitted; however, the clinician must be confident that the potential benefits significantly outweigh the risks.

- **Review of imaging**

  While typically scrutinised during the diagnostic process any imaging should be reviewed by the clinician beforehand. All cross-sectional imaging should be appropriately reported.

- **Medication check**

  Has any medication been administered that may make this procedure more dangerous e.g. by modifying clotting or risk of bleeding? The inherent procedural risk, the therapeutic agents used, and the urgency of the procedure should all be considered before starting the procedure. Expert advice should be sought as required.

- **Situational awareness**

  Right time – Is now the best time to do this, or should it be done only during core hours when there is more support available? Are there any procedural requirements? For example, xanthochromia in CSF should only be sampled 12 hours after the onset of symptoms.

  Right place – Is there an appropriate space/environment to perform this safely? Are there any specific equipments or monitoring requirements?

  Right person – The practitioner should have appropriate knowledge and skill in this procedure, know their limitations and the point at which they seek further advice, support or to terminate the procedure. There should be clear escalation in place in the event of complication.

Post Procedure

- **Clinical review**

  Check how the patient is after the procedure ensuring that they are clean and comfortable following the intervention. Ensure adequate monitoring and frequency of observations. Make sure all appropriate samples are labelled and sent.

- **Medication check**

  Consider the need for ongoing analgesia and prescribe accordingly. Check any anticoagulants/antiplatelets are held and then restarted as appropriate. Ensure any local anaesthetic and procedural medications such as heparinised priming for lines have been prescribed.

- **Documentation**

  Clearly document the consent process, the intervention including number attempts, the outcome (success/failure), and record any immediate complications. Ensure that parameters are set for escalation, referral, or discharge.

ANALGESIA AND ANAESTHESIA

Procedures are more painful and anxiety-inducing than most clinicians appreciate, indeed rolling a patient in the ICU has been found to be painful and distressing. Therefore, adequate analgesia or even anaesthesia is imperative for any procedure. While oral analgesic agents are appropriate for some minor procedures or examinations, the procedures considered in this chapter typically require at least local anaesthesia but consideration for regional anaesthesia or procedural sedation should be given. The latter is beyond the scope of this chapter but the interested reader may consider some of the texts listed at the end of this chapter.

Local anaesthetic (LA) is commonly used in the ED, acute care, and ICU environments. However, little consideration is given for the pharmacodynamics of the agent used or for modification of these factors with additives.

LA agents are classified as esters, e.g. cocaine and amides e.g. lidocaine. However, both groups primarily rely on the blockade of voltage-gated sodium channels preventing depolarisation and the generation of an action potential. The primary difference between the groups is stability in solution and therefore half-life. Amides are more stable and are more commonly encountered clinically (see Table 19.1).

TABLE 19.1   Characteristics of the amide local anaesthetic agents.

	Relative potency	Onset of action	Duration of action	Half life (min)	Maximum dose	Uses
Lidocaine	2	15 min	60–90 min	100	3 mg/kg or 7 mg/kg with adrenaline	Local infiltration Topically Nerve blocks
Bupivacaine	8	10–30 min	4–8 hours	210	2 mg/kg	Nerve blocks Local infiltration but slow onset
Levobupivacaine	8	10–15 min[a]	6–9 hours	80	150 mg	Nerve blocks
Ropivacaine	8	1–5 min	2–6 hours	120	200 mg	Nerve blocks
Prilocaine	2	15 min	60–90 min	120	6 mg/kg or 8 mg/kg with felypressin	Local infiltration IV anaesthesia

[a] Based on intrathecal administration.

The onset of action is determined by the pH at which the drug is 50% ionised and 50% unionised, known as pK_a, with only the latter fraction contributing to the drug's effect. Therefore, the closer the pK_a is to tissue pH, the faster the onset of action. Lidocaine has a pK_a of 7.9, so at a tissue pH of 7.4 a quarter of the drug is unionised whereas bupivacaine with pK_a of 8.1 would have only 15% available in unionised form. This also explains why most LA agents, which typically have pK_a greater than 7.6, work poorly when injected into infected tissue which is more acidic than healthy tissue.

The duration of action is determined by the degree of protein binding; greater binding equals longer action, as well as the inherent vasodilation effect of the drug and the local circulation. Adrenaline is frequently added to agents such as lidocaine, as 5 mcg/ml or 1:200000, and it reduces vascular reabsorption and bleeding while prolonging the duration of action. It has no meaningful effect on long-acting agents such as bupivacaine, and should not be used in blocks of terminal extremities or on flap repairs where the vasoconstriction can result in ischaemic necrosis.

Injection of LA can be very painful and the practitioner can take several steps to reduce the patient's discomfort:

- Reassure the patient and provide a distraction.
- Consider applying a topical anaesthetic first (e.g. eutectic mixture of local anesthetics [EMLA]) for intact skin or LAT gel for open wounds.[3]
- Warm the LA agent if possible.
- Buffering has been shown to improve discomfort and speed up the onset of action. Typically, 1 ml of 8.4% bicarbonate solution for injection is added to every 9 ml of lidocaine with or without adrenaline.
- Use a fine, long needle for the injection. Enter the skin once and, while periodically aspirating, advance the needle along the tract you wish to anaesthetise. Once at the proximal end slowly withdraw the needle while injecting the LA agent.
- Whenever possible use your anatomical knowledge to target specific nerves proximally to the site of interest thereby reducing the pain of multiple injections e.g. ring block.

COMPLICATIONS OF LOCAL ANAESTHESIA

Complications are grouped by those related to the technique and those related to the agents employed (see Table 19.2).

Local anaesthetic toxicity describes a syndrome where systemic side effects of the LA agent arise as the systemic concentration increases to toxic levels. It is characterised by CNS, respiratory, and cardiovascular manifestations that cannot be otherwise explained (see Table 19.3). Risk factors for LA toxicity include poor metabolic clearance (hepatic impairment, cimetidine therapy), cardiovascular compromise (elderly, low cardiac output, heart block, anti-arrhythmic, or beta-blocker therapy), or CNS impairment (epilepsy, myasthenia gravis), as well as small children or porphyria. In general, subcutaneous infiltration results in the lowest systemic concentrations and intercostal the highest, with brachial plexus, epidural, and caudal in between.

---

[3] Be aware, these contain LA and therefore the volume used should be included in the total dose calculation.

TABLE 19.2   Complications of local anaesthesia.

Technique-related	Drug-related
Direct trauma to the nerve	Inadvertent intravascular injection
Bleeding and/or haematoma	Toxicity due to systemic absorption
Damage to surrounding soft tissues e.g. tendons, lung parenchyma	Anaphylaxis
Infection	Methemoglobinemia

TABLE 19.3   Signs and symptoms of LA toxicity.

Timeline/serum concentration	CNS	Cardiovascular	Respiratory
Early/low	Light headedness Tinnitus Circumoral/tongue numbness	Tachycardia and hypertension (if adrenaline is used)	
	Abnormal taste Confusion	Bradycardia and hypotension	
Intermediate	Drowsiness Visual disturbance Muscular twitching	Conduction blocks	Respiratory depression
	Convulsions Reduced LOC	Cardiovascular collapse	
Late/high	Coma	Asystole and ventricular arrhythmias	Respiratory arrest

Treatment is predominantly supportive once the infusion has been stopped. Consult the Association of Anaesthetists of Great Britain and Ireland (AAGBI) guideline for severe local anaesthetic toxicity for further guidance.

LUMBAR PUNCTURE (DIAGNOSTIC)

Indications

The most common indications are suspicion of:

- Meningitis or encephalitis
- Sub-arachnoid haemorrhage
- Idiopathic intracranial hypertension

LP may be required, following specialist advice, for investigations of:

- CNS malignancy
- CNS vasculitis
- Multiple sclerosis
- Guillain-Barre syndrome

Contraindications

- Anticoagulation, antiplatelet therapy[4] and bleeding disorders
- Raised intracranial pressure
- Infection overlaying LP site
- Meningococcal sepsis
- Untreated shock
- Seizures until adequately controlled

Risks

Common risks from LP are:

- Pain
- Bruising/bleeding/infection at site
- Post-procedure headache
- Transient radicular pain or paraesthesia
- Failure of procedure

Rare but serious risks include:

- Prolonged radicular pain or paraesthesia and paraparesis
- Infection including meningitis and discitis
- Spinal haematoma (can cause cauda equina syndrome)
- Cerebral herniation
- Abducens or other cranial nerve palsy
- Epidermoid tumour

Process

Pre-procedure (In Addition to Above)

If there is clinical suspicion of raised intracranial pressure, ensure CT Head has been performed and reported. Rarely, clinically significant raised intracranial pressure can be present even with a normal CT scan, therefore fundoscopy should be performed routinely.

Equipment

- Procedure trolley
- Fenestrated sterile drape
- Gauze swabs

---

[4] This may be a relative contraindication, please see – The Association of Anaesthetists of Great Britain and Ireland, The Obstetric Anaesthetists Association and Regional Anaesthesia, UK. Regional Anaesthesia and Patients with Abnormalities of Coagulation. (2013). *Anaesthesia*. 68, pp. 966–972.

- Sterile towels
- 10 ml syringe
- Green needle
- Orange needle
- Drawing up needle
- Manometer (if performing opening pressures)
- Small self-adhesive dressing
- Paper bag (to protect xanthachromia sample from light)
- 4× universal specimen containers (this is a minimum requirement – check with microbiology laboratory beforehand)
- Yellow clinical waste bag
- Spinal needle – Atraumatic
- Non-sterile – 1× grey glucose bottle
- Local anaesthetic
- Appropriate skin disinfectant
- Sterile gloves
- Venesection equipment (in order to take one U&E bottle immediately post LP)

Procedure – Left Lateral Position

This is the position of choice as it allows opening pressures to be measured. If the patient is technically challenging (reduced mobility, obesity, etc.) consider procedure in the upright position, however be aware that opening pressures cannot be measured.

1. Lie the patient on the left side in the foetal position, ensuring correct alignment of the spine. Supporting the head with a pillow and putting a pillow between knees may improve position and patient comfort.
2. Expose lumbar spine.
3. Select site for LP.
   - Identify the highest point of the iliac crests. A direct line (commonly referred to as Tuffiers line) joining these landmarks should guide the identification of the fourth lumbar vertebral body.
   - Palpate to identify L3/4 or L4/5 space and mark (see Figure 19.2).
4. Thoroughly clean and sterilise with antiseptic spray, allow to dry and apply drape.
5. Use LA infiltration so that a small bleb is raised. Deeper infiltration can then be undertaken.
6. The introducer should then be inserted, angling slightly towards the head as if aiming for the umbilicus. The bevel should be positioned towards the patient's flanks to spread rather than cut the dural sac.
7. The LP needle should then be guided through the introducer and gently advanced towards the dural space. It should be introduced incrementally, and the stylet periodically removed to check for the presence of CSF flow. If no flow is demonstrated, reinsert the stylet until the subarachnoid space is entered.
8. Once CSF appears, the stylet should be removed, and if required the manometer attached and opening pressures recorded.

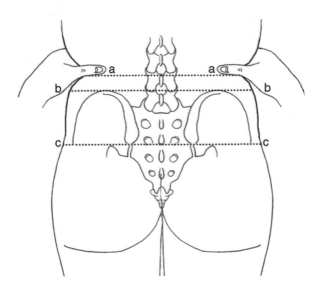

FIGURE 19.2   Identification of site for LP using anatomical landmarking. Line a-demonstrates the line between superior illiac crests which commonly sits at L4. Line b is a radiological Tuffiers line and identifies L4/5. *Source*: Chakraverty et al. (2007) / John Wiley & Sons.

9. 10–15 drops of CSF should be collected in sequentially numbered universal containers, and then the Glucose bottle.
10. Once the samples have been collected, the spinal needle can be gently removed until it is within the body of the stylet and then both stylet and needle can be removed together.
11. The insertion site should be covered with a dressing.

Post Procedure

- Complete LocSSIP paperwork and document according to local practice.
- The CSF samples must be transported to the laboratory in a timely fashion. Air Pod systems are not indicated for this due to theoretical impact on sample and potential system delay/failure.
- Xanthochromia degrades in light and therefore needs to be protected.
- A paired serum U&E should also be taken and sent to the biochemistry laboratory.
- The patient should be encouraged to drink plenty, and given simple analgesia as indicated.

Practical tips

- This should always be a two-person procedure with the non-operator primarily responsible for patient comfort and reassurance.
- Ensuring the patient position is correct and the operator height appropriate increases the success rate.
- Build into your routine, enough time to allow the local anaesthetic time to take effect; rushing at this point will cause the procedure to be more uncomfortable for the patient and reduce the chance of a successful procedure.

LARGE VOLUME PARACENTESIS (LVP)

Indications

- Symptomatic relief of severe ascites not controlled by diuretics

Contraindications

- Uncooperative patient
- Known bowel obstruction
- Pregnancy
- Skin infection at proposed puncture site
- Disseminated intravascular coagulation

Risks

- Bleeding and/or bruising
- Bowel perforation
- Pain
- Infection
- Failure

Process

Specific pre-procedure requirements (in addition to above)

- Record baseline observations
- Obtain IV access and ensure availability of 20% HAS
- Ask patient to empty bladder (reduces the risk of accidental perforation)
- Consider need for ultrasound site selection

Equipment

- Procedure trolley
- Sterile procedure pack
- Absorbent pad
- Appropriate drain (according to local protocol – commonly Rocket or Bonano catheter)
- Dressing to secure drain in place
- Scalpel
- Gauze swabs
- Sterile towels
- 10 ml syringe

- Green needle
- Orange needle
- Drawing up needle
- 1× universal specimen containers
- 1× set of blood culture bottles
- Yellow clinical waste bag
- Local anaesthetic
- Skin disinfectant
- Sterile gloves

Procedure

1. Lie the patient supine on examination couch or bed with head slightly raised and put absorbent pad under the drain side.
2. Select site for LVP
   - Percuss the abdomen for dullness to ensure appropriate ascites and that there is no organomegaly.
   - Preferably use the left lower quadrant as the abdominal wall is thinnest. The site should be approximately 2–4 cm superomedial to the anterior superior iliac spine (see Figure 19.3).
   - Avoid any obvious distended veins or sites of scar tissue.
3. Thoroughly clean and sterilise the skin around the proposed site.
4. Using local anaesthetic infiltrate the skin with local anaesthetic, raising a small bleb. Deeper injection can then be achieved using a 'Z-technique' (see Figure 19.4) through the abdominal wall using a 21G (green) needle, taking care to aspirate prior to injection, until straw-coloured ascitic fluid is aspirated.

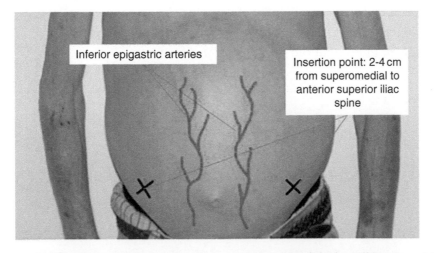

FIGURE 19.3   Anatomical locations of drain insertion. *Source*: Reuben (2016) / John Wiley & Sons. https://aasldpubs.onlinelibrary.wiley.com/doi/10.1002/cld.556 last accessed 22 February 2023.

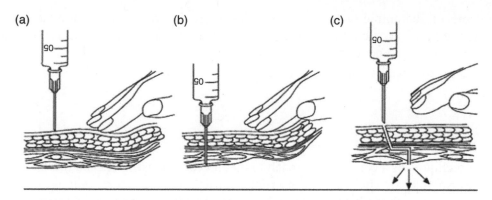

FIGURE 19.4 Z-injection technique. *Source*: Rodger and King (2008) / John Wiley & Sons.

5. Puncture the skin with the tip of the scalpel making a small incision. This reduces skin tenting on insertion of the drain and reduces the force required to breach the skin therefore reduces risk of perforation.

6. Insert the drain using the Z-technique.

7. Once the needle enters the peritoneal cavity, indicated by a loss of resistance and a 'flashback' of fluid into the cannula, advance a further 1–2 cm into the fluid before pushing the cannula off the needle then withdrawing the needle from the cannula. Fluid should then be draining freely from the catheter.

8. Take diagnostic ascitic samples as required (5 ml for urgent WBC to microbiology; 5–10 ml each into two blood cultures bottles; universal samples to biochemistry for albumin and protein levels; cytology if required).

9. Connect the cannula to the urinary catheter drainage tube and bag and ensure free drainage.

10. Secure the drain to the abdominal wall.

Post Procedure

- Complete LocSSIP paperwork and document according to local practice.
- Observations should be taken hourly to ensure no post-paracentesis hypotension.
- Catheter should be left on free drain until dry but for a maximum 6–8 hours. Longer than this increases the risk of infection.
- One unit of HAS 20% should be infused for every 2.5 l of ascitic fluid drained.

Removal of Drain

1. On completion of the procedure, the drain should be gently withdrawn, and the site covered with an adhesive dressing.

2. Patient can be discharged if, after 60 minutes, they are asymptomatic and observations are stable.

Practical Tips

- Ascitic fluid is an irritant to tissue – once this is aspirated during the infiltration of local anaesthetic do not inject further LA with this syringe.

- The depth of abdominal wall is estimated during the infiltration of local anaesthetic. If, when passing the drain, ascitic fluid is not obtained at a similar depth the drain has been inserted too obliquely and should be withdrawn and realigned.
- Ascitic tap – this can be done to exclude spontaneous bacterial peritonitis (SBP)

THE SELDINGER TECHNIQUE

The Seldinger technique is a common approach to the insertion of catheters and drains of a large diameter. The same principles are applied to the insertion of an arterial line, central venous catheter, or smaller bore intercostal drain. In the following section the general Seldinger technique is described, and the later sections highlight the particular considerations and modifications for each type of device. A commonly encountered modification is the use of an over-the-catheter needle whereby the needle is withdrawn before the guidewire is introduced.

Contraindications

- Puncture site with overlying infection or interruption
- Absence of collateral circulation
- Disorders of coagulation (relative)

Risks

- Thrombus and distal ischaemic injury
- Infection
- Arteriospasm
- Haematoma

Process

Equipment

- Skin cleaning swabs or solution
- Sterile field i.e. dressing pack including sterile gauze or central line pack
- Appropriate suture material, e.g. 2/0 silk on a colt or straight needle unless using a needle-driver when a small cutting needle can be used, or an adhesive securing device e.g. SecuraCath™ or StatLock™.
- Heparinised syringe (vascular access only)
- Appropriate Seldinger kit including needle, syringe, guide wire, scalpel, dilator(s) and cannula or drain
- Sterile ultrasound probe cover and sterile gel
- Appropriate local or regional anaesthesia – ensure all drugs are clearly labelled to prevent inadvertent intravascular injection and LA toxicity

Pre-procedure

- Identify an appropriate site after ruling out contraindications and position the patient in an optimal position.
- Position the ultrasound screen so you have the insertion site, your equipment, and the screen all in the same visual field with the consistent left-to-right orientation.
- Scan the selected insertion site before skin cleaning.
  - Check the probe orientation and optimise the depth and gain.
  - Look out for anatomical variation, nerve bundles, scarring, and signs of infection.
  - For vascular access: check for thrombus within the target vessel proximal and distal to the insertion site and use colour Doppler, if necessary, to differentiate between arteries and veins.
- Don a cap and mask, scrub your hands, and don a sterile gown and gloves.
- Clean the skin and allow the solution to dry. Once cleaned ensure all open containers of cleaning solution are discarded from the field.
- Place a fenestrated drape over the site to provide a sterile area with only the insertion site exposed.
- Apply a sterile cover to the ultrasound probe and secure it with the bands provided.
- Administer local anaesthetic prior to assembling the Seldinger device to allow sufficient time for the peak effect (see Anaesthesia section)
- After administering LA, prepare the equipment (see Figure 19.5):
  - Attach all three-way taps and/or needle-less connectors then flush all ports with sterile saline before locking closed.
  - Draw up 1–2 ml saline into the insertion syringe.
  - Attach the insertion needle checking the bevel faces up and flush with saline.
  - Prepare the guide wire by removing the cap and gently retracting the wire so the J-tip straightens and is ready to be inserted into the back of the needle.[5]

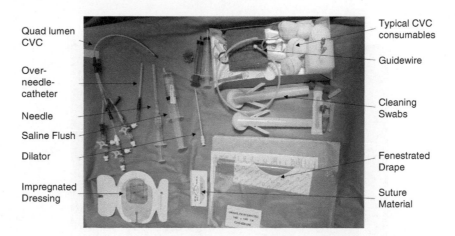

FIGURE 19.5 Typical sterile tray for Seldinger procedure – specifically CVC placement. Omitted is the local anaesthetic.

---

[5]Some kits allow the wire to be inserted through a hole in the syringe plunger thereby reducing the risk of entraining air into the needle and vascular, ensure you read the product literature before using a new kit.

- Position the ultrasound probe in the same orientation as before and identify the target for cannulation which should be kept in the middle of the screen.
- Using needle or forceps check that your anaesthesia is effective.

Procedure – Cannulation

- Insert the needle
  - Insert at 30°–45° with the bevel up and in-line with the target.
    - If targeting a superficial vessel, it may be necessary to tilt the probe at a fixed position on the skin to allow needle tip tracking rather than sliding the probe over the skin as for deeper targets.
    - Keep a perpendicular angle between the needle and probe.
  - Ensure you are guiding the tip of the needle to the target and not the shaft.
    - This is achieved by advancing the probe along the skin away from the needle until the needle signal disappears. Then advance the needle until it appears on the screen, once again slide the probe away from the needle, then advance the needle again.
    - The shaft looks identical to the tip, so strict discipline is required.
    - Do not aspirate continuously, rather occasional tests on each advance helps to determine whether the tip is in the tissues or a vessel.
    - If entering a high-pressure vessel, blood may flashback into the syringe, advance another 1–2 mm to ensure the entire bevel is within the vessel – this can be verified on ultrasound by visualising a length of needle inside the vessel (see Figure 19.6).
- Insert the guidewire.
  - Pass the wire gently through the needle with a back-and-forth motion until slightly more wire than the length of the Seldinger device is in the vessel.
    - At all times ensure that the end of the wire is free.
    - Confirm the guidewire is in the correct position on ultrasound and that it can be seen to move freely.

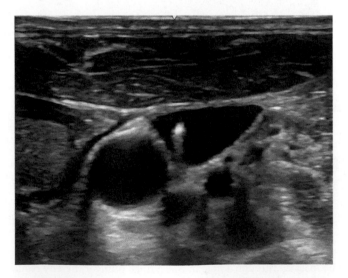

FIGURE 19.6   Needle length within the right IJV.

- ■ If any resistance is felt do not attempt to advance any further, consider the following or start again at a new site:
    - • Confirm that the needle/catheter is in the centre of the correct target in both short- and long-axis views – if not optimise the position or attempt a new site.
    - • Withdraw the wire completely and then rotate the needle 180° and/or slightly flatten the angle of the needle to the skin by 10°–15°. Do not attempt to reinsert the wire until you have checked you can still aspirate
- ○ When the guidewire is placed successfully then hold the free end of the guidewire and withdraw the needle along it until it is completely out of the skin
    - ■ With one hand hold the guidewire where it enters the skin and, with the other pull the needle off the free end.
- • Dilatation – as required for the particular device in use
    - ○ Using your ultrasound, confirm that the guidewire is within the vessel, and check it slides freely and does not penetrate the opposite wall of the vessel.
    - ○ Make a small nick in the skin no larger than the diameter of the dilator, cutting away from the guidewire, to allow the dilator to pass without tearing the skin.
    - ○ Only once the guidewire has been confirmed to be in the target then thread the dilator over the guidewire and ensure the wire exits the other end of the dilator before insertion.
    - ○ Gently but firmly advance the dilator over the wire using a slow rotation near to the skin. Continue to gently oscillate the guidewire in and out to prevent kinking the wire at the tissue interface.
    - ○ Once inserted to the appropriate depth allow to sit for a minute before gently withdrawing the dilator using the same motion.
    - ○ Firm pressure is now required over the site to prevent significant bleeding as the dilator is withdrawn.
- • Inserting the Seldinger device
    - ○ Load the device onto the guidewire. Ensure the wire's end passes out the back of the device, remembering that the port may need to be unlocked/opened, before the tip is inserted into the patient.
    - ○ Advance the catheter over the guidewire using a smooth, firm motion close to the skin while holding the end of guidewire with the other hand.
- • Remove the guidewire
    - ○ Once the device is completely inserted withdraw the guidewire. Put this aside for two-person confirmation of removal and later reloaded onto the dispenser for disposal.
    - ○ Vascular access only: Only once you and your assistant have both visually confirmed the guidewire is removed, then a blood sample should be taken in a heparinised syringe and run through a blood gas analyser to verify either arterial or venous access.

Post procedure

- • Secure the device
    - ○ Secure the device to the skin using sutures or according to your local protocols. Ordinarily, a typical IV dressing is not sufficient.
    - ○ Cap the access port being careful to prevent any entrainment of air.

- o Observe the monitor and ensure the trace depicts an appropriate systolic uptake, systolic decline, dicrotic notch, and diastolic runoff. If the trace is not adequate, the pressure reading cannot be relied upon and over-dampening may be present or the catheter may be in an adjacent vein. Review the blood gas sample.
- Clean the site
  - o Once secure and working, clean and dress as described above. Mark the line as Arterial.
- Documentation
  - o Document the procedure in the patient's notes as for all Seldinger insertions.

Practical Tips

- The trace will be different for each location e.g. the femoral arterial line typically has no dicrotic notch.
- If the trace looks over dampened, then check the lines for any air bubbles and remove any unnecessary three-way taps. Ensure all remaining taps and ports have been flushed.
- While the ulna artery is difficult to palpate, it is frequently larger than the radial and clear on ultrasound.
- Avoid the brachial artery as there is no collateral arterial supply to the distal limb.

CENTRAL VENOUS CATHETERS

Central venous catheters (CVC) are available in multiple configurations including single lumens, double-lumen dialysis catheters, and multi-lumen catheters.

Indications

- Administration of medications especially vasoactive
- Total parenteral nutrition
- Fluid status monitoring
- Continuous Renal Replacement Therapy
- Venous access for resuscitation

Contraindications

- Thrombus in the target vessel
- Local Infection

Relative Contraindications

- Coagulopathy and therapeutic anticoagulation
- Superior vena cava syndrome
- Patient is unable to tolerate position i.e. raised ICP or intraocular pressure

Risks

Risks and complications are largely determined by the site and type of device employed but may include:

- Infection
- Vascular injury including arterial puncture
- Pneumothorax/Haemothorax
- Haematoma
- Air embolism, thrombosis
- Catheter misplacement resulting in hydrothorax, hydromediatinum, or damage to the tricuspid valve.

Process

Pre-procedure

Site Selection: Major sites include the internal jugular vein (IJV) (see Figure 19.7), subclavian vein (SCV), external jugular vein (EJV), femoral vein, and antecubital vein. The ideal location provides access to the vein with minimal risk of puncturing the artery or damaging the nerve bundle. The SCV site also carries the greatest risk of pneumothorax but this is reduced when using ultrasound. The risk of infection is historically considered to be highest with the femoral site, but the implementation of central line bloodstream infection (CLABSI) bundles has resulted in lower rates overall and little difference between sites.

In all cases, maximal barrier precautions should be taken and WHO-type time out should be observed.

Positioning

See Table 19.4 for summary of patient positioning and anatomical landmarks for each of the target vessels for central venous catheters (CVC).

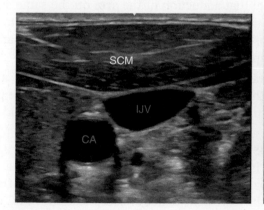
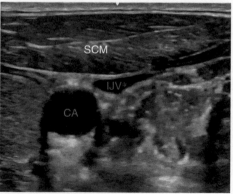

FIGURE 19.7   Ultrasound anatomy of internal jugular vein (IJV) in transverse view. The collapsibility of the IJV (IJV*) differentiates it from the rounder, firmer CA. CA – carotid artery, SCM – sternocleidomastoid muscle.

TABLE 19.4   Target vessel position and anatomical landmark.

Target Vessel	Position	Anatomical landmark
IJV	Position the patient in approximately 15° of Trendelenburg with the head partially rotated to the opposite shoulder.	The IJV runs below the confluence of the 2 heads of the sternocleidomastoid muscle and the clavicle. It lies 1–2 cm lateral of the palpable pulsations of the internal carotid.
EJV	Position in a low Trendelenburg position with head rotated away from the side of insertion.	Use your left index finger and thumb to anchor and distend this very superficial vessel.
Femoral	Generally performed in the supine position, in patients with a large amount of abdominal adipose tissue, it may be useful to keep the patient in low Trendelenburg with an assistant manually displacing the abdomen.	On the imaginary line joining the pubic tubercle and anterior superior iliac spine, the femoral artery is found at the medial border of the middle third. The needle should be inserted 2–3 cm inferior to the inguinal ligament, medially to the artery.
SCV	Place the patient in 15°–30° deg. Trendelenburg and their head turned to the opposing shoulder.	The SCV arises from the axillary vein as it crosses the first rib the arches cephalad under the medial clavicle before returning caudally to drain into the internal jugular vein posterior to the sternoclavicular joint.

Procedure

For all sites, the Seldinger technique described above is used. There are some specific considerations for certain sites:

- IJV: Limit depth of insertion of the guidewire and catheter to 15–20 cm on the right-hand side, or 19 to 24 cm on the left, to avoid arrhythmias.
- EJV: An often-overlooked option, especially for initial central venous access, the EJV can be cannulated with a simple over-the-needle 16G device. A guidewire is then introduced, and the first catheter is exchanged for a central line. Note that adduction of the arm on the same side while applying pressure to the clavicle may allow the catheter to transition from the EJV into the SCV towards the heart preventing hold-up or insertion towards the arm. If the appropriately sized equipment is available, this is a very useful approach for children.
- Femoral: It can also be useful to flex the knees, bring the ankles together in the midline, and allow the knees to fall outwards thereby opening the groin crease. 20 cm length catheters are preferred as there may be substantial tissue over the insertion point and the insertion site should be some distance distal to the groin crease.
- SCV: Shown to have the lowest rate of CLABSI, the SCV is the preferred first option for a CVC but is technically more difficult and may result in a pneumothorax. Due to its arching anatomy, the SCV may be cannulated at either the supra- or infraclavicular segments; however; the infraclavicular approach with ultrasound guidance has the lowest incidence of complications in RCTs.
  - Use the ultrasound to identify a straight segment of the SCV which overlies a rib, thereby offering protection to the underlying pleura – having the patient shrug his shoulders may open up new

windows for an optimal site. Insert the needle 2–3 cm below the midpoint of the clavicle while directing the tip towards the suprasternal notch and direct the needle to the identified segment.

   o If possible, insert the SCV line on the left using a 20-cm catheter, however, if there is already a chest drain in situ then use the same side if there are no contraindications.

Post Procedure

– Obtain and analyse a blood gas sample – ensure the oximetry values are consistent with venous blood.
– Transduce the catheter and ensure there is an appropriate CVP trace following calibration and zeroing.
– Order an x-ray to confirm the jugular or subclavian CVC lies in the junction of the superior vena cava and the right atrium. Carefully examine the film to ensure there is no pneumothorax. This is not necessary with femoral lines but should still be done for guided PICC lines.

Practical Tips

– Consider if your patient is likely to need ongoing dialysis for permanent renal failure – if so avoid the SCV as subclavian stenosis will adversely affect permanent haemodialysis options.
– If a central line is required only for vasopressors, consider starting peripheral vasopressors until the patient is more stable which will allow the line to be inserted under optimal conditions.
– The length of the catheter at the insertion site, in cm, can be estimated from the following formulae (accuracy varies from 90% to 97%):

Right IJV: (Height/10)

Left IJV: (Height/10) + 4 cm

Right SCV: (Height/10) – 2 cm

Left SCV: (Height/10) + 2 cm

THORACENTESIS

Drainage of air or fluid from the pleural space may be accomplished by using one of several techniques depending on the experience of the practitioner, the aetiology, and the urgency of the indication. For the patient with a symptomatic pleural effusion or primary spontaneous pneumothorax, simple needle aspiration is expedient and safe. It allows time to assemble the correct equipment and team to place a longer-term drain, such as a small gauge percutaneous device or a large bore open chest drain. While percutaneous, or over-the-needle systems, and Seldinger devices have become popular, safety reports indicate that they are associated with more incidents than open thoracostomy, and these were most often related to poor site selection and omitting the use of ultrasound.

Indications

- Tension pneumothorax
- Primary spontaneous pneumothorax
- Haemothorax
- Pleural effusion

A Seldinger-type drain may be placed to allow ongoing drainage of fluid or air. The procedure is similar to all Seldinger procedures discussed previously with the following modifications:

- Anaesthetise the tract as before and then ensure you have the correct combination of underwater drain connectors and adaptors as the sets frequently come with several options.
- Set the depth gauge on the dilator according to the measurements on the ultrasound.
- Prior to inserting the introducer needle make a 5 mm incision through the bleb raised previously by inserting the scalpel perpendicular to the skin, do not use a cutting motion.
- With the syringe attached to the introducer needle advance along the tract, as described above, until the pleural cavity is reached. Anchor the needle against the skin and detach the syringe. Note the depth of insertion – the dilator should be set to the same depth.
- Insert the guidewire as described previously and withdraw the needle. While anchoring the wire at the skin, feed the dilator onto the wire and hold it firmly at the depth identified on the needle. While holding the back of the wire, insert the dilator with a rotating motion. Larger gauge tubes may require several stepwise dilatations. Ensure the wire continues to move freely and does not change depth.
- Load the drain over the wire and insert it into the chest while holding the back of the wire.
  - o Aim the end of the drain towards the apex for a pneumothorax and towards the base for an effusion.
  - o Hold the drain near to the skin while advancing it, there should be minimal resistance after passing through the parietal pleura.
  - o Insert the tube to a depth of double the chest wall diameter or according to the manufacturer's instructions. Ensure no fenestrations remain outside.
- Remove the wire and attach the drain.
- Suture the drain
  - o Pass the suture through the skin above the drain and pull through equal lengths. The suture needle can be cut off before tying three knots which do not pull tightly against the skin.
  - o Wrap the remaining suture material, in an alternating fashion, around the drain. Keep the wraps tight to the tubing.
  - o After 5–10 wraps tie the material tight against the tube so that it kinks slightly. Place three knots in a similar manner close to one another. Trim any excess material.
- Dressing
  - o These devices typically have several hard plastic components tight to the skin which may cause pain or pressure damage.
  - o Place several pieces of sterile gauze between the chest wall and any components and then apply transparent adhesive dressing films over these.
  - o Do the same for the three-way tap, if used.

Thoracostomy

When presented with a patient in extremis due to a tension pneumothorax or a traumatic cardiac arrest, it is often most expedient to get definitive control by performing a simple (or finger) thoracostomy. This has the benefits of requiring very little equipment, immediately releasing the tension, if present, and completing the first step to either placing a tube thoracostomy or converting to an open thoracotomy as indicated.

- Identify the 4th or 5th intercostal space in the mid-axillary line. If you are lower than the inferior mammary fold then check your landmarks again, and if time allows use an ultrasound to confirm you are at the level of the pleural cavity.
- When prepping and draping include the nipple in your field.
- Anaesthetise the tract as described above but make a larger 4–5 cm bleb initially and provide parenteral analgesia and sedation.
- Make a 2–3 cm incision through the bleb and parallel to the ribs down to the subcutaneous tissues.
- Blunt dissect through the remaining tissues by inserting a curved Kelly, Spencer-Wells or similar clamp, over the inferior rib and angling slightly superior while avoiding the superior rib and its associated neurovascular bundle.
- Puncture the parietal pleura while holding the closed clamp near the tip to prevent inserting too deep when the resistance is lost. Open the clamp to widen the pleural opening.
- Insert a sterile gloved finger into the pleural cavity and sweep in a radial motion to clear any clots, ensure the lung parenchyma is clear of the opening and remove any adhesions.

In a traumatic cardiac arrest, this procedure would be performed bilaterally as localising a tension pneumothorax during cardiac arrest is unreliable. If the patient's condition does not improve, the bilateral thoracostomies may be used to perform a thoracotomy, but that procedure is beyond the scope of this chapter.

In other presentations or once ROSC is achieved, the simple thoracostomy is completed by placing thoracostomy drains.

- The depth of the drain is estimated by placing the tip of the tube at the clavicle and draping the tube over the chest wall to the incision. A clamp should be placed on the distal end of the tube prior to insertion.
- Use the clamp to guide the tip of the tube through the chest wall before removing the clamp and advancing posteriorly to the measured depth.
- Attach the underwater drain while anchoring the drain at the skin, then remove the distal clamp and assess for misting, draining of blood/fluid, and swinging of the underwater drain. Have an assistant hold the drain in position while you secure it.
- Secure the drain by passing a horizontal mattress suture across the incision and cut the needle off. This will be used to close the incision on removal of the tube, so leave long tails. Place a second suture at the edge of the incision closest to the anterior chest. Tie three simple knots but ensure the suture is not tight to the skin. After cutting off the needle secure the drain as described for the Seldinger procedure above.
- Take the long tails of the first suture and wrap these in a similar manner more distally along the drain before tying them off.
- Apply a transparent film dressing and pad all connectors as described previously.

Post Procedure

- Ensure air bubbles out of the underwater drain or pleural fluid/blood drains into it. Check that the fluid level rises with inspiration and drops with expiration.
- Obtain a chest x-ray immediately after the procedure and then at appropriate intervals to assess resolution.
- Document the procedure fully including the size and depth of the tube as well as the x-ray findings. If you have included a mattress suture to allow atraumatic closure (as described above) then document this accordingly.

Practical Tips

- As the collection resolves and the lung re-expands, the patient may experience more pain, consider patient-controlled analgesia immediately after the procedure to allow adequate tidal volumes and cough.
- If the drain and underwater drainage system do not have complementary couplings, it may be necessary to cut the one side off, join the tubes and secure with tape or zip-ties.

Case Study

Consider a 68-year old lady who was sustained a laceration to her forearm after falling onto a glass vase. She estimates her weight at 60 kg, has a history of hypertension but takes no beta-blockers, and is not allergic to any medication.

You wish to close the wound, which has stopped bleeding, after instilling LA. In the ED, you have lidocaine as a 1% solution or bupivacaine as a 0.25% solution. (a) Which LA agent is appropriate? (b) What is her maximum dose and (c) What volume should be drawn up?

- (a) 1% Lidocaine, as it has a rapid onset and will provide sufficient anaesthesia for the entire procedure.
- (b) No additive is required, so the maximum dose is 3 mg/kg, at 60 kg she should not receive more than 180 mg. Note the maximum dose irrespective of body weight is 200 mg.
- (c) 1 ml of 1% lidocaine $= 10$ mg lidocaine, therefore no more than 18 ml of 1% lidocaine should be drawn up.

Take Home Points

- Consent should be viewed as part of the procedure.
- Any procedure must be justified and appropriate.
- Practical skills and competence, once gained, must be maintained.

REFERENCES

Chakraverty, R., Pynsent, P., and Isaacs, K. (2007). Which spinal levels are identified by palpation of the iliac crests and the posterior superior iliac spines? *Journal of Anatomy* 210 (2): 232–236.

Health Education England (HEE). (2017). *Multi-professional Framework for Advanced Clinical Practice in England* [online]. Available from: https://www.hee.nhs.uk/sites/default/files/documents/multi-prof essionalframeworkforadvancedclinicalpracticeinengland.pdf [accessed 20 June 2023].

Health Education England (HEE). (2022). *Advanced Clinical Practice in Acute Medicine Curriculum Framework – Credentials* [online]. Available from: https://advanced-practice.hee.nhs.uk/our-work/credentials [accessed 20 June 2023].

NHS England patient Safety Domain. (2015). *National Safety Standards for Invasive Procedures.*

Reuben, A. (2016). Examination of the abdomen. *Clinical Liver Disease: A Multimedia Review Journal*, 7(6), 143–150. https://aasldpubs.onlinelibrary.wiley.com/doi/10.1002/cld.556 [last accessed 22 February 2023].

Rodger, M.A. and King, L. (2008). Drawing up and administering intramuscular injections: a review of the literature. *Journal of Advanced Nursing* 31 (3): 574–582.

The Faculty of Intensive Care Medicine. (2018). *Curriculum for Training for Advanced Critical Care Practitioners – Syllabus. V1.1* [online]. Available from: www.ficm.ac.uk/media/6896 [accessed 20 June 2023].

The Intensive Care Society, Critical Care Networks – *National Nurse Leads and The National Outreach Forum.* (2022). *Advanced Critical Care Outreach Competencies* [online]. Available from: https://ics.ac.uk/asset/43B8C11B-4512-41D0-B97768FABA2C30B2 [accessed 20 June 2023].

The Royal College of Emergency Medicine. (2022). *Emergency Medicine Advanced Clinical Practitioner Curriculum 2022 (Adult)* [online]. Available from: https://rcem.ac.uk/wp-content/uploads/2022/09/ACP_Curriculum_Adult_Final_060922.pdf [accessed 20 June 2023].

FURTHER READING

Intensive Care Society. (2022). *Guidance for the Use of Vasopressor Agents by Peripheral Intravenous Infusion in Adult Critical Care Patients. V 1.1 September 2022.*

Sharma, S. and Alijani, A. (2021). Insertion of chest drain for pneumothorax. *Anaesthesia and Intensive Care Medicine* 23 (3): 172–176.

Williams, S., Khalil, M., Weerasinghe, A. et al. (2017). How to do it: bedside ultrasound to assist lumbar puncture. *Practical Neurology* 17: 47–50.

RESUS & 1ST STAGE MX OF THE CRITICALLY UNWELL

CHAPTER 20

Advanced Life Support

Sadie Diamond-Fox and Alexandra Gatehouse

> **Aim**
> The aim of this chapter is to provide the reader with an overview of the principles applied to advanced resuscitation.

LEARNING OUTCOMES

After reading this chapter the reader will:

1. Have gained an understanding of the key life-threatening emergencies that may present within acute, emergency, and critical care environments (AECCE).
2. Understand the algorithm for adult in-hospital resuscitation and key elements of advanced life support.
3. Appreciate clinical signs and potential causes and associations leading to life-threatening emergencies.
4. Understand the key principles of management of cardio-pulmonary resuscitation (CPR) and life-threatening emergencies.

SELF-ASSESSMENT QUESTIONS

1. Describe the initial sequence for the management of an in-hospital cardiac arrest.
2. Name two causes of life-threatening emergencies for airway, breathing, circulation, disability, and exposure.
3. Differentiate between respiratory and cardiac arrest.
4. Based upon current evidence, critically discuss two drugs that may be sued in the treatment of cardiac arrest.
5. Discuss the importance of teamwork and human factors during cardiac arrest

The Advanced Practitioner in Acute, Emergency and Critical Care, First Edition. Edited by Sadie Diamond-Fox, Barry Hill, Sonya Stone, Caroline McCrea, Natalie Gardner, and Angela Roberts.
© 2024 John Wiley & Sons Ltd. Published 2024 by John Wiley & Sons Ltd.

INTRODUCTION

Emergencies can be a common occurrence within the AECCE. The following chapter outlines some of the common emergencies that may be encountered within the AECCE and provides an overview as to their recognition, potential causes, potential treatments, and relevant evidence-based guidance. There are a plethora of scenarios which may be encountered by the advanced practitioner; some of these scenarios are outlined within Figures 20.1–20.3.

As with any emergency scenario, regardless of the clinical area, assessment and immediate management by a suitably trained healthcare professional should follow the well-established A–E approach (see Figure 20.1).

Multi-professional Framework (MPF) for Advanced Clinical Practice in England (HEE 2017)

This chapter maps to the following statements within the MPF:

1. Clinical Practice:	1.2	1.4	1.5	1.6	1.7	1.8	1.10
2. Leadership:	2.1						
3. Education:	3.1	3.2					

Accreditation Considerations

This chapter maps to the following statements within the following national accreditation documents:

Curriculum for Training for Advanced Critical Care Practitioners Syllabus V1.1
(The Faculty of Intensive Care Medicine 2019):

4.1	

Advanced Critical Care Outreach Competencies
(The Intensive Care Society, Critical Care Networks – National Nurse Leads and The National Outreach Forum 2022):

A3	

Emergency Medicine Advanced Clinical Practitioner Curriculum 2022 – Adult
(The Royal College of Emergency Medicine 2022):

RP1–8	RC1–3	

Advanced Clinical Practice in Acute Medicine Curriculum Framework
(Health Education England 2022):

- Generic Clinical CiPs: 2
- Acute Medicine ACP Practical Procedures: Advanced cardiopulmonary resuscitation

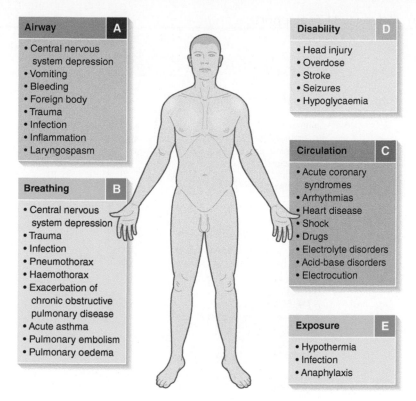

Airway A

- Central nervous system depression
- Vomiting
- Bleeding
- Foreign body
- Trauma
- Infection
- Inflammation
- Laryngospasm

Breathing B

- Central nervous system depression
- Trauma
- Infection
- Pneumothorax
- Haemothorax
- Exacerbation of chronic obstructive pulmonary disease
- Acute asthma
- Pulmonary embolism
- Pulmonary oedema

Disability D

- Head injury
- Overdose
- Stroke
- Seizures
- Hypoglycaemia

Circulation C

- Acute coronary syndromes
- Arrhythmias
- Heart disease
- Shock
- Drugs
- Electrolyte disorders
- Acid-base disorders
- Electrocution

Exposure E

- Hypothermia
- Infection
- Anaphylaxis

FIGURE 20.1   Causes of deterioration. *Source*: Holbery and Newcombe (2016) / John Wiley & Sons.

Airway

- Talking?
- Breathing?
- Noisy breathing?
- Respiratory distress?
- Obvious foreign body?
- Obvious facial injuries?
- Vomit/blood/secretions?
- Swelling?

Breathing

- Talking in sentences?
- Complaining of difficulty in breathing/shortness of breath?
- RIPPAS:
  - Respiratory rate?
    - tachypnoeic?
    - bradypnoeic?
  - Inspection
    - agitation?
    - drowsy?
    - cyanosis?
    - injuries?
    - equal chest expansion?
    - accessory muscle use?
  - Palpation
    - tenderness?
    - deformity?
    - crepitus?
    - surgical emphysema?
    - tracheal deviation?
  - Percussion
    - hyporesonance?
    - hyperresonance?
  - Auscultation
    - breath sounds?
    - equal air entry?
    - wheezing?
    - crackles?
  - Saturations?
    - hypoxic?

Circulation

- Palpable pulse?
- Pale?
- Cool?
- Sweaty?
- Bleeding?
- Heart rate?
- Blood pressure?
- Capillary refill time?
- Urine output?
- Arrhythmias?

Disability

- AVPU (alert, voice, pain, unconscious)/GCS?
- Pupils reacting?
- Blood glucose?
- Recent drugs?

Exposure

- Temperature?
- Tenderness?
- Wounds?
- Bleeding?
- Infection?
- Swelling?
- Rashes?

FIGURE 20.2   ABCDE approach to assessment. *Source*: Holbery and Newcombe (2016) / John Wiley & Sons.

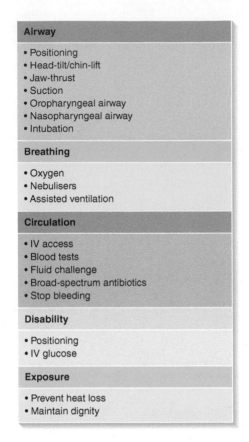

Airway

- Positioning
- Head-tilt/chin-lift
- Jaw-thrust
- Suction
- Oropharyngeal airway
- Nasopharyngeal airway
- Intubation

Breathing

- Oxygen
- Nebulisers
- Assisted ventilation

Circulation

- IV access
- Blood tests
- Fluid challenge
- Broad-spectrum antibiotics
- Stop bleeding

Disability

- Positioning
- IV glucose

Exposure

- Prevent heat loss
- Maintain dignity

FIGURE 20.3   ABCDE approach to management. *Source*: Holbery and Newcombe (2016) / John Wiley & Sons.

Life-threatening emergencies may require interventions such as those detailed within the Adult inhospital resuscitation algorithm (RCUK 2021a) (see Figure 20.4) and advanced life support (ALS) algorithms (see Figures 20.5 and 20.6) may need to be performed by appropriately trained members of the team. The ALS interventions performed within the emergency department and critical care unit may differ slightly compared to that of other clinical areas that do not routinely care for critically ill patients due to the rapid availability of diagnostic tools such as ultrasound, point-of-care testing, invasive monitoring, and alternative drugs not commonly used in areas outside of the emergency department or critical care unit.

A – Airway

Airway emergencies cover a wide spectrum of presentations within the AECCE that include airway obstruction, complications with endotracheal intubation as well as endotracheal tube, and tracheostomy difficulties. Chapter 7 explores the respiratory system pathologies associated with AECCE in more depth; however, Table 20.1 describes some of the common airway emergencies that may be encountered.

Within the UK, the Difficult Airway Society (DAS) in conjunction with the Royal College of Anaesthetists (RCoA), the Faculty of Intensive Care Medicine (FICM) and the Intensive Care Society (ICS) formulated guidelines for the management of tracheal intubation in critically ill adults (Higgs et al. 2017). They were based upon the findings of the 4th National Audit Project which reported higher rates of major complications and avoidable deaths due to deficient airway management, in this group of patients

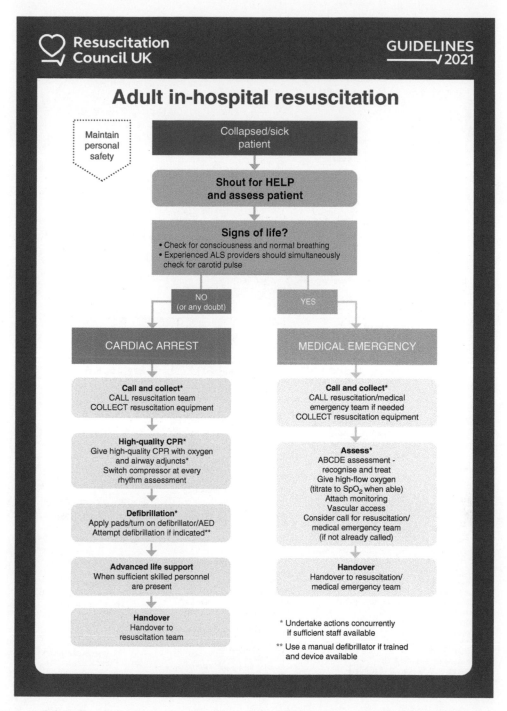

FIGURE 20.4   Adult in-hospital resuscitation algorithm. *Source*: Resuscitation Council (UK) (2021a).

(Cook et al. 2011). Commonly used algorithms for tracheal intubation of critically ill adults may be found in Figures 20.7–20.9. In addition, the National Tracheostomy Project (2023) produced guidance regarding the emergency management of tracheostomies and laryngectomies. All guidelines provide clinicians with a standardised approach to managing life-threatening airway emergencies.

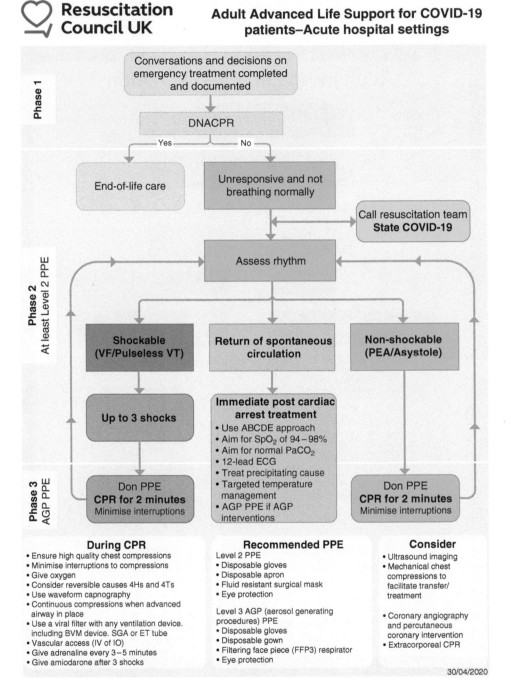

FIGURE 20.5   Adult advanced life support for COVID-19 patients – acute hospital settings. *Source*: Resuscitation Council (UK) (2021a).

intensive care society — *care when it matters*

Intubation Checklist: critically ill adults – to be done with whole team present.

The Faculty of Intensive Care Medicine · **RCOA** — *Royal College of Anaesthetists*

Prepare the patient

☐ **Reliable IV/IO access**

☐ **Optimise position**
- ☐ Sit-up?
- ☐ Mattress hard

☐ **Airway assessment**
- ☐ Identify cricothyroid membrane
- ☐ Awake intubation option?

☐ **Optimal preoxygenation**
- ☐ 3 minutes or ETO₂ > 85%
- ☐ Consider CPAP/NIV
- ☐ Nasal O₂

☐ **Optimise patient state**
- ☐ Fluid/pressor/inotrope
- ☐ Aspirate NG tube
- ☐ Delayed sequence induction

☐ **Allergies?**
- ☐ ↑ Potassium risk?
  - avoid suxamethonium

Prepare the equipment

☐ **Apply monitors**
- ☐ SpO₂/waveform ETCO₂/ECG/BP

☐ **Check equipment**
- ☐ Tracheal tubes × 2
  - cuffs checked
- ☐ Direct laryngoscopes × 2
- ☐ Videolaryngoscope
- ☐ Bougie/stylet
- ☐ Working suction
- ☐ Supraglottic airways
- ☐ Guedel/nasal airways
- ☐ Flexible scope/Aintree
- ☐ FONA set

☐ **Check drugs**
- ☐ Consider ketamine
- ☐ Relaxant
- ☐ Pressor/inotrope
- ☐ Maintenance sedation

Prepare the team

☐ **Allocate roles**

One person may have more than one role.
- ☐ Team Leader
- ☐ 1st Intubator
- ☐ 2nd Intubator
- ☐ Cricoid force
- ☐ Intubator's assistant
- ☐ Drugs
- ☐ Monitoring patient
- ☐ Runner
- ☐ MILS (if indicated)
- ☐ Who will perform FONA?

☐ **Who do we call for help?**

☐ **Who is noting the time?**

Prepare for difficulty

☐ **Can we wake the patient if intubation fails?**

☐ **Verbalise "Airway Plan is:"**

☐ **Plan A:**
Drugs and laryngoscopy

☐ **Plan B/C**
Supraglottic airway
Face-mask
Fibreoptic intubation via supraglottic airway

☐ **Plan D:**
FONA
Scalpel-bougie-tube

☐ **Does anyone have questions or concerns?**

FIGURE 20.6 Intubation checklist. *Source:* (i) Difficult Airway Society (ii) The Intensive Care Society (iii) Royal College of Anaesthetists.

TABLE 20.1 Airway emergencies that may be encountered within AECCE.

Scenario	Recognition	Potential causes and/or associations	Potential treatments	Relevant guidance

Airway obstruction	• Grunting
	• Snoring
	• Coughing, choking, drooling
	• Stridor
	• Voice change
	• Paradoxical breathing pattern
	• Neck swelling
	• Difficulty swallowing
	• Respiratory distress
	• Cyanosis
	• Epistaxis, haemoptysis
	• Trismus
	• Fever
	• Hypotension
	• Bradycardia
	• Poor or absent air entry and chest expansion
	• Anxiety
	• Soot in airway
	• Facial burns and/or swelling
	• Decreased level of consciousness
	• Cardiac arrest
		• Intrinsic –
		  – Tumour
		  – Foreign body
		  – Bleeding
		  – Vomit
		  – Infection
		  – Laryngospasm
		  – Oedema – burns, inhalation injury, upper airway manipulation or instrumentation, surgery, angio-oedema
		• Extrinsic –
		  – Haematoma – neck surgery or trauma, central venous catheter insertion,
		  – Neck trauma
		  – Tumour or mass
		• Neurological –
		  – Head injury
		  – Intracerebral bleed or thrombosis
		  – Drug overdose
		  – Alcohol intoxication
		  – Neurological pathology - Guillain–Barré, myaesthenia gravis
		  – Recurrent laryngeal nerve palsy or damage
		  – Inadequate muscle relaxant reversal
			• Open airway – manual in-line stabilisation in suspected cervical spine injury
			• Airway clearance
			• Airway adjuncts
			• Bag mask ventilation
			• Intubation
			• Specialist considerations –
			  – Bleeding – correct coagulopathy, transfuse, blood products
			  – Laryngospasm – low dose propofol 0.25mg/kg intravenous (IV), suxamethonium 1mg/kg IV, positive end-expiratory pressure, Larson's manoeuvre
			  – Oedema – IV steroids
			  – Swelling, physical obstruction or infection - Nebulised adrenaline 5 mg/5ml 1:1000
			  – Surgical haematoma – open sutures
			  – Drug overdose – reversal agent as appropriate
			  – Muscle relaxant reversal – neostigmine 2.5 mg with glycopyrronium bromide 0.5 mg intravenous (non-depolarising muscle agent), sugammadex 2–4 mg/kg intravenous (rocuronium)
				Adult Basic Life Support Guidelines, 2021d
				Adult Advanced Life Support Guidelines, 2021a
				Difficult Airway Society Guidelines, 2012

Condition	Signs/Symptoms	Causes/Triggers	Management	Reference
Anaphylaxis	• Skin and/or mucosal changes – urticaria, flushing, angioedema • Airway swelling • Hoarse voice • Stridor • Bronchospasm • Hypoxia • Respiratory distress • Respiratory arrest • Cardiovascular shock • Confusion or decreased level of consciousness • Cardiac arrest	• Food • Medication • Sting or bite • Latex	• Remove trigger • Intramuscular adrenaline 500 micrograms (0.5 millilitres 1:1000), up to two doses • Intravenous fluid challenge 500–1000 millilitres of crystalloid • Oxygen	Adult Advanced Life Support Guidelines, 2021a

Intubation complications	• Oesophageal intubation
	  – Hypoxaemia
	  – No chest wall movement
	  – No endotracheal tube misting
	  – Absence or diminishing end-tidal carbon dioxide waveform
	• Bronchial intubation
	  – Hypoxia
	  – Unilateral chest wall movement
	  – High airway pressures
	  – Length of endotracheal tube at the lips
		• Vocal cords not visualised on intubation
		• Difficult grade of intubation
		• Endotracheal tube dislodgement on patient positioning, loose tube ties
			• Follow 'Tracheal intubation of critically ill adults' algorithm (Higgs et al., 2017)
			• Remove endotracheal tube and reintubate
			• Reposition endotracheal tube
			• Secure tube ties
			• Anticipate complications – checklist including preparation of patient, equipment, team and difficulties
				Difficult Airway Society Guidelines, 2012
				Difficult Airway Society ICU intubation guidelines, 2017
				4th National Audit Project, 2011

(Continued)

TABLE 20.1 (Continued)

Scenario	Recognition	Potential causes and/or associations	Potential treatments	Relevant guidance
Can't Intubate, Can't Oxygenate (CICO)	• Profound hypoxaemia • Failed intubation – maximum three attempts • Failed rescue oxygenation with second-generation supraglottic airway – maximum three attempts	• Airway obstruction • Poor mouth opening, dentition and neck mobility • Reduced thyromental distance and sternomental distance • Distorted anatomy due to tumour, trauma, airway oedema, radiotherapy, previous tracheostomy and surgery • Body habitus • Pregnancy • Craniofacial pathology • Documented previous difficult intubation • Airway assessment indicative of difficult intubation – high Mallampati score	• Follow 'Can't Intubate, Can't Oxygenate' algorithm (Higgs et al., 2017) • Front of neck airway – scalpel cricothyroidotomy	Difficult Airway Society ICU intubation guidelines, 2017
Endotracheal complications	• Respiratory distress • Hypoxaemia • Cyanosis • Increasing ventilatory setting requirements • Poor tidal volumes associated with high ventilator pressures • Loss of end-tidal carbon dioxide waveform • Audible leak associated with ventilator leak alarm and loss of airway pressures • Decreased air entry or widespread crackles on auscultation	• Accidental extubation due to mobile, awake or delirious patient • Obstruction due to sputum, blood or foreign body • Cuff leak or herniation • Trachea mucosal ulceration or granulation due to high cuff pressures • Vocal cord damage • Aspiration of gastric contents	• Follow 'Tracheal intubation of critically ill adults' algorithm (Higgs et al., 2017) • Give 100% oxygen • Check endotracheal tube position • Pass suction catheter via the endotracheal tube • Manually ventilate with a waters circuit • Check cuff pressure and inflate as required • Bronchoscopy • Assisted ventilation with airway adjuncts as required in accidental extubation • Consider removing endotracheal tube and re-intubating	Difficult Airway Society ICU intubation guidelines, 2017 4th National Audit Project, 2011

Tracheostomy complication			National Tracheostomy Safety Project, 2012 4th National Audit Project, 2011 The Faculty of Intensive Care Medicine, 2020
• As for endotracheal complications • Haemoptysis, bleeding from airway or around tracheostomy • Cellulitis, erythema or pus from or around the tracheostomy • Subcutaneous surgical emphysema • Ability to vocalise with cuff inflated	• On insertion – – bleeding – loss of airway – misplacement – damage to neck structures • Post insertion - – Accidental dislodgement due to mobile, awake or delirious patient – Obstruction due to sputum, blood or foreign body – Cuff leak or herniation – Trachea mucosal ulceration or granulation due to high cuff pressures – Bleeding – Skin breakdown or infection – Fistulae – Aspiration of gastric contents	• Follow 'Emergency tracheostomy management – patent upper airway' (McGrath et al., 2012) • Give 100% oxygen via face and tracheostomy • Check tracheostomy position • Pass suction catheter via the tracheostomy • Attach waters circuit, gentle manual ventilation if no spontaneous breathing • Remove and check inner tube • Extremis or obstruction – deflate cuff, remove tracheostomy, apply occlusive dressing, bag mask ventilate with airway adjuncts as required, re-intubate with oral endotracheal tube or consider re-siting tracheostomy • Follow 'Emergency laryngectomy management' (McGrath et al, 2012) if no patent upper airway, ventilate via stoma and consider intubating via the stoma • Bleeding – – Minor – apply pressure, haemostatic dressing – Major – intubate orally cuff below tracheostomy stoma, digital pressure to stoma, fluid resuscitation and blood product transfusion – Sputum plugging – suction and chest physiotherapy • Infection - antibiotics	

Source: Adapted from Peate and Hill (2022).

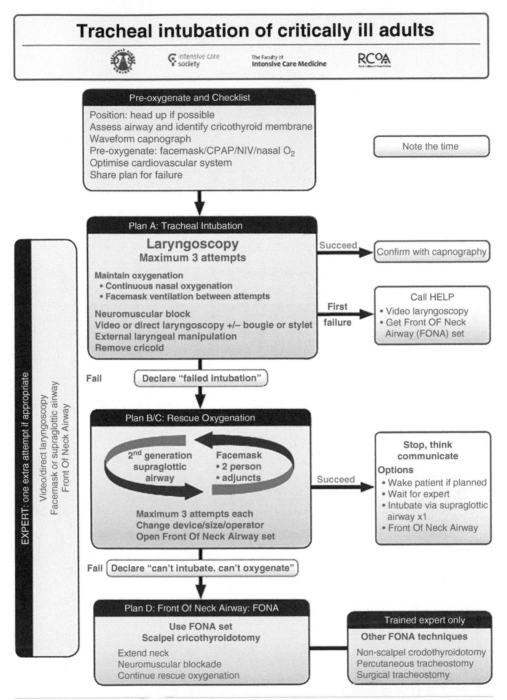

FIGURE 20.7 Tracheal intubation of critically ill adults. *Source*: Author: Higgs et al. (2017). Reproduced with the kind permission of the Difficult Airway Society.

Can't Intubate, Can't Oxygenate (CICO) in critically ill adults

 Intensive care society   **The Faculty of Intensive Care Medicine**   **RCoA**

CALL FOR HELP

Declare "Can't Intubate, Can't Oxygenate"

Plan D: Front Of Neck Airway: FONA

Extend neck
Ensure neuromuscular blockade
Continue rescue oxygenation
Exclude oxygen failure and blocked circuit

Scalpel cricothyroidotomy

Equipment: 1. Scalpel (wide blade e.g. number 10 or 20)
2. Bougie (≤ 14 French gauge)
3. Tube (cuffed) 5.0–6.0 mm ID)

Laryngeal handshake to identify cricothyroid membrane

Palpable cricothyroid membrane

Transverse stab incision through cricothyroid membrane
Turn blade through 90° (sharp edge towards the feet)
Slide coudé tip of bougie along blade into trachea
Railroad lubricated cuffed tube into trachea
Inflate cuff, ventilate and confirm position with capnography
Secure tube

Impalpable cricothyroid membrane

Make a large midline vertical incision
Blunt dissection with fingers to separate tissues
Identify and stabilise the larynx
Proceed with technique for palpable cricothyroid
membrane as above

Trained expert only

Other FONA techniques
Non-scalpel cricothyroidotomy
Percutaneous tracheostomy
Surgical tracheostomy

Post-FONA care and follow up
- Tracheal suction
- Recruitment manoeuvre (if haemodynamically stable)
- Chest X-ray
- Monitor for complications
- Surgical review of FONA site
- Agree airway plan with senior clinicians
- Document and complete airway alert

This flowchart forms part of the DAS, ICS, FICM, RCoA Guideline for tracheal in intubation in critically ill adults and should be used conjunction with the text.

FIGURE 20.8   Can't Intubate, Can't Oxygenate (CICO) in critically ill adults. *Source*: Reproduced with the kind permission of the Difficult Airway Society.

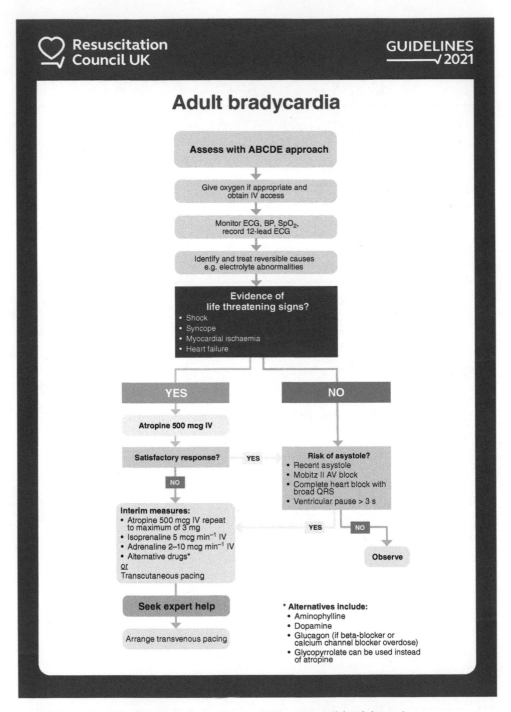

FIGURE 20.9   Adult bradycardia algorithm. *Source*: Resuscitation Council (UK) (2021a).

RED FLAGS – PATHOLOGICAL CONSIDERATIONS

End-tidal carbon dioxide is used to monitor patient's ventilatory status within critical care. Loss of, or diminishing, capnography waveform may indicate several life-threatening emergencies and warrants immediate attention. These include airway obstruction or dislodgement, detached airway circuit, inadequate ventilation, pneumothorax, respiratory, or cardiac arrest.

B – Breathing

Breathing emergencies cover a wide spectrum of presentations within the CCE. The overarching presentation is that of respiratory failure, which encompasses severe bronchospasm, tension pneumothorax, and pulmonary embolus. Chapter 16 explores respiratory system pathologies in more depth; however, Table 20.2 describes some of the common breathing emergencies that may be encountered.

The Resuscitation Council (2021a), in addition to the British Thoracic Society (BTS) (2019), Difficult Airway Society (2011), Difficult Airway Society (2015a,b), The Faculty of Intensive Care Medicine (2016, 2020), the Intensive Care Society (2019), and the Intensive Care Society & Faculty of Intensive Care Medicine (2019), have formulated evidence-based guidance regarding the management of life-threatening breathing emergencies. These guidelines are utilised within THE CCE. The British Medical Journal (BMJ) Best Practice online series (http://www.bestpractice.bmj.com) also provides quality-assessed evidence that informs clinical decision-making, giving a structured approach to diagnosis and treatment.

Examination Scenario – Tension Pneumothorax

Tension pneumothorax is a life-threatening emergency and requires time-critical treatment. Prompt needle decompression, and subsequent chest drain insertion, may prevent progressive intrathoracic air accumulation, haemodynamic compromise, and cardiac arrest. Recognition of tension pneumothorax is based upon clinical signs, unless cardiovascular stability allows for an urgent chest x-ray, chest ultrasound, or a computerised tomography (CT) scan to be performed.

Signs include:

- Tracheal deviation
- Diminished or absent unilateral air entry on auscultation
- Respiratory distress
- Hyper-resonance on percussion
- Increasing oxygen requirements
- Hypoxaemia
- Cardiovascular compromise
- Pulseless electrical activity cardiac arrest

TABLE 20.2 Breathing emergencies that may be encountered within AECCE.

Scenario	Recognition	Potential causes and/or associations	Potential treatments	Relevant guidance
Respiratory failure – • Type I respiratory failure – hypoxaemia • Type II respiratory failure – hypoxaemia and hypercarbia	• Respiratory distress • Cyanosis • Hypoxaemia and or hypercarbia on arterial blood gas • Reduced air entry on auscultation • Altered percussion note • Poor chest expansion • Decreased respiratory rate • Decreased level of consciousness • Cardiovascular compromise • Ventilator alarms	• Airway obstruction • Lung parenchymal pathology – adult respiratory distress syndrome, lung fibrosis, pneumonia, pulmonary oedema, lung contusion, inhalation injury haemorrhage, chronic lung disease • Pulmonary circulation pathology – pulmonary embolus, cardiac failure, vascular disease • Neurological compromise – head injury, intra-cranial bleed or ischaemia • Neuromuscular weakness or paralysis • Respiratory mechanical compromise – chest wall deformity, pleural effusion, fractured ribs, heamothorax, pneumothorax, ascites	• Oxygen • Airway clearance • Non-invasive ventilation • Bag mask ventilation • Direct laryngoscopy • Bronchoscopy • Intubation and mechanical ventilation • Cricothyroidotomy • Tracheostomy • Review of mechanical ventilator settings • Treatment of underlying cause	Adult Basic Life Support Guidelines, 2021d BTS/ICS Guidelines, 2017 Adult Advanced Life Support Guidelines, 2021a Difficult Airway Society Guidelines, 2012 The Faculty of Intensive Care Medicine, 2016 British Medical Journal (BMJ) Best Practice, 2020b
Severe bronchospasm	• Respiratory distress • Bilateral wheeze • Reduced peak expiratory flow rate • Cyanosis • Silent chest on auscultation • Altered conscious state • Cardiovascularly compromise • Normal or rising arterial carbon dioxide • Mechanical ventilation - increasing peak inspiratory pressures, decreasing tidal volumes, 'gas trapping'	• Asthma • Chronic obstructive pulmonary disease • Hay fever • Eczema	• Oxygen • Nebulised salbutamol (5 mg every 15–30 minutes) and ipratropium bromide (500 mcg 4–6 hourly) • Corticosteroids • Intravenous magnesium sulphate • Additional specialist treatment – ketamine, salbutamol and aminophylline infusions • Intubation and ventilation • Ventilator – remove positive end-expiratory pressure (PEEP), disconnect from ventilator circuit allowing chest to decompress, 'permissive' hypercapnia	Adult Advanced Life Support Guidelines, 2021a BTS/SIGN, 2019 BMJ Best Practice, 2020a

Condition	Signs/Symptoms	Causes/Risk factors	Treatment	Source
Tension pneumothorax	• Tracheal deviation • Diminished or absent unilateral air entry on auscultation • Respiratory distress • Hyper-resonance on percussion • Increasing oxygen requirements • Chest pain • Hypoxaemia • Cardiovascular compromise • Cardiac arrest	• Trauma to chest • High ventilator pressures • Central line insertion • Underlying lung disease – asthma, chronic obstructive pulmonary disease • Chest or abdominal surgery • Blocked chest drain	• Oxygen • Needle decompression • Chest drain	Adult Advanced Life Support Guidelines, 2021a British Thoracic Society, 2010 BMJ Best Practice, 2020c
Pulmonary embolism (PE)	• Dyspnoea • Hypoxaemia • Pleuritic chest pain • Haemoptysis • Syncope • Features of a deep vein thrombosis (DVT) • Cardiovascular compromise • Right ventricle heave • Raised jugular venous pressure • Cardiac arrest	• DVT or history of thromboembolic disease • Malignancy • Recent major surgery • Reduced mobility • Pregnancy • Orthopaedic pelvic or lower limb fractures • Coagulation disorders	• Oxygen • Thrombolysis for unstable massive PE –alteplase • Anticoagulation for stable patient with a PE – therapeutic low molecular weight heparin	Adult Advanced Life Support Guidelines, 2021a BMJ Best Practice, 2020d

Source: Adapted from Peate and Hill (2022).

C – Circulation/Cardiovascular

Circulatory emergencies within AECCE cover a large spectrum of presentations that may be due to a primary cardiac disorder, such as acute coronary syndrome with associated acute heart failure, or due to a secondary problem such as circulatory collapse because of major haemorrhage. Chapters 8 covers cardiovascular system (CVS) pathologies in more depth, however, Table 20.3 describes some of the common CVS emergencies which may be encountered.

The Resuscitation Council UK (2021a) produces evidence-based guidance and standardised training for the provision of resuscitation in the adult, paediatric, and neonatal population. Said guidance is based upon recommendations from the European Resuscitation Council (ERC 2021). The algorithms that are produced as part of said guidance provide clinicians with a standardised way in which to approach and subsequently treat life-threatening emergencies. These algorithms are utilised within the AECC settings. Two common cardiovascular emergencies that may be encountered are tachycardia and bradycardia; their respective algorithms can be found in Figures 20.10 and 20.11.

D – Disability

Neurological emergencies cover a wide spectrum of presentations within the AECCE, including decreased level of consciousness, seizures, meningitis, encephalitis, raised intracranial pressure (ICP), neuromuscular weakness, as well as agitation and delirium. There are a vast number of European and International clinical guidelines available, and these are utilised for management of specific life-threatening neurological emergencies, within the AECCE. Chapter 9 explores the neurological system pathologies in more depth; however Table 20.4 describes some of the common neurological emergencies that may be encountered.

Raised ICP and 'critical neuroworsening' is a life-threatening emergency and warrants immediate attention and management. The Seattle International Traumatic Brain Injury Consensus Conference (SIBICC) published a consensus-based algorithm (see Figure 21.11) for the management of severe traumatic brain injury patients with ICP monitoring (Hawryluk et al. 2019). The consensus-based management protocol (crevice protocol) for the treatment of severe traumatic brain injury based on imaging and clinical examination for use when ICP monitoring is not employed (Chesnut et al. 2020) has since been produced for those without intracranial monitoring in-situ (Figure 20.12). Each tier (1–3) incorporates treatments; the lower tiers should be employed first as the side effects have preferential and less detrimental side effects.

Recognition of the 'Cushing's Triad' is essential as this is a late sign of raised ICP and represents imminent brain herniation followed by death. The three physiological signs include:

1. Hypertension
2. Bradycardia
3. Irregular breathing or Cheyne-Stokes respiration

Immediate response to suspected herniation includes:

1. Hyperventilation (not limited to $PaCO_2$ 30 mmHg/4.0 kPa)
2. Bolus hypert.onic solution

(Hawryluk et al. 2019)

Definitive treatment requires management of the underlying cause of the raised ICP.

TABLE 20.3 Circulatory emergencies that may be encountered within AECCE.

Scenario	Recognition	Potential causes and/or associations	Potential treatments	Relevant guidance
Cardiac arrest (CA)	• Unexpected CA are rare in CC due, in part, to access to extensive monitoring and diagnostics • ECG trace change, e.g. VT or VF • Sudden loss of consciousness • Sudden loss of arterial trace, and/or impalpable pulse • Sudden loss of endtrial CO_2 trace	Hypoxia	• Airway adjuncts • Oxygen therapy	• RCUK, 2021a, 2021b • National Poisons Information Service, 2020
		Hypovolaemia	• Intravenous (IV) fluid • Blood products	
		Hypokalaemia	• Intravenous potassium infusion	
		Hyperkalaemia	• Intravenous calcium • Insulin/glucose infusion	
		Hypothermia	• Active internal re-warming via cardiopulmonary bypass • Forced air warming • Warm IV fluids	
		Hyperthermia (e.g serotonin syndrome)	• Stop triggering agent • Dantrolene IV	
		Tamponade	• Sternotomy • Pericardiocentesis	
		Tension pneumothorax	• Needle decompression • Chest drain insertion	
		Thrombosis – coronary or pulmonary	• Thrombolytic "clot busting" therapy	
		Toxins	• Reversal agents (e.g. naloxone for opioid overdose) • Support therapies (e.g. renal replacement therapy in metformin overdose)	
Cardiogenic shock	• Hypotension • ECG trace change, e.g. ST segment elevation • Sudden change in conscious level	'Pump failure' – acute coronary syndrome (ACS)	• Primary coronary intervention (PCI)	• NICE, 2020a • NICE, 2019
		Outflow obstruction – malignant hypertension	• Vasodilator medications	
		Valvular pathology – valvular rupture	• Valve replacement surgery	

(Continued)

TABLE 20.3 (Continued)

Scenario	Recognition	Potential causes and/or associations	Potential treatments	Relevant guidance
Hypovolaemic shock	• Hypotension • Increased lactate • Metabolic acidosis	• Major haemorrhage secondary to upper gastrointestinal bleed	• Massive transfusion – red cells, platelets, cryoprecipitate, etc. • IV calcium • Sengstaken tube placement	• JPAC, 2020
Bradycardia with haemodynamic instability/ symptomatic bradycardia	• Heart rate <60 beats/min • Systolic blood pressure <90 mmHg • Signs of ischaemia on ECG trace, e.g. ST segment depression	• ACS • Medications (e.g. beta-blockers) • Raised intracranial pressure	• PCI for ACS • Atropine IV • Glycopyrrolate IV • Isoprenaline IV • Transcutaneous pacing	• RCUK, 2021
Tachycardia with haemodynamic instability/ symptomatic tachycardia	• Heart rate >100 beats/min • Systolic blood pressure <90 mmHg • Signs of ischaemia on ECG trace, e.g. ST segment depression	• ACS • Pulmonary embolism • Haemorrhage • Electrolyte abnormalities	• PCI for ACS • Thrombolysis • Blood products • Rapid correction of electrolyte abnormalities	• RCUK, 2021
Hypertensive crisis	• Blood pressure (BP) ≥220/120 mmHg or high BP with 'emergency symptoms', also referred to as end-organ damage (i.e. retinal haemorrhage, papilloedema, newonset confusion, chest pain, heart failure, or acute kidney injury)	• Drugs (e.g. amphetamines, cocaine) • Endocrine emergencies (e.g. Cushing's syndrome) • Renal disease • Aortic dissection • Raised ICP • Preeclampsia/ eclampsia	• Systemic vasodilators • Beta-blockers • Calcium channel blockers	• NICE, 2019 • International Society of Hypertension, 2020

Source: Adapted from Peate and Hill (2022).

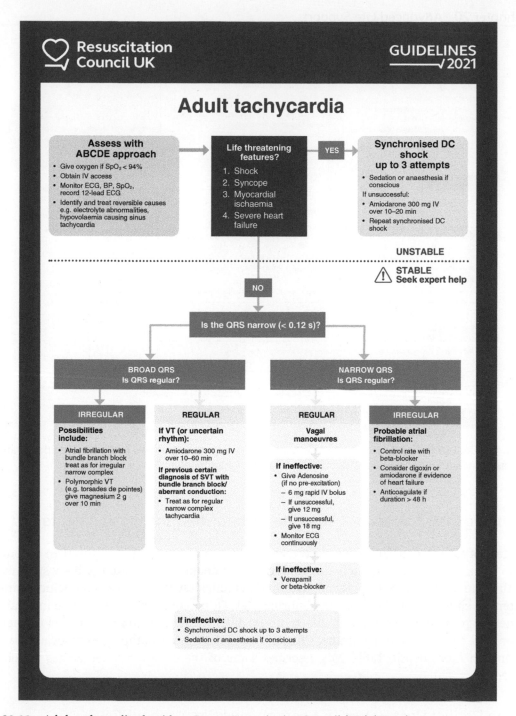

FIGURE 20.10 Adult tachycardia algorithm. *Source*: Resuscitation Council (UK) (2021a).

RED FLAG – HYPOGLYCAEMIA

Rapid recognition and correction of hypoglycaemia is vital to prevent seizures and coma which can lead to permanent brain damage. There are several cardinal symptoms of hypoglycaemia that may proceed seizures and coma; diaphoresis, tachycardia, confusion, visual changes, slurred speech, and dizziness.

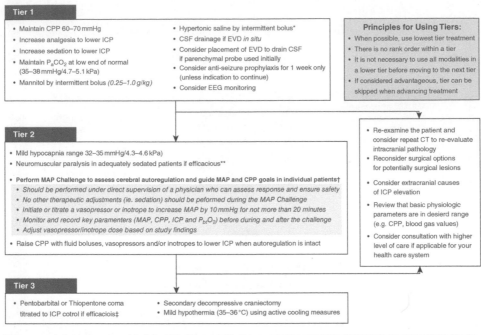

Tier 1

- Maintain CPP 60–70 mmHg
- Increase analgesia to lower ICP
- Increase sedation to lower ICP
- Maintain P_aCO_2 at low end of normal (35–38 mmHg/4.7–5.1 kPa)
- Mannitol by intermittent bolus *(0.25–1.0 g/kg)*

- Hypertonic saline by intermittent bolus*
- CSF drainage if EVD *in situ*
- Consider placement of EVD to drain CSF if parenchymal probe used initially
- Consider anti-seizure prophylaxis for 1 week only (unless indication to continue)
- Consider EEG monitoring

Principles for Using Tiers:
- When possible, use lowest tier treatment
- There is no rank order within a tier
- It is not necessary to use all modalities in a lower tier before moving to the next tier
- If considered advantageous, tier can be skipped when advancing treatment

Tier 2

- Mild hypocapnia range 32–35 mmHg/4.3–4.6 kPa)
- Neuromuscular paralysis in adequately sedated patients if efficacious**
- Perform MAP Challenge to assess cerebral autoregulation and guide MAP and CPP goals in individual patients†
  - *Should be performed under direct supervision of a physician who can assess response and ensure safety*
  - *No other therapeutic adjustments (ie. sedation) should be peformed during the MAP Challenge*
  - *Initiate or titrate a vasopressor or inotrope to increase MAP by 10 mmHg for not more than 20 minutes*
  - *Monitor and record key parameters (MAP, CPP, ICP and $P_{br}O_2$) before during and after the challenge*
  - *Adjust vasopressor/inotrope dose based on study findings*
- Raise CPP with fluid boluses, vasopressors and/or inotropes to lower ICP when autoregulation is intact

- Re-examine the patient and consider repeat CT to re-evaluate intracranial pathology
- Reconsider surgical options for potentially surgical lesions
- Consider extracranial causes of ICP elevation
- Review that basic physiologic parameters are in desierd range (e.g. CPP, blood gas values)
- Consider consultation with higher level of care if applicable for your health care system

Tier 3

- Pentobarbital or Thiopentone coma titrated to ICP cotrol if efficaciois‡
- Secondary decompressive craniectomy
- Mild hypothermia (35–36 °C) using active cooling measures

* We recommend using sodium and osmolality limits of 155 mEq/L and of 320 mEq/L respectively as administration limits for both mannitol and hypertonic saline.
**We recommend a trial dose of neuromuscular paralysis and only processing to a continuous infusion when efficacy is demonstrated.
† Rosenthal G. et al 2011
‡ Barbiturate administration shoud only be continued when a beneficiant effect on ICP is demonstrated.
Titrate barbiturate to achieve ICP control but do not exceed the dose which achieves bursr suppression.
Hypotension must be avoided when barbiturates are asministered.

FIGURE 20.11　Consensus-based algorithm for the management of severe traumatic brain injury guided by intracranial pressure measurements. *Source*: Author: Hawryluk et al. (2019). Reproduced with the kind permission.

E – Everything Else (Exposure, Endocrine, Electrolytes, and Environmental)

The 'E' section of an A–E clinical assessment can be referred to as 'everything else,' this then encourages the clinician to use a 'top-to-toe' approach after undertaking a detailed assessment of body systems encompassed within the A–D sections of the examination. Emergencies within this section include immediately life-threatening endocrine and electrolyte abnormalities. Other considerations include intra-abdominal catastrophes such as: bowel perforation due to ulcers, diverticulitis and tumours; bowel ischaemia, and intra-abdominal compartment syndrome. Chapters 10 and 11 cover pathologies associated with these body systems in more depth. Table 20.5 describes some of the common emergencies which may be encountered.

Care of the Patient Post Return of Spontaneous Circulation (ROSC)

The Resuscitation Council UK (2021b) have produced evidence-based guidance regarding post-resuscitation care. This is underpinned by recommendations for the European Resuscitation Council (2021), and the ILCOR. It begins immediately following sustained ROSC and can impact significantly upon patient outcome. An algorithm has been produced as part of this guidance, which provides a standardised approach to post-resuscitation care, and this is utilised within the AECCE. This can be found in Figure 20.11.

TABLE 20.4 Neurological emergencies that may be encountered within AECCE.

Scenario	Recognition	Potential causes and/or associations	Potential treatments	Relevant guidance
Decreased consciousness	• Falling Glasgow Coma Score (GCS) or Alert Voice Pain Unconscious (AVPU) score • Patient history – including loss of consciousness, mechanism of injury • Headache • Vomiting • Agitation • Incontinence • Loss of sensation, co-ordination, motor power, balance, gait • Abnormal reflexes • Seizures • Altered speech or vision • Abnormal pupil size or reaction • Partial or complete airway obstruction • Abnormal breathing pattern or rate • Cardiovascular compromise or cardiac arrest	• Seizures • Central nervous or systemic infection • Traumatic brain injury (TBI) • Intra-cranial haemorrhage including subarachnoid haemorrhage (SAH) • Thromboembolic stroke • Tumour • Agitation and delirium • Neuromuscular weakness • Drugs • Alcohol • Respiratory failure • Cardiovascular compromise • Liver or renal failure • Metabolic derangement including hypo- or hyperglycaemia	• Oxygen • ABCDE approach • Intubation for compromised airway, GCS ≤ 8 or rapidly falling GCS • Sedation for management of seizures, significant TBI, stroke, intra-cranial haemorrhage, neurological weakness • Hypertonic saline or mannitol for raised intra-cranial pressure (ICP) • Stroke – thromboembolic – aspirin if haemorrhage has been ruled out, thrombolysis (tissue plasminogen activator) • Neurosurgical management – clot evacuation, decompressive craniotomy, external ventricular drain, clipping or coiling of cerebral aneurysm • SAH – enteral nimodipine • Intravenous (IV) glucose or glucose gel for hypoglycaemia • Drug reversal agents • Treat the underlying cause	American Heart Association/ American Stroke Association, 2012 Brain Trauma Foundation, 2016 British Infection Association, 2016 NICE, 2019a NICE, 2019b NICE, 2021 SIGN, 2018 The Association of British Neurologists British Infection Association, 2012

(Continued)

TABLE 20.4 (Continued)

Scenario	Recognition	Potential causes and/or associations	Potential treatments	Relevant guidance
Status epilepticus and seizures	• Loss of consciousness • Vacant episode • Abnormal eye movements • Mydriasis • Tonic-clonic movements • Urinary incontinence • Teeth clenching • Tongue biting • Facial twitching • Hallucinations • Autonomic symptoms • Physiological manifestations – increased respiratory rate, tachycardia, hypertension, sweating, hyperthermia	• History of seizures • Intra-cerebral tumour • TBI • Stroke or intracranial haemorrhage • Hypoxia • Central nervous system infection • Metabolic or electrolyte derangement • Alcohol withdrawal • Eclampsia in pregnancy	• Oxygen • ABCDE approach • First-line treatment – rectal, buccal, intramuscular or IV benzodiazepines • Second line treatment – IV anti-epileptic drugs including levetiracetam, phenytoin or sodium valproate • Hypoglycaemia – give glucose • Alcohol withdrawal – give high potency thiamine	NICE, 2021 SIGN, 2018
Meningitis and encephalitis	• Headache • Vomiting • Neck stiffness • Photophobia • Decreased GCS • Altered mental state • Seizures • Focal neurological signs • Physiological signs of infection or sepsis • Rash • Respiratory or cardiovascular compromise	• Infection secondary to bacterial, viruses, tuberculosis or fungal • Head injury • Sinus or ear infection • Neurosurgery • Immunocompromised patients • Autoimmune disease • Malignancy	• Oxygen • ABCDE approach • Antibiotics • Antivirals • Steroids for meningitis	The Association of British Neurologists British Infection Association, 2012 British Infection Association, 2016

Condition	Signs/symptoms	Management	References
Raised intra-cranial pressure	• As for decreased consciousness • Late signs – bradycardia, hypertension, irregular breathing pattern • Increasing pressure as evidenced on ICP monitor or via an intraventricular drain	• TBI • Intra-cerebral haemorrhage • Space occupying lesions (SOLs) – tumour, abscess • Hydrocephalus • Cerebral oedema – hyponatraemia, eclampsia, infection, encephalopathy (hepatic/hypertensive), altitude • Intra-cranial hypertension	• Oxygen • ABCDE approach • Intubation and ventilation • Ventilated patient – adequate sedation and analgesia, IV paralysing agent, head up 30°, strict control of arterial oxygen and carbon dioxide levels, minimal obstruction of neck veins, cerebral perfusion pressure ≥ 60 mmHg. • IV mannitol or hypertonic saline • Avoid pyrexia • Treatment of underlying precipitant	Brain Trauma Foundation, 2016 NICE, 2019a
Neuromuscular weakness	• Inability to maintain airway • Respiratory failure or failure to wean from ventilation • Limb weakness • Loss of sensation, reflexes, co-ordination • Poor cough • Inadequate swallow • Presentation will be dependent upon cause	• TBI • Stroke or intra-cranial haemorrhage • SOLs • Spinal cord injury • Motor neuron disease • Guillain-Barré syndrome (GBS) • Myaesthenia gravis • Poliomyelitis • Critical illness polyneuropathy or myopathy • Electrolyte disorders • Metabolic disorders • Autoimmune disease • Congenital – muscular dystrophy	• Oxygen • ABCDE approach • Intubation and ventilation • Correction of electrolytes • Treatment of the underlying cause • GBS – IV immunoglobulins, plasmaphoresis • Myaesthenia gravis – acetylcholinesterase inhibitor, IV immunoglobulins, plasmaphoresis	NICE, 2016 NICE, 2019b NICE, 2021 SIGN, 2018

(Continued)

TABLE 20.4 (Continued)

Scenario	Recognition	Potential causes and/or associations	Potential treatments	Relevant guidance
Agitation and delirium	• Shouting out • Confusion • Pulling off or pulling out non-invasive or invasive monitoring • Inattention • Disorganised thinking • Fluctuating mental status • Assessment according to Richmond Agitation Scale, Confusion Assessment Method for the Intensive Care Unit, Clinical Institute Withdrawal Assessment for alcohol	• Drugs • Respiratory failure • Infection • Sleep or sensory deprivation • Elderly • Poor nutritional state • Surgery • Visual, cognitive or hearing impairment • Constipation • Urinary retention • Neurological insult • Metabolic or electrolyte derangement • Drug or alcohol withdrawal	• Oxygen • ABCDE approach • Antipsychotics – haloperidol, olanzapine, clonidine • Benzodiazepines – withdrawal or rescue therapy • Electrolyte replacement • Sleep hygiene	NICE, 2019c American College of Critical Care Medicine, 2018

Source: Adapted from Peate and Hill (2022).

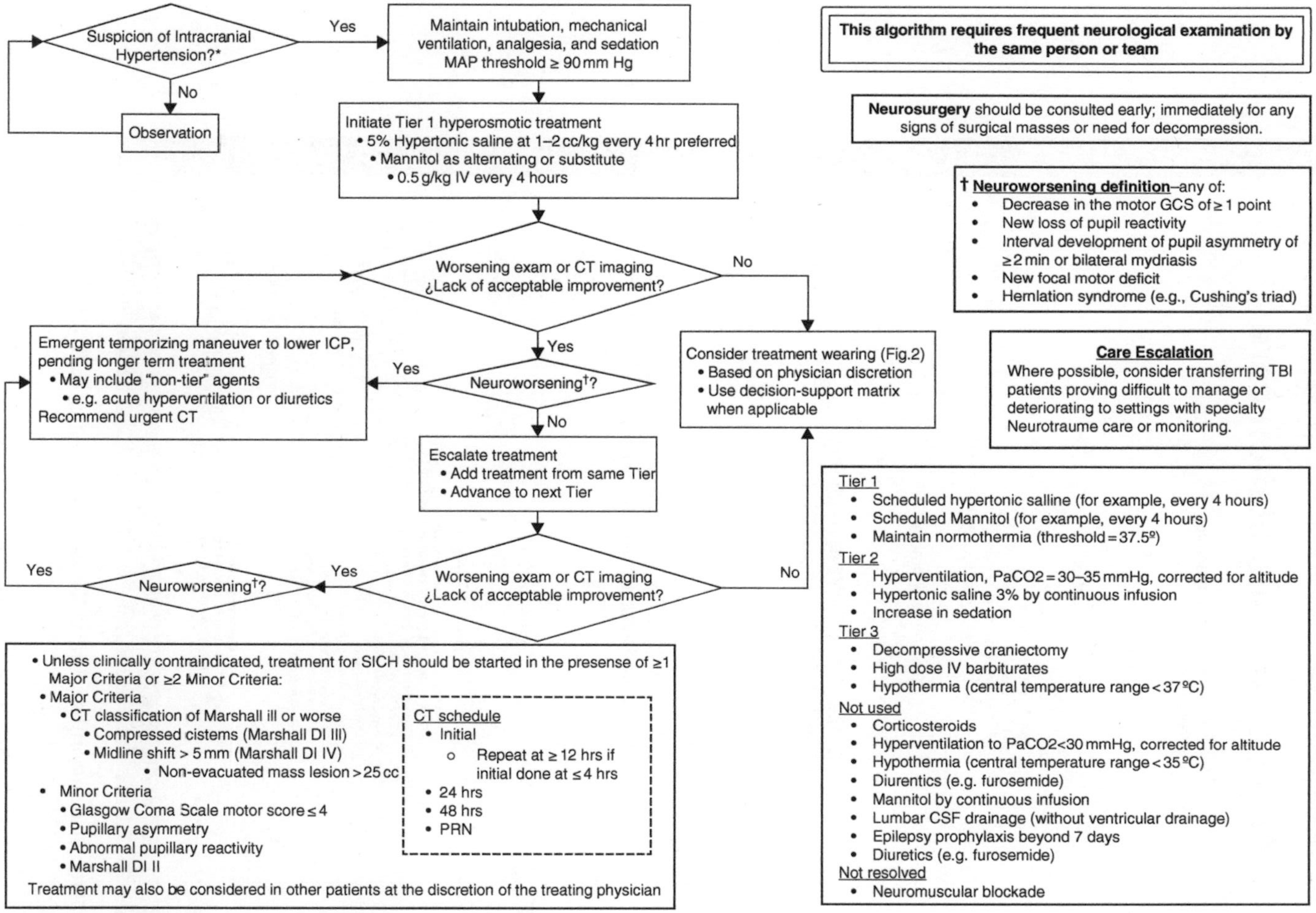
Suspicion of Intracranial Hypertension?*
Yes
No
Observation
Maintain intubation, mechanical ventilation, analgesia, and sedation MAP threshold ≥ 90 mm Hg
Initiate Tier 1 hyperosmotic treatment
• 5% Hypertonic saline at 1–2 cc/kg every 4 hr preferred
• Mannitol as alternating or substitute
• 0.5 g/kg IV every 4 hours
Worsening exam or CT imaging ¿Lack of acceptable improvement?
No
Yes
Neuroworsening†?
Yes
No
Emergent temporizing maneuver to lower ICP, pending longer term treatment
• May include "non-tier" agents
• e.g. acute hyperventilation or diuretics
Recommend urgent CT
Escalate treatment
• Add treatment from same Tier
• Advance to next Tier
Consider treatment wearing (Fig.2)
• Based on physician discretion
• Use decision-support matrix when applicable
Worsening exam or CT imaging ¿Lack of acceptable improvement?
Yes
No
Neuroworsening†?
Yes
• Unless clinically contraindicated, treatment for SICH should be started in the presense of ≥1 Major Criteria or ≥2 Minor Criteria:
• Major Criteria
• CT classification of Marshall ill or worse
• Compressed cistems (Marshall DI III)
• Midline shift > 5 mm (Marshall DI IV)
• Non-evacuated mass lesion > 25 cc
• Minor Criteria
• Glasgow Coma Scale motor score ≤ 4
• Pupillary asymmetry
• Abnormal pupillary reactivity
• Marshall DI II
CT schedule
• Initial
o Repeat at ≥ 12 hrs if initial done at ≤ 4 hrs
• 24 hrs
• 48 hrs
• PRN
Treatment may also be considered in other patients at the discretion of the treating physician
This algorithm requires frequent neurological examination by the same person or team
Neurosurgery should be consulted early; immediately for any signs of surgical masses or need for decompression.
† Neuroworsening definition–any of:
• Decrease in the motor GCS of ≥ 1 point
• New loss of pupil reactivity
• Interval development of pupil asymmetry of ≥2 min or bilateral mydriasis
• New focal motor deficit
• Hemlation syndrome (e.g., Cushing's triad)
Care Escalation
Where possible, consider transferring TBI patients proving difficult to manage or deteriorating to settings with specialty Neurotraume care or monitoring.
Tier 1
• Scheduled hypertonic salline (for example, every 4 hours)
• Scheduled Mannitol (for example, every 4 hours)
• Maintain normothermia (threshold = 37.5º)
Tier 2
• Hyperventilation, PaCO2 = 30–35 mmHg, corrected for altitude
• Hypertonic saline 3% by continuous infusion
• Increase in sedation
Tier 3
• Decompressive craniectomy
• High dose IV barbiturates
• Hypothermia (central temperature range < 37 ºC)
Not used
• Corticosteroids
• Hyperventilation to PaCO2<30 mmHg, corrected for altitude
• Hypothermia (central temperature range < 35 ºC)
• Diurentics (e.g. furosemide)
• Mannitol by continuous infusion
• Lumbar CSF drainage (without ventricular drainage)
• Epilepsy prophylaxis beyond 7 days
• Diuretics (e.g. furosemide)
Not resolved
• Neuromuscular blockade

FIGURE 20.12 Graphic representation of the Consensus REVised Imaging and Clinical Examination (CREVICE) protocol for the treatment of suspected intracranial hypertension (SICH). The flow chart represents individual steps involved in the decision to treat for SICH, the choice of therapeutic agents, and the evaluation of the need for treatment escalation. The definition of 'neuroworsening' is presented in a box at the upper right. The indications for initiating treatment for SICH are in the box at the lower left. The recommended therapeutic agents and their ranking into treatment tiers are contained in the box at the lower right. *Source*: Chesnut et al. (2020). Reproduced with kind permission.

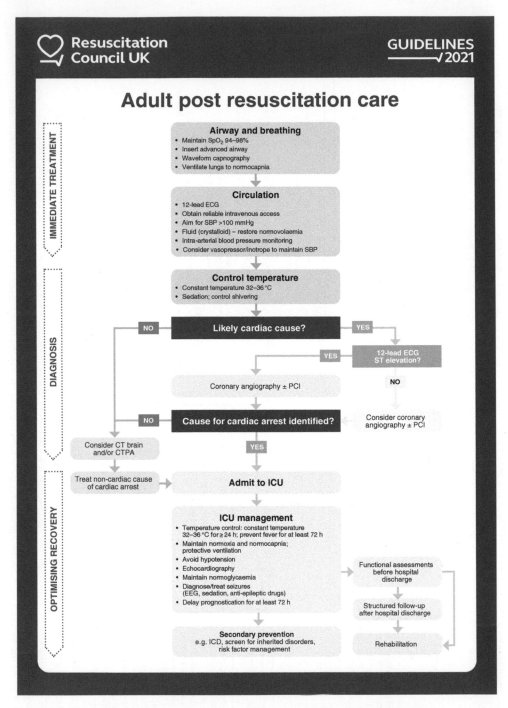

FIGURE 20.13   Post-resuscitation care algorithm. *Source*: Resuscitation Council (UK) (2021b).

Initial management includes assessment and management of airway, breathing, circulation, and temperature control (Figure 20.13). The cause of cardiac arrest needs to be established due to the time-critical nature of subsequent treatment, such as percutaneous coronary intervention. Respiratory or neurological causes, such as PE or stroke, will require further investigation including CT or CTPA.

TABLE 20.5   Emergencies concerning exposure, endocrine, electrolytes & environmental that may be encountered within AECCE.

Scenario	Recognition	Potential Causes and/or Associations	Potential Treatments	Relevant Guidance
Cardiac Arrest (CA)	• Unexpected CA are rare in CC due, in part, to access to extensive monitoring and diagnostics • ECG trace change, e.g. VT or VF • Sudden loss of consciousness • Sudden loss of arterial trace, and/or impalpable pulse • Sudden loss of end-trial CO_2 trace	**H**ypoxia	• Airway adjuncts • Oxygen therapy	RCUK, 2021[a,b] National Poisons Information Service, 2020
		Hypovolaemia	• Intravenous (IV) fluid • Blood products	
		Hypokalaemia	• Intravenous potassium infusion	
		Hyperkalaemia	• Intravenous calcium • Insulin/glucose infusion	
		Hypothermia	• Active internal re-warming via cardiopulmonary bypass • Forced air warming • Warm IV fluids	
		Hyperthermia (e.g Serotonin syndrome)	• Stop triggering agent • Dantrolene IV	
		Tamponade	• Sternotomy • Pericardiocentesis	
		Tension pneumothorax	• Needle decompression • Chest drain insertion	
		Thrombosis – coronary or pulmonary	• Thrombolytic "clot busting" therapy	
		Toxins	• Reversal agents (e.g. naloxone for opioid overdose) • Support therapies (e.g. renal replacement therapy in metformin overdose)	
Cardiogenic Shock	• Hypotension • ECG trace change, e.g. ST segment elevation • Sudden change in conscious level	"Pump failure" - Acute Coronary Syndrome (ACS)	• Primary coronary intervention (PCI)	NICE, 2020 NICE, 2019
		Outflow obstruction - Malignant hypertension	• Vasodilator medications	
		Valvular pathology - Valvular rupture	• Valve replacement surgery	

(Continued)

TABLE 20.5 (Continued)

Scenario	Recognition	Potential Causes and/or Associations	Potential Treatments	Relevant Guidance
Hypovolaemic Shock	• Hypotension • Increased lactate • Metabolic acidosis	• Major haemorrhage secondary to upper-gastrointestinal bleed	• Massive transfusion – red cells, platelets, cryoprecipitate, etc. • IV calcium • Sengstaken tube placement	JPAC, 2020
Bradycardia with haemodynamic instability/ Symptomatic bradycardia	• Heart rate <60 beats/min • Systolic blood pressure <90mmHg • Signs of ischaemia on ECG trace, e.g. ST segment depression	• ACS • Medications (e.g. beta blockers) • Raised intracranial pressure	• PCI for ACS • Atropine IV • Glycopyrrolate IV • Isoprenaline IV • Transcutaneous pacing	RCUK, 2021
Tachycardia with haemodynamic instability/ Symptomatic tachycardia	• Heart rate >100 beats/min • Systolic blood pressure <90mmHg • Signs of ischaemia on ECG trace, e.g. ST segment depression	• ACS • Pulmonary embolism • Haemorrhage • Electrolyte abnormalities	• PCI for ACS • Thrombolysis • Blood products • Rapid correction of electrolyte abnormalities	RCUK, 2021
Hypertensive crisis	• Blood pressure (BP) ≥220/120 mmHg or high BP with "emergency symptoms", also referred to as end-organ damage (i.e. retinal haemorrhage, papilloedema, new onset confusion, chest pain, heart failure, or acute kidney injury)	• Drugs (e.g. amphetamines, cocaine) • Endocrine emergencies (e.g. Cushing's syndrome) • Renal disease • Aortic dissection • Raised ICP • Pre-eclampsia/ Eclampsia	• Systemic vasodilators • Beta blockers • Calcium channel blockers	NICE, 2019 International Society of Hypertension, 2020

Source: Adapted from Peate and Hill (2022).

Physiological derangement is expected following cardiac arrest and other tests are required, such as full blood count, biochemistry, arterial blood gas, 12-lead ECG, chest x-ray, and echocardiography.

Optimisation of organ function is critical following stabilisation and transfer to a CCE, in order to prevent further secondary organ injury. This includes targeted temperature management, treatment of myocardial dysfunction, and neurological protective strategies such as normoxia, normocapnia, haemo-dynamic optimisation, normoglycaemia, and seizure control.

Prognostication following cardiac arrest is complex, multimodal, and tends not to be reliable until 72 hours following ROSC. It is dependent upon clinical examination, electroencephalography, biomarkers, and further imaging including CT and magnetic resonance imaging and assists in guiding targeted treatments in order to achieve a neurological meaningful recovery for the patient. Evidence of significant hypoxic brain injury with poor neurological recovery may lead to withdrawal of life-sustaining treatment and subsequent death. Organ donation should be considered (see Chapter 23).

In cardiac arrest survivors, screening for cognitive, emotional, and fatigue problems following hospital discharge is standard, and early rehabilitation may be indicated as a result of hospital functional assessments.

ORANGE FLAG – COMMUNICATION WITH RELATIVES DURING RESUSCITATION

Communication and providing support to patient's relatives during resuscitation is crucial and allows healthcare professionals to establish the wishes of both the patient and their relatives in terms of their presence during resuscitation. The advantages of relatives witnessing resuscitation includes being able to speak to their relative, reduced distress at being separated, observing optimal treatment given to the patient and the reality of the patient's death. Disadvantages include distress if the relatives are not fully informed, their expectations or cultural beliefs have not been considered, and relatives' emotional or physical hindrances to resuscitation.

CRITICAL CARE EMERGENCIES AND HUMAN FACTORS

The CCE is one of the highest risk environments within the healthcare setting. Managing time-critical emergencies requires multiple team members to manage often unrehearsed and complex situations. Acknowledgement of the way in which non-technical skills such as teamwork, communication, leadership, and decision-making have been acknowledged as having a potential impact on patient safety for over a decade (Odell 2011). The application of these non-technical skills is often referred to as 'human factors'. Human factors are key to all aspects of clinical practice and providing safe and effective care. Consequently, these are core strands of healthcare training and ongoing professional development.

Effective team-working, communication, leadership, and decision-making (all human factors) can lead to improvement in both treatment quality and safety metrics (Scalise 2006; Krug 2008; Brock 2013); conversely, poor communication, leadership, and teamwork have been highlighted as one of the main concerns that lead to complaints to the Parliamentary and Health Service Ombudsman (2021).

Human factors should always be a consideration during any high-stress, time-sensitive situation, particularly in the CCE where the cognitive load is high, and there are multiple team members and multiple decibels being emitted from an array of devices. Concepts applied in the combat field are often applied

TABLE 20.6   The SBAR tool.

SBAR	Overview
Situation	• Identify yourself • State the site or unit you are calling from • Identify the patient by name and the reason for your call • Briefly describe your concern.
Background	• Give the patient's reason for admission • Explain significant medical history • Briefly describe relevant recent events.
Assessment	• Provide key vital signs • Use ABCDE and NEWS • Suggest your clinical impression.
Recommendation	• Explain what you need • Be specific about request and time frame • Make suggestions • Clarify expectations.

Source: Adapted from Peate and Hill (2022).

to the resuscitation scenario, a concept which is now widely taught within resuscitation courses and has rather neatly been coined by Reid et al. (2018) as speaking 'Resuscitese'. Communication is 'Directive, descriptive, and informative' with a focus upon limiting non-essential communication to promote a 'sterile cockpit' (Lauria 2020). 'Resuscitese' also focuses upon loops of communication being closed, with communication between team members being reinforced, for example, 'Mark, please administer 300 mg of amiodarone IV', followed by a response from the person administering the medication, '300 mg of amiodarone administered' (Lauria 2020).

Several structured communication tools exist that can be used during time-critical emergency and resuscitation scenarios. The 'SBAR' tool is advocated by the Resuscitation Council UK (2021a) and NHS England & NHS Improvement (2021) (see Table 20.6). Further, extensive information can be found here: https://www.england.nhs.uk/improvement-hub/publication/safercare-sbar-situationbackground-assessment-recommendation-implementation-andtraining-guide.

The Department of Defence (DoD) and the Agency for Healthcare Research and Quality (AHRQ) have developed a comprehensive evidence-based teamwork system (TeamSTEPPS® 2.0) to improve communication and teamwork skills. TeamSTEPPS® 2.0 'Module 4: Leading Teams' is particularly useful when considering the intricacies of effective leadership and teamworking. Further details regarding the online training course may be found here: https://www.ahrq.gov/teamstepps/index.html.

DEBRIEFING

Dealing with emergency situations within the AECCE can be emotional and stressful. Debriefing is considered a powerful learning tool after emergency situations in the context of clinical education, quality improvement, systems learning, and team wellbeing (Kessler et al. 2014). It can prove to be a useful tool in all cases; where things went well, near misses. and where adverse events occurred. TeamSTEPPS® 2.0 advocates the use of an after-action review using a debrief for critical team events, which focuses upon the evaluation of the following:

1. Communication
2. Roles and responsibilities
3. Situational awareness
4. Workload distribution
5. Asking for or offering assistance (cross-monitoring)
6. Errors: made or avoided
7. What went well, what should change, and what could be improved?

Do-Not-Attempt-Cardiopulmonary-Resuscitation (DNACPR) and Recommended Summary Plan for Emergency Care and Treatment (ReSPECT)

A Do-Not-Attempt-Cardiopulmonary-Resuscitation (DNACPR) order is a sensitive advanced decision. Instituting DNACPR orders has been shown to be sub-optimal (Hawkes et al. 2020), as such the Recommended Summary Plan for Emergency Care and Treatment (ReSPECT) was developed (RCUK 2021c). It details a summary of recommendations tailored to the patient regarding care provision during an emergency. The document is completed through conversations between the patient and their healthcare team, at a time when the patient has the mental capacity to make such decisions. It aims to respect both patient preferences and clinical judgement (RCUK 2021c). An interactive learning web-application has been designed so that both healthcare professionals and patients can learn about the ReSPECT tool. This can be accessed via https://learning.respectprocess.org.uk. Not all healthcare providers within the UK utilise the ReSPECT tool, therefore it is advised that healthcare professionals familiarise themselves with local practice and policy.

Take Home Points
- Emergencies can be a common occurrence within the CCE and may require interventions such as those detailed within the adult in-hospital resuscitation and ALS algorithms (RCUK 2021a, b, d). They ensure that patients receive standardised, evidence-based, good quality care.
- The ABCDE approach is essential to the assessment and management of emergency situations, facilitating timely recognition and prompt treatment.
- Following CPR patients require post-resuscitation care to prevent secondary organ injury.
- Teamwork, human factors, debriefing, and team wellbeing are essential to creating learning opportunities, allowing constructive reflection, and recognising the delivery of excellent care.

REFERENCES

British Thoracic Society/Scottish Intercollegiate Guidelines Network. (2019). *British Guideline on the Management of Asthma* [online]. Available from: https://www.brit-thoracic.org.uk/quality-improvement/guidelines/asthma [accessed 25 June 2023].

Brock, D. (2013). Interprofessional education in team communication: working together to improve patient safety. *Postgraduate Medicine Journal* 89 (1057): 642–651.

Chesnut, R.M., Temkin, N., Videtta, W. et al. (2020). Consensus-based management protocol (CREVICE protocol) for the treatment of severe traumatic brain injury based on imaging and clinical examination for

FURTHER READING

The European Resuscitation Council Guidelines. *The European Resuscitation Council Guidelines for Resuscitation provide specific instructions for how resuscitation should be practiced and take into account ease of teaching and learning, as well as the science.* They were developed by Europeans and have been specifically written with European practice in mind [online]. Available from: `https://cprguidelines.eu` [accessed 25 June 2023].

International Liaison Committee on Resuscitation. *The International Liaison Committee on Resuscitation (ILCOR) was formed in 1992 to provide a forum for liaison between principal resuscitation organisations worldwide* [online]. Available from: `https://www.ilcor.org` [accessed 25 June 2023].

CHAPTER 21

Shock

Francesca Riccio and Phil Broadhurst

Aim

The aim of this chapter is to provide an overview of the recognition and management of the different types of shock, introduce the concept of haemodynamics, and provide an understanding of the key investigations and interventions to aid in diagnosis and treatment of shock.

LEARNING OUTCOMES

After reading this chapter the learner will:

1. Understand the underlying pathophysiology of shock.
2. Recognise the different presentations of shock and their causes.
3. Understand key haemodynamic variables that help to guide therapy.
4. Be able to consider appropriate interventions and goals in the management of shock.

SELF-ASSESSMENT QUESTIONS

1. What are the different types of shock? What are their presentations and how do they differ?
2. What are they key components in the management of sepsis?
3. What drugs should be considered for the management of sepsis? What are their modes of action?
4. What are the normal haemodynamic values? What happens to these in the different types of shock? How can these be supported to maintain normal ranges?

The Advanced Practitioner in Acute, Emergency and Critical Care, First Edition. Edited by Sadie Diamond-Fox, Barry Hill, Sonya Stone, Caroline McCrea, Natalie Gardner, and Angela Roberts.
© 2024 John Wiley & Sons Ltd. Published 2024 by John Wiley & Sons Ltd.

Multi-professional Framework (MPF) for Advanced Clinical Practice Guidance for Professional Development (HEE 2017)

This chapter maps to the following statements within the MPF:

1. Clinical Practice:	1.2	1.3	1.4	1.6	1.7	1.10	1.11
2. Leadership and Management:	2.7	2.8	2.9				
3. Education:	3.1	3.2					
4. Research:	4.1	4.7					

Accreditation Considerations

This chapter maps to the following statements within the following national accreditation documents:

Curriculum for Training for Advanced Critical Care Practitioners Syllabus V1.1
(The Faculty of Intensive Care Medicine 2018)

2.1	2.2	2.3	2.4	2.5	2.6	2.7	

Advanced Critical Care Outreach Competencies
(The Intensive Care Society, Critical Care Networks – National Nurse Leads and The National Outreach Forum 2022)

A1	A2	A3	

Emergency Medicine Advanced Clinical Practitioner Curriculum 2022 – Adult
(The Royal College of Emergency Medicine 2022)

RP3	RP6	RP7	

Advanced Clinical Practice in Acute Medicine Curriculum Framework
(Health Education England 2022)

Presentations and Conditions of Acute Medicine by System/Specialty: Emergency presentations

INTRODUCTION

Shock is a life-threatening condition of circulatory failure, leading to inadequate oxygen delivery to meet cellular metabolic needs and oxygen consumption requirements, producing cellular and tissue hypoxia. Initially shock is reversible, but quickly becomes irreversible, resulting in multi-organ failure and death. There are several different types of shock which will be discussed in this chapter. These include cardiogenic, hypovolaemic, distributive, and obstructive shock. Shock is defined as a state of cellular and tissue hypoxia due to either reduced oxygen delivery, increased oxygen consumption, inadequate oxygen utilisation, or a combination of the above.

CLASSIFICATION AND AETIOLOGY

Distributive Shock

Characterised by severe peripheral vasodilation, the molecules that mediate the vasodilation vary depending on the aetiology. See Table 21.1 for the different subtypes of distributive shock.

Cardiogenic Shock

Due to intracardiac causes of pump failure that result in reduced cardiac output (CO). Table 21.2 outlines the different causes of cardiogenic shock.

Hypovolaemic Shock

Reduced intravascular volume, which in turn leads to reduced CO. It can be divided into two types as described in Table 21.3.

Obstructive Shock

This is due to extracardiac causes of cardiac pump failure and often associated with poor right ventricular output. The causes of obstructive shock can be divided into pulmonary vascular and mechanical, as described in Table 21.4.

PATHOPHYSIOLOGY OF SHOCK

Mechanisms of Shock

Cellular hypoxia occurs because of reduced tissue/oxygen delivery and/or oxygen consumption, or from inadequate oxygen utilisation. This in turn causes the following biochemical processes:

- Cell membrane ion pump dysfunction
- Intracellular oedema
- Leakage of intracellular contents into the extracellular space
- Inadequate regulation of cellular pH

TABLE 21.1 Distributive shock.

Subtype of distributive shock	Definition
Septic shock	• Dysregulated host response to infection resulting in life-threatening organ dysfunction (Shankar-Hari et al. 2016) • It is the most common cause of distributive shock (Shankar-Hari et al. 2016) • It has a mortality of 40–50% (Smulders 2000) • It can be identified by the use of vasopressor therapy and the presence of elevated lactate levels (>2 mmol/l) despite adequate fluid resuscitation (Smulders 2000)
Systemic inflammatory response syndrome (SIRS)	• Clinical syndrome characterised by a robust inflammatory response, usually induced by a major body insult that can be infectious or non-infectious (Standl et al. 2018) • Examples of non-infectious conditions include • Pancreatitis • Burns • Hypoperfusion secondary to trauma • Blunt trauma and crush injury • Amniotic fluid embolism • Fat embolism • Post cardiac arrest syndrome (Standl et al. 2018)
Neurogenic shock	• Hypotension and in some cases overt shock are common in patients with severe traumatic brain injury and spinal cord injury (Standl et al. 2018) • Interruption of autonomic pathways, causing decreased vascular resistance and altered vagal tone are thought to be responsible for distributive shock in patients with spinal cord injury (Standl et al. 2018)
Anaphylactic shock	• Acute systemic reactions caused by direct release of mediators from mast cells and basophils produced by various triggers (Standl et al. 2018).
Drug and toxin-induced shock	• Drug and toxin reactions can be associated with shock or SIRS-like syndromes (Standl et al. 2018).
Endocrine shock	• Addisonian crisis (adrenal failure due to mineralocorticoid deficiency) and myxedema can be associated with hypotension and states of shock (Standl et al. 2018).

Subsequently if left unchecked the above lead to systemic dysfunction. This can be demonstrated by acidosis, endothelial dysfunction, and further stimulation of inflammatory and anti-inflammatory cascades. Serum lactate levels have been used as a surrogate marker for hypoperfusion and tissue hypoxia, and therefore can be a useful surrogate for hypoperfusion and tissue hypoxia.

Physiology

The delivery of oxygen (DO_2) to cells depends on the content of oxygen in the blood mainly combined with haemoglobin (Hb). This is regulated by both the respiratory system, and the transport in the blood. These are functions of the CO/mean arterial pressure/peripheral vascular resistance inter-relationship, and of the oxygen extraction/consumption rate at a cellular level.

TABLE 21.2 Cardiogenic shock.

Subtypes of cardiogenic shock	Definition
Cardiomyopathic	• Myocardial infarction involving >40% of the left myocardium (Standl et al. 2018). • Myocardial infarction of any size if accompanied by severe extensive ischaemia due to multi-vessel disease (Standl et al. 2018). • Acute exacerbation of cardiac failure with underlying dilated cardiomyopathy (Standl et al. 2018). • Myocardial depression due to advanced septic shock (Standl et al. 2018)
Arrhythmic	• Sustained tachy and brady arrhythmias leading to cardiogenic shock (Standl et al. 2018)
Mechanical	• Severe aortic or mitral valve insufficiency (Standl et al. 2018) • Severe VSD (Standl et al. 2018)

TABLE 21.3 Hypovolaemic shock.

Subtype of hypovolaemic shock	Description
Haemorrhagic	• Reduced intravascular volume due to blood loss, either blunt or penetrating (Standl et al. 2018)
Non-haemorrhagic	• Reduced intravascular volume from fluid loss other than blood e.g. gastrointestinal, skin, and renal loss (Standl et al. 2018)

TABLE 21.4 Obstructive shock.

Subtype of obstructive shock	Description
Pulmonary vascular	• Right ventricular failure from haemodynamically significant pulmonary embolism or severe pulmonary hypertension
Mechanical	• Usually present clinically as hypovolaemic shock because of reduced preload rather than pump failure e.g. tension pneumothorax, pericardial tamponade, constrictive pericarditis

Hypoxia, which is low oxygen to tissues, Bonanno (2011) classified this into three main categories:

1. Scarce oxygen offer from microcirculation
2. Maldistribution of offer
3. Incapacity of consumption

Shock, a cause of hypoxaemia pertains instead to their exchange in the target organs and tissues. The major physiological determinants of tissue perfusion (and systemic blood pressure [BP]) are CO and systemic vascular resistance (SVR):

$$BP = CO \times SVR$$

CO is the product of heart rate (HR) and stroke volume (SV)

$$CO = HR \times SV$$

The stroke volume is determined by:

1. Vessel length
2. Blood viscosity
3. Vessel diameter

Throughout all types of shock, CO is affected in a variety of ways. Cardiac reserve is the maximum quantity of blood that can be pumped above basal normal level during exercise or to compensate for basic deficits within physiological limits. The lower the myocardial functional reserve, the higher the chances of shock overlapping failure of the pump. Septic shock can differ to other forms of shock due to its initial hyperdynamic response. Lipopolysaccharide and other bacterial toxins are responsible for the initial hyperdynamic, physiologically compensatory, vasodilatory phase.

The cardiovascular system responds to hypotension and hypovolaemic shock by increasing the heart rate, increasing myocardial contractility, and constricting peripheral blood vessels. This is by a direct stimulation via the sympathetic nervous system on the heart and blood vessels by the cardiac and vasomotor centres. The sympathetic system releases catecholamines (noradrenaline and adrenaline), these are released from the adrenal medulla. Another hormone associated with shock is arginine vasopressin (AVP). There is an increase in the level of AVP in haemorrhagic shock, stimulated by low pressure and low atrial filling. Alongside this there are fluid readjustments between the three compartments (intravascular, extravascular, and intracellular). This leads to more fluid shifting via osmosis to the organs that require it the most. Decompensation occurs when the natural endogenous catecholamines fail to maintain compensatory vasoconstriction and manifests as hypotension. It has been shown that vascular reactivity and calcium sensitivity are increased in early shock and decreased in late shock. Moreover, atria and pulmonary artery have low-pressure baroreceptors responding to an increase of pressure with an increase in heart rate and decrease in ADH secretion by the hypothalamus. Hypoxaemia triggers a similar alarm reaction of hypotension by direct stimulation of the vasomotor centre in the medulla oblongata with a powerful increase in blood pressure, as well as an increase in ventilation by direct triggering of the peripheral PaO_2-sensitive chemoreceptors. Pulmonary artery floatation catheter devices can demonstrate different haemodynamic profiles depending on the type of shock (see Table 21.5).

Common to most forms of shock is diminished CO and/or SVR. Occasionally, the SVR is low relative to a high CO (e.g. Thyrotoxicosis), which can result in poor tissue perfusion. In general, severe hypovolaemia, cardiogenic shock, and late-stage obstructive shock are characterised by low CO and a compensatory increase in SVR to maintain perfusion to vital organs. Distributive shock, however, has a reduced SVR with an insufficient compensatory increase in CO to maintain oxygen delivery.

TABLE 21.5 Haemodynamic variables in shock.

Physiological variable	Preload	Pump function	Afterload	Tissue perfusion
Clinical measurement	Pulmonary capillary wedge pressure	Cardiac output	Systemic vascular resistance	Mixed venous oxyhaemoglobin saturations
Haemodynamic monitoring normal values:	SVV	CI/CO	SVR/SVRI	DO2
Hypovolaemic	Normal (early) Decreased (late)	Normal (early) Decreased (late)	Increased	>65% (early) or <65% (late)
Cardiogenic	Increased	Decreased	Increased	<65%
Distributive	Normal (early) Decreased (late)	Increased or decreased	Decreased	>65%
Obstructive				
• PE, PH, tension pneumothorax	Normal (early) Decreased (late)	Normal (early) Decreased (late)	Increased	>65%
• Pericardial tamponade	Increased	Decreased	Increased	<65%

Source: Adapted from Standl et al. (2018).

PATHOPHYSIOLOGY OF SEPSIS

Sepsis produces structural damages, derangements, and dysfunction in the microcirculation ecosystem. Specifically leading to a persistent and exaggerated local inflammatory reaction, coagulopathy in the direction of procoagulant state, endothelial dysfunction, overproduction of nitric oxide, oxygen maldistribution. These all result in dysoxic-hypoxia.

The term endothelial dysfunction refers to decreased endothelial-dependent vascular relaxation, associated with a decrease of nitric oxide formation and release. This is best highlighted by the phenomenon 'mottled cyanosis'. During the initial phase of sepsis there is a predominance of microcirculation dysfunction and later mitochondria fail, indicating a failure of compensation of microcirculation derangement.

The acute phase is marked by an abrupt rise in secretion of stress hormones and inflammatory mediators with an associated increase in mitochondrial and metabolic activity. This would highlight the flow-catabolic phase of the stress response. Finally, multi-organ dysfunction could be a protective mechanism because reduced cellular metabolism increases the chances of survival. It is thought that multi-organ dysfunction which then leads to multi-organ failure is initially a functional abnormality.

The pulmonary artery flotation catheter, as mentioned above, is one method of establishing cardiac function, the more recent evolution is the use of critical care ECHO.

The Role of Echo During Different Types of Shock

Echo is a rapid, non-invasive, comprehensive cardiac assessment option for patients presenting with haemodynamic instability. In septic shock, echo can be used to guide fluid therapy by measuring collapsibility of the inferior vena cava. Patients with persistent shock can be evaluated for right heart failure, dynamic left ventricular obstruction, or tamponade, if they do not respond to initial resuscitation or noradrenaline (Griffee et al. 2010). In recent years, there have been both increasing evidence and diffusion of the use of echo as a monitoring tool in patients with haemodynamic compromise. Septic shock is one of the most complex haemodynamic failure syndromes, as there may be derangement in all three of the mainstays of cardiovascular haemostasis. They include the following: absolute or relative reduction in central blood volume, peripheral vasodilatation, and myocardial failure. Echo offers the matchless advantage to perform both detailed functional and morphological assessment of the heart. Via et al. (2011) state that there is evidence to highlight that echo is more accurate than the standardised strategy demonstrated by surviving sepsis campaign. There are several different assessment targets when using focused echo to guide haemodynamic assessment:

1. Cardiac output
2. Volume status, volume responsiveness
3. Left ventricle (LV) systolic function
4. Right ventricle (RV) systolic function
5. Systemic arterial resistance
6. LV filling pressures

The above may then demonstrate the following at the point of shock onset:

1. Small LV
2. Small RV
3. LV and RV hyperkinesis
4. Small IVC
5. IVC respiratory collapse during spontaneous ventilation.

Although echo has been extensively validated as accurate and safe, there are limitations to its use (Cecconi et al. 2014). Whenever there are strict requirements for continual monitoring, clearly ECHO is not practical. It also requires a clinician to have sufficient competence in critical care ECHO.

STAGES OF SHOCK

Shock is a physiological continuum. It begins with an inciting eventing, triggering pathophysiological changes, which can then progress through several stages.

The early stages of shock are more amenable to treatment and therefore more likely to be reversible, compared with end-stage shock, which is associated with end-organ damage (see Table 21.6).

ASSESSMENT AND MANAGEMENT OF SHOCK

Airway and Breathing

The primary response to managing shock should follow the ABCDE approach, ensuring in the first instance that the patient's airway is safe. If there is any concern about patency, or the risk that the patient may not continue to maintain their airway, intubation and referral to ICU should be considered.

TABLE 21.6 Stages of shock.

Stage of shock	Definition	Signs and symptoms
Pre-shock (initial non-progressive)	• Known as compensated shock	• 15–25% fluid loss • Increased heart rate • Increased lactate • Increased or decreased BP (Tuchschmidt and Mecher 1994)
Shock (progressive)	• Compensatory mechanisms become overwhelmed	• 25–35% fluid loss • Tachycardia • Dyspnoea • Restlessness • Diaphoresis • Metabolic acidosis • Hypotension • Oliguria • Cool/clammy skin (Levy et al. 2003)
End-organ dysfunction (irreversible)	• Progressive shock leads to end-organ damage and multi-organ failure	• >35% fluid loss (Histopathology. guru) • Anuria • Acute renal failure • Acidaemia further reduces CO • Severe hypotension • Coma • Death (Levy et al. 2003)

Many patients in shock will experience respiratory distress due to increased oxygen uptake, reduced DO_2, or acidosis and clinicians need to ensure that appropriate interventions are utilised. Therapies including high-flow oxygen or non-invasive ventilation can often be helpful in the early stages of shock; however, if the patient's condition continues to worsen, intubation may need to be considered to facilitate positive pressure ventilation to reverse acidosis and improve oxygenation.

Circulation

After ensuring the safety of the airway and adequacy of breathing, clinicians should focus on managing the patient's circulation, with specific attention to the cause of shock, to aim to reverse hypoperfusion and restore effective circulation.

Where hypovolaemia exists, urgent fluid replacement is vital as the duration of fluid depletion directly impacts upon mortality. it is often accepted practice to use crystalloid for initial resuscitation, with the recommendation in cases of septic shock being to administer 30 ml/kg of crystalloid within the first three hours of management (Evans et al. 2021), with the use of blood products believed to offer little difference in mortality when the haemoglobin is maintained above 7 g/dl (Holst et al. 2014). Fluid management should be guided by haemodynamic monitoring and clinical examination as outlined within 'examination scenarios' later in this chapter, with close attention paid to CO and stroke volume variation (SVV) rather than physical examination or fixed parameters.

Vasopressor support may be required to support blood pressure (see 'Pharmacological Considerations' below). Although the target mean arterial pressure (MAP) is often decided locally based upon presentation, current guidelines recommend an initial target of 65 mmHg in cases of septic shock (Evans et al. 2021). Furthermore, it is believed that up to 90% of patients with cardiogenic shock will require vasopressor support, although clinicians should be aware of the increased myocardial oxygen requirement this can create, and aim to minimise this as much as possible. In cases of cardiogenic shock, the aim should be to manage or reverse the cardiovascular cause of shock. This may require cautious fluid resuscitation, the use of inotropes or thrombolysis, or onward referral to a cardiothoracic centre for PCI.

Disability

If the effects of shock progress, the continued fall in MAP and associated tissue hypoperfusion can lead to an altered level of consciousness, which may require practitioners to reconsider the need to protect the airway through intubation as well as appropriate sedation for the patient. If neurogenic shock is suspected, the clinician should focus upon management of the precipitating factor. Particularly at centres receiving trauma patients, spinal cord injury is a common presentation that should be excluded as a priority. Where diagnosis is confirmed, this should be managed within local trauma guidelines and appropriate specialist referrals considered. Other causes of neurogenic shock should also be considered and managed as appropriate, including reversal of toxins or management of Guillain Barre syndrome. As with other types of shock, fluid resuscitation and vasopressor support remain the key primary interventions in neurogenic shock, although phenylephrine should be avoided due to the risk of bradycardia.

Exposure

A thorough head-to-toe examination of a patient in shock can help practitioners to identify clues as to the cause, and therefore to subtype of shock, and lead to effective management of both the cause and the symptoms. A flushed appearance can present in distributive shock, which when combined with lingual, oropharyngeal or laryngeal oedema, itching or hives, can be suggestive of anaphylaxis. As well as rapid infusion of fluids, current UK guidelines advocate the administration of 500 µg IM adrenaline, repeated after five minutes if there is a poor response to the initial dose. When anaphylaxis is refractory to IM adrenaline, continuous administration should be started via the IV route, with ongoing fluid boluses titrated to clinical response (Resuscitation Council UK 2021).

Septic shock is another form of distributive shock, where head-to-toe examination can reveal indicators for suspected infection including rash, cellulitis, wound infection, fever, or flushing. Where sepsis is suspected as the cause of shock, it is recommended to commence antimicrobial therapy within the first hour of recognition due to the increased risk of mortality associated with delayed commencement of antibiotics. It is also advisable to ensure that blood cultures are obtained, and that serum lactate is measured to guide fluid resuscitation.

CLINICAL INVESTIGATIONS

Lactate

During cellular respiration, glucose is broken down by the process of glycolysis into pyruvate. This in turn then follows either the aerobic or anaerobic respiration pathways. During aerobic respiration, pyruvate is broken down into Acetyl-coenzyme A by reducing the enzyme NAD+ to NADH which then undergoes oxidative phosphorylation in the mitochondria, forming ATP, carbon dioxide, and water through the Krebs cycle and the electron transport chain (see Figure 21.1).

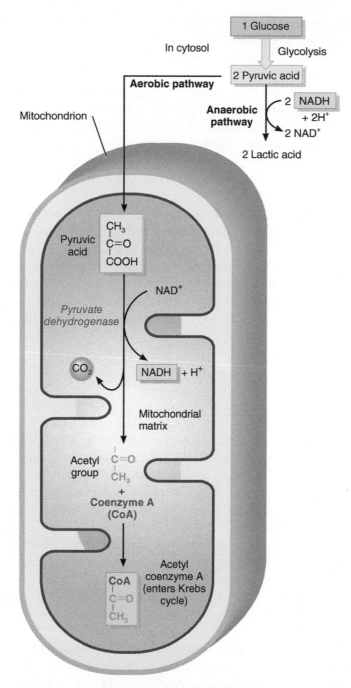

FIGURE 21.1   Cellular respiration. *Source*: Tortora and Derrickson (2006, figure 25.5, p. 957). / John Wiley & Sons.

In the absence of the oxygen required for oxidative phosphorylation, pyruvate is instead broken down into lactate via the anaerobic respiration pathway. During this reaction, LDH is used to catabolise pyruvate into lactate, the process of which creates the release of a hydrogen ion from the coenzyme NADH (which is the result of reducing the enzyme NAD+ during the process of oxidising Acetyl-CoA), therefore enabling this newly reoxidised NAD+ to continue the glycolysis process. Under normal physiological circumstances, lactate is often broken back down to pyruvate, allowing it to enter the aerobic respiration pathway, or is metabolised back to glucose by the liver through the process of gluconeogenesis.

The process of glycogenesis causes the release of ATP, although in a much lower quantity than through the Krebs cycle of aerobic respiration. As the anaerobic pathway follows only the first part of the aerobic pathway, this does mean that the process of energy creation can happen quicker. Due to lactate being the product of anaerobic respiration, raised levels can be an indicator of cellular hypo-perfusion and tissue hypoxia found in sepsis and shock, although clinical judgement and thorough assessment and examination of the patient should also be used to correlate findings, as lactate can also be raised secondary to other conditions, including depletion of pyruvate dehydrogenase (PDH) enzyme required to catabolise pyruvate to acetyl-CoA due to thiamine deficiency, or iatrogenic causes secondary to some medications.

The use of lactate in the recognition and management of septic shock features significantly within current international guidelines, with Surviving Sepsis Campaign guidelines (Evans et al. 2021) reminding clinicians that serum lactate measurement is a current recommendation within the first hour Sepsis-6 bundle, and that there is a direct correlation between raised lactate levels and mortality from sepsis. They recommend using serum lactate levels alongside other markers to guide fluid resuscitation in septic shock. Where serum lactate is >2 mmol/l, the one-hour sepsis care bundle recommends that it should be rechecked after two to four hours in order to guide fluid resuscitation, noting a reduction in mortality when this is done (Levy et al. 2018).

Urea and Electrolytes and Urine Output

Research has demonstrated that patients who develop acute kidney injury (AKI) secondary to hypo-perfusion from septic shock, experience worse outcomes and higher mortality when this is not recognised and reversed early. Indeed, AKI has been shown to occur in up to 65% of patients with severe sepsis or septic shock and was associated with a lower MAP at the time of diagnosis (Tarvasmäki et al. 2018). In cases of cardiogenic shock, an increased 30-day mortality has been associated with AKI, thought to be due to venous congestion and reduced venous perfusion (Fahad et al. 2020), with the incidence increasing with higher stages of shock and higher stages of AKI correlating with an increased mortality.

Current KDIGO guidelines (Kellum et al. 2012) define AKI as 'an abrupt decrease in kidney function' that is detected through an increase in serum creatinine to greater than 1.5 times the baseline creatinine within the last 7 days, an increase in serum creatinine by more than 0.3 mg/dl in 48 hours, or a urine output of less than 0.5 ml/kg/h over 6 hours.

AKI can be separated into three stages of increasing severity, with the higher stages suggesting increased mortality and a higher likelihood to require renal replacement therapy:

Stage 1: Serum creatinine >1.5× baseline or >0.3 mg/dl, or urine output <0.5 mg/kg/h for 6 hours.
Stage 2: Serum creatinine >2.0× baseline, or urine output <0.5 ml/kg/h for 12 hours.
Stage 3: Serum creatinine >3.0× baseline, or anuria for >12 hours. Patients in RRT are also considered to be in stage 3 AKI.

In cases of shock, clinicians should use U&Es to assess the risk of developing AKI, or to assist in its staging to provide effective preventative and management strategies. The use of both serum creatinine levels and urine output can help to understand risk earlier, and studies have shown that in cases of cardiogenic shock urine output can often be a more sensitive early indicator of kidney injury that would require intervention.

Examination Scenario

When assessing the patient with suspected shock, a full clinical examination should be completed and there should be specific attention paid to any abnormal findings. Table 21.7 highlights some of the key findings and variations that may be encountered between the different causes of shock, with proposed management being discussed throughout this chapter.

TABLE 21.7 Possible findings on CVS examination in shock.

Findings	Hypovolaemic	Cardiogenic	Distributive
HR	Raised	Can be raised, normal, or low	Raised
BP	Hypotensive	Hypotensive	Hypotensive
Pulse	Weak and thready	Weak and thready	Strong and bounding
JVP/CVP	Low	Raised	Low
Pallor	Pale/grey	Pale/grey	Flushed/pink
Temperature	Cool	Cool	Warm
CRT	Increased	Increased	Decreased

Examination Scenario

One significant variable that can help guide practitioners to an early diagnosis or cardiogenic shock, as opposed to other forms of shock, is jugular venous pressure (JVP). Although not a sensitive marker, a raised JVP can be an indicator for cardiogenic shock due to heart failure and can act as a prompt for practitioners to investigate further to confirm diagnosis. A sunken JVP can be a marker of fluid depletion and can be seen in hypovolaemic or distributive shock, again prompting further investigation.

FIELD OF PRACTICE: PAEDIATRICS

Introduction

The stages of shock still apply in children, but there are often more than one cause leading to a challenging diagnosis and management. There is an approach to the diagnosis of the cause of shock as outlined in Chart 21.1 (Waltzman et al. 2020).

Clinical and Physiological Targets

Early goals of therapy for shock aim to target improvement in clinical and physiological signs. The amount of intervention is guided by the degree of illness. There are several physiological parameters in children that assist in the treatment of shock (Waltzman et al. 2020):

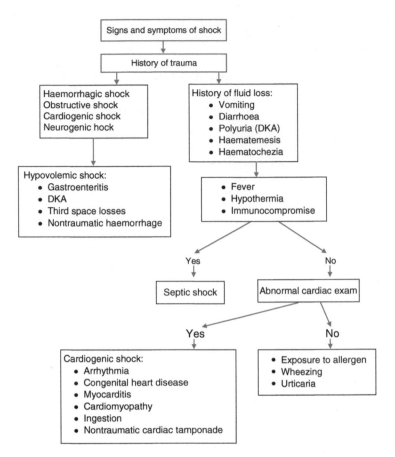

CHART 21.1   Diagnosis of shock in children.

1. Blood pressure
    - Systolic pressure at least fifth percentile for age
    - 60 mmHg <1 month of age
    - 70 mmHg + (2 x age in years) in children aged 1 month–10 years
    - 90 mmHg >10 years
2. Quality of central and peripheral pulses (distal versus central)
3. Skin perfusion (capillary refill time <2 seconds)
4. Mental status
5. Urine output (>1 ml/kg per hour once effective circulating volume is restored)

Heart rate can also be a useful indicator, in particular, a drop-in heart rate in response to an intervention such as fluid resuscitation. Table 21.8 below demonstrates normal values for children up to 12 years (American Academy of Pediatrics & American Heart Association 2016).

It is important to note that there are many factors that can influence heart rate (fever, drugs, hypoxia, and anxiety), therefore specific target goals are hard to define.

The above physiological indicators can be monitored non-invasively during the initial management of shock, and since children usually respond well, invasive monitoring can often be avoided.

TABLE 21.8   Normal heart rates in children.

Age	Awake rate	Asleep rate
Neonate (28 days or younger)	100–205	90–160
Infant (29 days to 1 year)	100–180	90–160
Toddler (1 to <3 years)	98–140	80–120
Preschool (3–5 years)	80–120	65–100
School aged (6–12 years)	75–118	58–90
Adolescent (>12 years)	60–100	50–90

In addition to the targets listed above, a raised serum lactate (>4 mmol/l) can also help identify the severity of shock. Although evidence is limited in children, a drop in serum lactate has been associated with improved survival in children with sepsis (Waltzman et al. 2020).

Initial Stabilisation

Within the first 5–15 minutes of shock recognition and treatment, the following actions should occur:

- Monitor heart rate, pulse oximetry, and blood pressure frequently.
- Establish vascular access (ideally two access sites, if unable then consider using interosseous).
- Rapid measurement of blood glucose and treat hypoglycaemia.
- For trauma patients ensure access to trauma surgeon.
- Identify any obstructive causes for shock.
- If possible, a focused ultrasound of the lungs, heart, and abdomen should be obtained.

Table 21.9 is a guide to what should occur in the first hour.

High Risk Conditions

There are some conditions where giving too much fluid can be harmful. Below is a list of some of the high-risk conditions where cautious fluid resuscitation needs to be employed:

- **Cardiogenic Shock**
  - Although some may have a degree of hypovolaemia, fluid should be omitted or administered slowly.
  - Boluses of 5–10 ml/kg should be given slowly.
  - Neonates with ductal dependent lesions the primary focus should be on reopening the ductus arteriosus with prostaglandin E1 (Waltzman et al. 2020)
- **Severe anaemia**
  - Rapid fluid administration in a child with haemoglobin <5 g/dl will further dilute leading to impaired oxygen delivery, and precipitate heart failure (Waltzman et al. 2020)

TABLE 21.9 First hour management of shock in children.

Time	Management
First 5–15 minutes	• Those without signs of fluid overload, give a rapid infusion of an isotonic crystalloid of 20 ml/kg over 5 minutes • Those with compensated shock should receive 10–20 ml/kg over 5–20 minutes • For those with cardiogenic shock who are hypovolaemic, fluid should be given cautiously and over a longer period • Complete remaining blood tests to include electrolytes, lactate, cultures, and crossmatch (Waltzman et al. 2020)
15–60 minutes	• Abnormalities in calcium and electrolytes should be identified and treated • Appropriate antibiotics should be initiated with suspected septic shock • Children, other than those with obstructive shock, cardiogenic shock, or DKA who have not improved to the initial fluid bolus should receive another 20 ml/kg to a total of 60 ml/kg • Vasoactive drugs may be initiated in children with neurogenic or cardiogenic shock who don't respond to fluid therapy (Waltzman et al. 2020)
>60 minutes	• If no improvement after 60 minutes, then other causes of shock should be considered • Consider colloid fluid such as blood • If fluid or catecholamine resistant shock, then should be admitted to a critical care unit for monitoring central venous oxygen saturations and central venous pressure (Waltzman et al. 2020)

- **Severe malnutrition**
  - The evidence of fluid resuscitation in children with severe malnutrition is controversial.
  - It is thought that malnutrition causes sodium and water retention and myocardial dysfunction.
  - Therefore, rapid infusion of fluids may lead to fluid overload, and then heart failure.
- **Syndrome of inappropriate antidiuretic hormone secretion (SIADH)**
  - Aggressive fluid therapy can cause cerebral oedema and significant changes in sodium balance.
- **Uncontrolled haemorrhage**
  - Delayed fluid resuscitation with controlled hypotension may be beneficial for some patients.

The Use of Vasoactive Agents During Shock

Table 21.10 demonstrates the vasoactive medication receptor activity and their clinical effects (Waltzman et al. 2020).

Mental Health

Within the context of critical care there is the emergence of a strong body of evidence linking the experience of critical illness to worsened mental health, with post-traumatic stress disorder and anxiety being widely researched. Indeed, studies suggest that between 25% and 50% of ICU survivors experience symptoms of PTSD, anxiety, or depression in the first 12 months following discharge, with septic shock believed to be one of the conditions with the highest reported rates of PTSD. Studies into the causality for this have made early hypotheses linking this to glucocorticoid receptors and cortisol production; however research

TABLE 21.10   Effects of vasoactive medication in children.

Drug	Alpha-1	Beta-1	Beta-2	Dopaminergic	Clinical effects
Phenylephrine	+++	0	0	0	SVR increased CO increased
Norepinephrine	+++	++	0	0	SVR increased CO increased
Epinephrine	+++	+++	++	0	CO increased SVR reduced at low dose SVR increased at high dose
Dopamine (mcg/kg/min)					
0.5–2	0	+	0	++	CO
5–10	+	++	0	++	CO increased SVR increased
10–20	++	++	0	++	SVR increased
Dobutamine	0/+	+++	++	0	CO increased SVR increased
Isoproterenol	0	+++	+++	0	CO increased SVR increased

Source: Waltzman et al. (2020) / Wolters Kluwer.

into this is ongoing (Hauer et al. 2014). There is an increasing acceptance of the role of patient diaries in the intensive care unit, which are often used by healthcare staff and patients' families to document a patient's stay, detail their illness, treatment, and progress, and help them to make sense of what has happened following their discharge from hospital. Studies have shown that these may lead to a reduction in depression and anxiety, although their role in reduction of PTSD and improved psychological recovery is still under debate (McIlroy et al. 2019; Ullman et al. 2015). Most importantly, however, research has demonstrated the value that patients place on their diaries following critical illness helps them to process their admission and subsequent recovery alongside gaining an understanding of their treatment in ICU through the multidisciplinary and family entries explaining daily their progress and setbacks during their ICU stay (Brandao Barreto et al. 2021).

Learning Difficulties

Within the UK, circulatory disorders are the second highest underlying cause of death amongst people with learning disabilities. Sepsis as a primary cause of death as recorded on a MCCD appears to have reduced over recent years from being the third most prevalent in 2017, to being the sixth in 2019 (LeDeR 2020); however, no statistics exist for shock, and therefore these mortality figures can only be used as a guide within this context. People with learning disabilities are more likely to have co-morbidities and therefore more likely to develop sepsis and require longer hospital stays, suffering longer-term effects from sepsis. Including the person's carer in communication and in the undertaking of care activities has been seen as helpful for purposes of consistency and reassurance to the patient (Grant et al. 2021).

Learning Event

A patient was brought into the emergency department with profound hypotension and tachycardia with a reduced urine output for 24 hours. Routine bloods revealed that he had raised inflammatory markers, stage 3 AKI and a metabolic acidosis with high lactate. He was later admitted to ICU, where he was commenced on haemodynamic monitoring which allowed practitioners to target fluid resuscitation and vasopressors to achieve their target MAP. He was also given a broad-spectrum antibiotic to treat his sepsis until a microbiological culture was grown, allowing treatment to be more targeted. Unfortunately, he did not respond sufficiently to treatment for his septic shock due to his late presentation, and he passed away four days later. Early recognition and management of sepsis is critical.

Learning Event

A patient returned to the surgical ward following an emergency laparotomy for a bowel perforation at the splenic flexure secondary to the ingestion of a foreign body. In the initial hours post-operatively he appeared to be comfortable and to be making a good recovery with IV fluids, antibiotics for peritonitis, and analgesia. Overnight, the nurse noted that he had become less responsive, and that his blood pressure was unrecordable. The emergency medical team were contacted, who prescribed fluid boluses and requested investigations. On the ABG, his haemoglobin was found to be 52 g/dl and he was returned to theatre with hypovolaemic shock secondary to a perforated spleen. Postoperatively he was admitted to the intensive care unit, where he received further blood products and vasopressors. He made a full recovery.

PHARMACOLOGICAL PRINCIPLES

The importance of fluid management in shock has already been discussed. In addition, and depending on the type of shock, various drugs may need to be considered as part of a management plan. Amongst the more common drugs, one may expect to find those that affect alpha-1 and beta-1 adrenergic receptors.

Alpha-1 Adrenergic Receptor Agonists

Vasopressors work by stimulating α_1 adrenergic receptors in blood vessels, thus causing vasoconstriction. This typically causes an increase in blood pressure and MAP through an increase in SVR, while having little-to-no effect on CO, although some vasopressors can also exhibit β_1 adrenergic receptor stimulation. In vasopressors that only stimulate α_1 adrenergic receptors, a reduction in CO can occur. This makes the use of vasopressors particularly beneficial in the management of distributive/dilatory shocks, and also as an adjunct in cardiogenic shock and hypovolaemic shock when intravascular space or cardiac work-load may benefit from reduction. Vasopressors are metabolised rapidly, with very short half-lives making them ideal for administration by continuous infusion.

Beta-1 Receptor Agonists

Positive inotropic drugs work by stimulating β_1 adrenergic receptors in the heart, causing an increase in myocardial contractility and SV through the opening of voltage-gated calcium channels. In terms of hae-modynamic monitoring, this increase in SV can lead to an increased CO, although allowances should also be made for fluid status and its effect on CO and therefore inotropes are particularly useful in managing patients who are displaying cardiac insufficiency; however, the increase in myocardial oxygen consumption may influence mortality (Amado et al. 2016). Although some inotropes work solely on β_1 adrenergic receptors, others may also affect α_1 adrenergic receptors causing vasoconstriction, while others can cause a mild vasodilation.

Within critical care, there are several inotropic and vasopressor drugs that are commonly used to help manage shock. These include:

- **Noradrenaline (Norepinephrine)** – Has an affinity for predominantly α_1 adrenergic receptors, although also affects β_1 adrenergic receptors to a lesser extent. It increases SVR while having little effect on CO. It is recommended as the first-line vasopressor for use in septic shock to achieve a target MAP of 65 mmHg (Surviving Sepsis Campaign 2021). Noradrenaline should be administered via central venous access and the patient should be monitored for peripheral ischaemia associated with peripheral vasoconstriction.

- **Dobutamine** – Works solely on β_1 adrenergic receptors, with no vasopressor action. It works by increasing cardiac contractility and therefore SV, which leads to an increase in CO, however it can also stimulate a sympathetic decrease in SVR. It has been shown to improve the efficiency of oxygen utilisation by improving mitochondrial function. It has a plasma half-life of two minutes. Although dobutamine can cause tachycardia, at low to moderate doses this is often not affected. In cases of septic shock, dobutamine should be considered when shock is refractory to noradrenaline alone (De Backer et al. 2021; Survivng Sepsis Campaign 2021; Zimmerman et al. 2019).

- **Adrenaline (Epinephrine)** – At lower doses, adrenaline has an affinity for β_1 adrenergic receptors, and at higher doses for α_1 adrenergic receptors. It also has some β_2 adrenergic receptor affinity, affecting smooth muscle in the lungs and vasculature, thus causing bronchodilation. It is predominantly recommended in anaphylactic shock due to its ability to increase MAP through vasoconstriction as well as reduce the release of histamine. Although there are some theoretical benefits to using adrenaline in smaller doses in cardiogenic shock, research has suggested that higher doses may increase tachycardia, myocardial ischaemia, and the effort of the left ventricle and therefore should be avoided, and it is recommended that noradrenaline would be a sensible alternative. In cases of septic shock that are refractory to fluid resuscitation and vasopressor support from dobutamine and noradrenaline, guidelines advocate switching to adrenaline (RCUK 2021; Surviving Sepsis Campaign 2021).

- **Phenylephrine** – Works solely on α_1 adrenergic receptors, and unlike noradrenaline, has no affinity for β_1 adrenergic receptors. This in turn means that CO may be sympathetically reduced through reduced heart rate. Whereas noradrenaline can often be the first choice of vasopressor due to its mild inotropic action, which minimises any sympathetic response by maintaining heart rate and CO, phenylephrine can provide some benefit in some cases of cardiogenic shock where tachycardias and arrythmias exist or myocardial oxygen consumption needs to be reduced. It is not routinely recommended in the management of septic shock. Due to its role in vasoconstriction, there is a risk of ischaemia or necrosis, and caution should be taken where this risk exists.

PATHOLOGICAL CONSIDERATIONS

In patients presenting with signs of shock, there are often warning signs that can assist practitioners to ascertain their diagnosis that can be found through effective history-taking and clinical examination.

Where history-taking exposes that the patient may be at risk of, or recently had, an episode of bleeding, investigations should be undertaken to establish the cause, and where necessary take preventative measures to minimise the risk of progression to hypovolaemic shock. There are many instances where clinicians may identify haemorrhage as a contributing factor to shock. Bleeding following non-cardiac surgery can occur in up to 17% of postoperative patients, with an associated mortality of 5.8% (Roshanov et al. 2020), and there is a strong association between GI bleed leading to shock and increased mortality (Siddiqui et al. 2019). Evidence has shown that early recognition, control of haemorrhage and other appropriate interventions to control bleeding can significantly reduce the risk of mortality, and clinicians should be aware of local major haemorrhage protocols and surgical escalation pathways.

Amongst patients admitted to hospital with acute myocardial infarction, cardiogenic shock is the leading cause of death, with 6.1% of patients progressing to cardiogenic shock. Studies have suggested that the 30-day mortality for this patient group is as high as 60%, compared to 8% for patients admitted with acute MI who do not progress to cardiogenic shock (Lauridsen et al. 2020). Clinicians should consider the need for revascularization and specialist referral in cases where this would be appropriate to prevent the development of cardiogenic shock, and early admission to ICU for vasopressors and inotropes where cardiogenic shock is believed to have manifested.

The incidence of sepsis is widely regarded to be rising worldwide. Furthermore, organ dysfunction from sepsis can be occult and practitioners should consider it a possibility in any patient who presents with a new infection that sepsis could be present. Where suspected this should be managed as per international guidelines, and clinicians should be vigilant for any progression of symptoms that are suggestive of septic shock.

ORANGE FLAG

It is thought that up to 40% of patients with septic shock can develop delirium secondary to cerebral hypoperfusion and dysregulation (Feng et al. 2021), which manifests as an altered level of consciousness with inattention and disorganised thinking and is linked to an increased length of stay and higher mortality. Some studies have suggested that ICU patients who have experienced delirium have an ongoing cognitive impairment following hospital discharge, however other studies have disputed this (Bruck et al. 2018; Green et al. 2018).

ORANGE FLAG

Following discharge from hospital, patients often suffer from a reduced quality of life secondary to the psychological impact of critical illness. Over recent years, a paradigm has developed focusing on peer support, both as a structured model facilitated by clinical psychologists and unstructured through shared spaces such as waiting rooms at follow-up clinics (Haines et al. 2019; McPeake et al. 2019). Early studies have suggested that survivors of critical illness who engage in volunteering with peer support groups find them beneficial for psychological recovery and clinicians could consider referral following discharge where access to these groups exist (Robinson et al. 2020).

GREEN FLAGS

Studies have found that socioeconomic status plays a large role in the development of sepsis, with those from poorer backgrounds or neighbourhoods, or lower levels of income or education experiencing higher levels of infection and sepsis leading to greater mortality, although further work is required to fully understand the correlation and produce recommendations for narrowing the gap (Sheikh et al. 2022; Galiatsatos et al. 2018).

GREEN FLAGS

Age also presents as a factor in both the onset and management of shock, with hospital mortality being higher in older patients presenting with cardiogenic shock than younger patients, with an increase in co-morbidities being a factor. It has also been proposed that treatment of older people can often be less aggressive, with a lower likelihood of receiving revascularisation therapy. When revascularisation is performed early, however, trials have concluded that survival benefit is similar to that of younger patients who also present with cardiovascular shock (Navarese et al. 2019; Padkins et al. 2020).

Case Study

A young male with no previous medical history has been admitted to the hospital for routine minor surgery. Today, he feels less well. His surgical wound is burning to touch, he is pyrexial, tachycardic, and hypotensive.

1. What is your differential diagnosis?
2. What findings would you expect from a physical examination?
3. What further assessments do you need?
4. What type of shock is he at risk of developing?
5. What is your initial management plan?

Case Study

A 64-year-old lady has presented to the Emergency Department with a seven day history of diarrhoea and vomiting. She was found at home by her neighbour with a reduced level of consciousness. The paramedic states that on their arrival she was hypotensive and pale, with a prolonged capillary refill time and a rapid, weak, and thready pulse.

1. What type of shock does this lady have?
2. What do you think her haemodynamic monitoring values would show?
3. What further investigations will you order? Why?
4. What is your initial management plan?

Case Study

An elderly gentleman has been in hospital for the last week for medical management of a STEMI. He had a coronary artery bypass graft 10 years ago and is a type 2 diabetic. Today, he has become acutely short of breath. He is hypotensive and tachycardic with a weak pulse. His urine output has reduced overnight and is now less than 0.5/ml/kg/h.

1. Is an echo indicated on him? What potential findings may there be? How would this relate to his expected haemodynamic values?
2. What clinical findings would you expect to see on examination?
3. What drugs would you consider using to help manage his hypotension? Why?
4. What type of shock does he have?
5. Are there any other interventions you would consider?

Take Home Points
- Shock can be hypovolaemic, cardiogenic, obstructive, or distributive in nature. They have similarities and differences between them that can help the advanced clinical practitioner to identify and manage them effectively.
- Left unrecognised, shock can lead to tissue hypoxia, end organ dysfunction, and increased mortality.
- The management of shock requires investigations including echocardiography, haemodynamic monitoring, and laboratory tests to help balance pharmacological and other interventions to support blood pressure and treat the source.

REFERENCES

Amado, J., Gago, P., Santos, W. et al. (2016). Choque cardiogénico – fármacos inotrópicos e vasopresores. *Revista Portuguesa de Cardiologia*. 15 (32): 681–695.

American Academy of Pediatrics & American Heart Association (2016). *Paediatric Advanced Life Support Provider Manual*. Dallas, TX: American Heart Association.

Bonanno, F.G. (2011). Physiopathology of shock. *Journal of Emergencies, Trauma, and Shock* 4 (2): 222–232. https://doi.org/10.4103/0974-2700.82210.

Brandao Barreto, B., Luz, M., Alves Valente do Amaral Lopes, S. et al. (2021). Exploring patients' perceptions on ICU diaries: a systematic review and qualitative data synthesis. *Critical Care Medicine* 49: e707–e718.

Bruck, E., Schandl, A., Bottai, M., and Sackey, P. (2018). The impact of sepsis, delirium, and psychological distress on self-rated cognitive function in ICU survivors – a prospective cohort study. *Journal of Intensive Care* 6 (2): 2.

Cecconi, M., De Backer, D., Antonelli, M. et al. (2014). Consensus on circulatory shock and hemodynamic monitoring. Task force of the European Society of Intensive Care Medicine. *Intensive Care Medicine* 40 (12): 1795–1815. https://doi.org/10.1007/s00134-014-3525-z.

De Backer, D., Arias Ortiz, J., and Levy, B. (2021). The medical treatment of cardiogenic shock: cardiovascular drugs. *Current Opinion in Critical Care* 27 (4): 426–432.

Evans, L., Rhodes, A., Alhazzani, W. et al. (2021). Surviving sepsis campaign: international guidelines for management of sepsis and septic shock 2021. *Criticval Care Medicine* 49 (11): e1063–e1143.

Fahad, F., Shaukat, S., Hamza, M., and Yager, N. (2020). Incidence and outcomes of acute kidney injury requiring renal replacement therapy in patients on percutaneous mechanical circulatory support with Impella-CP for cardiogenic shock. *Cureus* 12 (1): e6591.

Feng, Q., Ai, M., Huang, L. et al. (2021). Relationship between cerebral haemodynamics, tissue oxygen saturation, and delirium in patients with septic shock: a pilot observational cohort study. *Frontiers in Medicine* 641104.

Galiatsatos, P., Brigham, E.P., Pietri, J. et al. (2018). The effect of community socioeconomic status on sepsis-attributable mortality. *Journal of Critical Care* 46: 129–133.

Grant, N., Hewitt, O., Ash, K., and Knott, F. (2021). The experiences of sepsis in people with a learning disability – a qualitative investigation. *British Journal of Learning Disabilities* `https://doi.org/10.1111/bld.12500`.

Green, C., Bonavia, W., Toh, C., and Tiruvoipati, R. (2018). Prediction of ICU delirium: validation of current delirium predictive models in routine clinical practice. *Critical Care Medicine* 47 (3): 428–435.

Griffee, M.J., Merkel, M.J., and Wei, K.S. (2010). The role of echocardiography in hemodynamic assessment of septic shock. *Critical Care Clinics* 26 (2): `https://doi.org/10.1016/j.ccc.2010.01.001`.

Haines, K.J., McPeake, J., Hibbert, E. et al. (2019). Enablers and barriers to implementing ICU follow-up clinics and peer support groups following critical illness: the thrive collaboratives. *Critical Care Medicine* 47 (9): 1194–1200.

Hauer, D., Kaufmann, I., Strewe, C. et al. (2014). The role of glucocorticoids, catecholamines and endocanniboids in the development of traumatic memories and posttraumatic stress symptoms in survivors of critical illness. *Neurobiology of Learning and Memory* 112: 68–74.

Health Education England (HEE). (2017). *Multi-professional Framework for Advanced Clinical Practice in England* [online]. Available from: `https://www.hee.nhs.uk/sites/default/files/documents/multi-professionalframeworkforadvancedclinicalpracticeinengland.pdf` [accessed 20 June 2023].

Health Education England (HEE). (2022). *Advanced Clinical Practice in Acute Medicine Curriculum Framework – Credentials* [online]. Available from: `https://advanced-practice.hee.nhs.uk/our-work/credentials` [accessed 20 June 2023].

Holst, L.B., Wetterslev, J., Wernerman, J. et al. (2014). Lower versus higher hemoglobin threshold for transfusion in septic shock. *New England Journal of Medicine* 371 (15): 1381–1391.

Kellum, J.A., Lameire, N., Aspelin, P. et al. (2012). Kidney disease: improving global outcomes (KDIGO) acute kidney injury work group. KDIGO clinical practice guideline for acute kidney injury. *Kidney International Supplements* 2 (1): 1–138.

Lauridsen, M.D., Rørth, R., Lindholme, M.G. et al. (2020). Trends in first-time hospitalization, management, and short-term mortality in acute myocardial infarction-related cardiogenic shock from 2005 to 2017: a nationwide cohort study. *American Heart Journal* 229: 127–137.

LeDeR. (2020). *The Learning Difficulties Mortality Review (LeDeR) Programme Annual Report 2020* [online]. Available from: `https://leder.nhs.uk/images/annual_reports/LeDeR-bristol-annual-report-2020.pdf` [accessed 25 June 2023].

Levy, M.M., Fink, M.P., Marshall, J.C. et al., and SCCM/ESICM/ACCP/ATS/SIS(2003). 2001 SCCM/ESICM/ACCP/ATS/SIS international sepsis definitions conference. *Critical Care Medicine* 31 (4): 1250–1256. https://doi.org/10.1097/01.CCM.0000050454.01978.3B.

Levy, M.M., Evans, L.E., and Rhodes, A. (2018). The Survivng sepsis campaign bundle: 2018 update. *Critical Care Medicine* 46 (6): 997–1000.

McIlroy, P.A., King, R., Garrouste-Orgeas, M. et al. (2019). The effect of ICU diaries on psychological outcomes and quality of life of survivors of critical illness and their relatives: a systematic review and meta-analysis. *Critical Care Medicine* 47 (2): 273–279.

McPeake, J., Hirshberg, E., Christie, L.M. et al. (2019). Models of peer support to remediate post-intensive care syndrome: a report developed by the Society of Critical Care Medicine thrive international peer support collaborative. *Critical Care Medicine* 47 (1): e21–e27.

Navarese, E.P., Rao, S.V., and Krucoff, M.W. (2019). Age, STEMI, and cardiogenic shock. Never too old for PCI? *Journal of the American College of Cardiology* 73 (15): 1091–1094.

Padkins, M., Breen, T., Anavekar, N. et al. (2020). Age and shock severity to predict mortality in cardiac intensive care unit patients with and without heart failure. *ESC Heart Failure* 7 (6): 3971–3982.

Resuscitation Council UK. (2021). *Emergency Treatment of Anaphylaxis. Guidelines for Healthcare Providers* [online]. Available from: www.resus.org.uk/sites/default/files/2021-05/Emergency%20Treatment%20of%20Anaphylaxis%20May%202021_0.pdf [accessed 25 June 2023].

Robinson, C., Hibbert, E., Bastin, A.J. et al. (2020). An international study exploring the experience of survivors of critical illness as volunteers within ICU recovery services. *Critical Care Explorations* 2 (11): e0273.

Roshanov, P.S., Eikelboom, J.W., Sessler, D.I. et al. (2020). Bleeding independently associated with mortality after noncardiac surgery (BIMS): an international prospective cohort study establishing diagnostic criteria and prognostic importance. *British Journal of Anaesthesia* 126 (1): 163–171.

Shankar-Hari, M., Phillips, G.S., Levy, M.L. et al., and Sepsis Definitions Task Force(2016). Developing a new definition and assessing new clinical criteria for septic shock: for the third international consensus definitions for sepsis and septic shock (Sepsis-3). *JAMA* 315 (8): 775–787. https://doi.org/10.1001/jama.2016.0289.

Sheikh, F., Douglas, W., Catenacci, V. et al. (2022). Social determinants of health associated with the development of sepsis in adults: a scoping review. *Critical Care Explorations* 4 (7): e0731.

Siddiqui, S., Paul, S., Khan, Z. et al. (2019). Rising events and improved outcomes of gastrointestinal bleed with shock in USA: a 12-year national analysis. *Journal of Clinical Gastroenterology* 53 (5): e194–e201.

Smulders, Y.M. (2000). Pathophysiology and treatment of haemodynamic instability in acute pulmonary embolism: the pivotal role of pulmonary vasoconstriction. *Cardiovascular Research* 48 (1): 23–33. https://doi.org/10.1016/s0008-6363(00)00168-1.

Standl, T., Annecke, T., Cascorbi, I. et al. (2018). The nomenclature, definition and distinction of types of shock. *Deutsches Arzteblatt international* 115 (45): 757–768. https://doi.org/10.3238/arztebl.2018.0757.

Survivng Sepsis Campaign. (2021). *Vasoactive Agent Management* [online]. Available from: https://www.sccm.org/getattachment/d981da2d-c6b2-4ced-af18-bfcbbf859499/Surviving-Sepsis-Campaign-2021-Guidelines-Infographic_Vasoactive-Agent.pdf?lang=en-US [accessed 25 June 2023].

Tarvasmäki, T., Haapio, M., Mebazaa, A. et al. (2018). Acute kidney injury in cardiogenic shock: definitions, incidence, haemodynamic alterations, and mortality. *European Journal of Heart Failure* 20 (3): 572–581.

The Faculty of Intensive Care Medicine. (2018). *Curriculum for Training for Advanced Critical Care Practitioners – Syllabus. V1.1* [online]. Available from: www.ficm.ac.uk/media/6896 [accessed 20 June 2023].

The Intensive Care Society, Critical Care Networks – *National Nurse Leads and The National Outreach Forum*. (2022). *Advanced Critical Care Outreach Competencies* [online]. Available from: https://ics.ac.uk/asset/43B8C11B-4512-41D0-B97768FABA2C30B2 [accessed 20 June 2023].

The Royal College of Emergency Medicine. (2022). *Emergency Medicine Advanced Clinical Practitioner Curriculum 2022 (Adult)* [online]. Available from: https://rcem.ac.uk/wp-content/uploads/2022/09/ACP_Curriculum_Adult_Final_060922.pdf [accessed 20 June 2023].

Tortora, G.J. and Derrickson, B.H. (2006). *Principles of Anatomy and Physiology*. Wiley Balckwell.

Tuchschmidt, J.A. and Mecher, C.E. (1994). Predictors of outcome from critical illness. Shock and cardiopulmonary resuscitation. *Critical Care Clinics* 10 (1): 179–195.

Ullman, A.J., Aitken, L.M., Rattray, J. et al. (2015). Intensive care diaries to promote recovery for patients and families after critical illness: a cochrane systematic review. *International Journal of Nursing Studies* 52 (7): 1243–1253.

Via, G., Price, S., and Storti, E. (2011). Echocardiography in the sepsis syndromes. *Critical Ultrasound Journal* 3: 71–85. https://doi.org/10.1007/s13089-011-0069-0.

Waltzman, M., Torrey, S.B., Randolph, A.G., and Wiley, J.F. (2020). *Initial Management of Shock in Children* [online]. Available at: https://www.uptodate.com/contents/initial-management-of-shock-in-children [accessed 31 August 2022].

Zimmerman, J., Lee, J.P., and Clahan, M. (2019). Vasopressors and inotropes. In: *Pharmacology and Physiology for Anaesthesia: Foundations and Clinical Application*, 2e (ed. H. Hemmings and D. Egan). Philadelphia: Elsevier.

FURTHER READING

Chioncel, O., Parissis, J., Mebazaa, A. et al. (2020). Epidemiology, pathophysiology and contemporary management of cardiogenic shock – a position statement from the Heart Failure Association of the European Society of Cardiology. *European Journal of Heart Failure* 22 (8): 1315–1341.

Moranville, M.P., Mieure, K.D., and Santayana, E.M. (2011). Evaluation and management of shock states: hypovolaemic, distributive, and cardiogenic shock. *Journal of Pharmacy Practice* 24 (1): 44–60.

Stawicki, S.P. and Swaroop, M. (2020). *Clinical Management of Shock. The Science and Art of Physiological Restoration*. London: IntechOpen.

Singer, M., Deutchman, C.S., Seymour, C.W. et al. (2016). The third international consensus definitions for sepsis and septic shock (sepsis-3). *JAMA* 315 (8): 801–810.

Suh, G.J. (2018). *Essentials of Shock Management: A Scenario-Based Approach*. Singapore: Springer.

CHAPTER 22

Intra/Inter Hospital Transfers

Mark Cannan, Stuart Cox, and Kirstin Geer

Aim

To identify key considerations for advanced practitioners planning and delivering intra- and inter-hospital transfers of critically ill patients.

LEARNING OUTCOMES

After reading this chapter, the reader will be able to:

1. Identify rationale and risk assessment of both intra- and inter-hospital transfers provided by Advanced Practitioners.
2. Identify key patient safety considerations when preparing for transfer.
3. Identify importance of maximising communication to improve quality of the transfer.

SELF-ASSESSMENT QUESTIONS

1. How do you calculate oxygen required for transfer for both ventilated and non-ventilated patients?
2. What drugs can be discontinued and/or changed prior to transfer?
3. What are the minimum standards of monitoring for a ventilated patient?
4. Can you identify the process for transferring blood products between hospitals?

The Advanced Practitioner in Acute, Emergency and Critical Care, First Edition. Edited by Sadie Diamond-Fox, Barry Hill, Sonya Stone, Caroline McCrea, Natalie Gardner, and Angela Roberts.

INTRODUCTION

The aim of this chapter is to illuminate the significant considerations advanced practitioners must regard when organising and executing intra- and inter-hospital transfers of critically ill patients. A sophisticated understanding of such procedures is not merely a matter of logistics, but often involves life-critical decisions that necessitate a comprehensive understanding of the process. This includes cognizance of the rationale behind these transfers, risk assessments, and patient safety considerations that must be taken into account during the preparatory stages. Of utmost importance, too, is the effective utilisation of communication channels, a factor that greatly influences the quality of the transfer. By the conclusion of this chapter, readers will be equipped to identify the various elements that come into play during these transfers, thereby enhancing their preparedness for and execution of this critical task in their respective healthcare roles. The ultimate goal is to promote the safe, efficient, and effective transport of critically ill patients between and within healthcare institutions.

Multi-professional Framework (MPF) for Advanced Clinical Practice Guidance for Professional Development (HEE 2017)

This chapter maps to the following statements within the MPF:

1. Clinical Practice:	1.1	1.2	1.4	1.5	1.6	1.7	1.8	1.11
2. Leadership and Management:	2.1	2.3	2.8	2.11				
4. Research:	4.6							

Accreditation Considerations

This chapter maps to the following statements within the following national accreditation documents:

Curriculum for Training for Advanced Critical Care Practitioners Syllabus V1.1 (The Faculty of Intensive Care Medicine 2019)		
3.3	4.10	

GENERAL TRANSFER PRINCIPLES

Inter-hospital and intra-hospital transfers are important aspects for all acuity levels. Patient transfers are often to improve the existing management – for therapeutic/diagnostic purposes, unavailability of beds, or patient's end-of-life care. Transfers come with significant risk due to various physiological alterations which may affect the prognosis of the patient (Kulshrestha and Singh 2016). Transfer decisions should not be taken lightly, and be initiated systematically and in accordance with evidence-based guidelines. Intra-transfer adverse events are widely reported between 12.5% (Droogh et al. 2012) and 62% (Flabouris et al. 2006). Currently, there are no annual intra-hospital transfers data, however, ICS guidelines (2019) quote an 'under-reported' annual UK figure of 10 750 inter-hospital critical care transfers. It was noted that most transfers occur Monday through Friday; however, 56% occurred between 18:00 and 07:59. General critical care units accounted for 35.5% of inter-hospital transfers, the emergency room for 27.8%, 'other areas' for 25%, specialist critical care units for 11%, and repatriations for 13% (1.8% from abroad) (ICS 2019). Transfers are becoming more common due to centralisation of specialist centres, increase in demand, and the COVID-19 pandemic pressures. Previously, regional transfers were specific for paediatric patients; however, NHS England commissioned adult critical care transfers in 2022.

ADVANCED PRACTITIONERS LEADING TRANSFERS

Advanced practitioner (AP) transfers are becoming more common. Denton et al. (2021) reviewed ACCP-led inter-hospital transfers over a three-year period, capturing 934 high-acuity patients. This quality improvement review demonstrated 81.4% of transfers were uneventful with the main complication being hypotension. This highlights how a previously medical-led practice can be safely and effectively AP-led. Trust insurances currently do not cover inter-hospital transfer, it is therefore strongly recommended to APs undertaking transfers to employ professional indemnity insurance.

COMMUNICATION AND DOCUMENTATION

Transfers can be complex, often involving multiple healthcare professionals from a wide-ranging multidisciplinary team. Risks related to communication are common and account for 9% of all adverse events on transfers (Flabouris et al. 2006). Key communications are between the sending and receiving centre, inter-departments of the sending hospital (e.g. radiology and transfusion laboratory) and between the transfer team. Intra-hospital transfers can be daunting for relatives. To alleviate potential anxieties, early consultation including relevant contact numbers, visiting times, and directions of the receiving hospital are provided. To ensure there are no miscommunications, it is imperative that records are accurate and contemporary for all stages of the transfer, medical notes photocopied or printed, and any imaging made available to the receiving unit prior to transfer.

PREPARATION

The most important, but potentially stressful and demanding part of any transfer is the preparation stage. Using mnemonics aids individuals in considering all aspects of the task and minimises the risk of errors; however, in some situations, a 'scoop and run' approach may be necessary for time-critical transfers. This applies for both intra- and inter-hospital transfers. Table 22.1 highlights the MINT mnemonic to aid preparation.

Prior to departure it is important for the team to conduct an A–E assessment (see Table 22.2).

Patient stabilisation prior to transfer is essential, minimising any interventions en route unless an emergency arises. Any non-essential drug infusions must be disconnected (i.e. actrapid) and only necessary infusions must continue (i.e. sedation, vasopressors). Oxygen and drug calculations are paramount and the minimum amount to be taken should be twice the journey time (or a minimum of one

TABLE 22.1 MINT mnemonics (Malpass et al. 2012).

M	Medical	❖ Doctor ❖ AP ❖ Grade required (Consultant/Registrar/AP/Trainee AP)
I	Instrumentation	❖ Transfer bag – preferably set out in ABCDE approach ❖ Alternative oxygen delivery means (Bag-Valve Mask or a Mapleson Circuit) ❖ Oxygen cylinders (calculate requirements) ❖ Advanced airway (endotracheal tube/tracheostomy/surgical airway kit) ❖ Suction ❖ Invasive and non-invasive ventilator ❖ Monitors (ECG, NiBP, arterial, CVP, capnography, SpO_2, BG, temperature) ❖ Defibrillator (with externally pacing) ❖ Syringe drivers with a spare device ❖ Additional device batteries ❖ Drugs (both maintenance and emergency) ❖ Fluids (crystalloids including hypertonic saline or mannitol; colloids including blood products)
N	Nursing	❖ Nurse (ITU, ED, CCOR, CCU)? ❖ Operating Department Practitioner (ODP)? ❖ Paramedic?
T	Transportation	❖ Certified Bed/Trolley for transfer ❖ Patient Transport Service ❖ Blue Light Double crewed Ambulance ❖ Air Ambulance (including land ambulance transfer at base and destination)? ❖ Expected journey time?

TABLE 22.2 The A–E assessment for transfer (Malpass et al. 2012).

A	Airway
	(with C Spine)
		❖ Is the patient self-ventilating or invasively ventilated?
		❖ Is the endotracheal/tracheostomy secure and patent?
		  ➤ Migration (what level is the endotracheal at the lips)?
		  ➤ Cuff inflation pressure (is there a leak)?
		❖ Does the patient require immobilisation, with a vacuum mattress, scoop stretcher, or long spine board equivalent, cervical collar and/or head blocks and tape?

B	Breathing (with ventilation)	❖ Breathing assessment including auscultation and a chest x-ray ❖ Chest drains below the level of the heart and is secured? They are not pulling and ensuring they are swinging, draining or bubbling? ❖ What is the ventilation mode (BiPAP, SIMV, PS, CPAP)? Is the patient including settings (RR, Tidal/Minute volume, FiO_2)? ❖ Is ventilator tubing secured? ❖ Is there CO_2 capnography? ❖ Has there been a blood gas within the last 15 minutes before departure while on the transport ventilator? ❖ Does the blood gas show adequate oxygenation/ventilation (if not, can this be optimised?) ❖ What are the calculated oxygen requirements?

(Continued)

TABLE 22.2   (Continued)

C	Circulation (with haemorrhage control)	<ul><li>Cardiovascular assessment including inotropic support (which inotrope, strength, rate in mcg/kg/min)</li><li>What are the calculated infusion requirements?</li><li>Are there any haemorrhage concerns?<ul><li>Does any coagulopathy need to be reversed?</li><li>Does the patient require blood products for transfer?</li></ul></li><li>All monitoring leads (ECG, Invasive/Non-Invasive BP, SpO_2) are running centrally along the patient and will not cause skin damage?<ul><li>Are they on and all working?</li></ul></li><li>All IV, CVC, and Arterial lines secure and are accessible from the patient's right-hand side?<ul><li>at least two IVs accessible?</li></ul></li><li>Have all non-essential infusions been detached?</li><li>Are there IV bolus fluids attached?</li><li>Urinary catheter is running centrally down the patient?</li></ul>
D	Disability (with neurological control)	<ul><li>Neurological assessment including pupils, blood glucose and noting any seizure activity?</li><li>Is the patient 15–30° head up?</li><li>ETT ties appropriate if suspected raised intracranial pressure</li><li>Has secondary neurological injury prevention been considered?</li><li>Is the patient adequately sedated?</li><li>Are muscle relaxants required?</li><li>Are anticonvulsants required?</li></ul>
E	Exposure (with temperature regulation)	<ul><li>Are there any patient temperature concerns?</li><li>Does the patient require active or passive warming or cooling?</li><li>Have all attempts of minimising pressure damage been considered?</li><li>Have all wounds been dressed?</li><li>Is the patient secured to the stretcher, and stretcher secured to the ambulance?</li></ul>

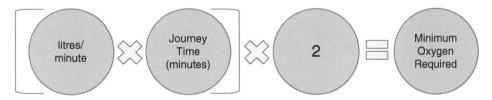

FIGURE 22.1   Oxygen calculations for the spontaneously breathing patient.

hour) to account for any unexpected delays or diversions. The patient's ventilation status (mechanical or self-ventilating) will decide how to calculate the oxygen requirement (see Figures 22.1 and 22.2a, b).

OXYGEN CALCULATIONS – SPONTANEOUSLY BREATHING PATIENT

A patient is requiring 40% (10 l/min) O_2 via venturi face mask. Journey time is one hour. Therefore: $(10 \, l/min \times 60 \, minutes) \times 2 = 1200$ litres of oxygen is required ($1 \times$ F size cylinder or $2 \times$ E size cylinders).

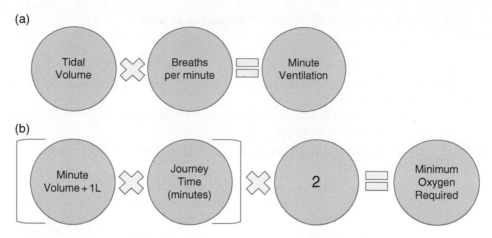

FIGURE 22.2   (a) Minute volume calculation. (b) Oxygen calculation for the ventilated patient.

OXYGEN CALCULATIONS – VENTILATED PATIENT

Calculate the Minute Ventilation (and add on the ventilator driving gas which is ventilator specific), e.g. 600 ml (Tidal Volume) $\times$ 15 bpm $=$ 9000 ml $+$ 1000 ml. Therefore, the minute ventilation will be 10 l per minute (Oxylog 2000 ventilators use approximately 1000 ml/min driving gas). Now that the MV is known, this needs to be calculated to double the journey time. e.g.: For a one-hour journey, this would be calculated as: (10 l $\times$ 60 min) $\times$ 2 $=$ 1200 l of oxygen will be required (1 $\times$ F size cylinder or 2 $\times$ E size cylinders).

The final consideration prior to departure relates to the transfer team conducting the transfer and can be remembered using the mnemonic PERSONAL (see Table 22.3).

HANDOVER/AUDIT

A comprehensive handover should take place at the receiving unit. Stable patients should have a 'hands off handover' approach so that both teams are undistracted. Questions from the receiving hospital must be answered prior to the transferring team leaving to ensure patient safety and continuity of care.

RED FLAGS

There are many red flag observations that can occur during transfer. These range from physiological changes, technical failure of equipment (e.g. loss of an endotracheal or chest tube), or communication failure. The occurrence of red flag events is proportional to the duration of the transfer. Transfers may have no or multiple occurrences which are proportional to the duration of the transport, severity of illness or injury – with longer transports, and higher patient acuity leading to an increase in red flags.

CLINICAL INVESTIGATIONS AND PROCEDURES

Prior to transfer it is important to undertake clinically necessary investigations or procedures based on the patients' acuity. Clinically necessary is a balance between purpose, method, reason for transfer, and acuity. FICM (2019) outline key considerations in their guidelines including tracheal tube position

TABLE 22.3   PERSONAL mnemonic for transfer (Malpass et al. 2012).

P	Phone	❖ Is it a personal mobile? ❖ Is it charged, and do you need a charging cable?
E	Enquiry Number and Name	❖ Do you have the receiving unit's phone number and the name of the receiving consultant? ❖ Do you have your consultants phone number in case of emergency and requiring advice/help en-route?
R	Revenue	❖ Has the transfer team got money in case of an emergency or a return taxi is required?
S	Safe Clothing	❖ Has everyone got high visibility clothing? ❖ Are there sufficient gloves, aprons, eye protection for personal protection? COVID PPE? ❖ Warm clothing?
O	Organised Route	❖ What is the route? ❖ Is there a backup route in case of obstruction? ❖ Do you have the correct hospital site?
N	Nutrition	❖ Is there food and water for the transfer team (if a prolonged transfer)?
A	A–Z Map	❖ Is there one? ❖ If using GPS do you have the correct postcode?
L	Lift Home	❖ Is the ambulance bringing the team home? ❖ Proposed method of returning to base location? ❖ What if the ambulance gets re-diverted on the way back?

confirmed on chest r-ray; adequate gas exchanged confirmed by an arterial blood gas; minimum of two routes of venous access; an arterial line and central venous access if appropriate; and if a pneumothorax is present or likely a chest drain should be inserted prior to departure.

Examination Scenarios

A 74-year-old female who has been in critical care for 12 days with community acquired pneumonia and multi-organ dysfunction. She has a high inotrope requirement, rising lactate, is deteriorating and has a distended abdomen with no bowel sounds. A computerised tomography (CT) scan is required to rule out bowel ischaemia/perforation.

Suitability for transfer/risk assessment – Transfer is justified to identify cause of deterioration, but is high risk.

Checklist – A transfer checklist based on an A–E approach must be utilised.

Preparation – Key considerations are optimising patient for transfer, timing of CT scan to allow adequate time for preparation of high-risk transfer including discontinuing Continuous Venovenous Haemofiltration (CVVH).

A – Ensure ETT is well secured.

B – Establish on a transfer ventilator and check ABG. Oxygen calculations and ensure adequate supply is available. When in CT scan, transfer to wall supply of oxygen to reserve cylinder supply.

C – Ensure all lines are secure. Administer fluid bolus. Drug calculations for noradrenaline, propofol, and alfentanil. Prepare boluses of neuromuscular blocker (NMB). Discontinue phosphate and Actrapid, ensure lines are flushed. Identify access for use in an emergency.

D – Ensure supply of sedation and NMB boluses. Accept blood glucose will rise while an Actrapid infusion is discontinued.

E – Recirculate CVVH and ensure vascath is flushed. Note time available on recirculation. Stop nasogastric (NG) feed and aspirate the NG tube.

Equipment – Transfer ventilator, transfer bag, emergency drugs, cage for oxygen cylinders, so they are not lying on the bed, portable drip stand that fits into bed, notes including details of allergies.

Staff – High-risk transfer requires an AP or Doctor and a Critical Care nurse or ODP who has had transfer training.

Key Learning Points

- Timing of CT scan to ensure adequate time to prepare for transfer
- Optimise patient for transfer, use a checklist
- Identify access for emergency drugs and where contrast can be administered
- Discontinue non-essential infusions, use bolus of muscle relaxants rather than infusions
- Check recirculation time of CVVH, will need ongoing CVVH particularly following contrast
- Top tips in CT scanner, ensure oxygen, ventilator, infusions and lines are not pulling. Using the straps on the CT scanner to secure them is useful. Do a 'run through' of the scan to be confident there is enough length on all devices. Place a monitor and ventilator, so you can see them from the scan room.

Examination Scenario

A 54-year-old male who has presented to ED in a District General Hospital following a collapse after severe back pain. CT scan confirms large Abdominal Aortic Aneurysm that requires urgent intervention at a tertiary centre.

Suitability for transfer/risk assessment – This is a time-critical scoop and run transfer. High risk but transfer is the only option for life-saving treatment.

Checklist – a checklist using an ABCDE approach should be used. This will require a team effort and must not delay the transfer.

Preparation – A–E assessment. Key considerations are intravenous access (two large bore venous access) and availability of blood products. Permissive hypotension and only transferring blood products for patients who require transfer en route are recommended by the National Blood Transfusion Committee (2021). One unit could be transfused rapidly while transferring onto an ambulance trolley ready for transfer. Paramedics will not administer blood products during transfer, and a 'medical' transfer may lead to delay. If blood products are required on transfer, the Regional Transfer of Blood Products Policy must be followed. Key points include ensuring maintenance of the cold chain, communication between the transferring and receiving hospital blood transfusion laboratories directly, completion of transfer of blood products document, appropriate transfer box sealed with a cable tie, transferring hospital transfusion lab must confirm dispatch with the receiving hospital laboratory.

(continued)

(continued)

When the transfer is completed transfusion lab staff must check the blood transfer box and complete documentation.

Equipment – Paramedic transfer within their competency with cautious infusion of crystalloids during transfer may be the most efficient transfer.

Learning Points

- Scoop and run time-critical transfers require team effort.
- Blood products should only be transferred with patients if they are going to be administered en route. Regional policies for the transfer of emergency blood products must be followed.
- Be sure the transferring team is sure of the exact location they are going to (e.g. straight to theatre in receiving hospital rather than going via ED).

Paediatric and Neonatal Retrieval and Repatriation Services

Paediatric and Neonatal transfer services are well-established with multiple dedicated services throughout the UK providing almost 11 000 transfers every two years (Seaton et al. 2021). Parents should be given the opportunity to travel with their child if clinically appropriate and the transferring vehicle allows.

Mental Health Transfers

Patients under the Mental Health Act (1983) Sections 2, 3, 37, and 47, who need to be transferred between hospitals or units approved to care for patients under the Mental Health Act must be transferred under Section 19. Transfers should be planned in advance, involve patients and their relatives if they give consent for them to be informed, and support from an Independent Mental Health Advocacy should be offered. The Responsible Clinician must hand over to the Responsible Clinician at the receiving unit prior to the transfer. As well as the patient and family, the Care Coordinator, and Mental Health Act office should be informed of transfer. Risk assessment of transfer must include the type of transport, and appropriate clinical that will accompany the patient. Form H4 must be completed prior to transfer, and the second part of Form H4 must be completed at the receiving unit. The Home Office must be informed if patients under section are crossing borders.

Learning Disabilities

Transfer to another part of the hospital or another unit could potentially be distressing for those with learning difficulties, who may feel more vulnerable. Transfers of care should only be done if there is a clear benefit to the patient. It is recommended good assessment of the patient's needs, encourages visiting and contribution from patients' family/usual carers (this may include them being with the patient when they are transferred between departments), remain calm and non-confrontational, and ensure patients have access to Independent Mental Capacity Advocate (IMCA).

PSYCHOLOGICAL, SOCIAL, AND CULTURAL CONSIDERATIONS

Patients and their relatives must be prepared psychologically for a transfer to another facility. Although it will be clinically assessed as required and deemed appropriate to undertake the transfer for specialist care such as trauma care, patients and their relatives' psychological considerations must be considered. This is multi-faceted ranging from the mode of transport (such as an ambulance, a plane, or a helicopter) not having space for a relative, and the location of care, which may be many miles away from a patient or a relative's support network. There is a paucity of evidence to quantify this psychological burden other than during the COVID pandemic. Some patients were cared for many miles from their home address or post-coded hospital. Despite this, even during a pandemic, an ethical framework was applied which protected individualised patient care decisions and prevented relatives from travelling to visit patients. Simple support can be undertaken in every case by the discharging (or transferring) facility and a receiving facility. Both facilities should be actively involved in supporting this by organising transport, providing accommodation, which should ideally be on site for a relative, providing contact information, and providing information for financial support. This financial support may come from specialist charities in the means of welfare benefits, grants, and other specific funding. Repatriation, when clinically appropriate to the discharging facility to support the patients and relatives psychological needs, should be arranged as soon as possible within the confines of an elective planned repatriation.

MEDICATION MANAGEMENT

Infusions required for transfer should be minimised to essential infusions only. In critical care transfers this includes sedation and vasopressors. Non-essential infusions e.g. electrolytes, insulin, antibiotics, enteral or parenteral feed can be stopped. Other drugs that may be given as an infusion, such as neuromuscular blocking agents can be given as a bolus. Most critical care transfer trolley only have room for up to four infusion devices. Drug calculations must be done prior to transfer to ensure there is no risk of running out. Some common medications can be:

- **Propofol** is a short acting intravenous general anaesthetic with a distribution half-life of 2–4 minutes. Common side effects are hypotension caused by vasodilation, and bradycardia. Emergency drugs to treat these complications must be readily available on transfer.
- **Atracurium and Rocuronium** are non-depolarising muscle relaxants. Elimination varies between NMB and it is not dependent on hepatic or renal metabolism or excretion. In specific patients cautions exist, which may include burns and cardiovascular disease.
- **Metaraminol and Phenylephrine** are vasoconstrictors and increase the force of myocardial contractility. A reflex bradycardia can occur after administering metaraminol.
- **Morphine and Fentanyl** are opioid analgesics which may be required during transfer. Naloxone should be available on all transfers in which opiates have been or may be administered.

Case Study

A 23-year-old patient requires transfer from the ED after sedation for shoulder manipulation to the orthopaedic ward. Full monitoring post-procedure has continued in the same clinical area (with the same facilities available including staffing) as per the Royal College of Emergency Medicine Best Practice Guidelines 2020, and transfer is required.

Key considerations:

- Have the vital signs returned to normal levels?
- Is the patient awake with intact protective reflexes and no longer at risk of reduced level of consciousness?
- Has nausea, vomiting, and pain been adequately addressed before transfer?
- Do you have appropriate monitoring and a checked transfer bag with basic airway adjuncts for transfer?

Case Study

A 62-year-old male presents to ED after an out of hospital Ventricular Fibrillation arrest, where return of spontaneous circulation was achieved after three shocks in accordance to the Advanced LifeSupport algorithm. The patient remains unconscious with an iGel that is not well seated; is cardio-vascularly stable; but has a Glasgow coma score of (E1, V1, M3) but requires transfer to a centre that can undertake Primary Percutaneous Coronary Intervention (PPCI) that is 45 minutes away.

Key considerations:

- Definitive airway before transfer that has been checked by x-ray and an arterial blood gas confirming ventilation.
- Appropriate sedation and paralysis before transfer.
- Appropriate critical care monitoring ensuring defibrillator pads are attached as preparing for rearrest is key.
- Consider advanced monitoring such as an arterial line if transfer is not delayed.
- Communication with the catheter laboratory team is paramount to ensure smooth transfer and early access to definitive treatment.

Case Study 3

A 75-year-old female presents to the ED with nausea and dizziness. 12-lead ECG confirms complete heart block. Transcutaneous pacing is established at a rate of 65, 70 joules, achieves mechanical and electrical capture. An isoprenaline infusion is also running.

Key considerations:

- Sedation boluses may be required to tolerate transcutaneous pacing. A–E assessment, monitoring and emergency equipment must be readily available during transfer.
- Positioning of defibrillator with pacing capabilities to ensure capture is not lost during transfer. Joules may need to be increased during transfer. Note 3 lead monitoring and defib pads must be in use for pacing.
- Ensure defibrillator in cath lab is compatible with defib pads in use, if not plan efficient change-over of pads to avoid interruptions to pacing.
- Communication with the catheter laboratory team is paramount to ensure smooth transfer and early access to definitive treatment.

Take Home Points
- Any transfers, especially critical care transfers are complex and high risk. Meticulous preparation, risk assessment, and communication are vital to providing safe high-quality transfers.
- Equipment and transfer checklists based on an A–E approach should be utilised to promote safety.
- Time-critical transfers require team working and clear communication. Procedures that are time-consuming should not delay transfer.
- Transfers links to the Advanced Practice framework and there is growing evidence APs provide high-quality transfers.

REFERENCES

Denton, G., Green, L., Palmer, M. et al. (2021). Evaluation of the safety of inter-hospital transfers of critically ill patients led by advanced critical care practitioners. *British Journal of Nursing* 30 (8): 470–476.

Droogh, J.M., Smit, M., Hut, J. et al. (2012). Inter-hospital transport of critically ill patients; expect surprises. *Critical Care* 16 (1): R26.

FICM (2019). Guidance for tracheostomy care. https://www.ficm.ac.uk/sites/ficm/files/documents/2021-11/2020-08%20Tracheostomy_care_guidance_Final.pdf

Flabouris, A., Runciman, W.B., and Levings, B. (2006). Incidents during out-of-hospital patient transportation. *Anaesthesia and Intensive Care* 34 (2): 228–236.

Government of the United Kingdom. (1983). *Mental Health Act* [online]. Available from: https://www.gov.uk/government/publications/of=practice-mental-health-act-1983 [accessed 11 October 2022].

Health Education England (HEE). (2017). *Multi-professional Framework for Advanced Clinical Practice in England* [online]. Available from: https://www.hee.nhs.uk/sites/default/files/documents/multi-professionalframeworkforadvancedclinicalpracticeinengland.pdf [accessed 20 June 2023].

Intensive Care Society (ICS) (2019). *Guidelines for the transport of the critically ill adult* [online]. London: The Intensive Care Society Available from: www.ics.ac.uk/Society/Guidance/PDFs/Patient_Transfer_Guidance [accessed 11 October 2022.

Kulshrestha, A. and Singh, J. (2016). Inter-hospital and intra-hospital patient transfer: recent concepts. *Indian Journal of Anaesthesia* [online] 60 (7): 451–457. Available from: `https://doi.org/10.4103/0019-5049.186012` [accessed 26 June 2023].

Malpass, H.C., Enfield, K.B., and Verghese, G.M. (2012). Interhospital intensive care transfer checklist facilitates early implementation of critical therapies and is associated with improved outcomes. *American Journal of Respiratory and Critical Care Medicine* 131 (23): 1–10.

National Blood Transfusion Committee. (2021). *Guidelines for the Emergency Transfer of Blood and Components with Patients Between Hospitals* [online]. Available from: `http://www.transfusionguidelines.org/document-library/documents/transfer-of-blood-pdf/download-file/Transfer%20of%20Blood.pdf` [accessed 11 October 2022].

Seaton, S.E., Draper, E.S., Pagel, C. et al. on behalf of the DEPICT Study Team(2021). The effect of care provided by paediatric critical care transport teams on mortality of children transported to paediatric intensive care units in England and Wales: a retrospective cohort study. *BC Paediatrics* 21: 217.

The Faculty of Intensive Care Medicine. (2019). *Curriculum for Training for Advanced Critical Care Practitioners – Syllabus. V1.1* [online]. Available from: `www.ficm.ac.uk/media/6896` [accessed 20 June 2023].

CHAPTER 23

Organ Donation and Optimisation

Jill Featherstone and Stevie Park

> **Aim**
> This chapter will enable the Advanced Practitioner to gain an understanding of the principles of organ and tissue donation care, the established pathways for this, and current best practice.

LEARNING OUTCOMES

After reading this chapter, the reader will:

1. Understand the role of the Specialist Nurse Organ Donation (SNOD) in this dynamic area of clinical practice.
2. Understand the organ donation pathways, process, and management and optimisation of a potential organ donor.
3. Understand the process and referral pathway of a potential tissue donor.
4. Understand how to respond to premature donation discussions.

SELF-ASSESSMENT QUESTIONS

1. Considering advanced clinical assessment skills, what key knowledge is required in the context of organ donation?
2. What are the benefits to early notification to the Specialist Nurse for Organ Donation?
3. Name the three characteristics of Cushing's reflex.

The Advanced Practitioner in Acute, Emergency and Critical Care, First Edition. Edited by Sadie Diamond-Fox, Barry Hill, Sonya Stone, Caroline McCrea, Natalie Gardner, and Angela Roberts.
© 2024 John Wiley & Sons Ltd. Published 2024 by John Wiley & Sons Ltd.

INTRODUCTION

Advanced practitioners (APs) play a vital role in supporting excellence in donation practice. Working collaboratively with the Specialist Nurse Organ Donation (SNOD) team enables a patient's end-of-life decisions to be sensitively explored and respected, any optimisation required made pre-emptively, proactively, and ethically, as well as lead to an effective and efficient process that can satisfy both the bereavement needs of a family and those of the busy clinical team.

According to NHS Blood and Transplant (NHSBT), the UK has the lowest rate of transplant consent in Europe. The UK may never achieve a world class donation and transplantation service if more than 4 out of every 10 families say no to donation. At present, 43% of families refuse to donate. Factors such as religion, culture, family influence, medical mistrust, and fear of early retrieval are recognised as the most important factors negatively affecting donation processes.

Multi-professional Framework (MPF) for Advanced Clinical Practice Guidance for Professional Development (HEE 2017)

This chapter maps to the following statements within the MPF:

1. Clinical Practice:	1.1	1.2	1.3	1.4	1.5	1.6	1.7	1.8	1.9	1.10	1.11
2. Leadership and Management:	2.1	2.2	2.3	2.4	2.6	2.7	2.8	2.10	2.11		
3. Education:	3.1	3.2	3.5								
4. Research:	4.3	4.7									

Accreditation Considerations

This chapter maps to the following statements within the following national accreditation documents:

Curriculum for Training for Advanced Critical Care Practitioners Syllabus V1.1
(The Faculty of Intensive Care Medicine 2018)

2.2	2.9	2.10	3.1	3.2	3.2	3.4	3.6	3.7	3.8	3.11	3.13	3.15	3.17	4.9

Advanced Critical Care Outreach Competencies
(The Intensive Care Society, Critical Care Networks – National Nurse Leads and The National Outreach Forum 2022)

METHODS OF ORGAN DONATION

Donation can occur in one of two ways, donation after brain death (or DBD) following diagnosis of death via neurological death testing (NDT), formally known as brain stem death testing, or via donation after a circulatory death (DCD). On occasions, the DCD route may be chosen for a DBD patient where a family's preference is to witness the cessation of their loved one's beating heart (see Table 23.1).

Following notification to the specialist nurse team, preliminary checks of suitability can be made, sensitive family discussions planned and carried out between the consultant, SNOD and bedside nurse with

TABLE 23.1 Pathophysiological response and the clinical consequences to neurological death.

1. Haemodynamic		Pathophysiological response		Clinical consequences
Pons	→Increasing ischaemia →	Vagal stimulation sympathetic stimulation	Bradycardia hypertension 'Cushing's reflex'	**Myocardial ischaemia (90%) ventricular dysfunction (45%) cardiac dysrhythmias (25%) pulmonary oedema (20%)**
Medulla		Sympathetic stimulation adrenergic storm	Blood pressure liability vasoconstriction	
2. Neuroendocrine				
Posterior pituitary		↓ ADH	Failure of urine concentration	**Diabetes insipidus (50–70%)**
Anterior pituitary		↓ T3 ↓ ACTH ↓ insulin	Hypotension cellular hypoglycaemia	**Haemodynamic instability (80%) metabolic acidosis (10%)**
Hypothalamus			Loss of thermoregulation	**Hypothermia (≈100%)**
3. Inflammatory				
Brain tissue		↑ Inflammatory cytokines and thromboplastin release	↑ Endothelial, leukocyte and platelet reactivity	**End organ dysfunction disseminated intravascular coagulation (30%)**

Source: Flemming and Thomson (2021) / with permission of Elsevier.

any consent/authorisation being established. Once a patient's whole health history has been ascertained and communicated by the SNOD to recipient centres and recipients found, a designated retrieval team attends the hospital to facilitate retrieval surgery before final cares are made in line with the family's expectations.

In DBD, the patient is prepared as a critical care transfer directly to theatre for the retrieval operation under the supervision of an anaesthetist. In DCD, where life sustaining treatment is withdrawn, the palliation care prior to death of these patients may occur either in the critical care area or in the theatre complex, depending on the circumstances of the hospital and the nature of donation itself. Once asystole is established and death is confirmed, prompt transfer into theatre for retrieval surgery occurs. For donation to be successful, in DCD, death must occur within a three-to-four-hour window and in a way that does not compromise the quality of the organs to be donated. Where there is a protracted time to asystole (PTA), palliation care continues in a designated place, such as the critical care unit or a prepared ward, with any tissue donation occurring in the mortuary suite following death.

EARLY NOTIFICATION TO THE SPECIALIST NURSE ORGAN DONATION SERVICE

Following national guidelines, early notification to the specialist nurse team is paramount, where a decision by the medical team is made to plan to withdraw life-sustaining treatment or recognised that testing for a neurological death can be made. Early notifications allow a collaborative approach that enables a family to feel safely supported, doing so with accurate contemporary information with which they can feel confident in their willingness to support the patient's donation decision, whatever that may be. Recent legislative changes within the UK, means many families, and clinical staff, are more aware of donation as an end-of-life option. This can lead to early, unscheduled conversations that can bring uncertainty for a family, if left unsupported by donation experts. For this reason, early mentions of organ donation by clinical staff are discouraged, and any discussions initiated by a family should be safely 'parked' with acknowledgement and thanks that it is important that they have raised the subject. A prompt and immediate referral to the specialist nurse team should be triggered to support the family's understanding of what donation may mean for them.

ROLE OF THE SPECIALIST NURSE FOR ORGAN DONATION

The SNOD's expert role is to verify suitability to donate, explore patient donation decisions, support donor management and optimisation, coordinate the teams involved, and organise the entire process. They provide expertise in bereavement support for the donor family during and after donation. The decision and discussion to withdraw life-sustaining treatment must be consultant–led, but the donation discussion is typically led by the SNOD. Notifications made via the national referral line result in one of three outcomes; rapid acceptance, where an SNOD will be mobilised to attend immediately; rapid decline, where a patient identified as unsuitable for donation can have palliation plans progressed with awareness of tissue donation potential to be discussed with the family; or thirdly, where a patient's potential to donate is uncertain, a suitable assessment plan can be put in place. This can take time to establish; APs can assist by providing a range of medical information.

DONOR PHYSIOLOGY

Pathophysiology resulting from a devastating brain injury and any subsequent neurological death can be profound. Any devastating brain injury results in cerebral oedema and can progress to a midline shift and herniation precipitating in further ischaemia. As this extends, intracranial pressure (ICP) rises.

TABLE 23.2   Hallmark signs of Cushing's reflex.

Side effect	Cause	Frequency (%)
Hypothermia	Hypothalamic dysfunction, vasoplegia	100
Hypotension	Vasoplegia, hypovolemia, myocardial dysfunction	80–97
Diabetes insipidus	Hypothalamic/pituitary dysfunction	65–90
Arrhythmias	Catecholamine release, myocardial injury	25–32
Pulmonary oedema	Injury to vascular endothelium	15–20
Cardiac arrest	Prolonged hypotension, arrhythmia	5–10

In response, the mean arterial pressure (MAP) rises to compensate and maintain cerebral perfusion pressure (CPP). The skull, as a fixed space, is restricting thus forcing the brain stem downward towards the spinal cord causing injury to the pons. Commonly known as the Cushing's Reflex, this process results in a triad of symptoms classically characterised by an initial sinus bradycardia, hypertension, and irregular or absence of breathing (see Table 23.2). Further, herniation involving the medulla oblongata, results in stimulation of the sympathetic system and an inflammatory response manifesting as hypertension with elevated cardiac output and cardiac stress leading to tachyarrhythmias, severe vasoconstriction, and poor organ perfusion as well as neuroendocrine effects, such as diabetes insipidus and hypothermia (see Figure 23.1).

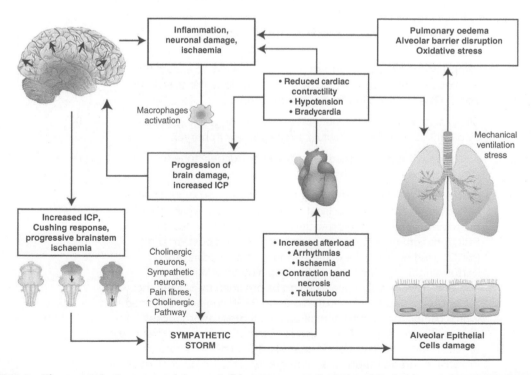

FIGURE 23.1   The sympathetic storm and the pro-inflammatory cascade. *Source*: Meyfroidt et al. (2019) / Springer Nature.

DIAGNOSIS OF DEATH

Whether made via neurological testing or circulatory criteria the diagnostic features of death are aligned because all death is anatomically located in the brain. The Academy of Medical Royal Colleges (2008), the Code of Practice for the Diagnosis and Confirmation of Death defines death as the irreversible loss of the capacity for consciousness, combined with the irreversible loss of the capacity to breathe unaided (see Tables 23.3 and 23.4).

TABLE 23.3   Confirmation of death – neurological and circulatory.

Test	Neurological death	Circulatory death
Loss of consciousness	Cranial nerve testing	Pupil responses are absent, no reaction to supraorbital pressure pain and no reaction to corneal stimulation.
Loss of capacity to breath	Apnoea test of 5 min observed respiratory arrest	Observed mechanical cardio-respiratory arrest 5 min

TABLE 23.4   Brain stem tests and cranial nerves.

Test	Procedure	Afferent	Efferent
Pupillary reflex	A bright light should be shone into each eye to observe for pupil constriction and consensual reaction.	II	III
Corneal reflex	Cornea is brushed with sterile gauze to assess for a blinking response.	V	VII
Response to painful stimuli	Supraorbital pressure to observe for facial grimacing.	V	VII
Vestibulo-ocular reflex	Tympanic membrane visualised prior to procedure to ensure no blockage followed by injecting 50 ml of ice-cold water over 1 min into each ear, observing for any eye nystagmus.	VIII	III, VI
Gag reflex	Direct stimulation of the pharynx to observe for gagging, usually by a Yankauer sucker or spatula on the posterior pharynx.	IX	X
Cough reflex	A suction catheter is placed down the endotracheal tube to stimulate the carina to observe for a cough.	IX	X
Apnoea test	Following cranial nerve testing at normocarbia, preoxygenation of the patient is made by placing them on FiO2 of 1.0 while adjusting the minute ventilation to allow the $PaCO_2$ to rise to at least 6.0 kPa PRIOR to commencing the apnoea test. Pre- and post-arterial $PaCO_2$ used as evidence of these markers being achieved. Performing the apnoea test while remaining on ventilation is not recommended. Oxygenation can be provided by placing the patient on a Mapleson C circuit, where a PEEP can be maintained which allows for a clear vision of any respiratory effort. Close observation for signs of breathing for 5 minutes is made at the end of which further arterial blood analysis should demonstrate an increase of greater than 0.5 kPa before re-establishing ventilation and normocarbia ahead of the second set of tests.		

Diagnosing circulatory death in expected deaths is permissible for APs. Where a Trust or Health Board has established the appropriate FICM/NHSBT approved training and assessment of competency, this can also be so in cases of DCD donation, once an AP is deemed competent and where an anaesthetist is not required for lung donation.

In neurological criteria, there is the proviso of two senior doctors alone, one of whom must be a consultant; however APs should have detailed knowledge of the features indicating when this diagnosis might be made, the preconditions required to be satisfied in order to make a correct diagnosis, and the requirement for stabilisation in order for the tests to be carried out, thereby providing an unequivocal diagnosis of death should the criteria be satisfied.

The strict criteria agreed by experts and endorsed for use by the Intensive Care Society, Paediatric Critical Care Society, and the Faculty of Intensive Care Medicine are reviewed regularly. The latest, full 'long version' guidance form (available online) should always be used to fully consider all factors that might influence a diagnosis unless where a consultant is both an expert in this testing procedure and in the patient group to be tested.

There are three distinct forms for three separate patient groups:

1. Over 18 years
2. Between 2 months and 18 years of age
3. Between 37 weeks corrected gestational age and 2 months

Further guidance is available where a patient is receiving extracorporeal membrane oxygenation (ECMO) treatment.

APs can play a vital role in supporting the stabilisation of a patient between where neurological death is suspected and the testing itself using the optimisation principles described in Section 23.7, but prior to testing, maintain a MAP consistently above 60 mmHg to support CPP, ensuring the diagnosis can be confidently embarked upon in a timely way without delay to a grieving family. Attention paid to physiological stability combined with prompt correction of electrolyte imbalances can prevent testing delays.

Spinal reflexes may be present resulting in limb movement that can mimic normal movement. These can be profound and challenging, but where there is any doubt over a diagnosis, caution prevails. Spinal reflexes are common, predictable, and repeatable to the same stimuli, a defining feature of these movements. To help families in their understanding of the situation, it is usual they are offered to witness the second set of tests with the SNOD to support them. Spinal reflex movements present during the first set of tests can be evaluated and explained to the family with expertise, prior to them witnessing the tests themselves.

Two sets of tests are required, ideally by the same two doctors. The first set of tests enables a diagnosis and is the time of death, the second confirms the first and completes the diagnosis. Family discussions are planned between the consultant, the bedside nurse and the SNOD prior to, between the sets of tests and after to lay clear the process and the diagnosis prior to any end-of-life discussions. Early notifications to the SNOD, therefore, enable a more seamless service of expertise for families during this unsettling period.

THE TESTS

The pre-conditions for NDT are set out as:

- A primary diagnosis with evidence of irreversible brain damage of known aetiology, a Glasgow Coma Score GCS of 3 and being mechanically ventilated.
- Exclusion of reversible causes of coma and apnoea including ensuring no residual effects of sedative agents or neuromuscular blockades.

'Red Flags', based on real cases, may trigger a delay in testing or suggest ancillary testing. The forms are updated following any landmark cases, therefore the most up to date form should always be consulted early to safely identify if any of these conditions are present. The SNOD can also offer quick access to medical expertise where there may be testing uncertainty.

OPTIMISATION AND THE DONOR OPTIMISATION CARE BUNDLE

High-quality management and optimisation of a potential donor (DBD or DCD) is critical to the outcomes of the donation and any subsequent transplantation outcome of those receiving organs. Instability of a donor can occur at any time, particularly prior to testing but is less frequent where detailed attention is made to a donor's physiological care prior to the donation procedure itself. No individual intends the gift of their organs to be then deemed unsuitable for transplant through poor attention to the care of those organs.

Until a potential donor's next of kin can confirm or establish the decision to donate, stabilisation prior to testing and optimisation should be instituted promptly, whether a potential DBD or DCD donor, until their decision can be understood. This prevents any deleterious effects from occurring in the interim, should their decision be to donate.

The structured, simple, and systematic ABCDE approach is advised, with life-threatening issues dealt with as a primacy. The aims of optimisation are to maintain normal physiology, anticipate physiological changes potentiated by any neurological testing, and to minimise any iatrogenic damage to organs.

Two documents support this work – the Donation Actions Framework guidance which supports the ethical decision-making around interventions made in the best interests of a donating patient, and NHSBT's Donor Care Bundle which guides DBD donation care.

FRM7261/1 – Donation After Death Using Neurological Criteria-Donor Optimisation Care Bundle - Adult

NHS
Blood and Transplant
Effective date: 13/06/2023

ADULT   PLEASE RETURN TO THE DFCS

Referral ID......................Donor No ....Age............ Weight .... Height ....

IMMEDIATELY AFTER DIAGNOSIS OF DEATH

- Perform lung recruitment manoeuvre.
- Set tidal volume to 4-8mls/kg (ideal body weight).
- Set optimum PEEP (5 to 10cm H20).
- Add vasopressin (0.48 to 4U/hr), where vasopressors are required. Wean noradrenaline.

Time of death.................... Signed..................... Name..................... GMC.....................

WITHIN 1 HOUR OF CONSENT/AUTHORISATION

- Administer methylprednisolone (15mg/kg, maximum 1G).
- Request an ECG.
- Request an echocardiogram.
- Request a CXR – post recruitment manoeuvre.

Time completed..................... Signed..................... Name..................... GMC.....................

WITHIN 4 HOURS OF CONSENT/AUTHORISATION

- ECG report complete.
- Echocardiogram report complete.
- CXR report complete.
- Site cardiac output monitoring, if able.

Time completed..................... Signed..................... Name..................... GMC.....................

DRUGS

- Vasopressin 20 units in 50mls 5% dextrose; rate 1.2 to 10mls/hour.
- DDAVP 1 TO 4mcg IV.
- Methylprednisolone 15mg/kg (max 1G).

CONTINUOUSLY

- Ensure ongoing lung protective strategy.
- Nurse 30-45 degrees' head up.
- Continue physiotherapy including suctioning.

- Review intravascular fluid status and correct hypovolaemia.
- Wean noradrenaline as able.
- Treat DI with DDAVP.

- Continue NG feed, as directed by SNOD.
- Monitor blood glucose and treat as per unit protocol.
- Monitor serum sodium concentration.

- Continue use of mechanical thromboprophylaxis.
- Ensure prophylactic low molecular weight heparin use.

- Continue hourly observations.
- Maintain normothermia.
- Stop all unnecessary medications.
- If not already present, insert a central line (right sided IJ or SC is preferable).

- Other tests or therapies may be indicated. SNOD to direct.

GOALS

PaO2 ≥ 10 kPa	U.O. 0.5 – 2 mls/kg/hr
PaCO2 5 – 6.5 kPa	Na < 150 mmol/L
pH >7.25	Glucose 4 – 10 mmol/L
MAP 60-80 mmHg	Temp 36 – 37.5 °

FRM7261/1 – Donation After Death Using Neurological Criteria-Donor Optimisation Care Bundle - Adult

NHS
Blood and Transplant
Effective date: 13/06/2023

ADULT

Referral ID.............................Donor No ....Age............. Weight .... Height ....

	Start	+1hr	+2hr	+4hr	+6hr	+8hr	+10hr	+12hr	+14hr	+16hr	+18hr	+20hr	+22hr	+24hr	+26hr	+28hr
PaO2 ≥ 10 kPa (FiO2 < 0.4 as able)																
PaCO2 5 – 6.5 kPa (or higher as long as pH >7.25)																
MAP 60 – 80 mmHg																
Cardiac index > 2.1 l/min/m² (if applicable)																
Urine output 0.5 – 2 mls/kg/hr																
Temperature 36 – 37.5 °C																
Blood glucose 4 – 10 mmol/L																
Signature																
Surname																
Date																
Time																

PLEASE RECORD ACTUAL VALUES
PAGE 1 TO BE PRINTED IN COLOUR AS PER ICS GUIDAN

PATIENT OPTIMISATION

A: Airway patency and positioning is assessed, maintained and optimised.

B: Breathing. Recruitment manoeuvres, particularly following the DNT apnoea test, followed by lung protective ventilation prevents atelectasis. The parameter goals of $PO_2 > 10\,kPa$, $FiO_2 < 0.4$ with a PEEP of 5–$10\,cmH_2O$ should be achieved where possible using positioning, good respiratory hygiene, 45° head tilt, physiotherapy as required, as for any critical care patient, to prevent hypoxaemia and maintain optimal conditions for organ metabolism.

C: Circulatory assessment of perfusion markers such as hourly urine output, MAP, and lactate reviews should be made regularly. Interventions should focus on the four areas of concern caused by a sudden catecholamine release. A reversal of hypovolaemia with suitable fluid resuscitation, reduction of low vascular tone with vasopressin, and low cardiac contractility reversed with dopamine as drugs of choice, along with restoration of normal sinus rhythm from the arrhythmia's underlying cause. Each element reversal limits these deleterious effects and those of alternative pharmaceutical agents, on organs to be donated. Desmopressin (DDAVP) or vasopressin may be used in instances of diabetes insipidus and cardiac output monitoring, if available, can be used to guide therapy.

D: Disability. In the DCD patient, neurological assessment should continue if there is a neurological component to their underlying deterioration. Attention should be paid to blood glucose, and maintenance of a target of 4–10 mmol/l with enteral feed continued and insulin as required.

E: Exposure. Hypothermia can occur in DBD and DCD patients secondary to loss of hypothalamic control, reduced metabolism, and vasodilation. Early active warming can prevent, coagulopathy, cardiac instability, and arrhythmias. Thromboembolic prophylaxis should continue for these procoagulant patients. Continued monitoring and care of electrolyte balance, haematological and infection markers with prompt attention to infection control should be continued for donor patients.

All DBD patients should be given methylprednisolone 15 mg/kg up to 1 g following DNT to stabilise organ function and reduce the inflammatory effects of harmful cytokines associated with neurological death.

TISSUE DONATION

Where solid organ donation is not suitable, tissue donation may still be considered from any clinical area. Most people can donate tissues, with some exceptions. Patient history, age, clinical requirement, and retrieval location will enable assessment for suitability. Corneas and heart valves are consistently in high demand with a range of other tissues, all offering transformational life change. As the retrieval may be undertaken up to 48 hours after death, the assessment process can be performed after the patient has died by specialist nurses in tissue donation following a referral to the individual referral service and local policy.

As only tissues that are required for clinical need at that time are retrieved, a referral should be made prior to offering the opportunity to a family, particularly in paediatrics.

Case Study
Overnight a 24-year-old woman is admitted into the intensive care unit, following a fall from a horse. Her GCS at the scene was 6/15, she was intubated at the scene. On arrival to hospital, she had a CT of her head, which showed a large subarachnoid haemorrhage with a severe midline shift. The next day, the bedside nurse caring for the patient, comes to tell you her pupils are fixed and dilated, and she is no longer coughing or taking any spontaneous breaths. On assessment of the patient, you find she is bradycardic and hypertensive. Her parents and 16-year-old brother are at the bedside and are asking what is wrong. • What are the priorities for this patient's care? • What would be your immediate next steps? • What you would tell her family? How might you approach any family questions around this change in condition?

Take Home Points
- Advanced Practitioners must use advanced assessment skills including effective communication and emotional intelligence when involved with organ donation.
- According to NHS Blood and Transplant, the UK has the lowest rate of transplant consent in Europe.
- The UK may never achieve a world class donation and transplantation service, if more than 4 out of every 10 families say no to donation. At present, 43% of families refuse to donate.
- Factors such as religion, culture, family influence, medical mistrust, and fear of early retrieval are recognised as the most important factors negatively affecting donation processes.

REFERENCES

Academy of Medical Royal Colleges. (2008). *A Code of Practice for the Diagnosis and Confirmation of Death* [online]. Available from: `https://aomrc.org.uk/wp-content/uploads/2016/04/Code_Practice_Confirmation_Diagnosis_Death_1008-4.pdf` [accessed 25 June 2023].

Flemming, G. and Thomson, E.M. (2021). Organ donation and management of the potential organ donor. *Anaesthesia and Intensive Care Medicine* 22 (8): 475–481.

Health Education England (HEE). (2022). *Advanced Clinical Practice in Acute Medicine Curriculum Framework – Credentials* [online]. Available from: `https://advanced-practice.hee.nhs.uk/our-work/credentials` [accessed 20 June 2023].

Health Education England (HEE). (2017). *Multi-professional Framework for Advanced Clinical Practice in England* [online]. Available from: `https://www.hee.nhs.uk/sites/default/files/documents/multi-professional framework for advanced clinical practice in england.pdf` [accessed 20 June 2023].

Meyfroidt, G., Gunst, J., MartinLoeches, I. et al. (2019). Management of the brain-dead donor in the ICU: general and specific therapy to improve transplantable organ quality. *Intensive Care Medicine* 45 (3): 343–353.

The Faculty of Intensive Care Medicine. (2018). *Curriculum for Training for Advanced Critical Care Practitioners – Syllabus. V1.1* [online]. Available from: `www.ficm.ac.uk/media/6896` [accessed 20 June 2023].

The Intensive Care Society, Critical Care Networks – *National Nurse Leads and The National Outreach Forum*. (2022). *Advanced Critical Care Outreach Competencies* [online]. Available from: `https://ics.ac.uk/asset/43B8C11B-4512-41D0-B97768FABA2C30B2` [accessed 20 June 2023].

The Royal College of Emergency Medicine. (2022). *Emergency Medicine Advanced Clinical Practitioner Curriculum 2022 (Adult)* [online]. Available from: `https://rcem.ac.uk/wp-content/uploads/2022/09/ACP_Curriculum_Adult_Final_060922.pdf` [accessed 20 June 2023].

FURTHER READING

As donation practice is constantly evolving, all current advice and resources can be found at `https://www.odt.nhs.uk/deceased-donation/best-practice-guidance` [accessed 25 June 2023].

Prefixes and Suffixes

Prefix: A prefix is positioned at the beginning of a word to modify or change its meaning. Pre means 'before'. Prefixes may also indicate a location, number or time.

  Suffix: The ending part of a word that changes the meaning of the word.

Prefix or suffix	Meaning	Example(s)
a-, an-	not, without	analgesic, apathy
ab-	from; away from	abduction
abdomin(o)-	of or relating to the abdomen	abdomen
acous(io)-	of or relating to hearing	acoumeter, acoustician
acr(o)-	extremity, topmost	acrocrany, acromegaly, acroosteolysis, acroposthia
ad-	at, increase, on, toward	adduction
aden(o)-, aden(i)-	of or relating to a gland	adenocarcinoma, adenology, adenotome, adenotyphus
adip(o)-	of or relating to fat or fatty tissue	adipocyte
adren(o)-	of or relating to adrenal glands	adrenal artery
-aemia	blood condition	anaemia
aer(o)-	air, gas	aerosinusitis
-aesthesi(o)-	sensation	anaesthesia
alb-	denoting a white or pale color	albino
-alge(si)-	pain	analgesic
-algia, -alg(i)o-	pain	myalgia
all(o-)	denoting something as different, or as an addition	alloantigen, allopathy
ambi-	denoting something as positioned on both sides	ambidextrous
amni-	pertaining to the membranous foetal sac (amnion)	amniocentesis
ana-	back, again, up	anaplasia

The Advanced Practitioner in Acute, Emergency and Critical Care, First Edition. Edited by Sadie Diamond-Fox, Barry Hill, Sonya Stone, Caroline McCrea, Natalie Gardner, and Angela Roberts.
© 2024 John Wiley & Sons Ltd. Published 2024 by John Wiley & Sons Ltd.

Prefix or suffix	Meaning	Example(s)
andr(o)-	pertaining to a man	android, andrology
angi(o)-	blood vessel	angiogram
ankyl(o)-, ancyl(o)-	denoting something as crooked or bent	ankylosis
ante-	describing something as positioned in front of another thing	antepartum
anti-	describing something as 'against' or 'opposed to' another	antibody, antipsychotic
arteri(o)-	of or pertaining to an artery	arteriole, arterial
arthr(o)-	of or pertaining to the joints, limbs	arthritis
articul(o)-	joint	articulation
-ase	enzyme	lactase
-asthenia	weakness	myasthenia gravis
ather(o)-	fatty deposit, soft gruel-like deposit	atherosclerosis
atri(o)-	an atrium (especially heart atrium)	atrioventricular
aur(i)-	of or pertaining to the ear	aural
aut(o)-	self	autoimmune
axill-	of or pertaining to the armpit (uncommon as a prefix)	axilla
bi-	twice, double	binary
bio-	life	biology
blephar(o)-	of or pertaining to the eyelid	blepharoplast
brachi(o)-	of or relating to the arm	brachium of inferior colliculus
brady-	slow	bradycardia
bronch(i)-	bronchus	bronchiolitis obliterans
bucc(o)-	of or pertaining to the cheek	buccolabial
burs(o)-	bursa (fluid sac between the bones)	bursitis
carcin(o)-	cancer	carcinoma
cardi(o)-	of or pertaining to the heart	cardiology
carp(o)-	of or pertaining to the wrist	carpopedal
-cele	pouching, hernia	hydrocele, varicocele
-centesis	surgical puncture for aspiration	amniocentesis
cephal(o)-	of or pertaining to the head (as a whole)	cephalalgy
cerebell(o)-	of or pertaining to the cerebellum	cerebellum
cerebr(o)-	of or pertaining to the brain	cerebrology
chem(o)-	chemistry, drug	chemotherapy
chol(e)-	of or pertaining to bile	cholecystitis
cholecyst(o)-	of or pertaining to the gallbladder	cholecystectomy

Prefix or suffix	Meaning	Example(s)
chondr(i)o-	cartilage, gristle, granule, granular	chondrocalcinosis
chrom(ato)-	colour	hemochromatosis
-cidal, -cide	killing, destroying	bactericidal
cili-	of or pertaining to the cilia, the eyelashes	ciliary
circum-	denoting something as 'around' another	circumcision
col(o)-, colono-	colon	colonoscopy
colp(o)-	of or pertaining to the vagina	colposcopy
contra-	against	contraindicate
coron(o)-	crown	coronary
cost(o)-	of or pertaining to the ribs	costochondral
crani(o)-	belonging or relating to the cranium	craniology
-crine, -crin(o)-	to secrete	endocrine
cry(o)-	cold	cryoablation
cutane-	skin	subcutaneous
cyan(o)-	denotes a blue colour	cyanosis
cyst(o)-, cyst(i)-	of or pertaining to the urinary bladder	cystotomy
cyt(o)-	cell	cytokine
-cyte	cell	leukocyte
-dactyl(o)-	of or pertaining to a finger, toe	dactylology, polydactyly
dent-	of or pertaining to teeth	dentist
dermat(o)-, derm(o)-	of or pertaining to the skin	dermatology
-desis	binding	arthrodesis
dextr(o)-	right, on the right side	dextrocardia
di-	two	diplopia
dia-	through, during, across	dialysis
dif-	apart, separation	different
digit-	of or pertaining to the finger (rare as a root)	digit
-dipsia	suffix meaning '(condition of) thirst'	polydipsia, hydroadipsia, oligodipsia
dors(o)-, dors(i)-	of or pertaining to the back	dorsal, dorsocephalad
duodeno-	duodenum	duodenal atresia
dynam(o)-	force, energy, power	hand strength dynamometer
-dynia	pain	vulvodynia
dys-	bad, difficult, defective, abnormal	dysphagia, dysphasia
ec-	out, away	ectopia, ectopic pregnancy

Prefix or suffix	Meaning	Example(s)
-ectasia, -ectasis	expansion, dilation	bronchiectasis, telangiectasia
ect(o)-	outer, outside	ectoblast, ectoderm
-ectomy	denotes a surgical operation or removal of a body part; resection, excision	mastectomy
-emesis	vomiting condition	hematemesis
encephal(o)-	of or pertaining to the brain; also see cerebr(o)-	encephalogram
endo-	denotes something as 'inside' or 'within'	endocrinology, endospore
enter(o)-	of or pertaining to the intestine	gastroenterology
eosin(o)-	red	eosinophil granulocyte
epi-	on, upon	epicardium, epidermis, epidural, episclera, epistaxis
erythr(o)-	denotes a red colour	erythrocyte
ex-	out of, away from	excision, exophthalmos
exo-	denotes something as 'outside' another	exoskeleton
extra-	outside	extradural hematoma
faci(o)-	of or pertaining to the face	facioplegic
fibr(o)	fibre	fibroblast
fore-	before or ahead	forehead
fossa	a hollow or depressed area; trench or channel	fossa ovalis
front-	of or pertaining to the forehead	frontonasal
galact(o)-	milk	galactorrhoea
gastr(o)-	of or pertaining to the stomach	gastric bypass
-genic	formative, pertaining to producing	cardiogenic shock
gingiv-	of or pertaining to the gums	gingivitis
glauc(o)-	denoting a grey or bluish-grey colour	glaucoma
gloss(o)-, glott(o)-	of or pertaining to the tongue	glossology
gluco-	sweet	glucocorticoid
glyc(o)-	sugar	glycolysis
-gnosis	knowledge	diagnosis, prognosis
gon(o)-	seed, semen; also, reproductive	gonorrhoea
-gram, -gramme	record or picture	angiogram
-graph	instrument used to record data or picture	electrocardiograph

Prefix or suffix	Meaning	Example(s)
-graphy	process of recording	angiography
gyn(aec)o-	woman	gynaecomastia
haemangi(o)-	blood vessels	haemangioma
haemat(o)-, hem-	of or pertaining to blood	haematology
halluc-	to wander in mind	hallucinosis
hemi-	one-half	cerebral hemisphere
hepat- (hepatic-)	of or pertaining to the liver	hepatology
heter(o)-	denotes something as 'the other' (of two), as an addition, or different	heterogeneous
hist(o)-, histio-	tissue	histology
home(o)-	similar	homeopathy
hom(o)-	denotes something as 'the same' as another or common	homosexuality
hydr(o)-	water	hydrophobe
hyper-	denotes something as 'extreme' or 'beyond normal'	hypertension
hyp(o)-	denotes something as 'below normal'	hypovolemia
hyster(o)-	of or pertaining to the womb, the uterus	hysterectomy, hysteria
iatr(o)-	of or pertaining to medicine, or a physician	iatrogenic
-iatry	denotes a field in medicine of a certain body component	podiatry, psychiatry
-ics	organized knowledge, treatment	obstetrics
ileo-	ileum	ileocecal valve
infra-	below	infrahyoid muscles
inter-	between, among	interarticular ligament
intra-	within	intramural
ipsi-	same	ipsilateral haemiparesis
ischio-	of or pertaining to the ischium, the hip joint	ischioanal fossa
-ismus	spasm, contraction	hemiballismus
iso-	denoting something as being 'equal'	isotonic
-ist	one who specializes in	pathologist
-itis	inflammation	tonsillitis
-ium	structure, tissue	pericardium
juxta- (iuxta-)	near to, alongside or next to	juxtaglomerular apparatus
karyo-	nucleus	eukaryote

Prefix or suffix	Meaning	Example(s)
kerat(o)-	cornea (eye or skin)	keratoscope
kin(e)-, kin(o)-, kinaesi(o)-	movement	kinaesthesia
kyph(o)-	humped	kyphoscoliosis
labi(o)-	of or pertaining to the lip	labiodental
lacrim(o)-	tear	lacrimal canaliculi
lact(i)-, lact(o)	milk	lactation
lapar(o)-	of or pertaining to the abdomen wall, flank	laparotomy
laryng(o)-	of or pertaining to the larynx, the lower throat cavity where the voice box is	larynx
latero-	lateral	lateral pectoral nerve
-lepsis, -lepsy	attack, seizure	epilepsy, narcolepsy
lept(o)-	light, slender	leptomeningeal
leuc(o)-, leuk(o)-	denoting a white colour	leukocyte
lingu(a)-, lingu(o)-	of or pertaining to the tongue	linguistics
lip(o)-	fat	liposuction
lith(o)-	stone, calculus	lithotripsy
-logist	denotes someone who studies a certain field	oncologist, pathologist
log(o)-	speech	logopaedics
-logy	denotes the academic study or practice of a certain field	haematology, urology
lymph(o)-	lymph	lymphedema
lys(o)-, -lytic	dissolution	lysosome
-lysis	destruction, separation	paralysis
macr(o)-	large, long	macrophage
-malacia	softening	osteomalacia
mammill(o)-	of or pertaining to the nipple	mammillitis
mamm(o)-	of or pertaining to the breast	mammogram
manu-	of or pertaining to the hand	manufacture
mast(o)-	of or pertaining to the breast	mastectomy
meg(a)-, megal(o)-, -megaly	enlargement, million	splenomegaly, megametre
melan(o)-	black colour	melanin
mening(o)-	membrane	meningitis
meta-	after, behind	metacarpus

Prefix or suffix	Meaning	Example(s)
-meter	instrument used to measure or count	sphygmomanometer
metr(o)-	pertaining to conditions of the uterus	metrorrhagia
-metry	process of measuring	optometry
micro-	denoting something as small, or relating to smallness	microscope
milli-	thousandth	millilitre
mon(o)-	single	infectious mononucleosis
morph(o)-	form, shape	morphology
muscul(o)-	muscle	musculoskeletal system
my(o)-	of or relating to muscle	myoblast
myc(o)-	fungus	onychomycosis
myel(o)-	of or relating to bone marrow or spinal cord	myeloblast
myri-	ten thousand	myriad
myring(o)-	eardrum	myringotomy
narc(o)-	numb, sleep	narcolepsy
nas(o)-	of or pertaining to the nose	nasal
necr(o)-	death	necrosis, necrotizing fasciitis
neo-	new	neoplasm
nephr(o)-	of or pertaining to the kidney	nephrology
neur(i)-, neur(o)-	of or pertaining to nerves and the nervous system	neurofibromatosis
normo-	normal	normocapnia
ocul(o)-	of or pertaining to the eye	oculist
odont(o)-	of or pertaining to teeth	orthodontist
odyn(o)-	pain	stomatodynia
-oesophageal, oesophag(o)-	gullet	gastroesophageal reflux
-oid	resemblance to	sarcoidosis
-ole	small or little	arteriole
olig(o)-	denoting something as 'having little, having few'	oliguria
-oma (*sing.*), -omata (*pl.*)	tumour, mass, collection	sarcoma, teratoma
onco-	tumour, bulk, volume	oncology
onych(o)-	of or pertaining to the nail (of a finger or toe)	onychophagy
oo-	of or pertaining to an egg, a woman's egg, the ovum	oogenesis

Prefix or suffix	Meaning	Example(s)
oophor(o)-	of or pertaining to the woman's ovary	oophorectomy
ophthalm(o)-	of or pertaining to the eye	ophthalmology
optic(o)-	of or relating to chemical properties of the eye	opticochemical
orchi(o)-, orchid(o)-, orch(o)-	testis	orchiectomy, orchidectomy
-osis	a condition, disease or increase	ichthyosis, psychosis, osteoporosis
osseo-	bony	osseous
ossi-	bone	peripheral ossifying fibroma
ost(e)-, oste(o)-	bone	osteoporosis
ot(o)-	of or pertaining to the ear	otology
ovo-, ovi-, ov-	of or pertaining to the eggs, the ovum	ovogenesis
pachy-	thick	pachyderma
paed-, paedo-	of or pertaining to the child	paediatrics
palpebr-	of or pertaining to the eyelid (uncommon as a root)	palpebra
pan-, pant(o)-	denoting something as 'complete' or containing 'everything'	panophobia, panopticon
papill-	of or pertaining to the nipple (of the chest/breast)	papillitis
papul(o)-	indicates papulosity, a small elevation or swelling in the skin, a pimple, swelling	papulation
para-	alongside of, abnormal	paracyesis
-paresis	slight paralysis	hemiparesis
parvo-	small	parvovirus
path(o)-	disease	pathology
-pathy	denotes (with a negative sense) a disease, or disorder	sociopathy, neuropathy
pector-	breast	pectoralgia, pectoriloquy, pectorophony
ped-, -ped-, -pes	of or pertaining to the foot; -footed	pedoscope
pelv(i)-, pelv(o)-	hip bone	pelvis
-penia	deficiency	osteopenia
-pepsia	denotes something relating to digestion, or the digestive tract	dyspepsia
peri-	denoting something with a position 'surrounding' or 'around' another	periodontal

Prefix or suffix	Meaning	Example(s)
-pexy	fixation	nephropexy
phaco-	lens-shaped	phacolysis, phacometer, phacoscotoma
-phage, -phagia	forms terms denoting conditions relating to eating or ingestion	sarcophagia
-phago-	eating, devouring	phagocyte
-phagy	forms nouns that denote 'feeding on' the first element or part of the word	hematophagy
pharmaco-	drug, medication	pharmacology
pharyng(o)-	of or pertaining to the pharynx, the upper throat cavity	pharyngitis, pharyngoscopy
phleb(o)-	of or pertaining to the (blood) veins, a vein	phlebography, phlebotomy
-phobia	exaggerated fear, sensitivity	arachnophobia
phon(o)-	sound	phonograph, symphony
phot(o)-	of or pertaining to light	photopathy
phren(i)-, phren(o)-, phrenico	the mind	phrenic nerve, schizophrenia
-plasia	formation, development	achondroplasia
-plasty	surgical repair, reconstruction	rhinoplasty
-plegia	paralysis	paraplegia
pleio-	more, excessive, multiple	pleiomorphism
pleur(o)-, pleur(a)	of or pertaining to the ribs	pleurogenous
-plexy	stroke or seizure	cataplexy
pneumat(o)-	air, lung	pneumatocele
pneum(o)-	of or pertaining to the lungs	pneumonocyte, pneumonia
-poiesis	production	haematopoiesis
poly-	denotes a 'plurality' of something	polymyositis
post-	denotes something as 'after' or 'behind' another	post-operation, post-mortem
pre-	denotes something as 'before' another (in [physical] position or time)	premature birth
presby(o)-	old age	presbyopia
prim-	denotes something as 'first' or 'most important'	primary
proct(o)-	anus, rectum	proctology
prot(o)-	denotes something as 'first' or 'most important'	protoneuron
pseud(o)-	denotes something false or fake	pseudoephedrine

Prefix or suffix	Meaning	Example(s)
psor-	itching	psoriasis
psych(e)-, psych(o)	of or pertaining to the mind	psychology, psychiatry
-ptosis	falling, drooping, downward placement, prolapse	apoptosis, nephroptosis
-ptysis	(a spitting), spitting, haemoptysis, the spitting of blood derived from the lungs or bronchial tubes	haemoptysis
pulmon-, pulmo-	of or relating to the lungs	pulmonary
pyel(o)-	pelvis	pyelonephritis
py(o)-	pus	pyometra
pyr(o)-	fever	antipyretic
quadr(i)-	four	quadriceps
radio-	radiation	radiowave
ren(o)-	of or pertaining to the kidney	renal
retro-	backward, behind	retroversion, retroverted
rhin(o)-	of or pertaining to the nose	rhinoplasty
rhod(o)-	denoting a rose-red colour	rhodophyte
-rrhage	burst forth	haemorrhage
-rrhagia	rapid flow of blood	menorrhagia
-rrhaphy	surgical suturing	nephrorrhaphy
-rrhexis	rupture	karyorrhexis
-rrhoea	flowing, discharge	diarrhoea
-rupt	break or burst	erupt, interrupt
salping(o)-	of or pertaining to tubes, e.g. Fallopian tubes	salpingectomy, salpingopharyngeus muscle
sangui-, sanguine-	of or pertaining to blood	exsanguination
sarco-	muscular, flesh-like	sarcoma
scler(o)-	hard	scleroderma
-sclerosis	hardening	atherosclerosis, multiple sclerosis
scoli(o)-	twisted	scoliosis
-scope	instrument for viewing	stethoscope
-scopy	use of instrument for viewing	endoscopy
semi-	one-half, partly	semiconscious
sial(o)-	saliva, salivary gland	sialagogue
sigmoid(o)-	sigmoid, S-shaped curvature	sigmoid colon
sinistr(o)-	left, left side	sinistrocardia

Prefix or suffix	Meaning	Example(s)
sinus-	of or pertaining to the sinus	sinusitis
somat(o)-, somatico-	body, bodily	somatic
-spadias	slit, fissure	hypospadias, epispadias
spasmo-	spasm	spasmodic dysphonia
sperma(to)-, spermo-	semen, spermatozoa	spermatogenesis
splen(o)-	spleen	splenectomy
spondyl(o)-	of or pertaining to the spine, the vertebra	spondylitis
squamos(o)-	denoting something as 'full of scales' or 'scaly'	squamous cell
stat.	statim	at once
-stalsis	contraction	peristalsis
-stasis	stopping, standing	cytostasis, homeostasis
-staxis	dripping, trickling	epistaxis
sten(o)-	denoting something as 'narrow in shape' or pertaining to narrowness	stenography
-stenosis	abnormal narrowing in a blood vessel or other tubular organ or structure	restenosis, stenosis
stomat(o)-	of or pertaining to the mouth	stomatogastric, stomatognathic system
-stomy	creation of an opening	colostomy
sub-	beneath	subcutaneous tissue
super-	in excess, above, superior	superior vena cava
supra-	above, excessive	supraorbital vein
tachy-	denoting something as fast, irregularly fast	tachycardia
-tension, -tensive	pressure	hypertension
tetan-	rigid, tense	tetanus
thec-	case, sheath	intrathecal
therap-	treatment	hydrotherapy, therapeutic
therm(o)-	heat	thermometer
thorac(i)-, thorac(o)-, thoracico-	of or pertaining to the upper chest, chest; the area above the breast and under the neck	thorax
thromb(o)-	of or relating to a blood clot, clotting of blood	thrombus, thrombocytopenia
thyr(o)-	thyroid	thyrocele

Prefix or suffix	Meaning	Example(s)
thym-	emotions	dysthymia
-tome	cutting instrument	osteotome
-tomy	act of cutting; incising, incision	gastrotomy
tono-	tone, tension, pressure	tonometer
-tony	tension	
top(o)-	place, topical	topical anaesthetic
tort(i)-	twisted	torticollis
tox(i)-, tox(o)-, toxic(o)-	toxin, poison	toxoplasmosis
trache(a)-	trachea	tracheotomy
trachel(o)-	of or pertaining to the neck	tracheloplasty
trans-	denoting something as moving or situated 'across' or 'through'	transfusion
tri-	three	triangle
trich(i)-, trichia, trich(o)-	of or pertaining to hair, hair-like structure	trichocyst
-tripsy	crushing	lithotripsy
-trophy	nourishment, development	pseudohypertrophy
tympan(o)-	eardrum	tympanocentesis
-ula, -ule	small	nodule
ultra-	beyond, excessive	ultrasound
un(i)-	one	unilateral hearing loss
ur(o)-	of or pertaining to urine, the urinary system; (specifically) pertaining to the physiological chemistry of urine	urology
uter(o)-	of or pertaining to the uterus or womb	uterus
vagin-	of or pertaining to the vagina	vagina
varic(o)-	swollen or twisted vein	varicose
vasculo-	blood vessel	vasculotoxicity
vas(o)-	duct, blood vessel	vasoconstriction
ven-	of or pertaining to the (blood) veins, a vein (used in terms pertaining to the vascular system)	vein, venospasm
ventricul(o)-	of or pertaining to the ventricles; any hollow region inside an organ	cardiac ventriculography
ventr(o)-	of or pertaining to the belly; the stomach cavities	ventrodorsal
-version	turning	anteversion, retroversion

Prefix or suffix	Meaning	Example(s)
vesic(o)-	of or pertaining to the bladder	vesical arteries
viscer(o)-	of or pertaining to the internal organs, the viscera	viscera
xanth(o)-	denoting a yellow colour, an abnormally yellow colour	xanthopathy
xen(o)-	foreign, different	xenograft
xer(o)-	dry, desert-like	xerostomia
zo(o)-	animal, animal life	zoology
zym(o)-	fermentation	enzyme, lysozyme

Normal Values

There are a variety of techniques that those who analyse blood use in the laboratory to identify the various components. These techniques can differ from laboratory to laboratory, it is essential that when assessment of blood results is undertaken, referral to the local laboratory's normal values is made. Variation occurs across the UK, Europe, and globally. Clinicians should adhere to local policy and guidelines and refer to biomedical scientists and clinical experts when requires.

Haematology
Full blood count
Haemoglobin (males) 13.0–18.0 g/dl
Haemoglobin (females) 11.5–16.5 g/dl
Haematocrit (males) 0.40–0.52
Haematocrit (females) 0.36–0.47
MCV 80–96 fl
MCH 28–32 pg
MCHC 32–35 g/dl
White cell count (4–11) × 109 l

White cell differential
Neutrophils 1.5–7 × 10^9 l
Lymphocytes 1.5–4 × 10^9 l
Monocytes 0–0.8 × 10^9 l
Eosinophils 0.04–0.4 × 10^9 l
Basophils 0–0.1 × 10^9 l
Platelet count 150–400 × 10^9 l
Reticulocyte count (25–85) × 10^9 l or 0.5–2.4%

Erythrocyte sedimentation rate
Westergren
Under 50 years:
   Males 0–15 mm/1st hour
   Females 0–20 mm/1st hour
Over 50 years:
   Males 0–20 mm/1st hour
   Females 0–30 mm/1st hour

The Advanced Practitioner in Acute, Emergency and Critical Care, First Edition. Edited by Sadie Diamond-Fox, Barry Hill, Sonya Stone, Caroline McCrea, Natalie Gardner, and Angela Roberts.
© 2024 John Wiley & Sons Ltd. Published 2024 by John Wiley & Sons Ltd.

Plasma viscosity 1.50–1.72 mPa s[1] (at 25 °C)

Coagulation screen
Prothrombin time 11.5–15.5 seconds
International normalized ratio < 1.4
Activated partial thromboplastin time 30–40 seconds
Fibrinogen 1.8–5.4 g/l
Bleeding time 3–8 minutes

Coagulation factors
Factors II, V, VII, VIII, IX, X, XI, XII 50–150 IU/dl
Factor V Leiden Present or not
Von Willebrand factor 45–150 IU/dl
Von Willebrand factor antigen 50–150 IU/dl
Protein C 80–135 IU/dl
Protein S 80–120 IU/dl
Antithrombin III 80–120 IU/dl
Activated protein C resistance 2.12–4.0
Fibrin degradation products <100 mg/l
D-dimer screen <0.5 mg/l

Haematinics
Serum iron 12–30 µmol/l
Serum iron-binding capacity 45–75 µmol/l
Serum ferritin 15–300 µg/l
Serum transferrin 2.0–4.0 g/l
Serum B$_{12}$ 160–760 ng/l
Serum folate 2.0–11.0 µg/l
Red cell folate 160–640 µg/l
Serum haptoglobin 0.13–1.63 g/l

Haemoglobin electrophoresis
Haemoglobin A > 95%
Haemoglobin A2 2–3%
Haemoglobin F < 2%

Chemistry
Serum sodium 137–144 mmol/l
Serum potassium 3.5–4.9 mmol/l
Serum chloride 95–107 mmol/l
Serum bicarbonate 20–28 mmol/l
Anion gap 12–16 mmol/l
Serum urea 2.5–7.5 mmol/l
Serum creatinine 60–110 µmol/l
Serum corrected calcium 2.2–2.6 mmol/l
Serum phosphate 0.8–1.4 mmol/l
Serum total protein 61–76 g/l

Serum albumin 37–49 g/l
Serum total bilirubin 1–22 μmol/l
Serum conjugated bilirubin 0–3.4 μmol/l
Serum alanine aminotransferase 5–35 U/l
Serum aspartate aminotransferase 1–31 U/l
Serum alkaline phosphatase 45–105 U/l (over 14 years)
Serum gamma glutamyl transferase 4–35 U/l (<50 U/l in males)
Serum lactate dehydrogenase 10–250 U/l
Serum creatine kinase (males) 24–195 U/l
Serum creatine kinase (females) 24–170 U/l
Creatine kinase MB fraction <5%
Serum troponin I 0–0.4 μg/l
Serum troponin T 0–0.1 μg/l
Serum copper 12–26 μmol/l
Serum caeruloplasmin 200–350 mg/l
Serum aluminum 0–10 μg/l
Serum magnesium 0.75–1.05 mmol/l
Serum zinc 6–25 μmol/l
Serum urate (males) 0.23–0.46 mmol/l
Serum urate (females) 0.19–0.36 mmol/l
Plasma lactate 0.6–1.8 mmol/l
Plasma ammonia 12–55 μmol/l
Serum angiotensin-converting enzyme 25–82 U/l
Fasting plasma glucose 3.0–6.0 mmol/L
Haemoglobin A1 C 3.8–6.4%
Fructosamine <285 μmo/l
Serum amylase 60–180 U/l
Plasma osmolality 278–305 mosmol/kg

Lipids and lipoproteins
Target levels will vary depending on the patient's overall cardiovascular risk assessment
Serum cholesterol <5.2 mmol/l
Serum LDL cholesterol <3.36 mmol/l
Serum HDL cholesterol >1.55 mmol/l
Fasting serum triglyceride 0.45–1.69 mmol/l

Blood gases (breathing air at sea level)
Blood H^+ 35–45 nmol/l
pH 7.36–7.44
PaO_2 11.3–12.6 kPa
$PaCO_2$ 4.7–6.0 kPa
Base excess ±2 mmol/l

Carboxyhaemoglobin
Non-smoker <2%
Smoker 3–15%

Immunology/rheumatology
Complement C3 65–190 mg/dl
Complement C4 15–50 mg/dl
Total haemolytic (CH50) 150–250 U/l
Serum C-reactive protein <10 mg/l

Serum immunoglobulins
IgG 6.0–13.0 g/l
IgA 0.8–3.0 g/l
IgM 0.4–2.5 g/l
IgE <120 kU/l
Serum β_2-microglobulin <3 mg/l

Cerebrospinal fluid
Opening pressure 50–180 mmH$_2$O
Total protein 0.15–0.45 g/l
Albumin 0.066–0.442 g/l
Chloride 116–122 mmol/l
Glucose 3.3–4.4 mmol/l
Lactate 1–2 mmol/l
Cell count ≤5 mL^{-1}

Differential
Lymphocytes 60–70%
Monocytes 30–50%
Neutrophils None
IgG/ALB ≤0.26
IgG index ≤0.88

Urine
Albumin/creatinine ratio (untimed specimen) <3.5 mg/mmol (males)
<2.5 mg/mmol (females)
Glomerular filtration rate 70–140 ml/min
Total protein <0.2 g/24 hours
Albumin <30 mg/24 hours
Calcium 2.5–7.5 mmol/24 hours
Urobilinogen 1.7–5.9 μmol/24 hours
Coproporphyrin <300 nmol/24 hours
Uroporphyrin 6–24 nmol/24 hours
δ-Aminolevulinate 8–53 μmol/24 hours
5-Hydroxyindoleacetic acid 10–47 μmol/24 hours
Osmolality 350–1000 mosmol/kg

Feces
Nitrogen 70–140 mmol/24 hours
Urobilinogen 50–500 μmol/24 hours
Fat (on normal diet) <7 g/24 hours

Index

Please note that page references to Figures will be followed by the letter 'f', to Tables by the letter 't'

blood dyscrasias, 258
blood flow, 138, 139*f*, 141, 399, 401
  hepatic, 403
  hepatopetal, 277
  liver, 407
  obstruction to, 333
  renal, 403
blood gas analysis
arterial blood gases (ABGs), 120, 121, 122*t*, 124,
      363, 372*t*, 396
    Chronic Obstructive Pulmonary Disease
        (COPD), 119, 120
    respiratory failure, 121, 122*t*
blood glucose, 512, 515, 529
blood loss *see* bleeding
blood tests, 14, 120, 124, 152*t*, 204
blood transfusions, 259
blood-brain barrier, 402
bone cortex abnormalities, 315
bone fractures, 184
bone fragments, 315
bone marrow, 247, 248, 258, 259, 363
bone metastases, 134
bone structures, 184
bore cannula, 237
brachial artery, 433
bradycardia
  adult bradycardia algorithm, 460*f*
  as emergency, 464
  medication management, 517
  reflex, 517
  risk of, 492
  sinus, 525
brain
  axial MRI slices, 186*f*
  examining, 182
  injury/trauma, 315, 316*t*
  meningitis/encephalitis, effects on, 175
  sagittal MRI slices, 185*f*
  Seattle International Traumatic Brain Injury
      Consensus Conference (SIBICC), 464
  tumours of, 314
    metastases, 244–245
brain stem death, 56, 526*t*
  see also death; NDT (brain stem death testing)
breathing, 237, 461–463, 490, 491
  emergency situations, 462–463*t*

shock, 490–491
shortness of breath *see* dyspnea; shortness
    of breath
tension pneumothorax, 312, 339*f*, 441, 461
British Lung Foundation (BLF), 112
British Medical Journal (BMJ), 461
British National Formulary (BNF), 403, 404, 407
British Nuclear Medicine Society, 320
British Society for Haematology, 409
British Thoracic Society (BTS), 461
bronchitis, 118
bronchoscopy, 132
BTS *see* British Thoracic Society (BTS)
B-type natriuretic peptide (BNP), 153
Budd-Chiari syndrome, 232

C
calcium, 211, 373*t*
calcium antagonists, 158*t*
cancer *see* oncological presentations
candour *see* duty of candour
cannulation
  bore cannula, 237
  disseminated intravascular coagulation
      (DIC), 251
  dyspnoea, 101
  large volume paracentesis (LVP), 427, 430
  Seldinger technique, 430–431
  vascular access, 343
capabilities
  and competences, 8, 10, 23–25
  core and specific, 9
  and credentials, 23–25
capabilities in practice (CiPs), 9, 24
capillaries, 138, 139*f*
CAR T-cell therapy, cancer, 254–255
carboxyhaemoglobin, 372*t*
cardiac imaging, 153–165
  cardiac catheterisation, 157
  cardiac MRI, 155–156
  chest x-ray (CXR), 154, 155*f*
  computed tomography coronary angiography
      (CTCA), 155, 156*f*
  echocardiography, 154–155
  myocardial perfusion, 157
  see also cardiac presentations; cardiovascular
      system (CVS)